OPERATIVE SKULL BASE SURGERY

OPERATIVE SKULL BASE SURGERY

Edited by
MICHAEL TORRENS
M.B., B.S., B.Sc., M.Phil., Ch.M., F.R.C.S.
Chairman, Division of Neurosurgery
Consultant Neurosurgeon
Ygeia Hospital
Marousi, Athens, Greece
Honorary Consultant Neurosurgeon
Frenchay Hospital
Bristol, England

OSSAMA AL-MEFTY, M.D.
Professor and Chairman
Department of Neurosurgery
University of Arkansas College of Medicine
Little Rock, Arkansas

SHIGEAKI KOBAYASHI, M.D.
Professor and Chairman
Department of Neurosurgery
Shinshu University School of Medicine
Matsumoto, Japan

With illustrations by
PETER COX, R.D.D., M.M.A.A.

CHURCHILL LIVINGSTONE

New York, Edinburgh, London, Madrid, Melbourne, San Francisco, Tokyo

CHURCHILL LIVINGSTONE

Medical Division of Pearson Professional Limited

Distributed in the United States of America by Churchill Livingstone Inc., 650 Avenue of the Americas, New York, N.Y. 10011, and by associated companies, branches, and representatives throughout the world.

First published 1997

ISBN 0-443-05079-1

British Library Cataloguing in Publication Data
A catalogue record for this book is available from the British Library

Library of Congress Cataloging in Publication Data
A catalog record for this book is available from the Library of Congress

Project Editor: *Deborah Russell*
Production Editor: *Donna C. Balopole*
Production Supervisor: *Sharon Tuder*
Cover Design: *Charlie Lebeda*

Printed in the United States of America

Contributors

Ossama Al-Mefty, M.D. *Professor and Chairman, Department of Neurosurgery, University of Arkansas College of Medicine, Little Rock, Arkansas*

Vinod K. Anand, M.D. *Professor and Program Director, Department of Surgery, University of Mississippi School of Medicine, Jackson, Mississippi*

Peter J. Catalano, M.D. *Associate Professor, Department of Otolaryngology, The Mount Sinai School of Medicine of the City University of New York, New York, New York*

H. Alan Crockard, M.D. *Consultant Neurosurgeon, Department of Surgical Neurology, The National Hospital for Neurology and Neurosurgery, London, England*

Vinko V. Dolenc, M.D., Ph.D. *Professor and Chairman, Department of Neurosurgery, University Medical Center, Ljubljana, Slovenia*

Rudolf Fahlbusch, M.D. *Director, Department of Neurosurgery, University of Erlangen-Nürnberg, Erlangen, Germany*

Kazuhiko Fujitsu, M.D. *Director, Department of Neurosurgery, National Hospital of Yokohama, Yokohama, Japan*

Masashi Fukui, M.D. *Chairman and Professor, Department of Neurosurgery, Faculty of Medicine, Kyushu University, Fukuoka, Japan*

Atul Goel, M.Ch. *Associate Professor, Department of Neurosurgery, K.E.M. Hospital and Seth G. S. Medical College, Bombay, India; Consultant Professor, Department of Neurosurgery, Shinshu University School of Medicine, Matsumoto, Japan*

Georges F. Haddad, M.D. *Division of Neurosurgery, Department of Surgery, American University of Beirut, Beirut, Lebanon*

Akira Hakuba, M.D., D.M.Sc. *Professor and Chairman, Department of Neurosurgery, Osaka City University Medical School, Osaka, Japan*

H. Louis Harkey, M.D. *Associate Professor, Department of Neurosurgery, and Assistant Professor, Department of Orthopedic Surgery, University of Mississippi School of Medicine, Jackson, Mississippi*

Jürgen Honegger, M.D. *Neurosurgeon, Department of Neurosurgery, University of Erlangen-Nürnberg, Erlangen, Germany*

Ricardo Izquierdo, M.D. *Clinical Associate Professor of Surgery, Division of Plastic and Reconstructive Surgery, Department of Surgery, Loyola University of Chicago Stritch School of Medicine, Maywood, Illinois; Partner, Plastic Surgeons Associated, S.C., Palos Heights, Illinois*

Ivo P. Janecka, M.D., F.A.C.S. *Director, Longwood Skull Base Program, Departments of Otolaryngology, Neurosurgery, and Plastic Surgery, Children's Hospital, Brigham & Women's Hospital, and Beth Israel Hospital, Harvard Medical School, Boston, Massachusetts*

Takeshi Kawase, M.D. *Professor, Department of Neurosurgery, School of Medicine, Keio University, Tokyo, Japan*

Savvas Kazanas, M.D. *Consultant Ear, Nose, and Throat Surgeon, Skull Base Surgery Group, Ygeia Hospital, Marousi, Athens, Greece*

T. T. King, F.R.C.S. *Consulting Neurosurgeon, Department of Neurosurgery, The Royal London Hospital, Whitechapel, London, England*

Shigeaki Kobayashi, M.D. *Professor and Chairman, Department of Neurosurgery, Shinshu University School of Medicine, Matsumoto, Japan*

Kazuhiko Kyoshima, M.D. *Associate Professor, Department of Neurosurgery, Shinshu University School of Medicine, Matsumoto, Japan*

Spiros A. Lazarou, M.D. *Consultant Plastic, Reconstructive, and Craniomaxillofacial Surgeon, Skull Base Surgery Group, Ygeia Hospital, Marousi, Athens, Greece*

Kiyoshi Matsuo, M.D. *Professor and Chairman, Department of Plastic and Reconstructive Surgery, Shinshu University School of Medicine, Matsumoto, Japan*

Toshio Matsushima, M.D. *Associate Professor, Department of Neurosurgery, Faculty of Medicine, Kyushu University, Fukuoka, Japan*

A. Fitzgerald O'Connor, F.R.C.S. *Consultant Surgeon, Department of Ear, Nose and Throat Surgery, St. Thomas's Hospital, Lambeth, London, England*

Kenji Ohata, M.D., D.M.Sc. *Assistant Professor, Department of Neurosurgery, Osaka City University Medical School, Osaka, Japan*

Hideyuki Ohnishi, M.D., D.M.Sc. *Assistant Professor, Department of Neurosurgery, Nara Medical University, Kashihara, Nara, Japan*

Albert L. Rhoton, Jr., M.D. *R. D. Keene Professor and Chairman, Department of Neurological Surgery, University of Florida College of Medicine, Gainesville, Florida*

Chandranath Sen, M.D. *Professor, Department of Neurosurgery, The Mount Sinai School of Medicine of the City University of New York, New York, New York*

Ryuzo Shiobara, M.D. *Assistant Professor, Department of Neurosurgery, School of Medicine, Keio University, Tokyo, Japan*

Sadao Tajima, M.D. *Professor, Department of Plastic Surgery, Osaka Medical College, Osaka, Japan*

Yoshio Tanaka, M.D. *Associate Professor, Department of Plastic Surgery, Osaka Medical College, Osaka, Japan*

Yuichiro Tanaka, M.D. *Assistant Professor, Department of Neurosurgery, Shinshu University School of Medicine, Matsumoto, Japan*

Michael Torrens, M.B., B.S., B.Sc., M.Phil., Ch.M., F.R.C.S. *Chairman, Division of Neurosurgery, and Consultant Neurosurgeon, Ygeia Hospital, Marousi, Athens, Greece; Honorary Consultant Neurosurgeon, Frenchay Hospital, Bristol, England*

Gerald F. Tuite, M.D. *Neurosurgeon, Department of Neurosurgery, All Children's Hospital, St. Petersburg, Florida*

Foreword

Very limited skull base surgery was possible more than 50 years ago when, as a medical student in Paris, I became interested in the anatomy of the parasellar region known as the cavernous sinus.

My numerous dissections led to conclusions very different from the classical descriptions. There was no large trabeculated sinus through which the internal carotid artery passed freely but a venous network draining mainly the orbital blood toward the petrosal sinuses. The oculomotor nerves crossing the region had meningeal sheaths. The oculomotor nerves and the vascular elements were all in an interduroperiosteal parasellar space communicating anteriorly with the orbit through the superior orbital fissure.

This new description visualizing the region was published in Paris in 1949 and 1961 but had a very limited acceptance. It became recognized and partly accepted much later on after Parkinson's publications in the 1960s. Parkinson also described and performed the first transdural approach to the parasellar space in order to treat a carotid-cavernous fistula.

The controversy and antagonism nevertheless continued. The precise knowledge of the complex anatomy of the region has important neurosurgical implications. If indeed "injury to the parasellar venous pathway is rare and generally does not present a serious surgical problem" (Taptas, 1982) then cavernous sinus surgery is possible.

During the years following these publications a few neurosurgeons led by Dolenc and Sekhar and colleagues, after studying the anatomy of the region, started to perform direct surgery of vascular and tumorous lesions developing in or invading the cavernous sinus. This important new chapter in the history of skull base surgery, together with the complementary balloon and embolization techniques, allowed the treatment of large aneurysms of the internal carotid artery, giant ophthalmic aneurysms, meningiomas, trigeminal neurinomas, and parasellar extensions of pituitary tumors.

At the same time as the above developments, the surgical anatomy of other areas of the skull base was being analyzed by surgeons and neuroanatomists. All this pioneering work has brought us to the point where a synthesis of techniques can be published in books designed for all specialists interested in the subject.

Operative Skull Base Surgery presents the techniques of specific operative and reconstructive surgery of all the skull base as well as the optimal approaches. The 23 chapters, written by experts in the field, cover surgery of the anterior fossa, the orbit, the clivus, the middle temporal fossa, the posterior fossa, and the foramen magnum. The complexity and variety of most of the techniques require not only well-organized medical centers but the collaboration of neurosurgeons, ophthalmologists, otolaryngologists, plastic surgeons, and neuroanesthesiologists. This multidisciplinary action has made possible the treatment of a great number of lesions, tumorous or vascular, many of which not so long ago were considered to be inoperable.

The editors, Michael Torrens, Ossama Al-Mefty, and Shigeaki Kobayashi, must be praised for the selection of topics and authors, which makes the volume indispensable to all surgeons concerned with cranial base pathology.

John N. Taptas, M.D.
Neo Psychiko, Athens, Greece

Reference

Taptas JN (1982) The so-called cavernous sinus: a review of the controversy and its implications for neurosurgeons. Neurosurgery 11:712-717

Preface

Skull base surgery is changing from a discipline involving procedures undertaken at considerable risk in highly specialized centers to a recognized subspecialization in most centers dealing with head and neck surgery.

This evolution has been enabled by the pioneering work of certain individuals, by improvements in technology relating to both surgical equipment and earlier diagnosis, and by the development of the concept of teamwork between specialties.

What should be done and by which approach or technique remains a debated area. *Operative Skull Base Surgery* is intended as a practical manual to assist those being trained (or training themselves by experience) to undertake the more appropriate procedures with a better understanding of the practical problems and therefore, hopefully, better results.

The book is concerned principally with the anatomy and surgery of approaches to the skull base. The multiplicity of approaches is such that only the more common and characteristic have been chosen. These, as noted in Chapter 1, can be extended, combined, or varied in particular circumstances. The target pathology will demand modifications and therefore the approach should be individually designed for each patient. This emphasizes the need for teamwork in planning, conduct of surgery, monitoring, repair procedures, and follow-up.

Chapter 1 discusses the factors influencing the choice of approach. This is followed by chapters, written by surgeons rather than anatomists, describing skull base anatomy. The most common approaches are described in the next chapters, and the final chapters discuss repair procedures.

It is hoped that the emphasis on practicality, not only in specific procedures but also in the area of operative "design," will help to remove the stigmata of danger and peculiarity from skull base procedures and further assist the dissemination of high quality surgical practice.

Michael Torrens, M.B., B.S., B.Sc., M.Phil., Ch.M, F.R.C.S.

Contents

1

Factors Influencing the Choice of Approach

Michael Torrens

Over the last 30 years, since the operating microscope became widely used, many surgeons have designed and promoted their approaches to the skull base. Others have modified and added to these approaches to the point where there are now a large variety of ways to reach the same targets. This gives the impression that skull base surgery is an extremely complex subspecialty. This may not be a fair conclusion.

Familiarity with the surgical approach is essential for good results. Thus different specialties may achieve similar results by using entirely different routes. Some surgeons are specialists in their own approaches. Some departments will have an anterior skull base team and a posterior skull base team. What is clear, however, is that the most effective innovations and outstanding results come from centers that are able to bring together the expertise of a number of specialties in order to choose what is best from each area of experience.

It was stated in the preface that each patient undergoing skull base surgery should have a personally designed operation. With such a variety of procedural possibilities in a small area, each with its own variations and extensions, this process may seem bewildering. This introductory chapter compares the merits of the various approaches, including some not otherwise described in this book.

Evaluation of Surgical Approaches

Optimal surgical access depends on matching the anatomic location and pathologic character of the target to the versatility of a particular approach. Therefore, before discussing approaches in relation to targets, the potential approaches will be evaluated in a topographic sequence.

When considering exposure the following general factors are relevant:

1. Take the shortest route from the skin to the target, bypassing structures essential for the satisfactory functional survival of the patient.

2. Use pre-existing or potential "surgical avenues" if possible. These include the spaces in the face, the skull bone (which can be removed and replaced), the epidural/subdural space, and areas of muscle that can be retracted.
3. Use osteotomy to reduce brain retraction.
4. Avoid neurovascular pedicle areas and consider previous incisions and radiotherapy in relation to vascularity of flaps.
5. Respect cosmesis.
6. Control feeding arteries to reduce bleeding.
7. Plan access in relation to reconstruction, especially to maintain compartmentalization (isolation of intradural space and nasopharynx in particular).
8. Consider the possibility of future surgery.

Anterocentral Approaches

The advantages and disadvantages of various anterocentral approaches are summarized in Table 1-1.

Transfrontal and Extended Transfrontal Approaches

The traditional transcranial approach to the anterior fossa skull base has been used by Derome (1983, 1988) to reach the sphenoid sinus and clivus. This allows access to the ethmosphenoidal complex and, laterally, to the optic canal, orbit, superior orbital fissure, and cavernous sinus. Even the first two cervical vertebrae have been reached, with preservation of an intact pharyngeal wall anteriorly. Extensions of clival lesions into the area hidden by the pituitary fossa cannot be resected without adding another approach (e.g., transnasal).

The disadvantages of the narrow oblique approach and the necessary retraction of the frontal lobes can be partly overcome by performing a frontal osteotomy. This extended subfrontal approach is described by Sen and Catalano in Chapter 4. By lowering the angle of view it also allows more of the clivus to be seen below the pituitary fossa (Fig. 1-1). A similar approach with a more restricted osteotomy, the "telecanthal approach" has been described by Fujitsu et al. (1991).

Table 1-1. Advantages and Disadvantages of Anterocentral Approaches

Approach	Disadvantages	Advantages
Transfrontal	Oblique angle Deep approach Brain retraction Loss of smell	May be combined with anterolateral craniotomy and orbital approaches
Transethmoidal	Limited access unless extended Facial scar	Short approach Versatile Extensible
Transnasal-transseptal	Narrow exposure Deep approach	Minimally invasive No scar
Transmaxillary (Le Fort 1)	Messy, prolonged, and invasive	No scar
Transoral	Limited to midline Very deep approach May destabilize	No scar Direct approach

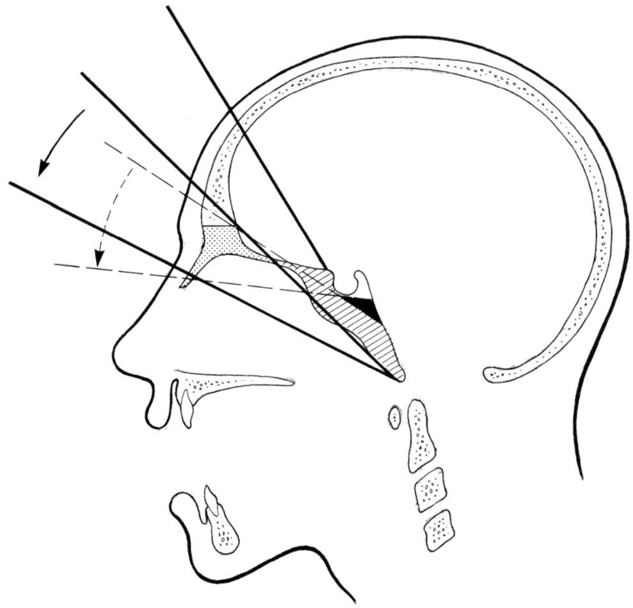

Figure 1-1. Transfrontal and extended transfrontal exposure of the clivus. The addition of a supra-orbital osteotomy (solid arrow) reduces the need for frontal lobe retraction, reduces the depth and obliquity of the approach, improves space for instrumental access, and, by lowering the inferior visual angle (dashed arrow), increases the exposure of the posterior clivus upward (solid black shading).

Transethmoidal and Extended Transethmoidal Approaches

The transethmoidal approach (Fig. 1-2) as described in Chapter 6 is a very simple and direct route to the anterocentral skull base but one that has lost favor recently

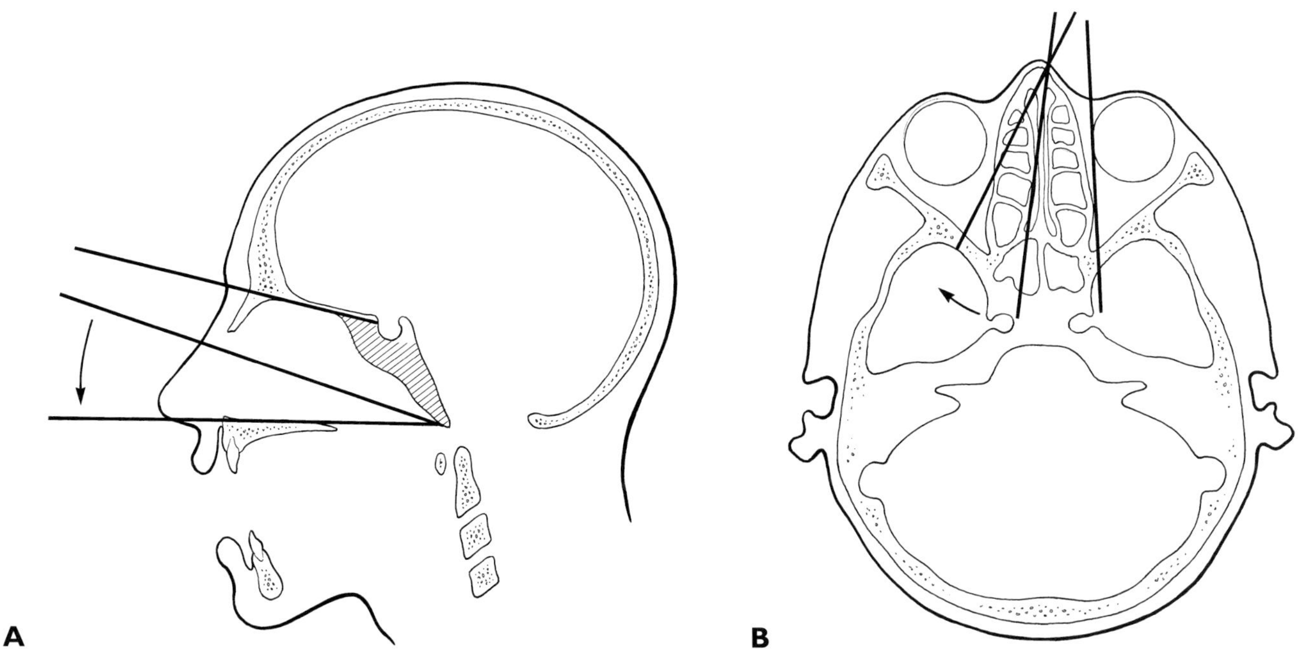

Figure 1-2. Transethmoidal and extended transethmoidal approaches. *(A)* The addition of a lower lateral rhinotomy (arrow) improves the instrumental access but does not alter the potential exposure of the clivus in the midline. *(B)* Removal or displacement of the nasal septum allows access to the contralateral petrous apex and even the contralateral orbit.

because of a desire to avoid incisions in the face for cosmetic reasons. Unless extended, the space for instrumental access is restricted. Extension is complicated by the position of the nasolacrimal apparatus.

Extension may be made upward (frontal sinus), laterally (medial orbit, maxillary sinus), and inferomedially (nasal cavity) and then posteriorly to the sphenoid and pituitary, clivus, pterygopalatine fossa, and petrous apex (especially contralaterally).

The extended transethmoidal approach is known also as Moure's operation (Moure, 1922). The approach described by Janecka (Ch. 8) as minifacial translocation–central is very similar. Janecka avoids problems with the nasolacrimal system by keeping the osteotomized nasomaxillary fragment attached to the medial canthal ligament, lacrimal duct, and skin. His chapter gives an excellent overview of the principles of access through the face.

Trans-Septal and Transnasal Approaches

The most simple approach to the pituitary and upper clivus is by utilizing the nares and proceeding transnasally, either microscopically or endoscopically (Fig. 1-3) (Ch. 6). The instrumental access is naturally very restricted in this approach and, until ultraminimally invasive surgery becomes more widely accepted, many may prefer the more traditional trans-septal approach (Ch. 5). This also has the theoretic advantage of remaining submucosal.

The transnasal or trans-septal approach can be extended downward and, if appropriate, combined with the transoral approach to expose the whole of the clivus. The limitation is more significant in the lateral extent than rostrocaudally.

Transmaxillary Approaches

Transmaxillary approaches (Fig. 1-4) may be undertaken without or with the mobilization of the lower maxilla by osteotomy. A simple extension of the paranasal

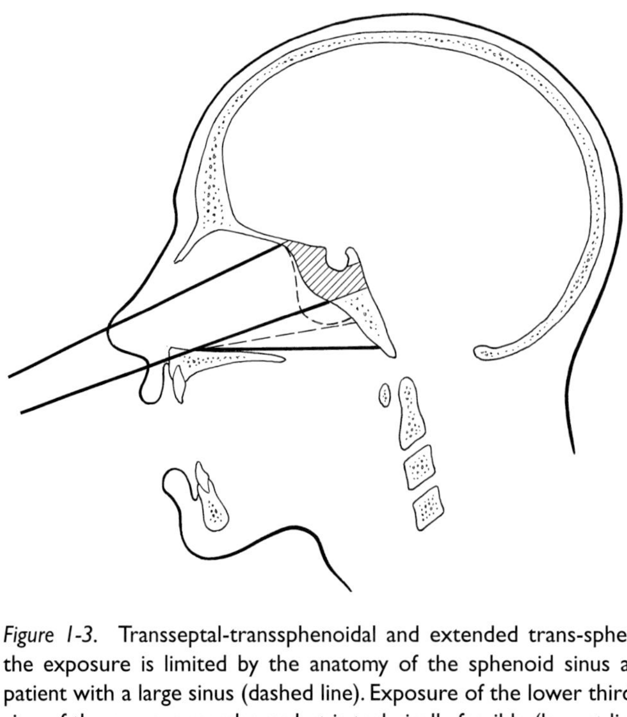

Figure 1-3. Transseptal-transsphenoidal and extended trans-sphenoidal approach. The extent of the exposure is limited by the anatomy of the sphenoid sinus and can be more extensive in a patient with a large sinus (dashed line). Exposure of the lower third of the clivus involves transgression of the mucous membrane but is technically feasible (lowest line).

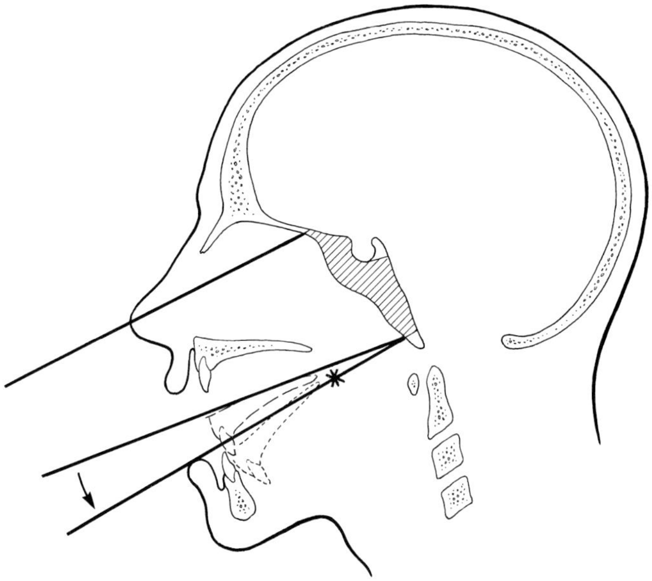

Figure 1-4. Le Fort I osteotomy approach. The ease of access to the clivus is determined particularly by the height of the posterior palate (*). This in turn is determined by the efficiency of the palatal retractor and the degree of stretching possible in the palatine vascular pedicles. For the same reason, although mandibulotomy allows further depression of the maxillary fragment (finely dashed line), the subsequent increased opening anteriorly (arrow) may not be reflected in much greater inferior exposure of the clivus unless one palatine vascular pedicle is also cut.

approach into the pterygoid region through the maxillary sinus requires no osteotomy. However, for more extended access various osteotomies have been described. These include a simple Le Fort 1 osteotomy (Ch. 7); Le Fort 1 plus mandibular section, which allows greater opening anteriorly (Ch. 11); and Le Fort 1 osteotomy with midline palatal split (Ch. 10), which exposes the whole clivus. A mandibulotomy can be added to this, which allows exposure down to C3.

The initial width of exposure at the clivus provided by these approaches is no greater than that allowed by the transnasal, trans-septal, or transoral routes but the wider instrumental access allows safer operative extension laterally when necessary. However, significant lateral extension of the pathology may require a separate lateral exposure or a combined anterolateral exposure. The problem is that the parapharyngeal structures of crucial anatomic importance (e.g., the cavernous sinus and structures along the jugulo-stylo-hamular line, see Ch. 2), are not well visualized by these anterior transpharyngeal approaches.

Transoral Approach

The simple transoral approach (Fig. 1-5) (Crockard, 1988; see Ch. 10) is confined to strictly midline lesions. The rostrocaudal extent of exposure is from the lower clivus to C2-C3. Its importance stems from the frequency of degenerative lesions at the C1-C2 level that are best managed by this route (Crockard, 1991). The access can be extended upward by a palatal division and downward by appropriate angulation of the tongue depressor. If the mouth will not open widely a maxillotomy or mandibulotomy may occasionally be necessary. Total division of the anterior arch of the atlas will tend to destabilize the craniocervical junction and requires a synchronous fusion procedure, which greatly limits mobility.

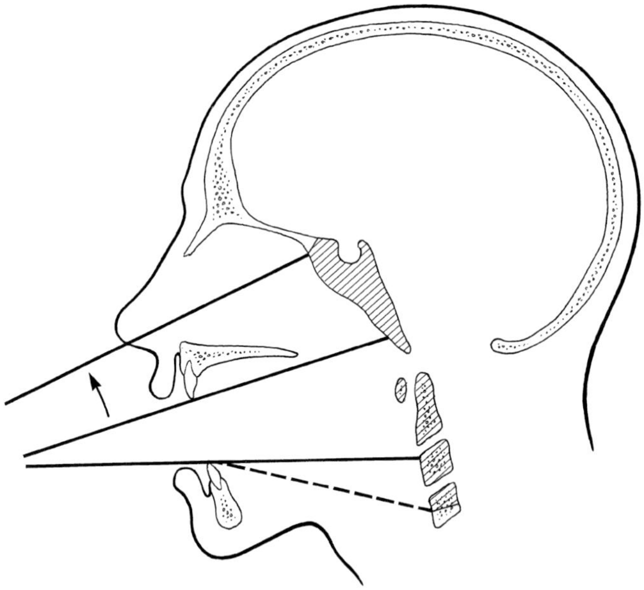

Figure 1-5. Transoral and extended transoral C3 approach. The standard access is from the lower clivus to C2-C3. Tilting the handle of the tongue retractor away from the body depresses the tongue more (dashed line) and may improve access to C3 or even C4. Splitting the soft and posterior hard palate gains 5 mm more upward exposure. With transverse (Le Fort I) and midline osteotomies of the maxilla, and lateral displacement of the two maxillary halves, the exposure can be extended to the top of the clivus (arrow).

Transmandibular (Central) Approach

When a very extended access to both the skull base and the cervical spine is needed, a transmandibular approach may be appropriate. Its chief advantage, apart from a very extensive central exposure, is the ability to deal with lesions extending laterally on the side of the incision. Therefore, the method is discussed in more detail in the section on anterolateral approaches.

Anterolateral Approaches

Frontotemporal Craniotomy and Its Extensions

An anterolateral craniotomy or one of its many modifications and extensions is the most common approach to much of the skull base (Fig. 1-6). The range of territory covered includes the orbit, sphenoid bone, cavernous sinus, petrous apex, infratemporal region, and anterior two-thirds of the clivus.

A significant proportion of this area is accessible with an unextended craniotomy (Ch. 13) perhaps with the removal, by drilling, of the anterior clinoid process (Fig. 1-7A). When appropriate the removal of the zygomatic arch alone or in combination with the orbital margin (Fig. 1-7B & C) greatly improves the access and reduces retraction of the brain without adding significant morbidity or unduly prolonging the operating time (Uttley et al., 1991; see Ch. 12). When access through the greater wing of the sphenoid is required, the use of an osteoplastic craniotomy that includes the roof of the orbit in one fragment together with the greater wing of the sphenoid helps to prevent postoperative enophthalmos that otherwise occurs after periorbital and transorbital approaches (Ch. 14).

Extending a craniotomy approach into the infratemporal fossa can be assisted, after removal of the zygomatic arch, by outfracture of the coronoid process of the

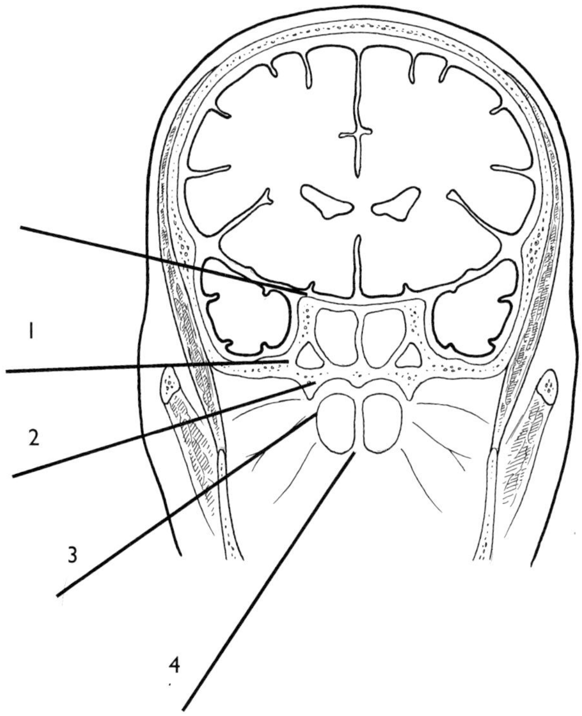

Figure 1-6. Anterior and lateral approaches. Craniotomy alone (1) inevitably requires significant retraction of the temporal lobe to reach the area of the posterior cavernous sinus and clivus. The addition of an osteotomy of the zygoma or even of only the zygomatic arch (2) improves the situation but some retraction is still required. Outfracture of the coronoid process/osteotomy of the condylar process (3) of the mandible greatly improves this access. Through an approach involving division of the mandible (4) the retropharyngeal craniocervical region can be widely exposed.

mandible. Even greater access is obtained by resection of the condylar process as well. This is often suggested (Sekhar et al., 1993) but is accompanied by a morbidity that can be avoided by the alternative of mandibular osteotomy and osteotomy of the condylar fossa with preservation of the temporomandibular joint (Ch. 15).

The approach described by Ohata and Hakuba as the lateral extensive middle fossa approach (Fig. 1-7D) and by Sekhar et al. (1993) as the subtemporal infratemporal approach (Fig. 1-7E) can be combined, on one hand, with the basal frontal approach (Fig. 1-7F; see Ch. 4) and, on the other, with a transpetrosal approach (Fisch et al., 1984; see Ch. 18), a far lateral/transcondylar approach (Ch. 21), or both. This makes it a particularly versatile approach. The basic access of lateral craniotomy to the petrous apex and the upper two-thirds of the clivus (Ch. 16) can be extended by mobilization of the carotid and facial nerve and by division of the mandibular nerve. The fifth complex can also be split through the ganglion between V2 and V3. These maneuvers provide access from the jugular foramen and lower clivus to the sphenoid, opposite petrous apex, cavernous sinus, and the infratemporal and pterygopalatine fossas.

Subcranial Approaches

It may be appropriate to approach a skull base lesion by a primary subcranial, transbasal route using craniotomy for extension as necessary, rather than by craniotomy using basal bone resection as the means of extension.

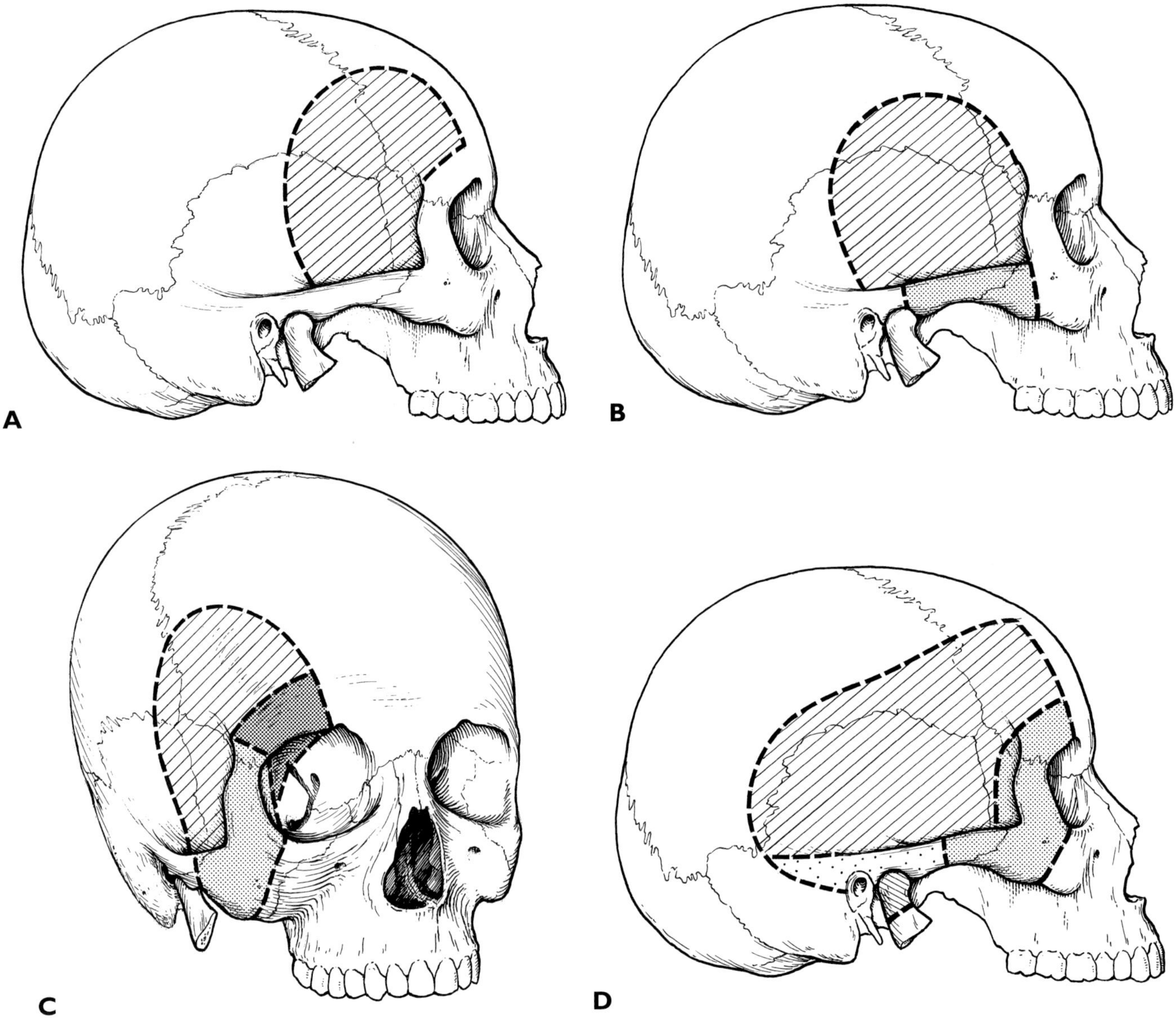

Figure 1-7. Anterior and lateral approaches, the extent of bone removal. *(A)* Unextended frontotemporal craniotomy through which can be reached a large proportion of lesions from the orbit back to the petrous apex. *(B)* The addition of an osteotomy of the zygomatic arch greatly aids access to the middle fossa base and reduces temporal lobe retraction. *(C)* Cranio-orbito-zygomatic approach (Ch. 12). *(D)* Lateral extensive middle fossa approach (Ch. 15). The areas of bone around the temporomandibular joint are preserved as osteoplastic flaps and replaced. *(Figure continues.)*

The facial translocation approach (lateral) of Janecka (Ch. 8) emphasizes the primary access through the zygomaticomaxillary complex, to which a craniotomy or craniectomy is added as necessary (Fig. 1-7G). This gives very good access to the lateral nasopharynx and is extensible to the whole area under consideration.

For lesions more posteriorly, particularly those involving the petrous apex, the facial approach may not be necessary and the transpetrous-infratemporal approach may be preferable (Fisch et al., 1984). This basically involves removal of the zygomatic arch and coronoid/condylar mandibular osteotomy to allow an approach through the petrous and sphenoid bones while minimizing the craniectomy.

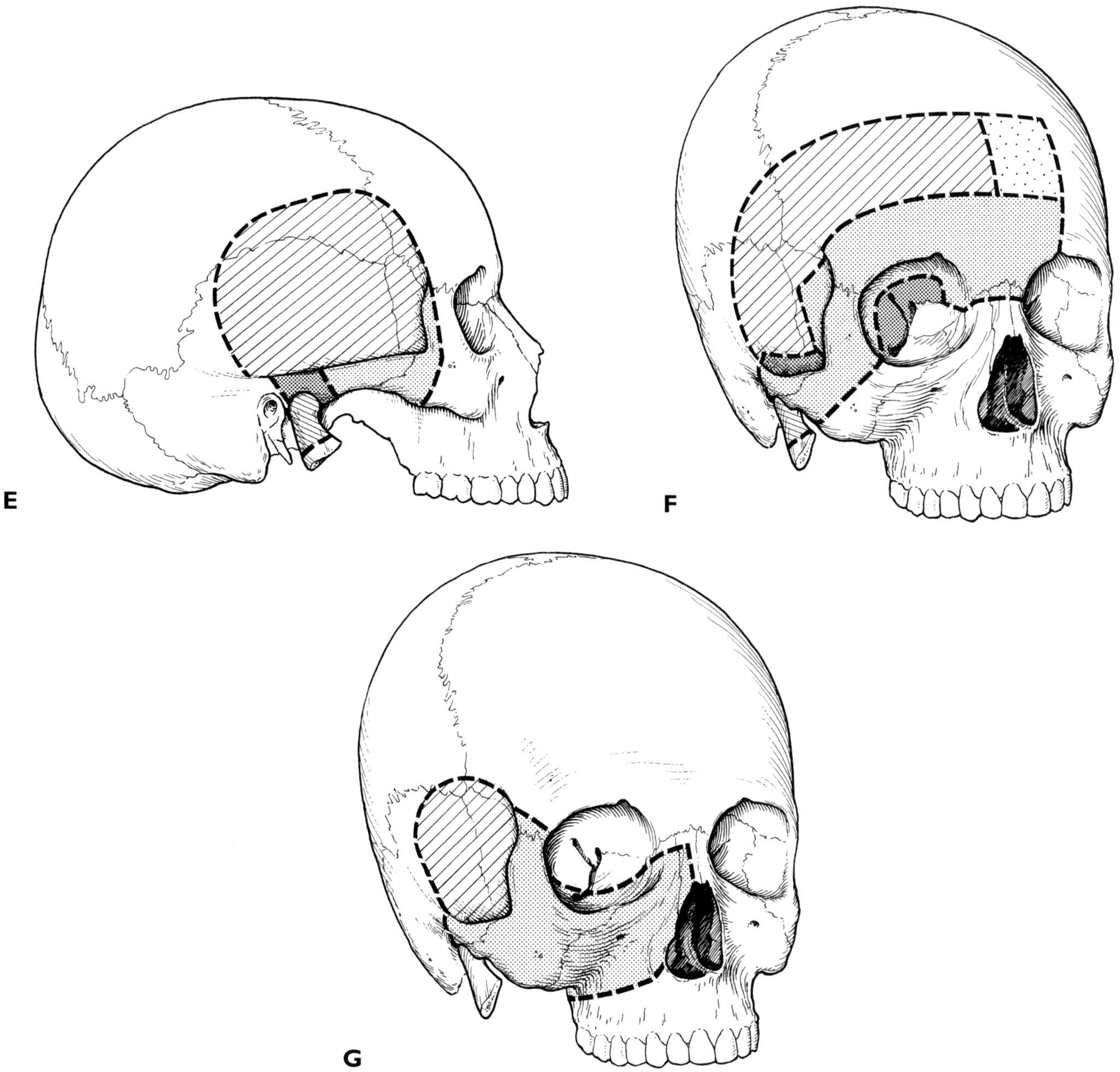

Figure 1-7 (Continued). (E) Subtemporal-infratemporal approach. In cases where the resection of the mandibular condyle is not required, the osteotomy of the zygomatic arch stops short of the condylar fossa. *(F)* The combination of anterior and lateral approaches allows exposure and resection of very large clival tumors. *(G)* The lateral facial translocation approach (Ch. 8).

Transmandibular Approaches

Transmandibular approaches (Krespi and Simon, 1984) allow access to the skull base and cervical region without the disadvantage of narrow exposure associated with the lateral rhinotomy and transoral operations. This is particularly useful for large lesions extending laterally in that vascular control is obtained early in the procedure. The mandibulotomy may be midline or laterally, just in front of the mental foramen. It is a very satisfactory inferolateral approach when the maxillary region is not involved, and is especially appropriate for problems extending to involve the cervical spine.

Posterolateral Approaches

The posterolateral approaches could also be called transpetrosal and peripetrosal approaches.

Middle Fossa Transpetrosal Approach

The most anterior of the transpetrosal approaches has already been mentioned above as a lateral approach (Fig. 1-8). The subtemporal transpetrous apex approach (Ch. 16) allows access to the upper two-thirds of the clivus and anterolateral brain stem, the internal acoustic meatus, and forward to the posterolateral cavernous sinus. The visibility upward can be improved by resection of the zygomatic arch. Downward visibility depends, after maximum possible petrous apex drilling, on the amount of temporal retraction that can be performed safely.

Transcochlear and Petrosectomy Approaches

These approaches (Fig. 1-9) involve the probable transposition, grafting, or sacrifice of the facial nerve and the destruction of the inner ear mechanism. They are indicated in three main circumstances: malignant lesions in the petrous bone for en bloc resection, benign lesions that involve the inner ear structures, and cases that need a wider transpetrosal access than can be provided by trans- or retrolabyrinthine routes. The typical example of glomus jugulare tumors is described by Anand and Al-Mefty (see Ch. 18). The transcochlear approach is appropriate for other conditions involving the medial third of the petrous region and can be extended forward into the infratemporal region as noted above (Fisch et al., 1984). Generally, however, more anterolateral approaches that do not destroy the internal ear are preferable.

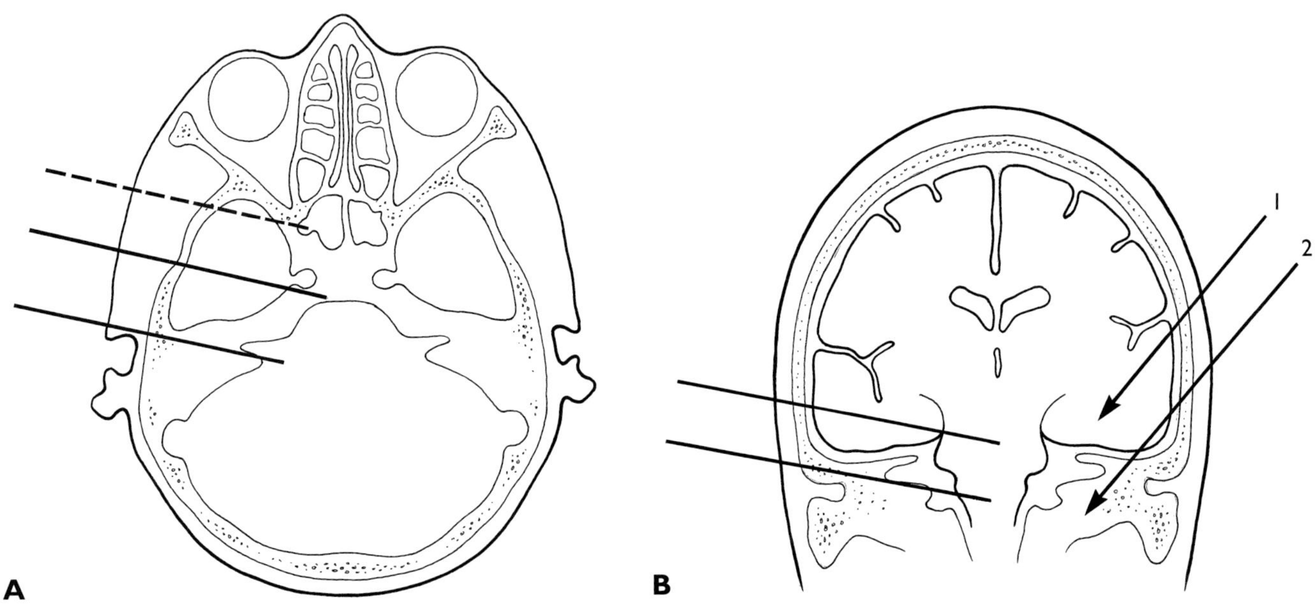

Figure 1-8. Middle fossa transpetrous apex approach; **(A)** transverse access and **(B)** coronal access. The access is limited anteriorly by the carotid artery but can be extended forward into the cavernous sinus especially for lesions such as neurinomas, which are well defined (dashed line). A good view of the prepontine clivus is obtained and the exposure reaches back to the internal auditory meatus. Extended visibility downward into the posterior fossa requires significant temporal lobe retraction (arrow 1) unless more petrous bone can be removed inferiorly (arrow 2).

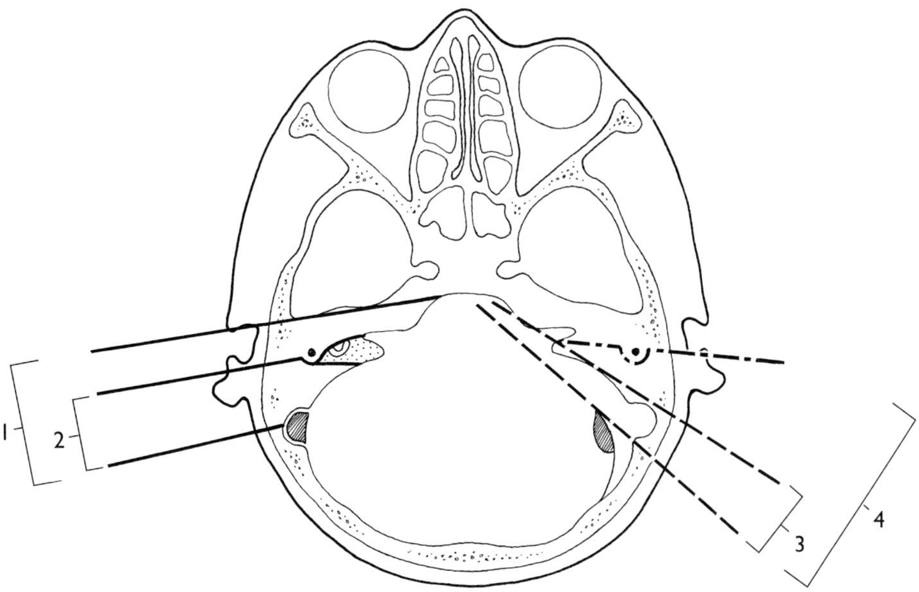

Figure 1-9. Trans- and peripetrous approaches. The drilling of the entire petrous bone (1), variously called the transcochlear, transotic, transpetrosal, and petrosectomy approach, is directed toward lesions in front of the internal auditory meatus and on the clivus. The more restricted translabyrinthine and retrolabyrinthine routes (2) preserve the seventh nerve. The translabyrinthine route includes the semicircular canals (dotted area) and therefore allows access to the middle third of the petrous surface including the meatus. The retrolabyrinthine approach preserves this area and therefore allows access only to the posterior third of the petrous and to the jugular foramen. A parapetrosal route to the clivus (3) requires very little bone removal if the sinus is displaced. Additional translabyrinthine drilling (4) does not improve the exposure of the clivus but allows a better view of the lateral side of the brain stem.

Should en bloc resection of the petrous bone be required, the extent of surgery will normally be decided by the physical extent of the malignant tumor. If the radiologic studies suggest that total resection is possible then it should be undertaken. The relation between the extent of tumor and type of operation is summarized in Table 1-2.

Table 1-2. The Extent of Petrous Bone Resection in Malignant Tumors

Operation	Indication	Sacrificed	Retained
Partial	Tumor around EAM only, local invasion	EAM TM joint Involved skin Middle ear	VII Labyrinth Carotid artery Jugular vein Stapes
Subtotal	Tumor deeply but not along carotid canal or eustachian tube	As above plus petrous bone (except apex) VII[a] Involved dura Involved sinus	Carotid artery
Total	Tumor along carotid canal or eustachian tube but not through dura	As above plus carotid[a]	

Abbreviations: EAM, external auditory meatus; TM, temporomandibular.

[a]The facial nerve and carotid artery may be reconstituted with grafts but the radiotherapy that is usually necessary is likely to interfere with functional recovery.

Translabyrinthine Approach

In the translabyrinthine approach (Fig. 1-9) the facial nerve is left, protected by a shell of bone, in its canal. The labyrinth is destroyed in order to provide access to the middle third of the petrous bone including the internal auditory meatus. The use of this route for removal of acoustic neuromas is described by King and O'Connor (Ch. 17). The outcome for facial nerve function is much better than for the more extensive transcochlear approach and, for this reason, Desgeorges (1994) has recommended approaching the medial third of the petrous bone via an anterior extended translabyrinthine approach.

Retrolabyrinthine and Presigmoid Approaches

The true retrolabyrinthine approach preserves hearing and therefore must protect both the labyrinth and the endolymphatic sac (Fig. 1-9). The antrum is the site of elective closure of the mastoid cavity to prevent eustachian cerebrospinal fluid leaks. The direct medial access is limited to the posterolateral third of the petrous bone but drilling anteriorly below the labyrinth leads directly to the jugular fossa. The mastoid tip and the posterior part of the occipital condyle require removal. Craniectomy is extended over the sigmoid sinus. Mobilization and medial displacement of the sigmoid sinus allows a wider exposure. It is possible to work on both sides of the sinus to deal with intracranial extensions.

Exposure forward to the petrous apex and clivus usually involves more extensive petrous bone removal together with temporal and occipital craniotomy, as in the technique described by Haddad and Al-Mefty (Ch. 19), which is closer to a wider translabyrinthine approach and to the method of Desgeorges mentioned above. When a more narrow access is technically acceptable the parapetrosal approach of Fukushima (1993) requires the drilling of only a small amount of posterior petrous bone, enough to expose a 4 mm × 10 mm area of presigmoid dura. Otherwise his intracranial approach is similar to that of Al-Mefty.

Retrosigmoid and Suboccipital Approaches

The traditional posterior approach inevitably involves significant retraction of the cerebellum. However, the route has regained popularity, especially for smaller acoustic nerve tumors where there is a chance of preserving hearing. The technical experience gained from cases of microvascular decompression may have helped to improve the results of this approach for other lesions. Usually the cranial opening is kept small to protect the cerebellum, but Tanaka and Kobayashi (Ch. 20) suggest a more generous medial opening in order to obtain the right angle of approach to the internal meatus. This needs to be adequately oblique to drill open the whole meatus without damaging the adjacent semicircular canal. In each case the exact internal anatomy of the petrous bone needs to be checked on high-resolution scans.

Conversely, adequate medial visibility into the cerebellopontine angle may require the lateral displacement of the sigmoid sinus into a space prepared by drilling in the posterior petrous bone (Fig. 1-10).

Transcondylar/Far Lateral Approach

Direct posterior access to the foramen magnum region is obstructed by the medulla and spinal cord. The oblique lateral approach involves the removal of some posterior bony structures and sometimes, laterally, part of the mastoid, the occipital condyle, and the lateral mass of the atlas and axis (Fig. 1-11). The vertebral artery may need temporary transposition. The approach is described by Tuite and Crockard (Ch. 21). It can be combined with other anterior and superior approaches to treat more exten-

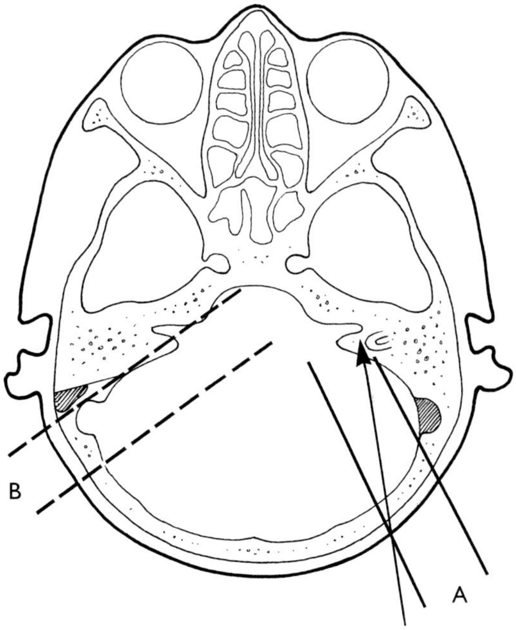

Figure 1-10. Suboccipital approaches. A retrosigmoid approach to the cerebellopontine angle (A) may require a more medially extended craniotomy if the line of view laterally (arrow) is to reach the lateral end of the internal auditory meatus without a medially placed semicircular canal being opened. A better view of the medial surface of the brain stem (B) can be obtained by drilling the presigmoid petrous bone and retracting the sigmoid sinus forward into the space so provided.

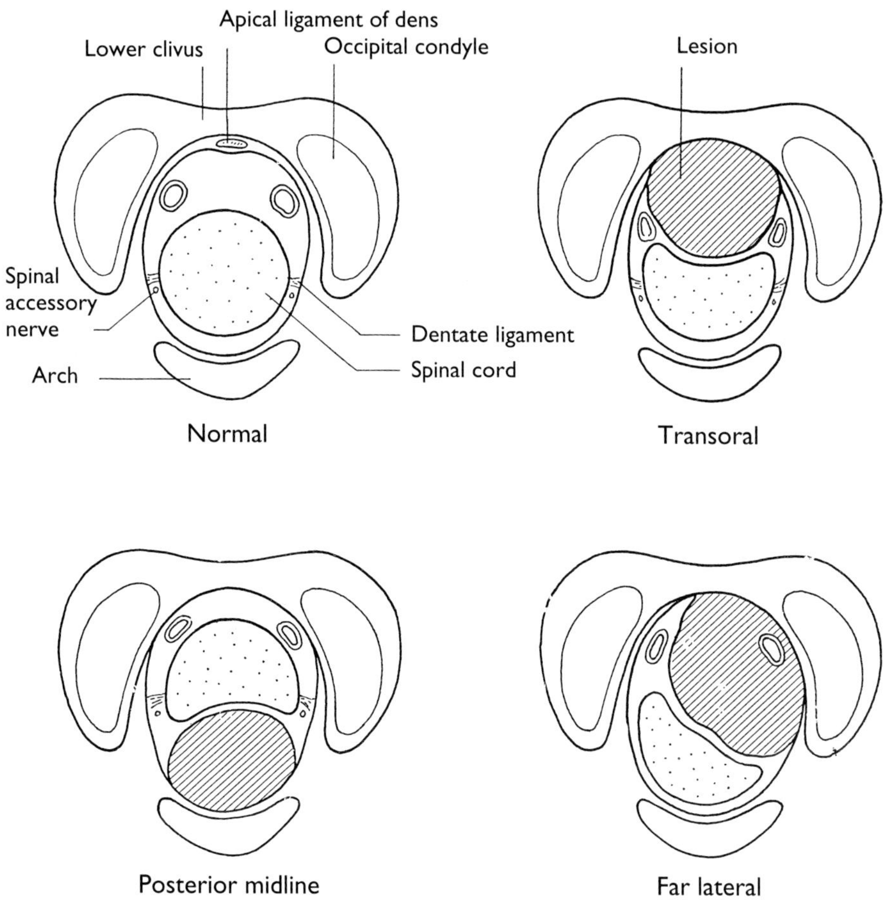

Figure 1-11. The anatomy of the craniocervical junction and the approaches appropriate for tumors in different anatomic locations. The approaches are described by Tuite and Crockard in Chapter 21.

sive skull base lesions. Removal of more than a small part of the condyle will destabilize the craniocervical junction and require some form of fusion. Fortunately such extensive bone removal is not usually necessary.

Target Areas for Surgical Approaches

Approaches to some of the regions of the skull base have been adequately summarized above. For other areas where access may be multidirectional the approaches are discussed below.

Clivus

It is appropriate to describe the clivus in four areas for the purpose of surgical access (Fig. 1-12, Table 1-3). At the upper end of the clivus the retrosellar area should be distinguished from the area behind the sphenoid sinus because the presence of the pituitary restricts anterior access to the retrosellar part. The midclivus extends from the lower margin of the sphenoid sinus (which is at a variable level) to the level of the jugular foramen. Below this the lower clivus includes the occipital condylar area and the anterior half of the foramen magnum.

The optimal approach is governed by the anatomic location of the lesion in relation to the clivus and to the dura. Any lesion that extends laterally into the skull base will require a more extensive and extensible approach, perhaps a combination of approaches. The anterior central approaches have a restricted role in the management of intradural lesions because the approach width is limited (the lesion must therefore be small) and because a watertight repair of the dura in this situation is technically difficult. Nevertheless the route has been used for aneurysms and tumors (Crockard et al., 1991).

The application of the various possible approaches is summarized in Table 1-3.

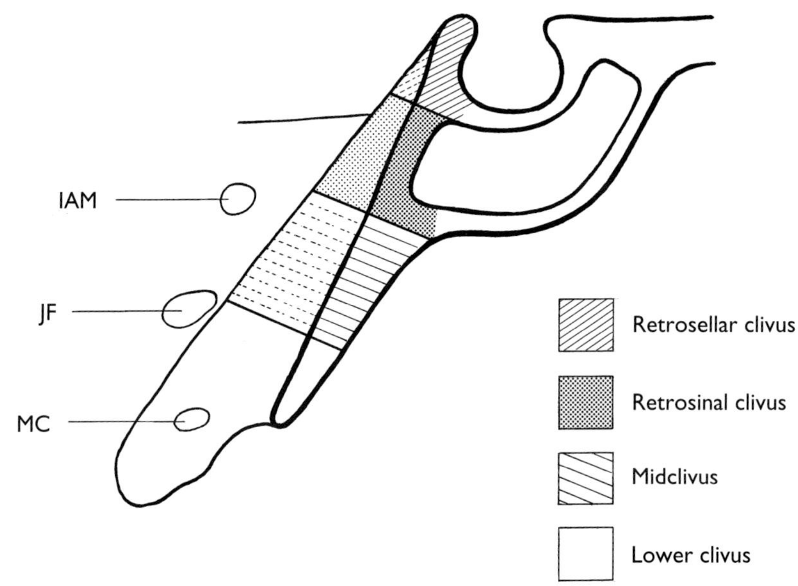

Figure 1-12. The areas of the clivus for the purpose of defining the surgical approaches in Table 1-3. (For explanation of abbreviations see Appendix 1, p. 373.)

Table 1-3. Approaches to the Clivus

	Midline Extradura	Extradural Extending Laterally	Intradural[a]
Retrosellar	Subtemporal Transcavernous	Subtemporal Transcavernous	Subtemporal Trans-Sylvian Presigmoid/parapetrosal
Retrosphenoid	Trans-sphenoidal Basal frontal Transethmoidal	Subtemporal transpetros apex Transcavernous Extended transethmoidal	Subtemporal transpetrous apex Presigmoid/parapetrosal
Midclivus	Basal frontal Le Fort 1 maxillotomy Extended transethmoidal Transoral/transpalatal	Subtemporal-infratemporal Extended transmaxillary Facial translocation	Transcochlear Transpetrous Presigmoid/parapetrosal
Lower clivus	Transoral	Subtemporal-infratemporal Transcondylar/transjugular Transmandibular	Extreme lateral

[a]For small intradural lesions an anterior transclival approach may be appropriate (see text).

Cavernous Sinus

The described approaches to the cavernous sinus are from medial, lateral, superior, and inferior directions (Fig. 1-13). Lesions arising medially may be accessed by the trans-sphenoidal route (Ch. 5) and removed if they have displaced the sinus or invaded only locally medial to the carotid artery.

All the other approaches require a craniotomy from an anterolateral direction. This may involve an orbitozygomatic osteotomy (Chs. 12, 14, and 15) or may not (Ch. 13). By this route, which may be oriented more frontally or more temporally as required, any or all of the other approaches to the cavernous sinus may be undertaken. Inoue et al. (1990) and Sekhar et al. (1987) came to the same conclusion, from studies of microsurgical anatomy, that one single-directional approach was not able to provide adequate access to all parts of the sinus. It is therefore logical to approach the area with a technique versatile enough to provide surgical access for all circumstances. A well-illustrated and in-depth account of this is given by Dolenc (Ch. 13).

Orbit

A comprehensive description of approaches to the orbit is given by Lazarou (Ch. 9).

Internal Auditory Meatus and Posterior Petrous Surface

The common lesions in this area are acoustic neurinomas and meningiomas.

The three approaches used for acoustic neurinomas, the middle fossa, translabyrinthine, and suboccipital routes, have been subjected to cumulative case analysis and discussed by Moskowitz and Long (1991). They showed that for larger tumors where hearing preservation was not an issue there was very little difference between the results of translabyrinthine and suboccipital procedures. The middle fossa approach seemed to have an advantage in very small tumors, allowing serviceable hearing preservation in one-third of cases. However, the same results can be obtained by the suboccipital route in comparable cases (Kemink et al., 1990) and even with larger tumors (Torrens et al., 1994). The conclusion, therefore, is that the surgeon should use the route with which he or she is most comfortable. It contrasts with a commonly held opinion that larger tumors are more safely removed by the trans-

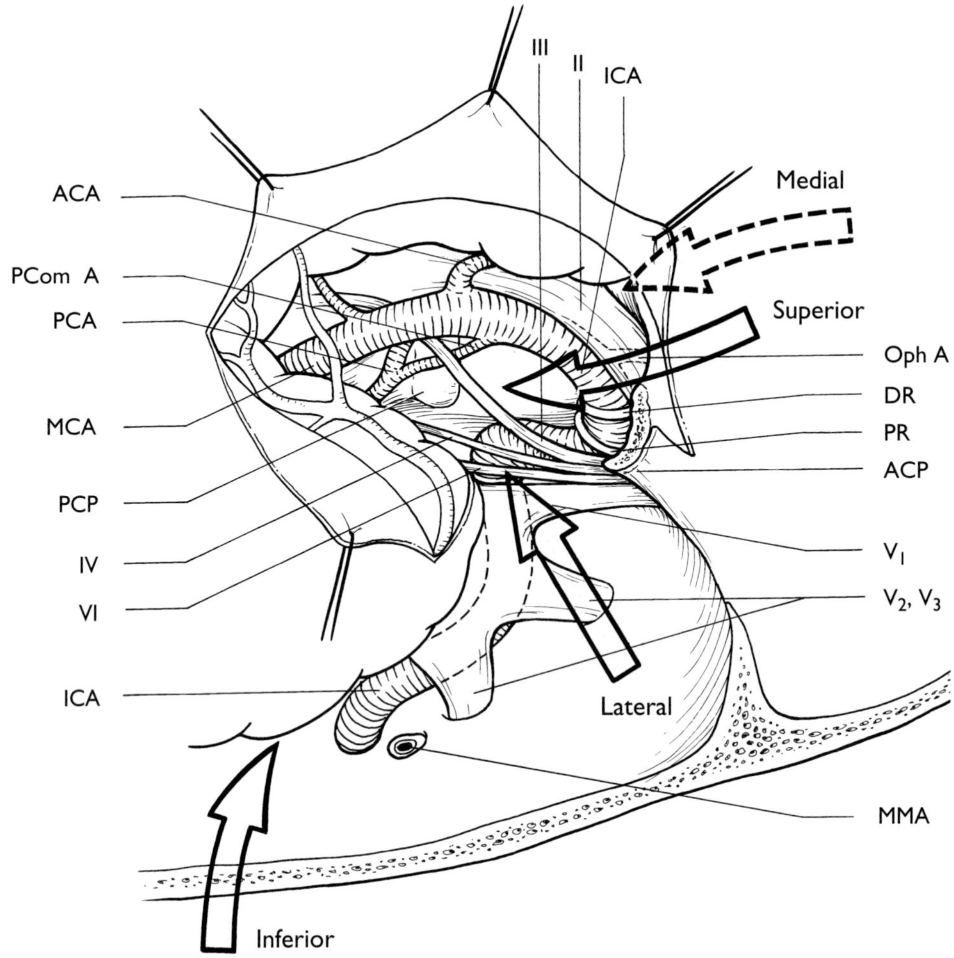

Figure 1-13. The surgical approaches to the cavernous sinus. The medial approach may be trans-sphenoidal via the nose or through the planum sphenoidale. The intracranial approaches can all be conducted through a single anterolateral craniotomy. When necessary the Gasserian ganglion can be split between its divisions.

labyrinthine route. This may in part be due to the advent of atraumatic debulking by ultrasonic aspiration.

Meningiomas are a different matter. Ultrasonic aspirators are not always effective. The lesions may be invasive and their blood supply is from the dural base. Small lesions can be totally removed by the suboccipital route but for larger or invasive lesions removal by this route is likely to be incomplete, leading to recurrence. Because the first operation is the one most likely to be curative it is necessary to design an approach that will succeed. Desgeorges (1994) has produced an elegant classification of petrous meningiomas according to their position, size, and extension; this is shown in Figure 1-14. The appropriate approaches for each position are summarized in Table 1-4.

Jugular Fossa

From the jugular foramen a lesion may extend intracranially, subcranially, or in both directions. The most common tumors in this area are meningiomas, chemodectomas, and neurinomas. Those that extend only intracranially can be removed through a suboccipital craniotomy. Those that extend only subcranially can be approached by the lateral cervical route.

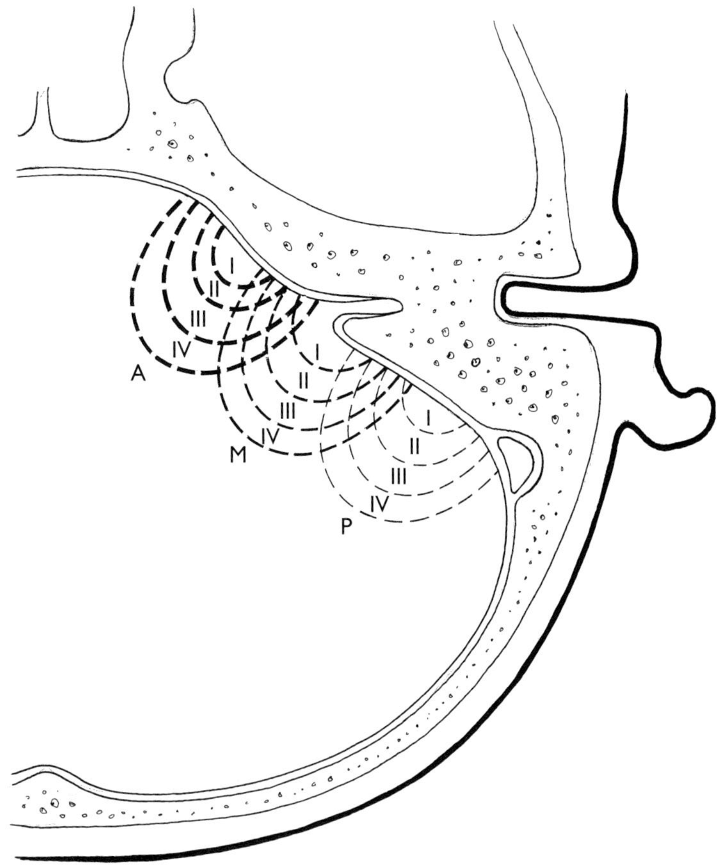

Figure 1-14. The areas of the petrous bone used to classify meningiomas by Desgeorges (1994). A, anterior; M, middle; P, posterior; I, less than 1 cm; II, 1 to1.9 cm; III, 2 to 2.9 cm; IV, 3 cm or greater. Extension may be to the tentorium, clivus, jugular foramen, or foramen magnum. (Adapted from Desgeorges, 1994, with permission.)

For those tumors that extend in both directions a two-stage procedure has sometimes been recommended. The disadvantage of this is that the plane of separation between the two procedures is normally at the jugular foramen and this creates great difficulty with dissection at the second procedure, thus compromising the preservation of nerves. The one-stage procedure is therefore preferable. The technique may require the combination of the infralabyrinthine approach (to preserve hearing), the suboccipital approach (for the intracranial component), the extreme lateral/

Table 1-4. Approaches to Petrous Meningiomas

	Anterior	Middle	Posterior
Transpetrous apex	+	(+)	–
Transcochlear	+	+	+
Anterior extended translabyrinthine[a]	+	+	+
Translabyrinthine	–	+	+
Retrolabyrinthine	–	–	+
Parapetrosal	(+)	+	+
Suboccipital	(+)	(+)	+

+, applicable; –, not applicable; (+), applicable only for small lesions.
[a]Approach described by Desgeorges (1994).

transcondylar approach (to open the posterior wall of the foramen) together with dissection of the neck as far down as necessary. An anterior invasive component is difficult to reach from this posterolateral approach and may need the addition of an infratemporal approach after mobilization of the facial nerve. Kveton and Cooper (1988) provide a colorful illustration of the microsurgical anatomy of this region.

Conclusion

There are certain basic rules for any surgical procedure in this area. I hope readers will forgive their restatement. They may seem obvious but are often overlooked, perhaps because of enthusiasm.

1. Treat the patient and not the computer-produced images. The patient's quality of life is more important than your surgical glory.
2. Know the anatomy and its variations. Anatomy is three-dimensional. Until technology produces widely available three-dimensional reference sources, which no doubt is imminent with CD-ROM, the best sources of knowledge are the cadaver and the patient.
3. Do not mutilate unnecessarily. A combination of two less-invasive approaches may be as good as one more extensive operation (e.g., the combination of transseptal and transoral, rather than the mobilization of the maxilla, to approach the clivus).
4. Know your own abilities and your results. Personal audit is essential. It enables you to tell the truth, to yourself as well as to others.
5. Downward extension of the approach may minimize brain retraction, but do not make life difficult for yourself and the patient by trying to do everything without encroaching on the cranial cavity. The brain withstands controlled retraction up to a point and sometimes even the resection of a noneloquent area of the brain is justified in order to ensure a better outcome.

Surgeons enjoy technical challenges. For neurosurgeons, as the status of aneurysm surgery declines, skull base surgery is attracting attention. No doubt in the next decade some other technical challenge such as endoscopy will supersede. For other surgical specialties dealing with the head and neck the dura remains a frontier to be respected, but not avoided to the detriment of the patient. Each specialty needs to cooperate in order to provide the most effective management of skull base problems.

References

Crockard HA (1988) Anterior approaches to lesions of the upper cervical spine. Clin Neurosurg 34:389–415

Crockard HA (1991) Atlanto-axial subluxation: anterior and posterior approaches. pp. 9–26. In Torrens MJ, Dixon RA (eds): Operative Spinal Surgery. Churchill Livingstone, Edinburgh

Crockard HA, Koksel T, Watkin N (1991) Transoral transclival clipping of anterior inferior cerebellar artery aneurysm using a new rotating applier. J Neurosurg 75:483–485

Crockard HA, Sen CN (1991) The transoral approach for the management of intradural lesions of the craniovertebral junction: a review of 7 cases. Neurosurgery 28:88–98

Derome P (1983) Chirurgie des tumeurs osseuses de la base du crane. Rev Laryngol 104:283–286

Derome P (1988) The transbasal approach to tumors invading the skull base. pp. 619–633. In Schmidek HH, Sweet WH (eds): Operative Neurosurgical Techniques. Grune & Stratton, Orlando

Desgeorges M (1994) Posterior skull base meningiomas. pp. 240–251. In Portmann M, Richards A, Sterkers J-M (eds): Rhino-otological Microsurgery of the Skull Base. Churchill Livingstone, Edinburgh

Fisch U, Fagan P, Valavanis A (1984) The infratemporal approach for the lateral skull base. Otolaryngol Clin North Am 17:513–552

Fujitsu K, Saijole M, Aoki F (1991) Telecanthal approach for meningiomas in the ethmoid and sphenoid sinuses. Neurosurgery 28:714–719

Fukushima T (1993) Combined supra- and infra-parapetrosal approach for petroclival lesions. pp. 661–669. In Sekhar LN, Janecka IP (eds): Surgery of Cranial Base Tumors. Lippincott-Raven, Philadelphia

Inoue T, Rhoton AL Jr, Theele D, Barry ME (1990) Surgical approaches to the cavernous sinus, a microsurgical study. Neurosurgery 26:903–932

Janecka IP, Nuss DW, Sen CN (1991) Midfacial split for access to the central base. Acta Neurochir suppl. 53:199–203

Kemink JL, LaRouere MJ, Kileny PR et al (1990) Hearing preservation following suboccipital removal of acoustic neuromas. Laryngoscope 100:597–602

Krespi YP, Simon GA (1984) Transmandibular exposure of the skull base. Am J Surg 148:534–538

Kveton JF, Cooper MH (1988) Microsurgical anatomy of the jugular foramen region. Am J Otol 9:109–122

Moskowitz N, Long DM (1991) Acoustic neurinomas. Historical review of a century of operated cases. Neurosurg Quart 1:2–18

Moure EJ (1922) Techniques Chirurgicales Oto-rhino-laryngologiques. Libraire Oc Douin, Paris

Sekhar LN, Burgess J, Akin O (1987) Anatomical study of the cavernous sinus emphasizing operative approaches and related neural and vascular reconstruction. Neurosurgery 21:806–816

Sekhar LN, Sen C, Snyderman CH, Janecka IP (1993) Anterior, anterolateral and lateral approaches to extradural petroclival tumors. pp. 157–223. In Sekhar LN, Janecka IP (eds): Surgery of Cranial Base Tumors. Lippincott-Raven, Philadelphia

Torrens M, Maw R, Coakham H et al (1994) Facial and acoustic nerve preservation during excision of extracanalicular acoustic neuromas using the suboccipital route. Br J Neurosurg 8:655–665

Uttley D, Archer J, Marsh HT, Bell BA (1991) Improved access to lesions of the central skull base by mobilization of the zygoma: experience with 54 cases. Neurosurgery 28:99–104

2

Surgical Anatomy of the Sphenoid Bone and Cavernous Sinus

Atul Goel
Michael Torrens
Savvas Kazanas

An excellent knowledge and understanding of anatomy and its possible variations is especially important in skull base surgery. It may be that the new technologic developments relating to three-dimensional imaging and image-directed surgery will assist the surgeon in the exact intraoperative location but it will still be necessary to know the details of the anatomy to be expected in that locality. Authors have stressed the importance of cadaveric dissections for postgraduate surgical training in this subject (Patel et al., 1993).

In these two introductory chapters on surgical anatomy of the skull base we relate the anatomy to two specific bones. The sphenoid bone has been chosen as the key to anterior and anterolateral approaches. Similarly, the petrous temporal bone is the key to posterolateral approaches.

The anatomy of the sphenoid region will be described in three sections: the lateral aspect (cavernous sinus), anterior aspect (paranasal sinuses, nasopharynx, orbit), and the inferior aspect (infratemporal and pterygopalatine fossas).

Surgical Anatomy of the Cavernous Sinus

Speculations on the Physiology of the Cavernous Sinus

The embryologic primary head vein persists and becomes modified to form the cavernous sinus on either side. This sinus has the distinction of draining the ocular tissues. Cavernous sinuses, venous sinusoids or plexuses are likely not to be vestigial but to have a specialized function to perform. The pathos of the eye when the cavernous sinuses are thrombosed emphasizes the important role they must play during physio-

logic states. Its relative capaciousness, distensibility, and interconnections are essential elements that the hydrodynamics of the fluid-filled anterior and posterior chambers of the eyeball may need to thrive. The fluid turnover in both the chambers must be rapid, fairly constant, and at "normal" pressure. A cavernous sinus related to each eye provides it with a large efferent area into which it can quickly drain fluid and any excess blood, allowing optimum function. It may also protect the delicate retinal artery from rupture by pressure due to venous congestion. The sinusoidal dilatation of the venous circuitry in the region of the cavernous sinus appears to be functionally necessary for the performance of the function of a "sponge" or a "shock absorber" to the eyeball.

Why should the cavernous sinus be the only one among all cranial sinuses to be cavernous, similar to the corpus cavernosum of the female or male erectile tissue? A possible reason is that both the cavernous sinus and the corpus cavernosum are the only venous channels designed to allow hemostasis without precipitating clotting. Future research may reveal that this is due to their caverna being endowed with a quantum of cells that secrete anticoagulant substances.

The sphenoid bone is formed from an island of ossification spread over a wide sphenoidal area. As this enlarges the juxtaposed primary head veins, later to become cavernous sinuses, get pushed laterally with the sella turcica rising in between. A plane of cleavage exists between the cavernous sinus and the underlying bone, a plane not easily demonstrated but a distinct embryologic and anatomic reality.

The crowding of structures on either side of the sella turcica and sphenoid sinus has misled anatomists into describing the cavernous sinus as an area through which cranial nerves and the carotid artery course. A little embryologic retrospection will clarify the issue. The cavernous sinuses are venous in origin. The carotid artery and the cranial nerves are in close relationship with this venous structure. This statement implies that the artery and nerves are paracavernous in nature. Any description that suggests that these structures are intracavernous is therefore embryologically incorrect. The venous structure enlarges and dilates and covers the artery and nerves, giving an appearance that these may be intracavernous. The cranial nerves have well-defined dural and arachnoid coverings that keep them isolated from direct contact with the venous blood in their course along the cavernous sinus.

Surgical Anatomy

The cavernous sinuses are situated in the center of the cranial base. The surgical treatment of intra- and paracavernous lesions has been the subject of many conferences and workshops held in the last few years, and also of many articles published in leading journals (Al Mefty and Smith, 1980; Dolenc et al., 1987; Patel et al., 1993). Various approaches have been described to deal with these lesions (Hakuba et al., 1982; Perneczcky et al., 1988; Sekhar et al., 1987). With the advancements in microneurosurgical technology and techniques, more and more of these lesions, which were previously considered inoperable, are being treated surgically.

The anatomy of this region, described by Parkinson (1979) as an "anatomical jewel box," is relatively complex. It is clear that only by perfect understanding of the local anatomy, in a three-dimensional perspective, can one attempt to treat peri- and intracavernous lesions surgically.

Dural Walls. The cavernous sinus extends from the superior orbital fissure anteriorly to the petrous apex posteriorly. It has posterior, medial, superior, inferior, and lateral dural walls (Figs. 2-1 and 2-2). The latter four walls merge at the anterior clinoid process giving the cavernous sinus a conical shape. It measures approximately 2 cm (length) × 1 cm (width) × 1 cm (height). Cranial nerves III and IV enter the dural

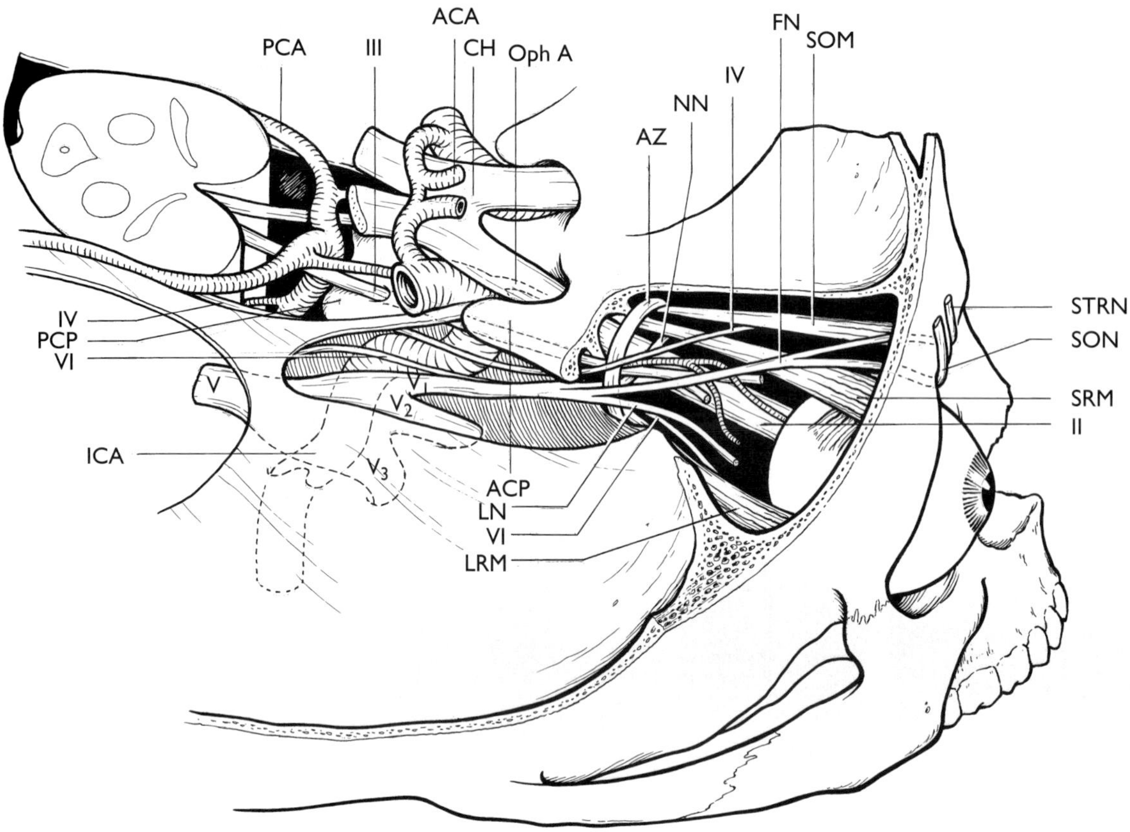

Figure 2-1. An expanded and semidiagrammatic anterolateral view of the anatomy of the sphenoid region and orbit. (For explanation of abbreviations see Appendix 1, p. 373.)

covering of the cavernous sinus through its superior wall and course in the superior aspect of its lateral wall. The Gasserian ganglion with its ophthalmic (V_1) and maxillary (V_2) divisions are located in the dural sheath of the lateral wall. The 6th cranial nerve, on gross observation, traverses within the cavernous sinus.

The dural envelope of the cavernous sinus is complex to understand. The lateral wall of the cavernous sinus has three well-defined and manually separable layers of dura. The internal two layers are formed by the in-curving of layers of the dura along the cranial nerves III, IV, and V as they enter the cavernous sinus in the 3rd nerve cave (discussed later), 4th nerve dural sheath, and in Meckel's cave, respectively. The dural coverings of each of these nerves (thick around the 5th nerve and thin around other nerves) are continuous with each other by a reticular membrane that varies in its thickness. An arachnoid layer is also identified as accompanying the cranial nerves, being better defined around the Gasserian ganglion and the 3rd cranial nerve.

The outer dural layer of the lateral wall of the cavernous sinus is thick and, by sharp dissection, can often be separated into two or more layers. This thick dural layer can be dissected off the inner dural layers covering cranial nerves III, IV, and V and the reticular layer between them by careful sharp dissection in a relatively bloodless plane. Brisk venous bleeding can, however, occur in the region of Parkinson's triangle (defined below) as the reticular membrane is often deficient at this site.

The two-layered middle fossa dura divides to encase the cavernous sinus, the inner (cerebral) layer forming the outer layer of the lateral wall and the outer (endosteal) layer forming the inferior wall of the cavernous sinus, and later continuing as its

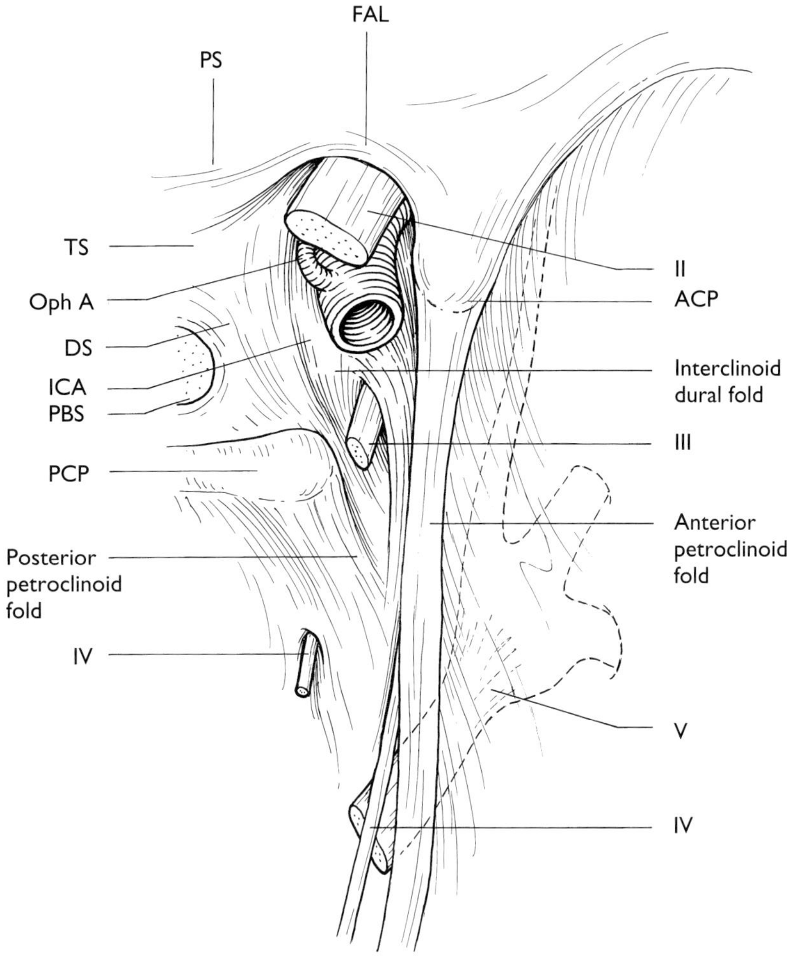

Figure 2-2. The anatomic structure and dural folds of the walls of the cavernous sinus as viewed from above.

medial wall. This description of the dural layers suggests that the cavernous sinus is like other venous sinuses (e.g., superior sagittal sinus) with the exception that cranial nerves and the carotid artery traverse in close proximity during their course in the base of the skull.

The dura of the medial wall of the cavernous sinus is very thin and closely adherent to the body of the sphenoid bone. The sphenoid bone separating the pituitary gland from the cavernous sinus is also thin. This explains the frequent spread of pituitary tumors into the cavernous sinus. The lateral wall of the cavernous sinus, being thick and resilient, restricts further lateral spread of pituitary tumors. The thinner outer layer of the middle fossa dura separates from the thicker inner layer at the lateral aspect of the Gasserian ganglion and its divisions. At the various foramina, this layer folds out with the nerves and the carotid artery. It thickens in the form of a firm ring at the entry of the carotid artery into the cavernous sinus. It also curves along the carotid artery into its petrous segment and forms the "periosteal sheath."

The outer thicker layer of dura forming the lateral wall of the cavernous sinus continues laterally as the inner layer of the middle fossa dura and medially as the superior wall of the cavernous sinus. The superior wall dura continues medially as the dura over the planum sphenoidale, wraps around the anterior clinoid process, covers the tuberculum sellae, and forms the diaphragma sellae. It also forms the roof of the

proximal part of the optic canal in the form of a thick dural fold called the *falciform ligament*. The dura layer is markedly thick at the anterior and posterior petroclinoid folds and moderately thick at the interclinoid dural folds. It is firmly adherent at the tip of the clinoid processes but is separable by blunt, or occasionally sharp, dissection. The same layer of dura is also continuous with the dura of the tentorium and the clivus.

The superior wall of the cavernous sinus is triangular in shape, the sides of the triangle being formed by thickened dural folds, which are anterior extensions of the dura of the tentorium and the dura of the lateral wall of the cavernous sinus. The apex of the triangle is formed by the anterior clinoid process. The short posterior side is formed by the posterior petroclinoid fold extending from the petrous apex dura to the posterior clinoid process. The lateral side is formed by the anterior petroclinoid dural fold, extending from the petrous apex to the anterior clinoid process, whereas the medial side is formed by the interclinoid dural fold. The space enclosed by these three dural folds is also called the *oculomotor trigone*.

Third Cranial Nerve. In the center of the oculomotor trigone the 3rd, or oculomotor, nerve enters the dural wall of the cavernous sinus (Figs. 2-1 and 2-3A & C). The 3rd nerve forms a smooth crater for itself along the superior wall of the cavernous sinus and posterior petroclinoid dural fold. The dura of the superior wall curves with and traverses along the 3rd nerve. A relatively large subarachnoid space covers the 3rd nerve for about 6 mm after its entry into the superior wall. The appearance of the nerve at its entry into the cavernous sinus from a superior view suggests that it is entering into a dural cave. One of the authors (A.G.) has observed, in his series of cases, entry of tumors in this region along the 3rd nerve into the cavernous sinus. The dura, being separate from the nerve in this region, also provides for the surgeon a plane to make an incision into the lateral wall of the cavernous sinus. The 3rd nerve itself (and similarly the other cranial nerves of the cavernous sinus that are surrounded by dural layers) is not in direct contact with the venous blood in the cavernous sinus. The direction of the 3rd nerve and the anterior clinoid process are important surgical landmarks. The inferolateral surface of the anterior clinoid process is in direct contact with and frequently grooved by the 3rd nerve. The nerve can therefore be injured during procedures involving drilling of the anterior clinoid process.

Fourth Cranial Nerve. The 4th, or trochlear, nerve enters the oculomotor trigone at its lateral angle (Figs. 2-1 to 2-3A & C). After its course in the ambient cistern just beneath the tentorial edge, it enters between the leaves of tentorial dura at 10 to 18 mm distance from the posterior clinoid process. To save the 4th cranial nerve during sectioning of the tentorium, the tentorium should be incised at least 15 mm posterior to the posterior clinoid process, keeping the 4th nerve in view during this process. The 4th nerve then traverses in the walls of the edge of the tentorium for 8 to 10 mm and turns to course parallel to the 3rd nerve. Just before entry of the nerve into the superior orbital fissure, it turns superiorly to cross the 3rd nerve.

Fifth Cranial Nerve. The two dural layers that enclose the Gasserian ganglion and its three divisions (after the 5th nerve enters Meckel's cave) are separate and easily dissectable from it until the semilunar-shaped ganglion divides into the three divisions, the space between the dura and ganglion being occupied by cerebrospinal fluid during life (Figs. 2-1 and 2-3A & C). Beyond the semilunar ganglion, the accompanying arachnoid layer becomes thinned out, and the dura is relatively firmly fixed to the divisions of the nerves and becomes continuous with the epineurium. The dura is

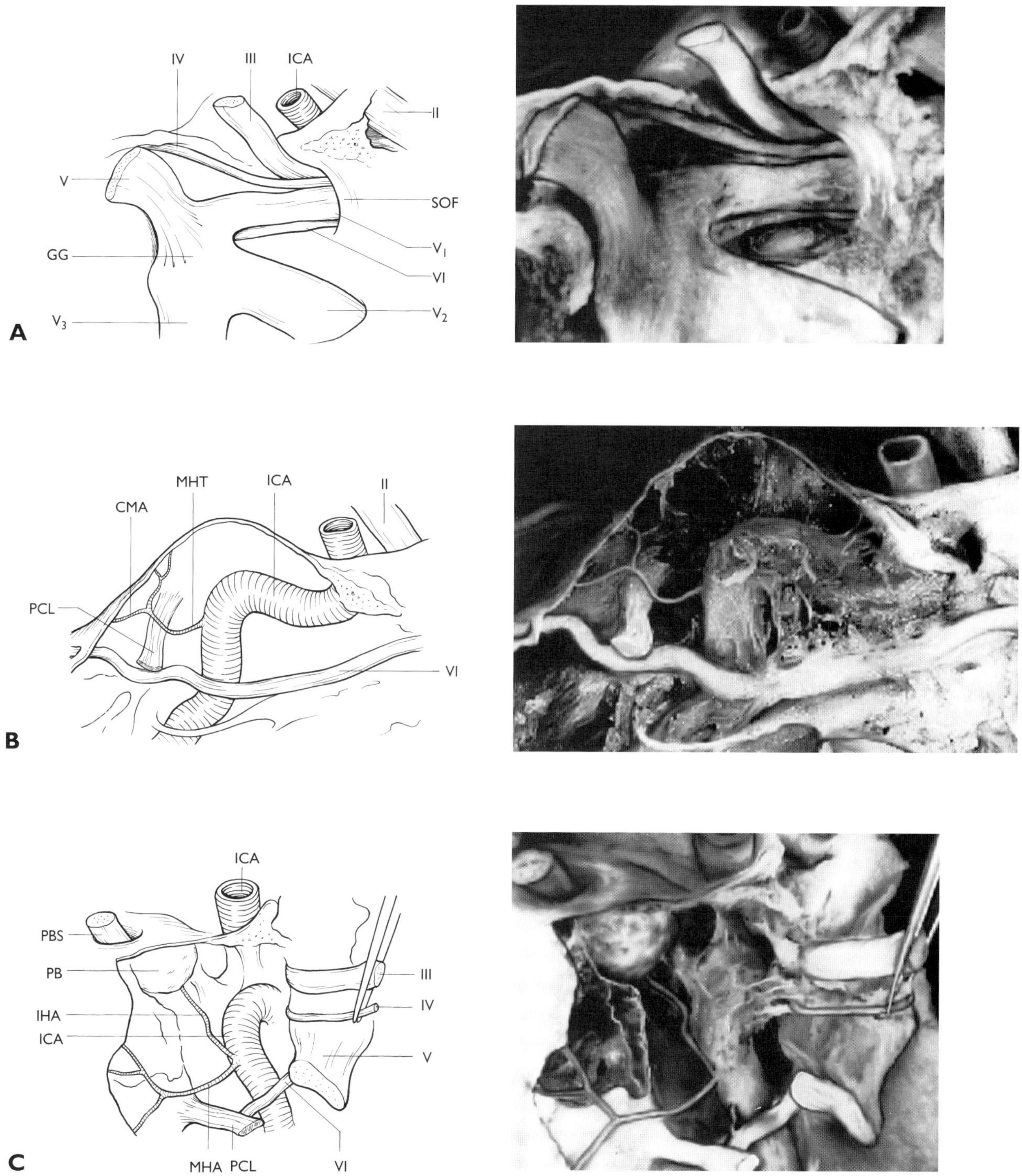

Figure 2-3. Retouched photographs of dissections of the cavernous sinus. *(A)* The lateral aspect after removal of the dura mater. *(B)* Lateral view following removal of the structures in the lateral wall (III, IV, V nerves) illustrating the course of nerve VI. *(C)* View from a posterior perspective. Nerves III, IV, and V are displaced laterally. The posterior loop of the intracavernous carotid artery and its branches are visualized.

more densely stuck to the first division (V_1) of the nerve, from which it is difficult to dissect free. The upper two-thirds of the Gasserian ganglion and its V_1 division, and often the upper part of the second division (V_2), are located in the lateral wall of the cavernous sinus. The third division (V_3) separates off from the ganglion and, after a short intracranial course, exits via the foramen ovale. V_2 exits via the foramen rotundum and its initial segment forms the lateral wall of the cavernous sinus. The foramena rotundum, ovale, and spinosum (the foramen of the middle meningeal artery) are important surgical landmarks. V_1 forms the lateral wall of the cavernous sinus and is the longest segment of the 5th cranial nerve in direct relation with the cavernous sinus. The superior ophthalmic vein drains into the cavernous sinus through the angle between V_1 and V_2 nerves.

Sixth Cranial Nerve. The 6th, or abducens, nerve enters the cavernous sinus via Dorello's canal. This canal is situated in the two layers of the dura of the petroclival region. It is located between the petroclinoid ligament and the superior surface of the medial part of the clivus, which is covered by the dural layer forming the medial wall of the cavernous sinus. The entry point of the nerve into the clival dura is situated about 15 mm below the tip of the posterior clinoid process. The two nerves enter the dura parallel to each other at a distance of 12 to 15 mm apart. The nerve enters the clival dura carrying along with it a very thin dural and an arachnoid sheath. It courses superiorly in the basilar venous sinus of the clivus, then takes a smooth bend over the petrous apex. At the petrous apex it traverses under the medial part of the petroclinoid ligament (Gruber's ligament), which is a bow-tie–shaped ligament extending from the petrous apex to the clival dura. It is wider at its attachments and relatively thinner at its center. This ligament is situated in a venous pool at the region demarcating the cavernous sinus from the large basilar venous plexus. There are multiple rootlets of the 6th nerve that join into a single bundle at its entry into the clival dura. These rootlets may separate again in Dorello's canal into two to five elements. Some of these rootlets may even course above the petroclival or petrosphenoid ligament (Gruber's ligament), which can always be identified by its large size, tough and elastic character (unlike relatively weak dural folds in the surroundings), and shiny, silvery appearance. Dorello's canal is an osteofibrous conduit located over the clivus measuring about 3 to 4 mm in length (its floor being formed by the lateral edge of the clival bone and its roof by Gruber's ligament) and is about 3.5 mm anteromedial to the petrous apex.

The 6th nerve traverses Dorello's canal to reach the cavity of the cavernous sinus. After the 6th nerve has passed under the petroclinoid ligament, it turns superolaterally to traverse lateral to the carotid artery at its posterior ascending segment. It is sometimes important to identify and dissect the 6th nerve during surgery. It can be traced during its course medial to Meckel's cave and the inferior aspect of the first division of the 5th nerve. It is usually situated in the axilla between the horizontal segment of the intracavernous carotid artery and the artery of the inferior cavernous sinus. The nerve traverses lateral to the carotid artery at its posterior ascending segment, and is then inferolateral to it.

The average distance between the points of entry of the cranial nerves into the cavernous sinus was found to be as follows: between III and IV, 6.16 mm; between III and V, 12.34 mm; between IV and V, 10.52 mm; and between V and VI, 6.50 mm. The mean length of intracavernous cranial nerves was as follows: III, 12.26 mm; IV, 14.40 mm; V, 16.38 mm; and VI, 20.44 mm.

Venous Sinuses. There has been considerable controversy as to whether the cavernous sinus is made up of large sinusoidal venous spaces or of a plexus of veins

(Taptas, 1982). The recent opinion based on histoarchitectural studies confirms the plexiform pattern. However, in cadaveric studies large sinusoidal venous spaces are seen. The description of the plexiform venous pattern does not appear to be clinically relevant. The plexus pattern is more distinct in fetal cavernous sinus and in the cavernous sinus of lower animals. The main venous entry to the cavernous sinus comes through the superior ophthalmic veins via the superior orbital fissure draining into the cavernous sinus between nerves V_1 and V_2. The cavernous sinus also communicates anteriorly with the sphenoparietal sinus and the superficial sylvian vein, laterally with the venous sinuses accompanying the middle meningeal artery, and posteriorly with the basilar sinus. The pterygoid venous plexus communicates with the cavernous sinus via the emissary sphenoidal foramen situated medial to the foramen ovale.

The anterior and posterior intercavernous sinuses, closely related to the pituitary gland, connect the two cavernous sinuses. The posterior intercavernous sinus is larger than the anterior. These interconnections are situated between two layers of dura. There is a large venous connection between the two cavernous sinuses via the basilar clival venous plexus. The basilar venous plexus contains a large pool of venous blood. This pool of blood can significantly affect transclival surgical approaches. The basilar venous plexus has a major communication with the cavernous sinus at the petrous apex. There is a larger superior petrosal sinus and smaller inferior petrosal sinus draining the cavernous sinus. The superior petrosal sinus is situated over the petrous ridge. It traverses over the root of the 5th nerve within two layers of dura. The inferior petrosal sinus travels inferior to the root of the 5th nerve. The venous spaces in the cavernous sinus have been named by Harris and Rhoton (1976) based on their relationship to the carotid artery. The main venous spaces are the medial, lateral, anteroinferior, and posterosuperior venous spaces. The medial and posterosuperior venous spaces are larger than the lateral and anteroinferior venous spaces, respectively, in most specimens.

Carotid Artery and Branches. The carotid artery traverses the petrous apex region underneath the Gasserian ganglion (Figs. 2-1, 2-3, and 2-4). A dural ring under the Gasserian ganglion marks the entry point of the artery into the cavernous sinus. The artery under this dural ring is relatively fixed and the segment in the cavernous sinus beyond this ring is relatively mobile. The carotid artery is also fixed to the skull base at the anterior clinoid process by dural rings. In about 70 percent of specimens the bone separating the carotid artery from the lateral half of the Gasserian ganglion is absent. It was seen during our dissections that there are membranous adhesions attached to the carotid artery, 6th nerve, and 3rd and 4th nerves. The artery makes several twists around its longitudinal axis during its course in the cavernous sinus, which may in some way be responsible for the temperature regulation of cerebral blood flow (Dolenc, 1983).

The intracavernous carotid artery has been divided into a posterior ascending segment, posterior genu, horizontal segment, anterior genu, and anterior ascending segment. The dome of the posterior genu can sometimes, particularly in elderly patients with atherosclerotic vessels, be very close to the posterior clinoid process. The distal part of the anterior ascending segment of the carotid artery is situated medial to the anterior clinoid process. Removal of the anterior clinoid process permits an additional exposure of approximately 6 mm of the internal carotid artery without entering into the cavernous sinus.

The juxtaclinoid carotid artery is surrounded by bone almost in its entire circumference. Laterally it is related to the medial surface of the anterior clinoid process, anteriorly it is in close proximity of the posterior surface of the optic strut, whereas

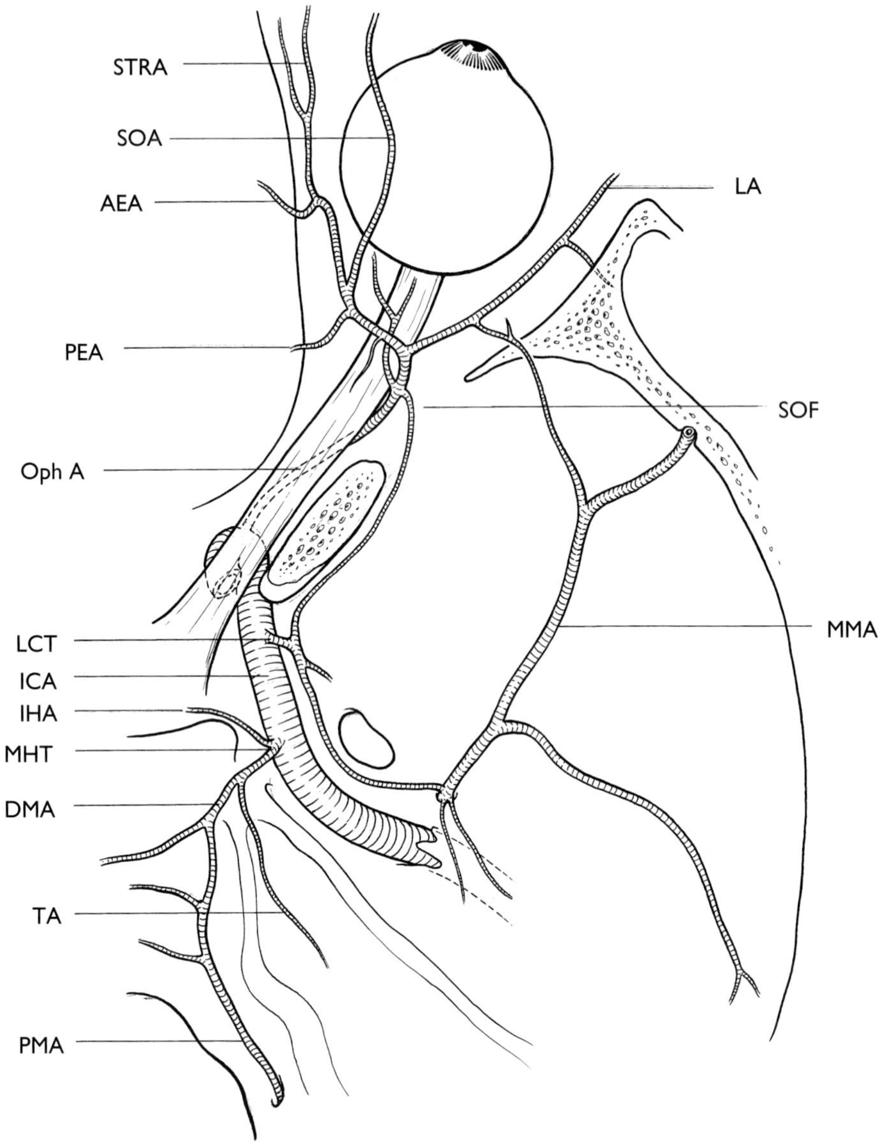

Figure 2-4. A typical distribution of arteries in relation to the cavernous sinus and orbit.

medially it lies on the body of the sphenoid bone. The posterior border of this segment of the carotid artery is in relation to the cavity of the cavernous sinus. However, sometimes the middle clinoid process may form a bony divide between the artery and the cavernous sinus.

The anterior clinoid process is separated from the carotid artery by a dural sheath. There are two prominent dural folds lateral to the carotid artery after the anterior clinoid process is drilled off. These are called the *proximal* and *distal dural rings* of the carotid artery. The dural sheath covering the artery is continuous with the dura covering the nerves of the superior orbital fissure and the dura over the planum sphenoidale and tuberculum sellae and with the lateral wall of the cavernous sinus. There is controversy as to whether the "clinoidal segment" of the carotid artery is intracavernous or extracavernous. In our study it was seen that the segment of the dura covering the artery may be separated from it for the initial part and then be continuous with the cavernous sinus. It appears that there is a potential space between the dura and the artery at this site that is, or may become, continuous with the cavernous

sinus in certain situations. The supraclinoid carotid artery courses over the superior wall of the cavernous sinus. Lateral or medial retraction of this segment of the carotid artery can lead to exposure of the superior wall. The exposure of the intracavernous lesions via the superior wall is an important surgical avenue.

There are two main branches of the intracavernous carotid artery. The posterior caroticocavernous or meningohypophyseal trunk emerges from the posterior aspect of the ascending segment of the cavernous carotid artery about 4 to 6 mm below the dome of the posterior genu of the artery. In our study the artery was seen to divide into multiple branches immediately after its origin. Of these the tentorial artery (of Bernasconi and Cassineri), after its short course in the cavernous sinus, enters into the tentorial dural fold. The dorsal meningeal artery and inferior hypophyseal artery have a relatively long course in the venous pool. The dorsal meningeal artery traverses in a posteromedial direction near the clival end of the petroclival ligament, courses over the clival dural surface, and then divides into superior and inferior clival branches. Branches of this artery anastomose with the branches of the contralateral artery and with the posterior meningeal artery. The inferior hypophyseal artery runs medially, in a relatively straight course, to the posterior lobe of the pituitary gland. Branches of the meningohypophyseal trunk were seen going to cranial nerves III to VI.

The lateral caroticocavernous trunk or artery of the inferior cavernous sinus (inferolateral trunk) is the other branch of the intracavernous carotid artery. This artery arises from the horizontal segment of the carotid artery and traverses over the 6th cranial nerve. It corresponds to the proximal remnant of the embryonic dorsal ophthalmic artery. In one specimen, however, the artery coursed under the 6th nerve. It supplies the dura of the inferior wall of the cavernous sinus and also small branches supply the intracavernous cranial nerves. McConnel's capsular artery has been seen to arise in 18 percent of specimens from the medial surface of the distal half of the horizontal segment of the carotid artery, supplying the dural sheath around the pituitary gland. The ophthalmic artery has sometimes been seen to arise from the intracavernous carotid.

A sympathetic plexus of nerves accompanies the carotid artery in the petrous bone. After the artery enters the cavernous sinus by passing under the dural ring, the sympathetic nerves separate off the carotid. Some branches join initially the 6th nerve, and then the V_1 division of the 5th nerve, and ultimately leave the cavernous sinus, with each division of the trigeminal nerve providing sympathetic innervation in the respective territory. A ganglion of the sympathetic nerve was seen between the 6th cranial nerve and the carotid artery.

Occasionally some fat globules may be seen in the cavernous sinus. The fat is commonly situated at the anterolateral end adjoining the orbital adipose tissue and at the posterior end near the petrous margin of the cavernous sinus. In the middle part scattered fat deposits around the pituitary fossa are often seen. It is frequently difficult to differentiate fat globules from sympathetic fibers and ganglia with the surgical microscope.

Triangles. Various triangles have been described by Dolenc et al. (1987) and others to make understanding of the anatomy of the cavernous sinus more clear. These triangles often get distorted by the presence of intracavernous pathology. However, the entry points of the nerves and artery into the cavernous sinus are via relatively fixed sites and, even if the triangles may get distorted, orientation during surgery can be gained from the fixed entry points of these nerves.

Parkinson (1979) described an important triangle for approaching the cavernous sinus through its lateral wall. The boundaries of this triangle are the 3rd–4th nerve complex superiorly, the first division of the 5th nerve inferiorly, and the clival dura

posteriorly. The maximum distance between V_1 and the 4th cranial nerve was 4 mm. The 6th nerve is not seen in this triangle. V_1 must be retracted inferiorly to expose the 4th nerve. Occasionally the medial surface of V_1 may be indented by the 6th nerve. The posterior ascending segment of the carotid artery and its meningohypophyseal trunk can be exposed in this triangle. Parkinson described this triangle for exposure of the carotid artery and the meningohypophyseal trunk, because this is an important site of development of intracavernous carotid artery aneurysm and caroticocavernous fistula. The triangle is thus an important landmark for exposure of intracavernous lesions.

Prior to actually incising the walls of the cavernous sinus it is important to get oriented to the local anatomy. Important bony landmarks are the anterior clinoid process, posterior clinoid process, foramen ovale, foramen rotundum, superior orbital fissure, and petrous apex. Soft tissue landmarks are the exit point of the carotid artery from the roof of the cavernous sinus, optic nerve, divisions of the 5th nerve, greater superficial petrosal nerve, and the entry points and directions of the various oculomotor nerves.

Anterior Relations of the Sphenoid Bone

Orbit

The orbit is in the shape of a tilted cone with the apex posterior and medial. Within the bony cone is the muscle cone, arising at the apex mostly from the annulus of Zinn (Fig. 2-5). This annulus surrounds the optic canal (pars optica) and the medial end of the superior orbital fissure (pars oculomotoria). The contents of these foramina are also shown in Figure 2-5 and the superior orbital fissure has been described by Morard et al. (1994). The most variable structure is the ophthalmic vein (or veins). The optic canal is approximately 10 mm long and 5 mm in diameter and contains the optic nerve with the ophthalmic artery below it, very occasionally in a separate bony canal.

Surgical exploration within the orbit requires the surgeon to have an image of the expected anatomy (Figs. 2-4 and 2-6). The nervous anatomy is less variable than the vascular. In addition to the larger nerves shown in Figure 2-6 there are also the small branches of the oculomotor nerve to the appropriate muscles and the long and short ciliary nerves. When necessary the surgical anatomy is easier to trace from the apex outward, thus making the superolateral approach the most preferable.

Nasal Cavities

The two nasal cavities are separated by the nasal septum. This is formed by the septal cartilage anteriorly, the vomer posteroinferiorly, and the perpendicular plate of the ethmoid posterosuperiorly. The ala of the vomer fits into the groove formed by the vaginal processes at the base of the sphenoid.

The lateral nasal wall is an anatomically complicated area (Fig. 2-7). It bears the three or four prominent nasal turbinates (conchae) named inferior, middle, superior, and supreme. The air passages between the lateral nasal wall and the lateral aspect of these turbinates are named the inferior, middle, superior, and supreme meatae, respectively. The space above and behind the turbinates is called the sphenoethmoidal recess and contains the opening of the sphenoidal sinus. The inferior meatus receives the nasolacrimal duct; the opening is 2 to 3 cm posterior to the vestibule. The middle meatus contains the openings of the frontal sinus, anterior ethmoidal cells, and maxillary sinus. Secretions from these sinuses pass through the infundibulum, a complicated cleft-like canal ending near the superior surface of the inferior turbinate.

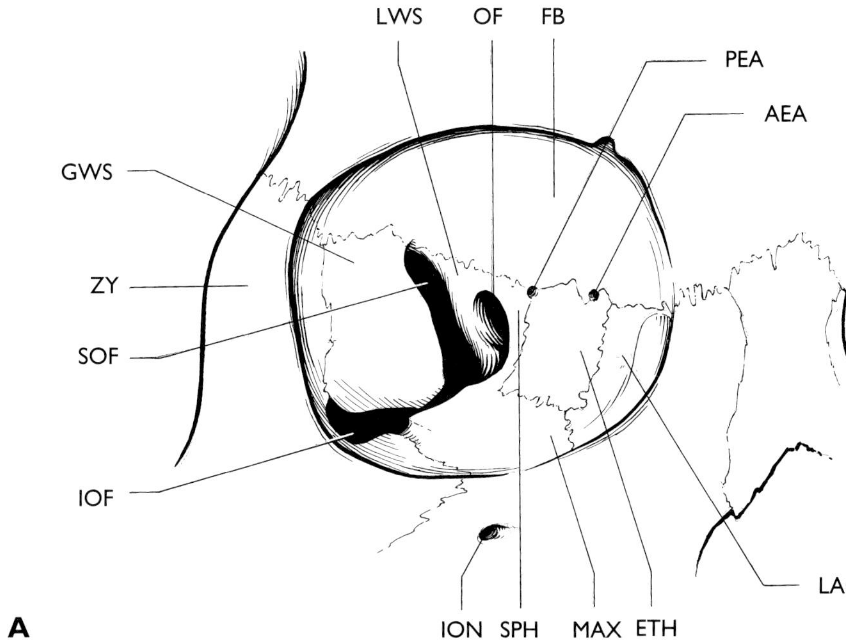

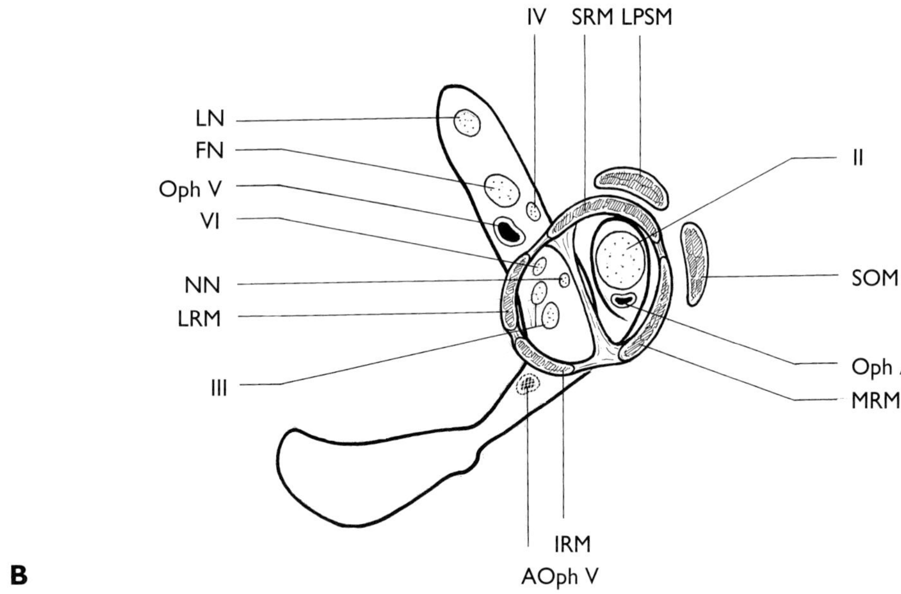

Figure 2-5. The anatomy of the orbit. *(A)* The bony structure. *(B)* The orbital fissures and the structures arising from the apex of the orbit. The annulus of Zinn, from which the majority of ocular muscles originate, is divided into two parts: the medial pars optica and the lateral pars oculomotoria.

Blood Supply of the Nasal Cavity. A number of arteries form a rich anastomotic network. The sphenopalatine artery (maxillary artery branch) enters through the sphenopalatine foramen, branches to form the lateral nasal and septal arteries, and supplies most of the posterior part of the nose, the turbinates, and the posterior septum. The septal branch crosses the anterior wall of the sphenoid sinus where it is vulnerable to surgical injury. The anterior and posterior ethmoidal arteries (ophthalmic) supply the upper part of the cavity. The descending palatine artery (maxillary)

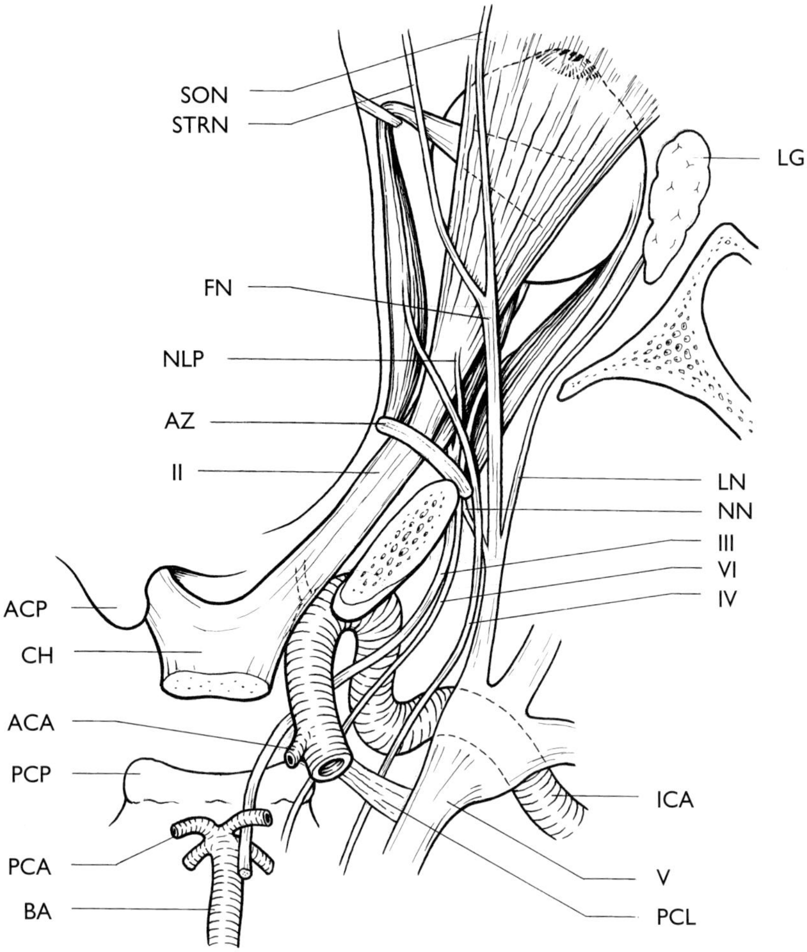

Figure 2-6. The distribution of nerves in relation to the cavernous sinus and orbit.

divides into greater and lesser palatine branches, which supply the soft and hard palate. The superior labial artery (facial) supplies the vestibule and anterior septum.

Paranasal Sinuses

The morphology of the paranasal sinuses is so variable that, before a surgical transgression, the surgeon needs to establish the individual anatomy in each patient using computed tomography and magnetic resonance imaging. In this section we concentrate only on those details that may aid in the interpretation of these scans.

Ethmoid Sinus. In the ethmoid sinus certain areas are of particular importance to the surgeon. The highest point of the roof is usually above the level of the cribriform plate. According to Kainz and Stammberger (1989) there are three types of olfactory fossa. In type 1 (12 percent) the lamina cribrosa is almost level with the roof of the ethmoid and the fossa is shallow or hardly existent. In type 2 (70 percent) the roof of the ethmoid is higher than the lamina cribrosa, the olfactory fossa is deeper, and its lateral wall, which is the medial wall of the upper ethmoidal cells, is thin (the thinnest area of the skull base). In type 3 (18 percent) the crista galli is lower than the ethmoid roof and the fossa is as deep as the height of the crista galli. This type is the most dangerous for the surgeon.

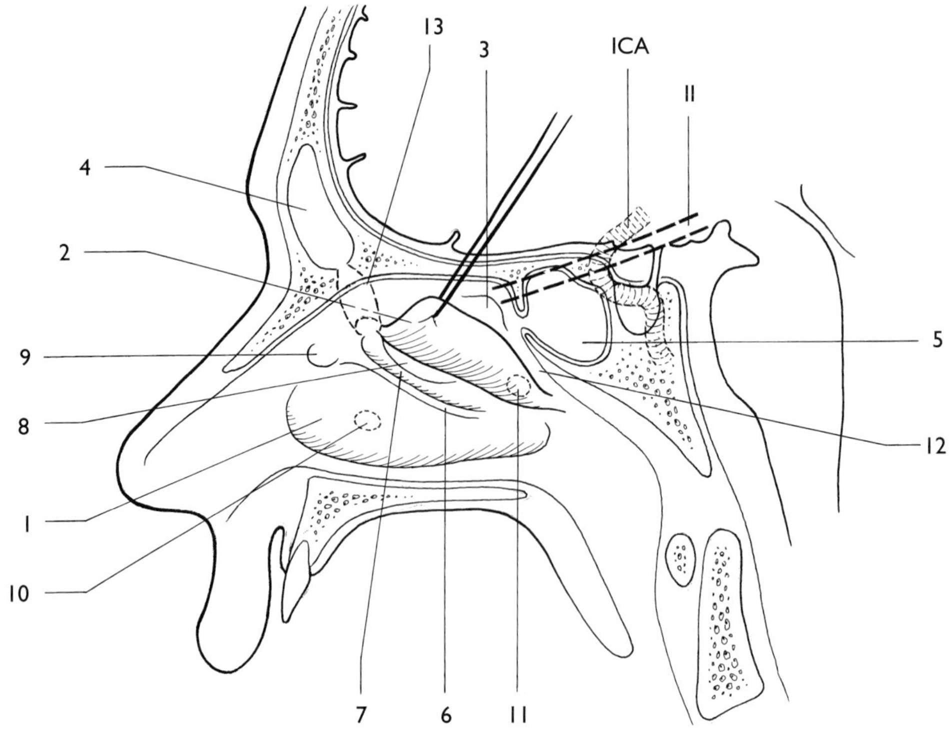

Figure 2-7. The lateral wall of the nasopharynx. 1, Inferior turbinate: 2, middle turbinate (held up by traction stitch); 3, superior turbinate; 4, frontal sinus; 5, sphenoid sinus; 6, uncinate process; 7, semilunar hiatus leading to infundibulum; 8, bulla ethmoidalis; 9, agger nasi; 10, opening of nasolacrimal duct; 11, position of sphenopalatine foramen; 12, sphenoethmoidal recess; 13, frontonasal duct.

The anterior ethmoidal artery passes through the anterior ethmoidal foramen to run anteromedially through the sinus in the anterior ethmoidal canal. This canal may hang from the roof of the sinus on a bony mesentery. It is usually at about the same level as the cribriform plate (2 mm below to 4 mm above) and is easily injured. Its terminal branch runs through the cribriform plate to the anterior fossa dura.

The posterior ethmoidal artery enters through the posterior ethmoidal foramen, which is very close to the orbital end of the optic canal. It also runs anteromedially in a bony canal, the posterior ethmoidal canal, which is usually slightly (1.5 mm) above the level of the cribriform plate. In one-third of cases (Lang, 1989) there are tertiary ethmoidal canals to be found between the anterior and posterior canals.

In some cases the posterior ethmoidal cells extend lateral to, or above, the sphenoid sinus. These are called Onodi cells and often the bony canals of the optic nerve and carotid artery can be seen in their lateral walls. Both structures are liable to injury here.

Sphenoid Sinus. The sphenoid sinus opens by a canal-like ostium through the upper lateral part of the anterior sphenoidal wall into the sphenoethmoidal recess. The sphenoid sinus may have extremely variable forms and can extend into the clivus, around the optic canal into the wings of the sphenoid bone, into the ethmoid and palatine bones, and even into the vomer. Average dimensions are therefore meaningless and individual anatomy must be obtained from scans. The two halves rarely communicate and in only one-quarter of cases is the septum in the midline. Accessory septa exist in 75 percent of cases.

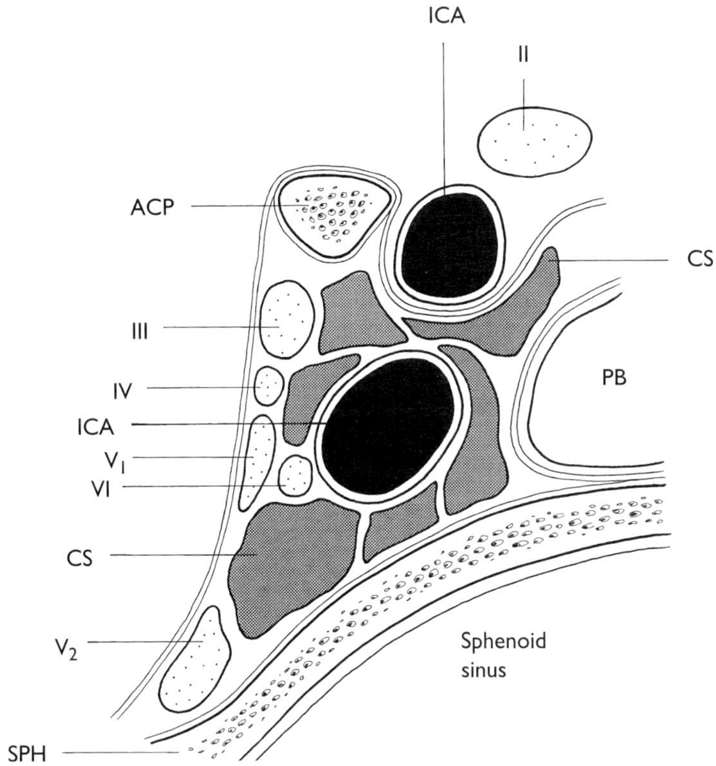

Figure 2-8. A coronal section at the level of the anterior clinoid process showing the superolateral relations of the sphenoid sinus.

The relations of the sphenoid sinus are illustrated in Figures 2-8 and 2-9. The most surgically vulnerable structure is the carotid artery. In 65 percent a carotid canal projects into the sinus (Van Alyea, 1941), and occasionally the carotids meet in the midline. The optic canal projects into the sinus in 7 percent (Dixon, 1937) to 40 percent (Van Alyea, 1941) of cases and the bone may be very thin or have dehiscences. A projection from the lateral side into the sinus may also be an ethmoidal Onodi cell.

In a small sphenoid sinus there may be no bulge of the pituitary fossa visible. It is important to be aware of this beforehand and avoid either too high or too low an approach, opening either the anterior or posterior fossa.

Nasopharynx

The nasopharynx is situated below the sphenoid sinus and basisphenoid, bounded laterally by the pharyngeal recesses and inferiorly by the upper surface of the soft palate and the pharyngeal isthmus. Just below and anterior to the pharyngeal recess, the opening of the eustachian tube can be seen. Lymphoid tissue (adenoids) can extend over the roof, posterior wall, and pharyngeal recess, especially in children.

At the junction between the roof and posterior wall can be found, in the mucosa and periosteum of the sphenoid bone, a pharyngeal hypophysis that corresponds to the lower end of Rathke's pouch. A little lower in the midline there is a small depression, the pharyngeal bursa, often covered by lymphoid tissue. This may be the site of cystic infection (Tornwaldt cyst).

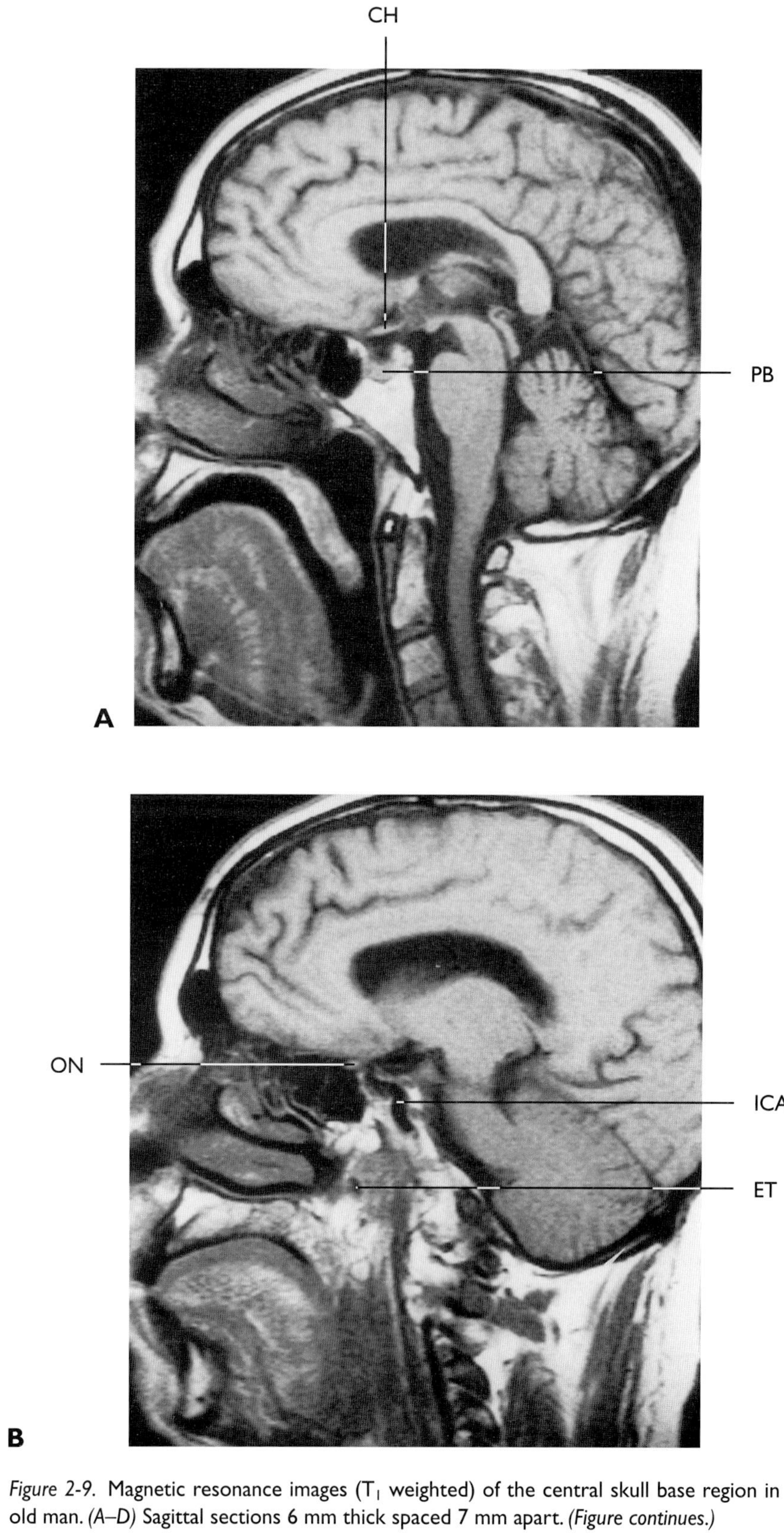

Figure 2-9. Magnetic resonance images (T_1 weighted) of the central skull base region in a 58-year-old man. *(A–D)* Sagittal sections 6 mm thick spaced 7 mm apart. *(Figure continues.)*

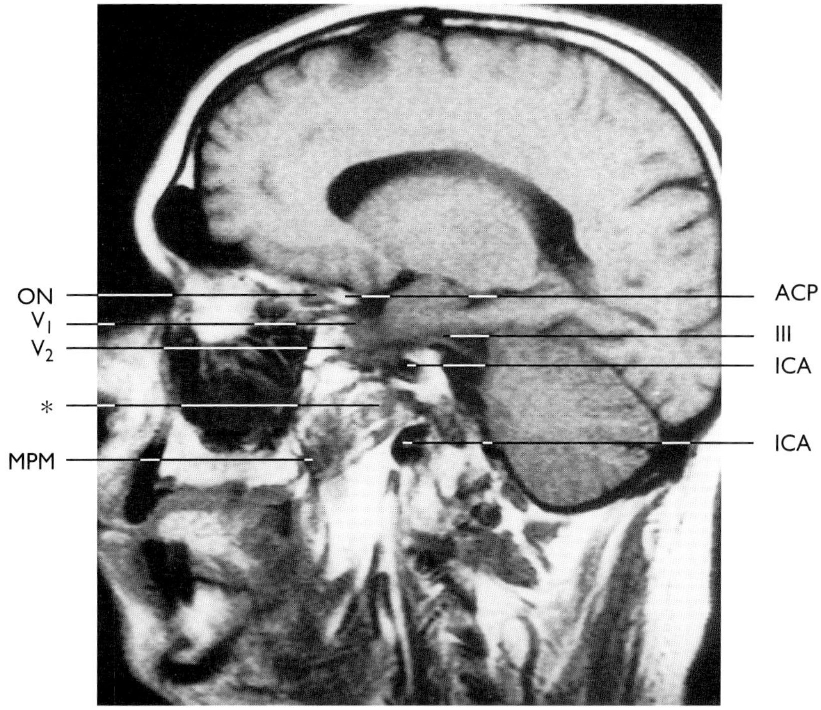

C

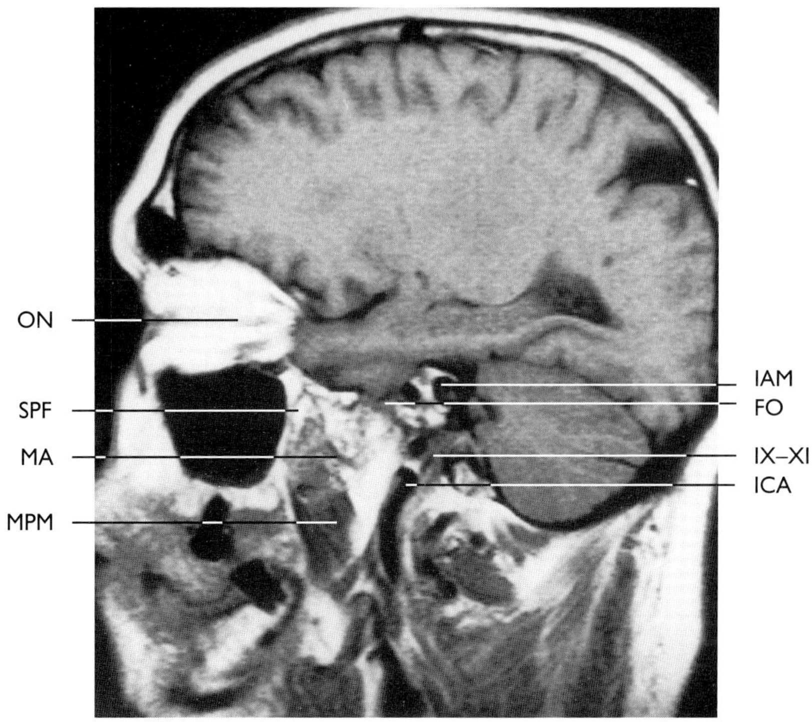

D

Figure 2-9 (Continued). (Figure continues.)

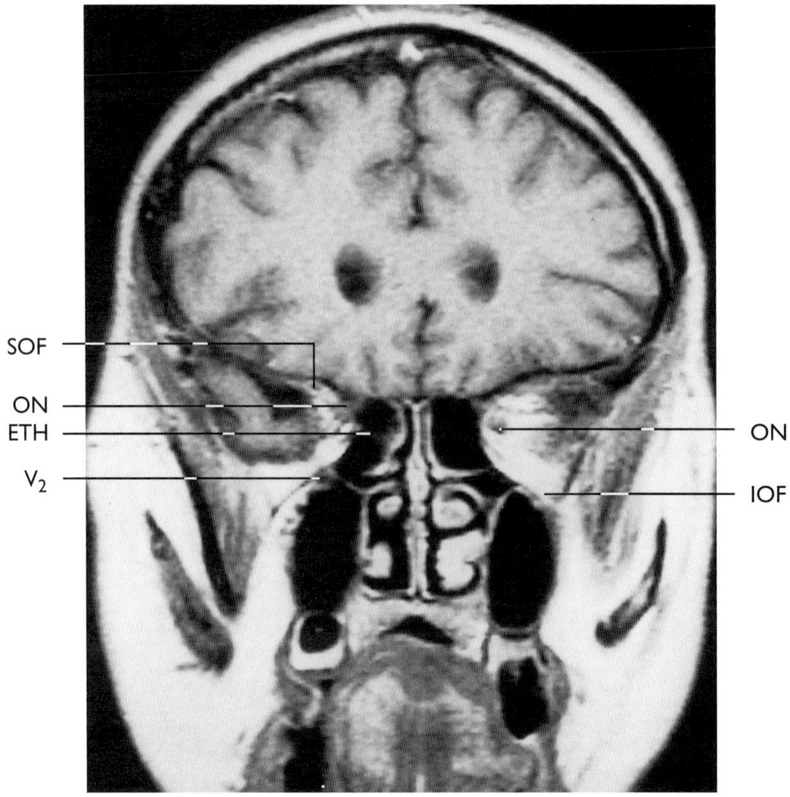

E

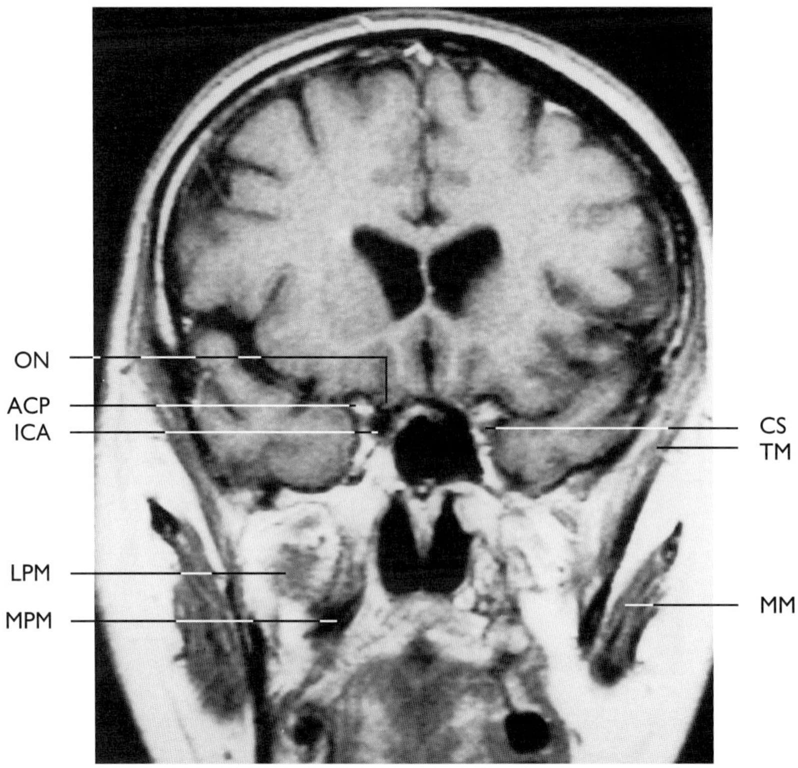

F

Figure 2-9 (Continued). (E–G) Coronal sections 6 mm thick spaced 12 mm apart. *(Figure continues.)*

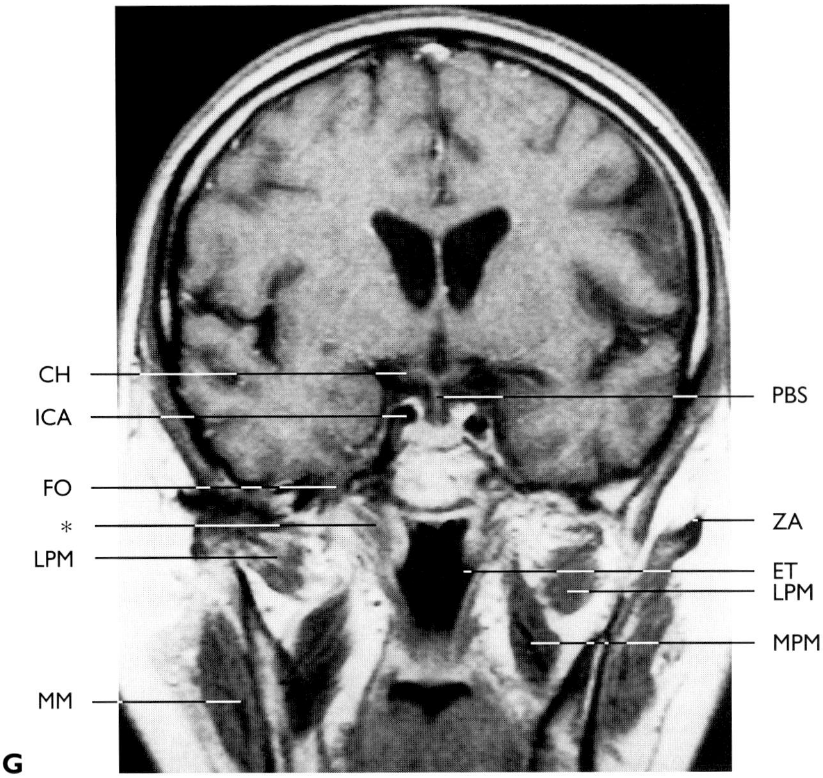

Figure 2-9 (Continued).

The Infratemporal Region

The infratemporal region (see Figs. 2-9 to 2-12) extends from the inferior orbital fissure anteriorly to the jugular foramen posteriorly. It is the area underneath both the cavernous sinus and the petrous temporal bone. Its anatomy is relevant to any lateral approach to the skull base. From the surface inward this area will be described in three layers. The inner layer contains the structures of most crucial functional, and therefore surgical, importance.

Outer Layer

The outer layer structures can be removed and replaced in any infratemporal operative approach. They include the zygomatic arch, temporomandibular joint and mandibular ramus, masseter and temporalis muscles, and the associated superficial vessels and nerves. The frontalis branch of the facial nerve is preserved by dissecting deep to the temporal fat pad (see Ch. 9) when raising the skin flap.

Intermediate Layer

The central part of the infratemporal fossa is occupied largely by the medial and lateral pterygoid muscles. The lateral pterygoid runs almost horizontally backward and has two heads: the superior or infratemporal head, which arises from the inferior surface of the greater wing of the sphenoid, and the inferior or pterygoid head, which arises from the outer surface of the lateral pterygoid plate. The insertion is into the neck of the mandible and part of the capsule of the temporomandibular joint, and the function is to pull the mandible and the articular disc forward. The medial ptery-

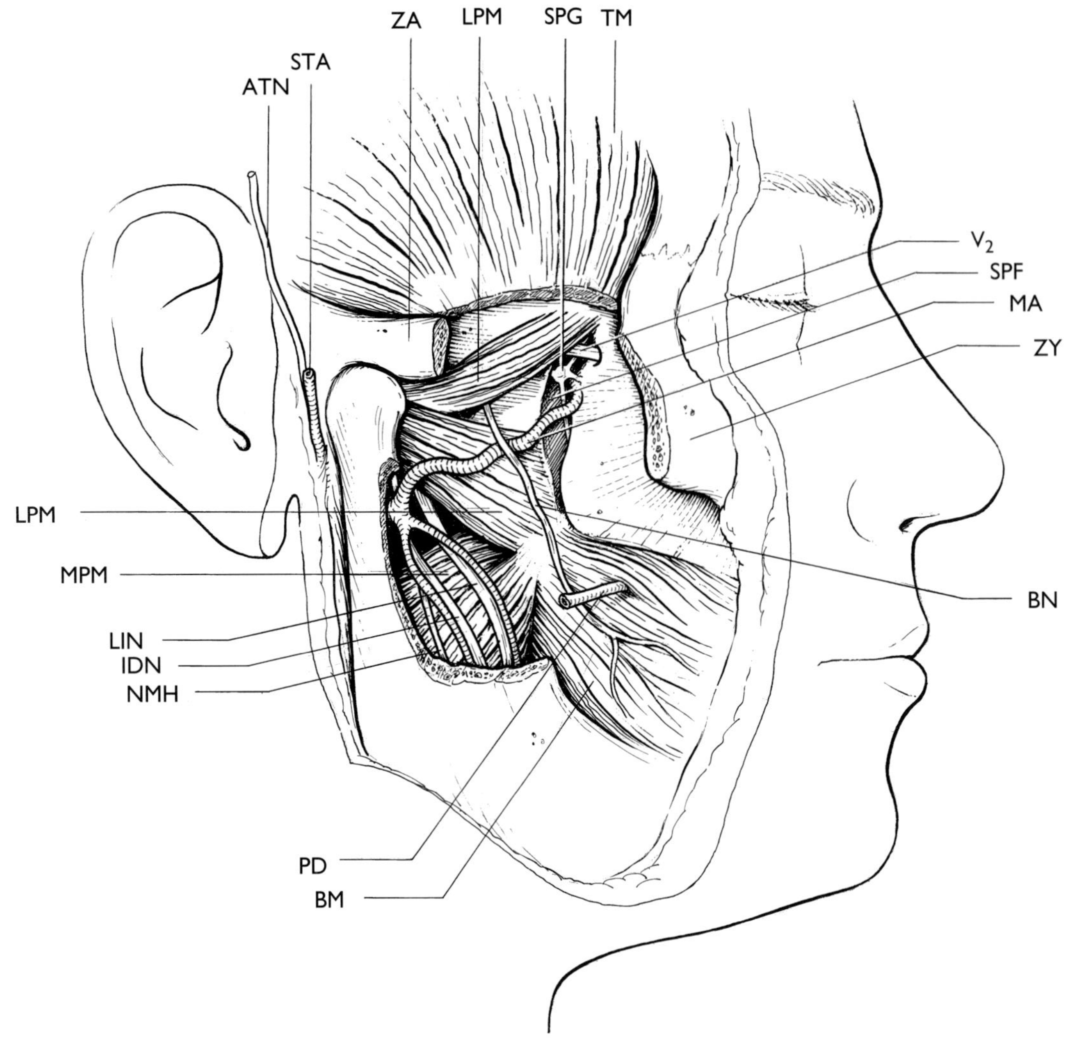

Figure 2-10. An external view of the anatomy of the middle layer of the right infratemporal fossa.

goid muscle arises from the pterygoid fossa between the pterygoid plates and runs obliquely backward and downward to insert at the angle of the mandible, thus rotating and assisting closure.

Between the pterygoid muscles is the pterygoid hiatus, a triangle bounded posteriorly by the ramus of the mandible. Through this hiatus runs the maxillary artery and the lingual, inferior dental, and mylohyoid nerves (Fig. 2-10). The chorda tympani separates from the lingual nerve at about this point and passes upward and backward to enter the petrotympanic fissure. Between the two heads of the lateral pterygoid muscle runs the buccal nerve, and the maxillary artery sometimes takes this route.

The maxillary artery gives off its first branches (deep auricular, tympanic, and middle meningeal) in its retromandibular course. Once superficial to the pterygoid muscles, it provides inferior dental, masseteric, pterygoid, and deep temporal arteries. It runs forward to the pterygopalatine fossa where it gives off the superior dental, infraorbital, greater palatine, and sphenopalatine branches. Also entering the pterygopalatine fossa are the maxillary nerve and the nerve of the pterygoid canal, both connected to the sphenopalatine ganglion. The anatomy of the pterygopalatine fossa is described by Turvey and Fonseca (1980) and Wentges (1975).

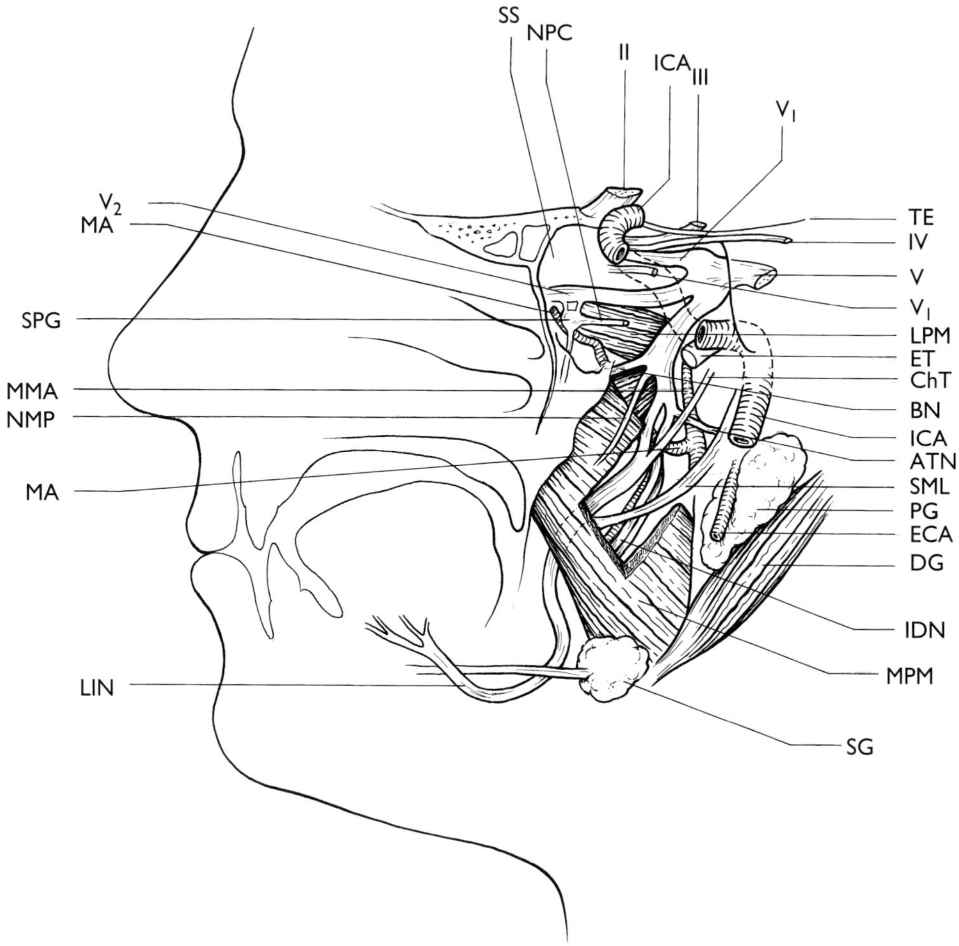

Figure 2-11. An internal view of the anatomy of the inner and middle layers of the right infratemporal fossa.

Inner Layer

Important anatomic structures (Fig. 2-11) run in a line from the stylomastoid foramen to the hook of the hamulus—the stylohamular line (Fig. 2-12). They may be listed from posterior forward as:

Stylomastoid foramen (facial nerve)
Styloid process (stylopharyngeus m., stylohyoid m., stylohyoid ligament, styloglossus m., stylomandibular ligament; there is also a stylopharyngeal septum extending from the process to the lateral pharyngeal wall)
Jugular foramen (internal jugular vein, nerves IX–XI)
Carotid canal (carotid artery)
Petrotympanic fissure (chorda tympani)
Sphenoid spine
Foramen spinosum (middle meningeal artery)
Eustachian tube
Foramen ovale (mandibular nerve)
Levator and tensor velum palatini muscles

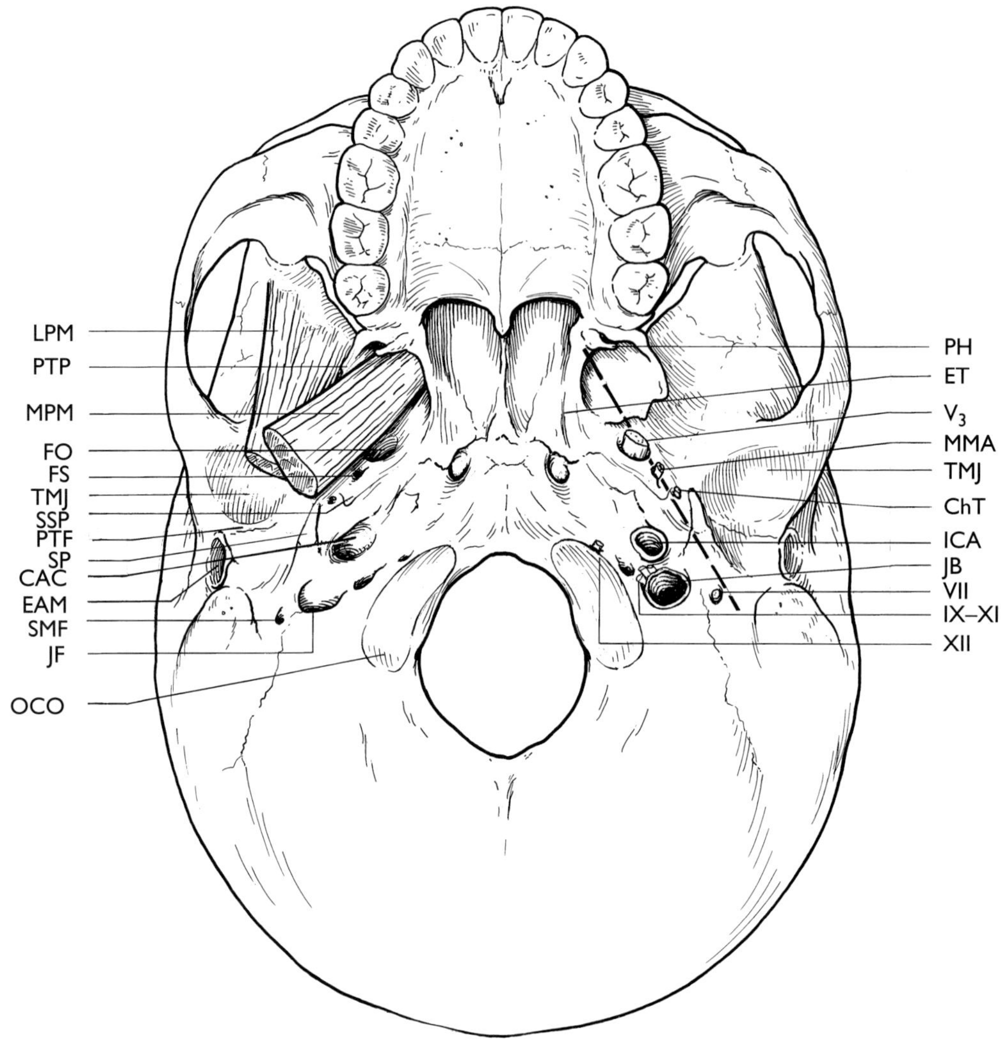

Figure 2-12. The most important anatomic structures in the infratemporal fossa are located medial to the stylohamular line, which is indicated here by solid dashes.

It is clearly better to stay lateral to this plane if at all possible. Practical landmarks are the styloid process and the sphenoid spine. Anteriorly is the pterygoid process, and in this region the pterygoid plexus of veins, fed from the cavernous sinus, can give troublesome bleeding.

For a more detailed analysis of the surgical anatomy of the infratemporal region, readers are referred to Goldenberg (1984), Fisch et al. (1984), Bosley and Martinez (1986), and Rosenblum et al. (1990).

Acknowledgments

Dr. Goel, author of the section on the cavernous sinus, acknowledges with respect and gratitude the help of Dr. Manu L. Kothari, Professor of Anatomy. The speculative issues discussed in the chapter are the products of his thoughts. Dr. S.K. Pandya, Professor of Neurosurgery, also provided support. We also thank Dr. John Andreou and the Magnetic Tomography Department of Hygeia Hospital, Athens, for the images used in Figure 2-9.

References

Al Mefty O, Smith RR (1980) Surgery of tumors invading the cavernous sinus. Surg Neurol 30:370

Bosley JH, Martinez DM (1986) Practical surgical anatomy of the skull base. Ear Nose Throat J 65:16–23

Dixon FW (1937) A comparative study of the sphenoid sinus. A study of 1600 skulls. Ann Otol Rhinol Laryngol 46:687

Dolenc VV (1983) Direct microsurgical repair of intracavernous vascular lesions. J Neurosurg 58:824

Dolenc VV, Kregar T, Ferluga M et al (1987) Treatment of tumors invading the cavernous sinus. p. 377. In Dolenc (ed): The Cavernous Sinus. A Multidisciplinary Approach to Tumorous and Vascular Lesions. Springer-Verlag, New York

Fisch U, Fagan P, Valavanis A (1984) The infratemporal approach for the lateral skull base. Otolaryngol Clin N Am 17:513–552

Goldenberg RA (1984) Surgeon's view of the skull base from the lateral approach. Laryngoscope 94/1211 suppl. 36

Hakuba A, Nishimura S, Tsukanoto M (1982) Surgical approaches to the cavernous sinus: report of 19 cases. Neurol Med Chir 22:295

Harris FS, Rhoton AL Jr (1976) Anatomy of the cavernous sinus: a microsurgical study. J Neurosurg 45:169

Holinshead WH (1982) Anatomy for Surgeons. Vol. 1. The Head and Neck. Harper & Row, Philadelphia

Kainz J, Stammberger H (1989) The roof of the anterior ethmoid, a place of least resistance in the skull base. Am J Rhinol 4:191–199

Lang J (1989) Clinical Anatomy of the Nose, Nasal Cavity and Paranasal Sinuses. Thieme, New York

Lang J (1993) Anatomy of the paranasal sinuses. pp. 123–130. In Sekar LN, Janecka IP (eds): Surgery of Cranial Base Tumors. Lippincott-Raven, Philadelphia

Morard M, Tcherekayev V, de Tribolet N (1994) The superior orbital fissure: a microanatomical study. Neurosurgery 35:1087–1093

Parkinson D (1979) Anatomy of the cavernous sinus. p. 62. In Pia HW, Langmaid C, Zierski J (eds): Cerebral Aneurysms: Advances in Diagnosis and Therapy. Springer Verlag, New York

Patel SJ, Sekhar LN, Wright DC (1993) Surgery for cavernous sinus meningiomas. Neurosurg Q 3:155–164

Perneczcky A, Knosp E, Matula CH (1988) Cavernous sinus surgery approach through the lateral wall. Acta Neurochir (Wien) 92:76

Rosenblum BN, Katsantonis GP, Cooper MH, Friedman WH (1990) Infratemporal fossa and lateral skull base dissection: long term results. Otolaryngol Head Neck Surg 102:106–110

Sekhar LN, Burgess J, Akin O (1987) Anatomic study of the cavernous sinus emphasizing operative approaches and related vascular and neural reconstruction. Neurosurgery 21:806

Taptas JN (1982) The so-called cavernous sinus: a review of the controversy and its implications for neurosurgeons. Neurosurgery 11:712

Turvey TA, Fonseca RJ (1980) The anatomy of the internal maxillary artery in the pterygopalatine fossa. Its relation to maxillary surgery. J Oral Surg 38:92–95

Umansky F, Nathan H (1982) The lateral wall of the cavernous sinus, with special reference to nerves related to it. J Neurosurg 56:228

Van Alyea OE (1941) Sphenoid sinus, anatomic study with consideration of the clinical significance of the structural characteristics of the sphenoid sinus. Arch Otolaryngol 34:225

Wentges RT (1973) Surgical anatomy of the pterygopalatine fossa. J Laryngol Otol 89:35–45

3

Surgical Anatomy of the Temporal Bone

Toshio Matsushima
Masashi Fukui
Albert L. Rhoton, Jr.

There are three principal approaches to lesions in or around the temporal bone (Matsushima et al., 1994; Pait et al., 1977). One type is the lateral suboccipital approach from the posterior fossa (see Ch. 20) (Rhoton, 1974; Tatagiba et al., 1992). A second is the middle fossa approach, such as the anterior transpetrosal approach or the extended middle cranial fossa approach (see Chs. 15 and 16) (House, 1961, 1964; Kanzaki et al., 1977; Kawase et al., 1985; Shiobara et al., 1988). The last type is a lateral approach to the temporal bone such as the posterior transpetrosal (see Ch. 19) (Al-Mefty et al., 1988; Hakuba et al., 1988; Malis, 1985), translabyrinthine (see Ch. 17) (Nelson, 1984), or the infralabyrinthine approach (Matsushima and Fukui, 1994). In performing all these approaches it is important to understand accurately the structures of the temporal bone, including the internal auditory canal, cochlea, vestibule, three semicircular canals, facial canal, 7th and 8th cranial nerves, and internal carotid artery. When their anatomic relationship to one another is clearly understood, the advantages and disadvantages of each approach can easily be comprehended.

Basic Structure

The temporal bone has three surfaces. The anterior surface forms the posterior floor of the middle cranial fossa while the posterior surface forms the lateral wall of the posterior cranial fossa (Fig. 3-1). The internal auditory canal is located in the center of the temporal bone and opens into the posterior fossa. Its length is about 1.0 cm. The cochlea is located within the floor of the middle fossa anterolateral to the internal auditory canal and medial to the geniculate ganglion. The three semicircular canals are situated either lateral or posterior to the internal auditory canal, and they extend from the middle fossa side to the posterior fossa side. The superior semicircu-

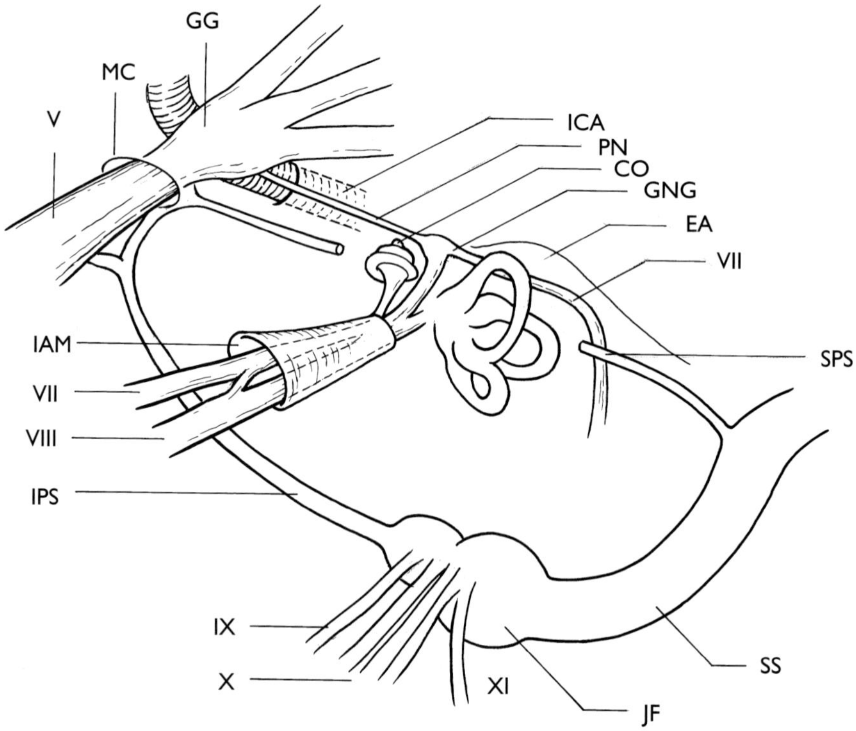

Figure 3-1. Schematic posterolateral view of the basic internal structure of the right temporal bone. (For explanation of abbreviations, see Appendix 1, p. 373.)

lar canal makes a bony bulge called the *arcuate eminence* on the posterior floor of the middle fossa near the petrous edge. The 7th and 8th cranial nerves pass through the internal auditory canal, and the cochlea and vestibular nerves end in the cochlea and vestibule, respectively. The facial nerve, however, crosses through the temporal bone to the geniculate ganglion in the floor of the middle fossa, and then runs downward around the posterior wall of the external auditory canal in the lateral part of the temporal bone from the facial hiatus toward the stylomastoid foramen. Meckel's cavity is located at the most anteromedial petrous edge under the trigeminal impression, while the jugular foramen is situated at the most posteroinferior portion of the temporal bone below the internal auditory canal (Fig. 3-1).

The trigeminal nerve passes through Meckel's cavity, and forms the trigeminal ganglion in the middle fossa. The internal carotid artery passing through the foramen lacerum runs under the ganglion. The sigmoid sinus and inferior petrosal sinus drain into the jugular bulb at the jugular foramen, and the 9th, 10th, and 11th cranial nerves also pass through the foramen.

Three Approaches

Posterior Fossa Approach (Lateral Suboccipital Approach)

The facial and acoustic nerves in the porus acousticus are located in the center of the cerebellopontine angle, and the trigeminal nerve and the glossopharyngeal, vagal, and accessory cranial nerves are situated above and below them, respectively (Fig. 3-2A). The anterior inferior cerebellar artery (AICA) passes between the 7th and 8th cranial nerves after forming the meatal loop in front of the porus acousticus. The artery and nerves have been called the arterial-nerve complex (Maitlin et al., 1980; Matsushima et al. 1992) (Fig. 3-3B). The subarcuate artery originating from the AICA is buried into the dura mater of the posterior edge of the porus acousticus. When the dura mater lateral to the porus acousticus is removed, the vestibular aqueduct appears (Fig. 3-2B). During surgery for acoustic neurinomas the posterior lip of the internal auditory canal is opened. When the bone lateral to the canal is drilled too far laterally, the common crus and posterior semicircular canal are exposed (Fig. 3-2B). They should not be destroyed if the patient still has some useful hearing ability. The common crus is the nearest structure to the lateral end of the internal auditory canal (Pait et al., 1977; Rhoton, 1974). The mean length between the lateral end of the internal auditory canal and the common crus is 4.0 mm. The air cells or the jugular bulb sometimes exist in the posterior wall, inferior wall, or both of the internal auditory canal (Fig. 3-2B). In the medial direction, the anatomic landmarks near the brain stem are the flocculus and the choroid plexus protruding from the

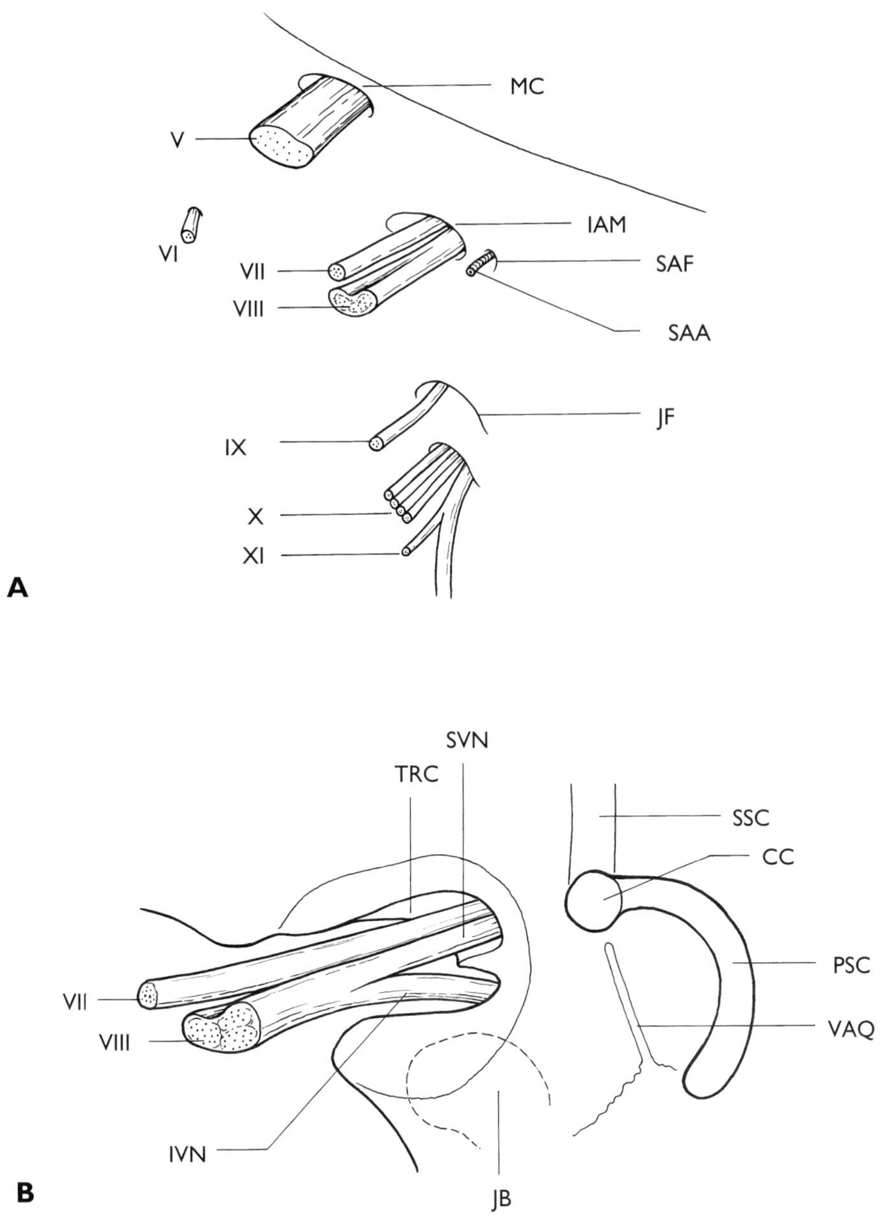

Figure 3-2. Posterior fossa approach. *(A)* Right cerebellopontine angle. *(B)* Structures surrounding the right internal auditory canal; the posterior lip of the canal is removed and the vestibule, posterior semicircular canal, and common crus are exposed.

foramen of Luschka. (Rhoton, 1986). The facial and acoustic nerves are situated anterior to the flocculus.

The lateral end of the internal auditory canal is divided into four parts by the transverse and vertical crests (Fig. 3-3A). The facial canal, connecting with the groove for the greater petrosal nerve in the middle fossa, occupies the anterosuperior part of the four. In accordance with this arrangement, four cranial nerve divisions, the facial, cochlear, and superior and inferior vestibular nerves, course in the internal auditory canal (Fig. 3-3B & C). The nervus intermedius and singular nerve are also present. The former, which consists of the central processes of the unipolar cells of the geniculate ganglion, leaves the trunk of the facial nerve in the internal auditory canal and enters the brain stem at the lower border of the pons usually together with the vestibulocochlear nerve. Therefore, it crosses between the facial and the acoustic nerves. The singular nerve joins the inferior vestibular nerve below the transverse crest.

The facial nerve is smaller than the acoustic nerve. When viewed from posterior it is hidden by the acoustic nerve. It runs laterally, and then enters the facial canal at the lateral end of the internal auditory canal. The 8th cranial nerve contains three divisions but actually appears to be one nerve in the cerebellopontine cistern and in most of the internal auditory canal. The three nerves, consisting of the cochlear, superior vestibular, and inferior vestibular nerves, join together a few millimeters medial to the transverse crest and form one large nerve (Matsushima et al., 1992) (Fig. 3-3C). The cochlear nerve originating from the cochlea area runs in the anteroinferior part of the 8th cranial nerve even after joining the other two nerves. The superior and inferior vestibular nerves course in the posterosuperior and posteroinferior portions of the 8th cranial nerve, respectively. This situation corresponds with the divisions of the lateral end of the canal.

The arteries running around the porus acousticus include (1) the meatal segment of the AICA or of the posteroinferior cerebellar artery (PICA), (2) the internal auditory artery (IAA), (3) the subarcuate artery (SA), and (4) the perforating arteries, particularly the recurrent perforating artery (RPA) (Martin et al., 1980; Matsushima et al., 1992). The meatal segment of the AICA or the PICA is the largest of these arteries and passes in front of the porus acousticus and forms the arterial-nerve complex with the 7th and 8th cranial nerves (Fig. 3-3B & C). The meatal arterial segment abruptly changes its course and forms a loop called the meatal loop. When the meatal segment crosses the 7th and 8th cranial nerve complex, about half of the loops course below the two nerves while the other half pass between the two nerves. In cases of acoustic neurinoma this artery encircles the tumor.

The IAAs originate from the meatal segment and enter the porus from anterior. They supply not only the 8th cranial nerve but also the 7th cranial nerve and the dura mater inside the internal auditory canal. Based on autopsy findings, the mean number of these arteries was two on each side. The subarcuate artery entering the subarcuate fossa is buried in the dura mater on either the superior or the posterior edge of the porus acousticus. Therefore, it may often be sacrificed when the posterior lip of the internal auditory canal is drilled. Because the artery is sometimes related to hearing, it should be carefully preserved as far as possible (Rhoton, 1974). These internal auditory and subarcuate arteries are too small to identify during the dissection of the arachnoid membrane in the cistern. Regarding the perforating arteries, attention should be paid to the recurrent perforating artery. The artery originates from the meatal loop around the porus acousticus and courses in a reverse direction to the brain stem between the 7th and 8th cranial nerves, and thus supplies the two cranial nerves. In the lateral suboccipital approach it is hidden by the 8th cranial nerve and cannot be seen.

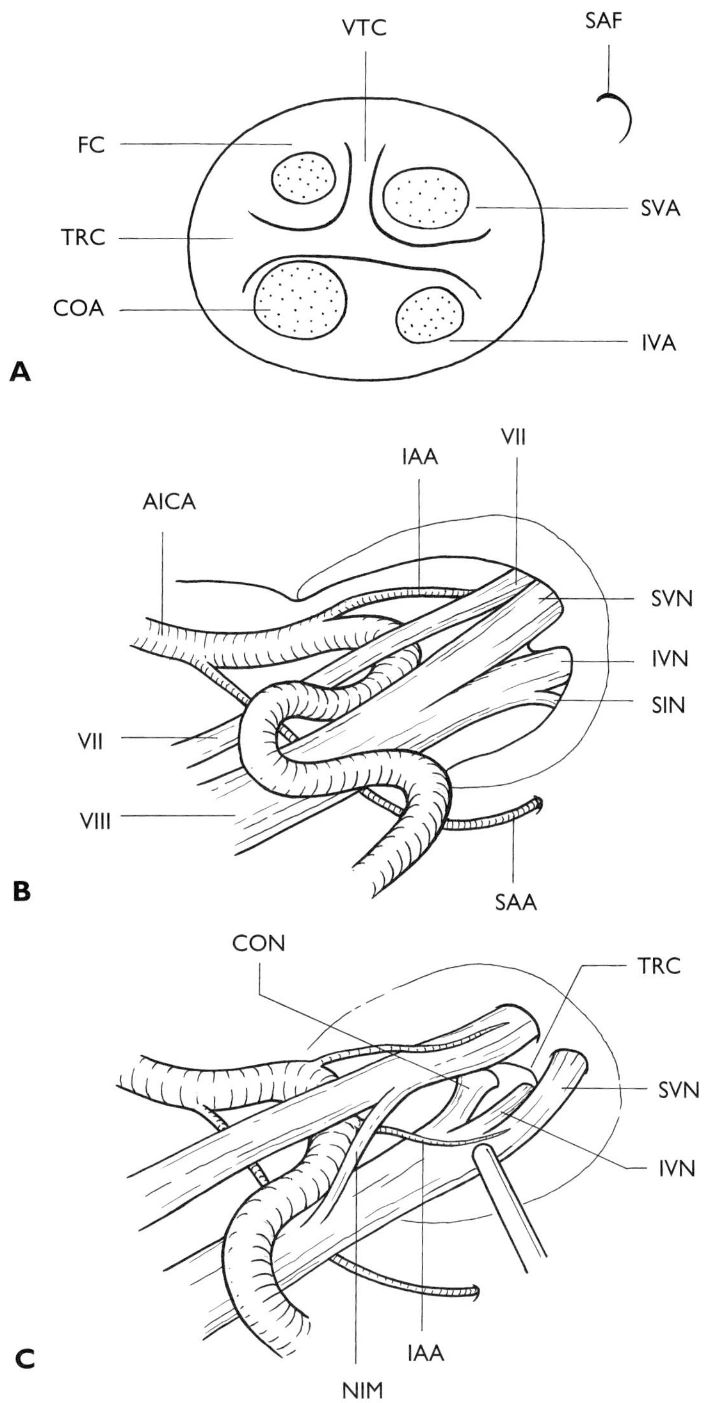

Figure 3-3. Contents of the internal auditory canal. *(A)* Lateral end of the bony structure of the right internal auditory canal. *(B)* Relationships between the 7th and 8th cranial nerves and the meatal loop, which form the so-called arterial-nerve complex. *(C)* The superior vestibular nerve is retracted to show the transverse crest, cochlear nerve, inferior vestibular nerve, and internal auditory artery.

Neurosurgeons should be familiar not only with the normal but also with the pathologic anatomy. To preserve facial nerve function and hearing during surgery for acoustic neurinoma, it is necessary to know both the anatomic relationship of the facial nerve to the acoustic tumor and that of the common crus to the internal auditory canal. In many cases the facial nerve is found to course anteroinferior to the acoustic tumor (Rhoton, 1974). These facts seem reasonable when the normal anatomic relationship of the facial nerve to the superior and inferior vestibular nerves are considered. Recently the proportion of acoustic tumors with postoperative hearing preservation have rapidly increased. Tatagiba et al. (1992) reported that postoperative hearing disturbance was intimately related to an injury of the common crus. In the lateral suboccipital approach the posterior wall of the internal auditory canal should be opened, avoiding injury to the common crus. In addition, the facial nerve should be sought in the light of the anatomic knowledge described above utilizing electric stimulation.

Middle Fossa Approach (Anterior Transpetrosal Approach, Extended Middle Cranial Fossa Approach)

The middle fossa approach includes all approaches that pass through the posterior part of the floor of the middle fossa extending from Meckel's cavity to the arcuate eminence. They include Kawase's approach (see Ch. 16) (Kawase et al., 1985) and the extended middle cranial fossa approach (see Ch. 15) (Kanzaki et al., 1977). On the posterior surface of the middle fossa the Gasserian ganglion and arcuate eminence are the most prominent structures (Fig. 3-4).

During this approach two bony bulges can be seen on the floor in the surgical view. The closer bulge is the arcuate eminence whereas the farther one is the bulging of the petrous apex. Between the two structures a cave can be observed (Figs. 3-4 and 3-5A). There are two petrosal grooves at the bottom of the cave where the major (greater) and minor (lesser) petrosal nerves and the petrosal and superior tympanic arteries run. Because the two nerves are connected laterally with the geniculate ganglion of the facial nerve, their retraction may cause facial nerve palsy (Pait et al., 1977). The petrous portion of the internal carotid artery, running away from the foramen lacerum, courses just in front of the Gasserian ganglion (Fig. 3-4). An

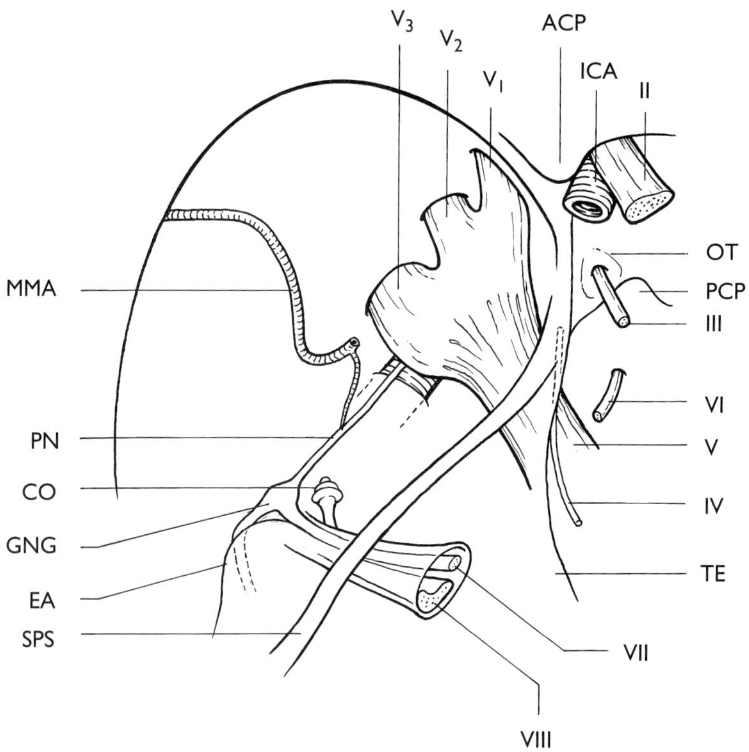

Figure 3-4. Left middle fossa, particularly the structures near the petrous ridge.

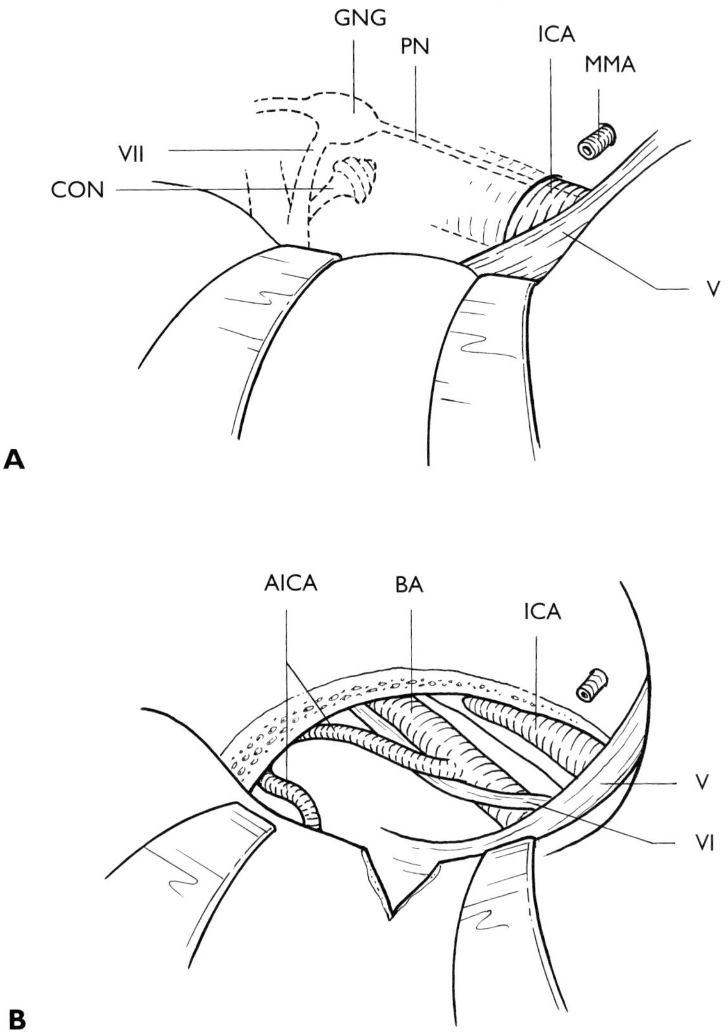

Figure 3-5. Kawase's approach (left side). *(A)* The middle meningeal artery has been cut and the trigeminal nerve is exposed through the extradural anterior transpetrosal approach. *(B)* Kawase's triangle is removed and the basilar artery, anterior inferior cerebellar artery, and abducens nerve are visible.

absence of bone over the medial part of the carotid canal may expose the carotid artery inferior or lateral to the ganglion. Kawase's triangle is the area surrounded by the trigeminal ganglion medially, the sphenopetrosal groove anteriorly, and the cochlear organ and internal auditory canal laterally (Kawase et al., 1985) (Fig. 3-5A & B). There are no important structures in the triangle. The area lateral to the trigeminal nerve should be drilled and the petrous portion of the internal carotid artery found.

The arcuate eminence is one of the best anatomic landmarks for finding the internal auditory canal from the side of the middle fossa (Fig. 3-6A). The canal is located just medial to the eminence. The facial nerve forms the geniculate ganglion just anteromedial to the medial surface of the arcuate eminence, so it is necessary to avoid injuring it when drilling here (Figs. 3-4 and 3-6B). Sometimes the geniculate ganglion is not covered with bone (Pait et al., 1977). In a case without hearing the arcuate eminence containing the superior semicircular canal may be destroyed, but in a case with hearing preserved the superior semicircular canal should be kept intact. When the dura mater is opened after unroofing the internal auditory canal, the 7th and 8th cranial nerve complex and the meatal loop of the AICA can be seen

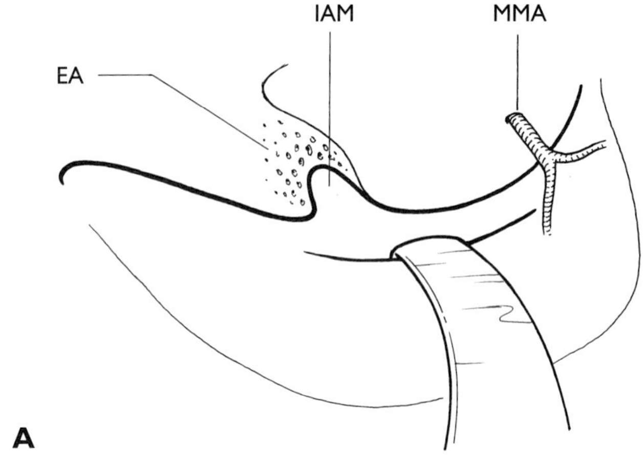

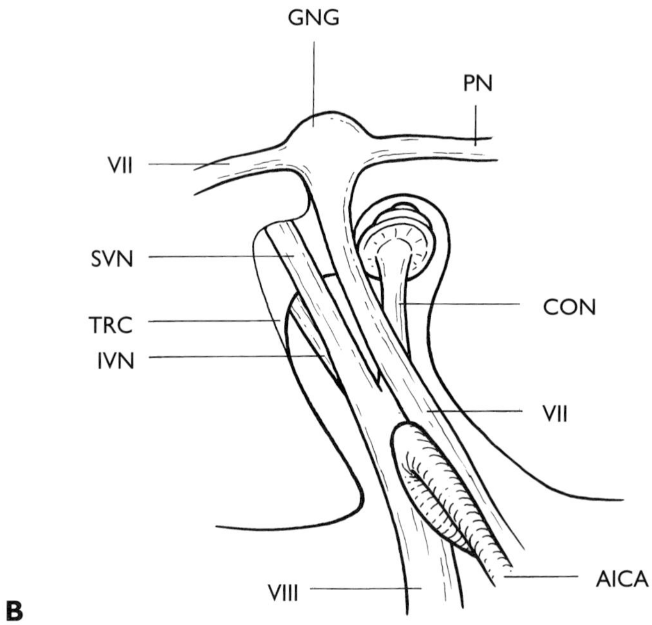

Figure 3-6. Modified extended middle fossa approach. *(A)* The anterior part of the arcuate eminence is removed to expose the internal auditory canal. *(B)* The roof of the internal auditory canal is opened and the geniculate ganglion is also exposed.

(Fig. 3-6B). The facial and the superior vestibular nerves appear first. The cochlea is present in the deep area just anterior to the internal auditory canal. In the middle fossa approach, the extent of removal of the petrous bone depends on the condition of the patient's hearing preoperatively.

Lateral Approaches (Posterior Transpetrosal, Translabyrinthine, and Infralabyrinthine Approaches)

The translabyrinthine approach has been frequently used by otorhinolaryngologists and has not been popular with neurosurgeons. It has some advantages, in particular it is not necessary to retract the cerebellum, and the facial nerve is identified early (House, 1964; Nelson, 1984). In this approach, however, there are also certain disadvantages. Three semicircular canals are destroyed and hearing is lost postoperatively. The approach may be applied when an acoustic tumor is small and hearing is completely lost preoperatively. Currently the posterior transpetrosal approach is becoming popular among neurosurgeons as skull base surgery advances. Because mastoidectomy is involved in both the posterior transpetrosal and infralabyrinthine approaches, the surgical anatomy of mastoidectomy and the translabyrinthine approach is described here.

Anatomic landmarks on exposure of the lateral surface of the mastoid bone include the external acoustic meatus (ear canal) anteriorly, the suprameatal spine (Henle's spine) at the superior posterior portion of the canal, and the temporal line, which is the posterior extension of the zygomatic arch (Fig. 3-7A). The area behind Henle's spine actually overlies the mastoid antrum. The mastoid antrum should be exposed before searching for the hard bone of the labyrinth and for the facial nerve. When first removing the mastoid cortex, a straight cut should be drilled along the temporal line posteriorly and another cut made immediately posterior to the external

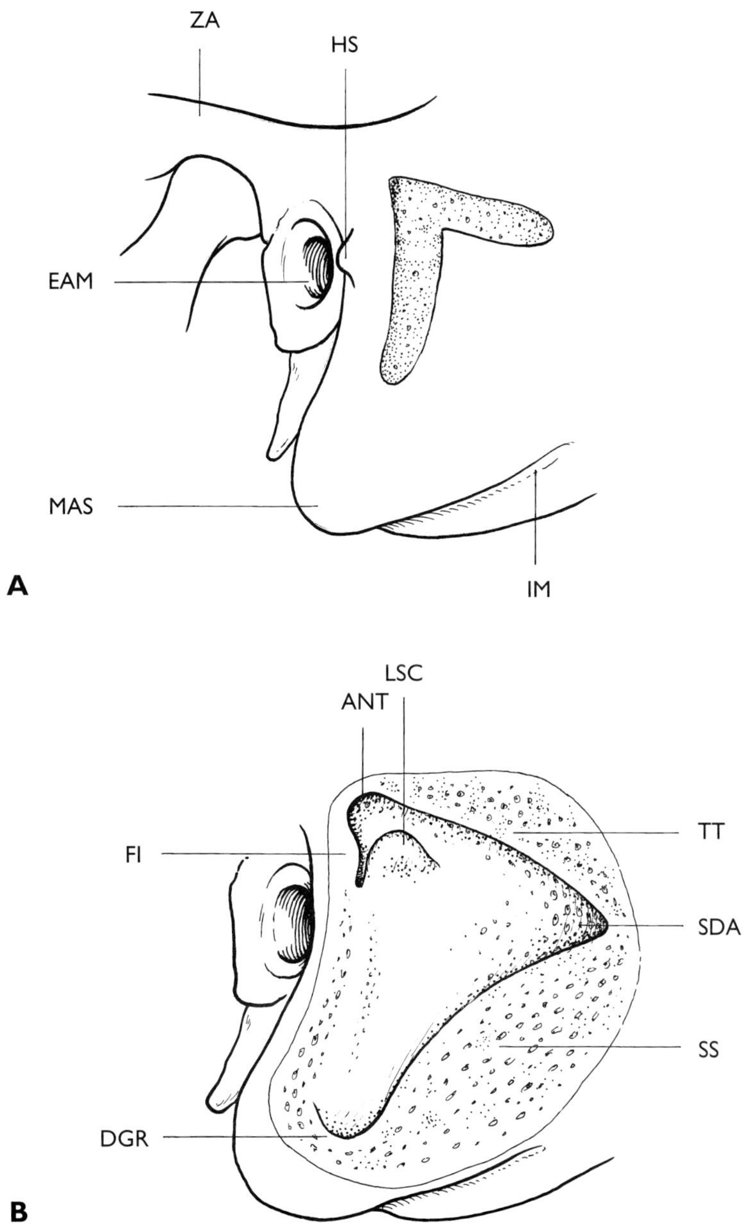

Figure 3-7. Mastoidectomy. *(A)* Removal of the cortex. *(B)* Identification of the sigmoid sinus, middle fossa plate, and mastoid antrum. *(Figure continues.)*

auditory canal and Henle's spine (Fig. 3-7A). Continue to drill the cortex, and then the sigmoid sinus and the dura mater covering the middle fossa appear posteriorly and superiorly, respectively (Fig. 3-7B). The middle fossa dural plate is the best landmark for gaining access to the antrum. The mastoid antrum is identified as a large air-containing space. The hard bone of the labyrinth appears inferoposterior to the mastoid antrum. Identification of the hard bone, especially the horizontal (lateral) semicircular canal, allows exposure of the fossa incudis. The facial recess is situated inferior to the fossa incudis. A careful dissection of the facial recess allows the surgeon to expose the external genu and the descending portion of the facial nerve just inferior to the horizontal (lateral) canal (Fig. 3-7C). The mastoidectomy will have a triangular shape. The more inferiorly the facial nerve descends, the closer it comes to the sigmoid sinus, which drains into the jugular bulb. The nerve finally passes the

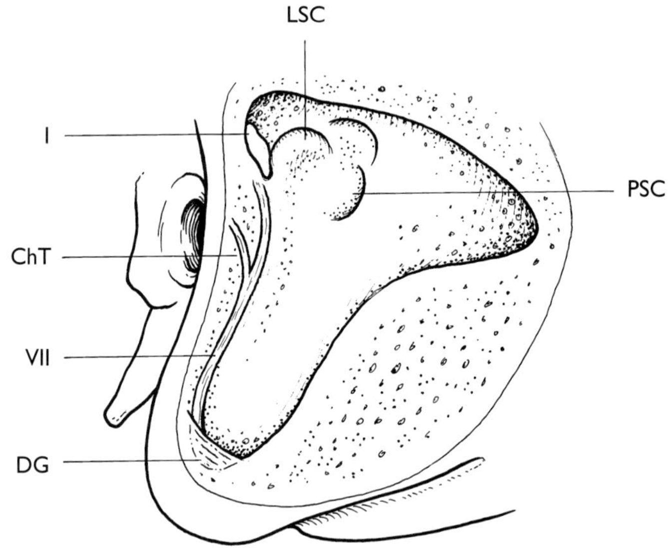

C

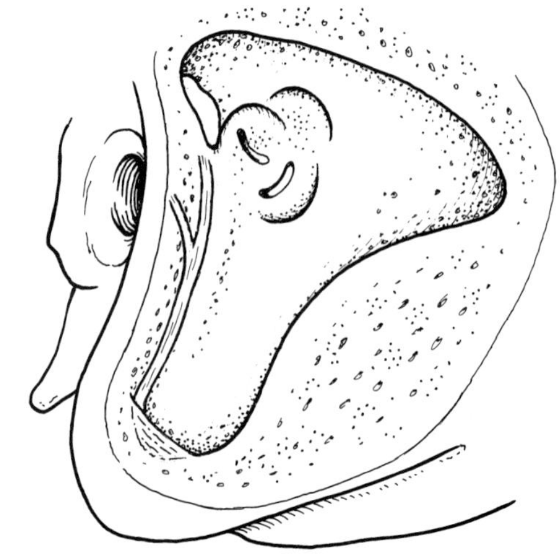

D

Figure 3-7 (Continued). (C) Completing the basic mastoidectomy and skeletonizing the descending portion of the facial nerve. The body of the incus can be seen in the antrum. The digastric muscle is also exposed. *(D)* Opening the lateral and posterior semicircular canals.

stylomastoid foramen at the most anterior portion of the digastric groove. Drilling the hard bone exposes the three semicircular canals (Fig. 3-7D). The chorda tympani runs just anterior to the descending facial nerve. The dura mater in the internal auditory canal appears when the hard bone, particularly the posterior semicircular canal, is removed. The superior and the inferior vestibular nerves are visible superior and inferior to the transverse crest, respectively. In addition, the facial nerve is also visible behind them.

In the posterior transpetrosal approach the upper part of the mastoid bone is removed, and then the petrous edge is drilled anteriorly as far as Meckel's cavity (Al-Mefty et al., 1988; Hakuba et al., 1988). In the infralabyrinthine approach the inferior part of the mastoid bone is removed to expose the inferior portion of the sigmoid sinus and the jugular foramen (Matsushima and Fukui, 1994). In all lateral approaches it is very important to understand the anatomic relationship between such structures as the middle fossa plate, sigmoid sinus, mastoid antrum, hard bone of the labyrinth, fossa incudis, facial nerve, internal auditory canal, and jugular foramen.

References

Al-Mefty O, Fox JL, Smith RR (1988) Petrosal approach for petroclival meningiomas. Neurosurgery 22:510–517

Hakuba A, Nishimura S, Jang BJ (1988) A combined retroauricular and preauricular transpetrosal-transtentorial approach to clivus meningiomas. Surg Neurol 30:108–116

House WF (1961) Surgical exposure of the internal auditory canal and its contents through the middle cranial fossa. Laryngoscope 71:1363–1385

House WF (1964) Monograph I. Transtemporal bone microsurgical removal of acoustic neuromas. Arch Otolaryngol 80:597–756

Kanzaki J, Kawase T, Sano F, et al (1977) A modified extended middle cranial fossa approach for acoustic tumors. Arch Otorhinolaryngol 217:119–121

Kawase T, Toya S, Shiobara R, Mine T (1985) Transpetrosal approach for aneurysms of the lower basilar artery. J Neurosurg 63:857–861

Malis LI (1985) Surgical resection of tumors of the skull base. pp. 1011–1021. In Wilkins RH, Rengachary SS (eds): Neurosurgery. Vol. 1. McGraw-Hill, New York

Martin RG, Grant JL, Peace D et al (1980) Microsurgical relationships of the anterior inferior cerebellar artery and the facial vestibulocochlear nerve complex. Neurosurgery 6:483–507

Matsushima T, Fukui M (1994) Suboccipital craniectomy combined with infralabyrinthine approach through mastoidectomy for jugular foramen neurinomas. pp. 331–336. In Hakuba H, Yamaura H (eds): Skull Base Surgery—Standard and Modified Techniques. Igaku-Shoin, Tokyo

Matsushima T, Fukui M, Rhoton AL Jr (1994) Microsurgical anatomy for acoustic tumor surgery—with special reference to three approaches. Neurosurgeons 13:83–90

Matsushima T, Inoue T, Natori Y et al (1992) Microsurgical anatomy of the region near the porus acusticus internus; arteries around the facial and acoustic nerves. Neurol Surg 20:409–415

Nelson RA (1984) Temporal Bone Surgical Dissection Manual. House Ear Institute, Los Angeles

Pait TG, Harris AZFS, Paullus WS (1977) Microsurgical anatomy and dissection of the temporal bone. Surg Neurol 8:363–391

Rhoton AL Jr (1974) Microsurgery of the internal acoustic meatus. Surg Neurol 2:311–318

Rhoton AL Jr (1986) Microsurgical anatomy of the brainstem surface facing an acoustic neurinoma. Surg Neurol 25:326–339

Shiobara R, Kanzaki J, Toya S (1988) A modified extended middle cranial fossa approach for acoustic nerve tumors. Results of 125 operations. J Neurosurg 68:358–365

Tatagiba M, Samii M, Matthies C (1992) The significance for postoperative hearing of preserving the labyrinth in acoustic neurinoma surgery. J Neurosurg 77:677–684

4

Extended Subfrontal Approach to the Anterior Skull Base and Clivus

Chandranath Sen
Peter J. Catalano

The extended frontal approach allows access to tumors of the anterior skull base, sphenoid sinus, and central clivus. It is based on the transbasal approach of Derome et al. (1972), but with additional bone removal from the supraorbital rim, orbital roofs, and ethmoid sinuses to permit an even lower trajectory (Raveh et al., 1993; Sekhar et al., 1992). It is suitable for both intra- and extradural tumors of the anterior fossa, but only for predominantly extradural tumors of the central portion of the middle and posterior skull base. Extensive tumors may require a transfacial or a lateral approach either at the same or a separate sitting. Intracavernous tumor extensions usually require an intradural operation. The procedure in most instances leads to anosmia. Reconstruction of a barrier between the dura and nasopharynx is performed predominantly by the pericranial flap; bony reconstruction is usually not required (Snyderman et al., 1990, Yamamoto et al., 1993).

Selection of Patients

The types of tumors appropriate for this approach have been identified previously (Catalano et al., 1994; Sekhar et al., 1992).

Intradural Tumors

Meningiomas of the anterior cranial floor as far back as the tuberculum sella are well suited for this procedure. In addition to early interruption of the tumor blood supply that comes from the ethmoidal vessels, the approach provides excellent exposure for resecting the abnormal bone and tumor extensions into the paranasal sinuses.

Extradural Tumors

Chordomas, chondrosarcomas, fibrous dysplasia, ossifying fibroma, and osteogenic sarcoma form the spectrum of bony and cartilaginous tumors that are encountered. Infiltration of the bones at the skull base is a special problem in chordomas and chondrosarcomas and requires aggressive bone drilling beyond the gross margins of the tumor. The wide and shallow exposure provided by this approach facilitates bone removal at such depth. Although these two tumors are malignant, they are slow growing, and piecemeal removal is an acceptable strategy.

On the other hand, high-grade malignancies arising from the paranasal sinuses and the nasal cavity require en bloc resection. Esthesioneuroblastoma, squamous cell carcinoma, adenocarcinoma, adenoid cystic carcinoma, and various sarcomas constitute this group and often invade the dura and brain.

Preoperative Investigations

Because they complement each other, both forms of imaging, high-resolution magnetic resonance imaging (MRI) and computed tomography (CT), are performed in all cases. The CT scan in coronal and axial planes provides bony definition of the tumor. If present, bone destruction, whether smooth or irregular, must be carefully noted in relation to the various foramina at the skull base. Minute calcifications are best detected by CT scan. Opacification of paranasal sinuses seen on CT scans may be from tumor involvement or from obstruction of their outflow, which is best differentiated by MRI. Bony hyperostosis and the degree of pneumatization of the sinuses (e.g., frontal and sphenoidal sinuses that may extend into the orbital roofs, anterior clinoid process, or pterygoid plates) are seen on CT and are useful for surgical planning. Three-dimensional reconstruction of the images with modern software can be used to study the tumor from different perspectives and may help in approach selection.

T_1 and T_2 weighted MRIs provide the soft tissue definitions of the tumor and its relations to the brain, meninges, and vasculature. The change in signal characteristics with the administration of gadolinium-diethylenetriamine pentaacetic acid (Gd-DTPA) can provide important clues to the identity of the tumor (e.g., meningioma and esthesioneuroblastoma will become uniformly hyperintense whereas chordoma and chondrosarcoma will show a heterogeneous enhancement). Presence of brain invasion or the status of the optic nerves is better appreciated by the MRI. MR angiography has replaced a formal arteriogram for evaluation of the normal vasculature and its distortion and displacement by the tumor in many instances.

Arteriography is occasionally useful in diagnosing tumors such as juvenile angiofibroma or in assessing the vascularity of certain tumors. Preoperative embolization is an important adjunct to surgery and is routinely performed where possible. Arteriography may also indicate vessel wall invasion.

Anesthesia and Positioning

Under general anesthesia with orotracheal intubation, the patient is positioned supine with the head, fixed in a three-point pin head rest, slightly extended. If intraoperative head repositioning is anticipated or a transfacial approach is to be performed, the head is placed on a horseshoe head rest and the endotracheal tube is sutured or wired in place to the teeth or the mandible. Muscle relaxants are used unless cranial nerve monitoring is anticipated. Electrophysiologic monitoring has not been helpful in the purely anterior approach. However, it is routinely used when a lateral approach is used or manipulation of the internal carotid artery is planned. Intra-arterial and central venous catheters are used and 1 g/kg body weight of mannitol is administered at the time of the skin incision. Although dehydration is used initially for brain relaxation, the patient is maintained euvolemic during and after the operation unless postoperative brain edema is anticipated due to direct manipulation of the brain when invaded by the tumor. The thigh is also prepared for fascial and fat grafts if needed. Insertion of a spinal drain is usually not necessary preoperatively for brain relaxation.

Incision and Bony Exposure

Although a bicoronal incision is preferred, the extent of the underlying craniotomy can be tailored to the size and side of the tumor. After infiltration with 1 percent xylocaine with epinephrine (1:100,000), a straight bicoronal incision is made from zygoma to zygoma about 15 cm above the nasion instead of following the hairline. This permits a greater length of pericranium to be available for reconstruction. Additional length of pericranium, if anticipated, can be raised from the posterior scalp which is then elevated with the frontal scalp in one layer down to the nasion. On the sides the pericranium, the superficial temporalis fascia and the adipose tissue are elevated in one layer by establishing a plane between them and the deep temporalis fascia to avoid injury to the frontal branch of the facial nerve. The periorbita at the roof and upper parts of the medial and lateral walls are elevated in continuity with the pericranium, with care given at the orbital rims where the tissue may be markedly adherent to the underlying bone. If present, the supraorbital foramina are converted into notches by fracturing the floor with a ¼-in. osteotome and the neurovascular bundles are carefully dissected inferiorly with the periorbita. These vascular pedicles serve as the principal source of blood supply to the pericranial flap. The periorbita are elevated for 2 to 3 cm posteriorly from the rims, and this includes the trochlea. The anterior ethmoidal arteries, which serve as an external landmark to indicate the floor of the cribriform plate, are coagulated and divided. If the orbital fat protrudes from lacerations of the periorbita, they can be closed or simply protected with a cottonoid strip. The temporalis muscles are elevated from the anterior portions of the temporal fossa, leaving a small cuff for their reattachment.

The bifrontal craniotomy is usually made in two pieces by doing the craniotomy on one side first and then the other side after separating the midline and opposite dura under direct vision (Figs. 4-1 and 4-2). This is facilitated by using a high-speed drill system such as the Midas Rex and only one burr hole is made at the "key hole." The craniotomy is made as low as possible on the orbital roofs. The procedure from here on varies depending on the particular pathology.

Nasopharyngeal Malignancy Invading the Skull Base

In cases such as esthesioneuroblastomas and sinus cancers, en bloc removal of the tumor with a surrounding margin of normal tissues is ideally desired. The anterior, posterior, and lateral limits of the tumor in the anterior fossa floor are noted on the preoperative scans including involvement of the dura and brain so that all subsequent dissection may avoid violating the tumor. The supraorbital rims are removed with as much normal bone of the orbital roofs as possible, which may then be replaced at the end of the operation. The subfrontal dura is elevated on either side of the cribriform plates to the lateral limits of the anterior fossa, and osteotomies are made at the lateral limits of the supraorbital rims with a reciprocating saw while pro-

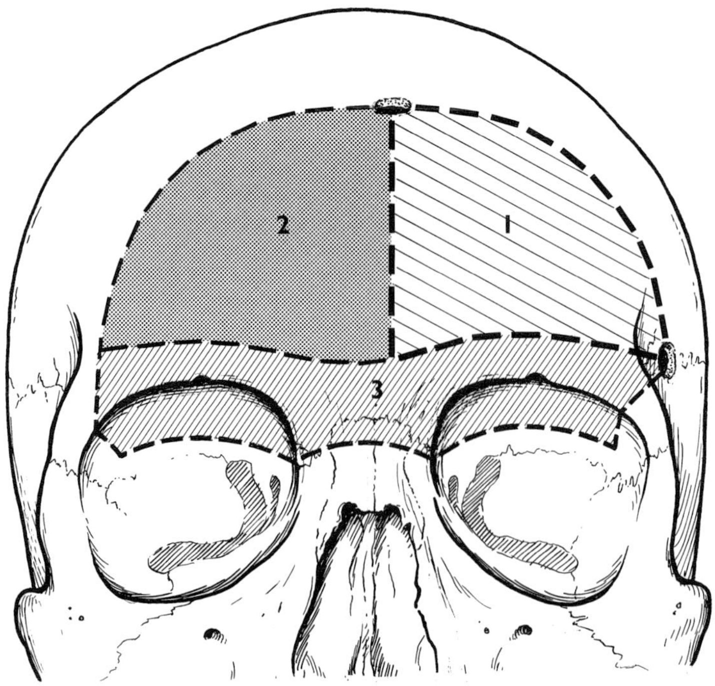

Figure 4-1. The bifrontal craniotomy is made with two separate flaps (1, 2) to allow separation of the dura under direct vision and minimize dural tears. The supraorbital bar of bone (3) is removed separately.

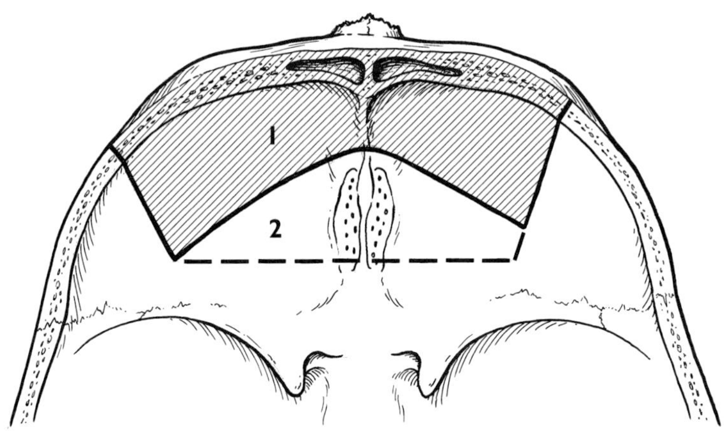

Figure 4-2. Intracranial view of the supraorbital osteotomy to show the cuts through the roofs. It should include as much of the orbital roofs as possible so that it may be replaced. In case of malignant sinus tumors the osteotomy is carried in front of the cribriform plate (1), whereas in the middle fossa and clival tumors the cut is carried through the ethmoid cells posterior to the cribriform plate (2).

tecting the dura and periorbita with malleable retractors. Coronal cuts are made using the high-speed drill, from lateral to medially across the orbital roofs to meet anterior to the cribriform plate (Figs. 4-1 and 4-2). The osteotomy is completed by making a horizontal cut with the saw from the outside across the nasion, at the level of the anterior ethmoidal arteries. The entire piece of bone is dislodged and removed with the help of a small osteotome.

The frontal lobes are elevated after opening the dura and ligating the superior sagittal sinus. The dura of the base is incised skirting the tumor. If there is brain invasion, a portion of the frontal lobe is also excised over the tumor. The bony cuts in the anterior fossa floor follow the dural incisions (Fig 4-3). The posterior limits of the bone cuts are determined by the optic nerves and the planum sphenoidale. The planum is entered with a high-speed drill and the extradural portions of the optic nerves are decompressed anteriorly out to the orbits with a diamond burr. This allows delineation of the medial walls of the orbits that extend forward from the medial wall of the optic canal. The lateral cuts are made intracranially with the reciprocating saw. Mobilization of the inferior parts of the tumor is best performed through a transfacial approach after which the tumor can be delivered inferiorly, although in some instances when the tumor is only in the ethmoid sinus the entire tumor may be removed transcranially (Blacklock et al., 1989).

Watertight dural closure is performed with a fascia lata or a pericranial patch harvested from the posterior scalp. Fibrin adhesive has not been found to be particularly useful in this repair. A wide strip of pericranium is raised from the frontal scalp, pedicled on the supraorbital vessels, and turned under the subfrontal dura and secured to the edges of the bone defect through small drill holes. This flap may be passed above or below the supraorbital bone piece, which is replaced with a titanium miniplate fixation system. It is important not to devitalize the pericranial flap by compression between free bone segments. The bone flaps are also secured with miniplates and subgaleal suction drains are left in place.

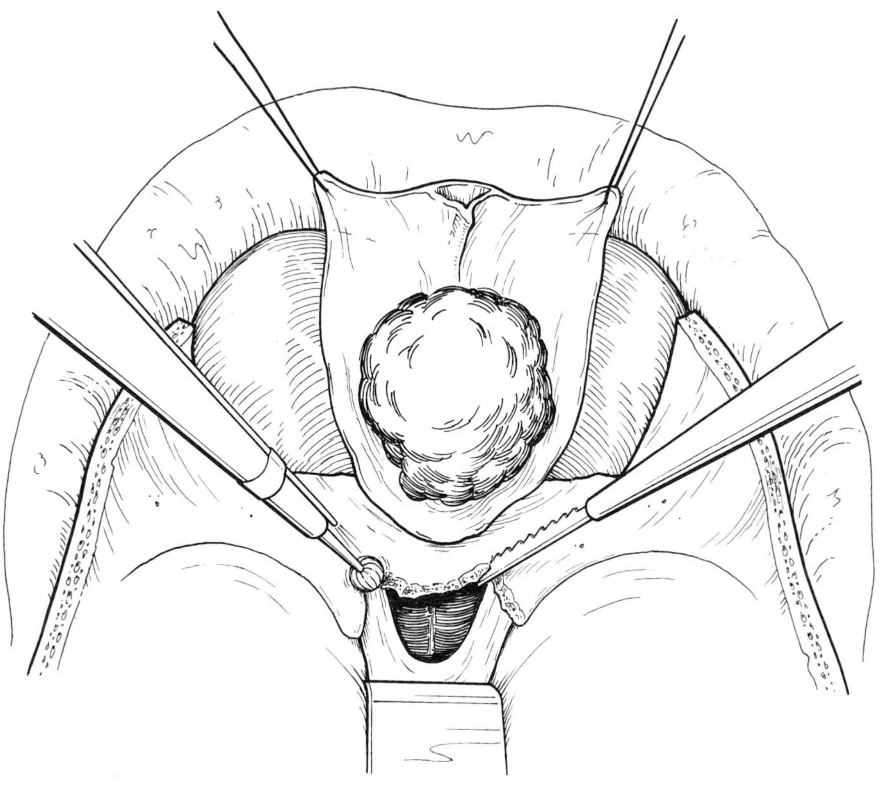

Figure 4-3. Intracranial view of en bloc resection of a tumor in the anterior fossa. After completing the dural incisions skirting the tumor from intradurally, the optic nerves are unroofed extradurally to allow delineation of the medial wall of the orbits and also the posterior limit of resection at the planum sphenoidale.

Extradural Tumors of the Central Portion of the Middle and Posterior Skull Base

Chordomas and low-grade chondrosarcomas form the majority of tumors for which this approach has been used. The lateral limits of tumor resection by this approach are the medial aspects of the cavernous internal carotid arteries (ICAs), Dorello's canal, and inferiorly the hypoglossal canals (Figs. 4-4 and 4-5). Tumor extension into the cavernous sinus, petrous bone, or lower clivus lateral to the above limits requires the use of other lateral approaches used in conjunction, at the same or a later sitting (Catalano and Biller, 1993; Cocke et al., 1990; Lanzino et al., 1993; Sekhar et al., 1988). Significant intracavernous extension may require an intradural approach.

Prior to the supraorbital osteotomy the olfactory nerves are divided at the cribriform plate and the entire subfrontal dura is elevated. The supraorbital osteotomy includes a larger portion of the orbital roofs and the cribriform plate to be replaced later (Fig. 4-2). Olfaction-sparing measures described by Spetzler et al. (1993) can also be used, which consist of making cuts on all four sides of the cribriform plate and

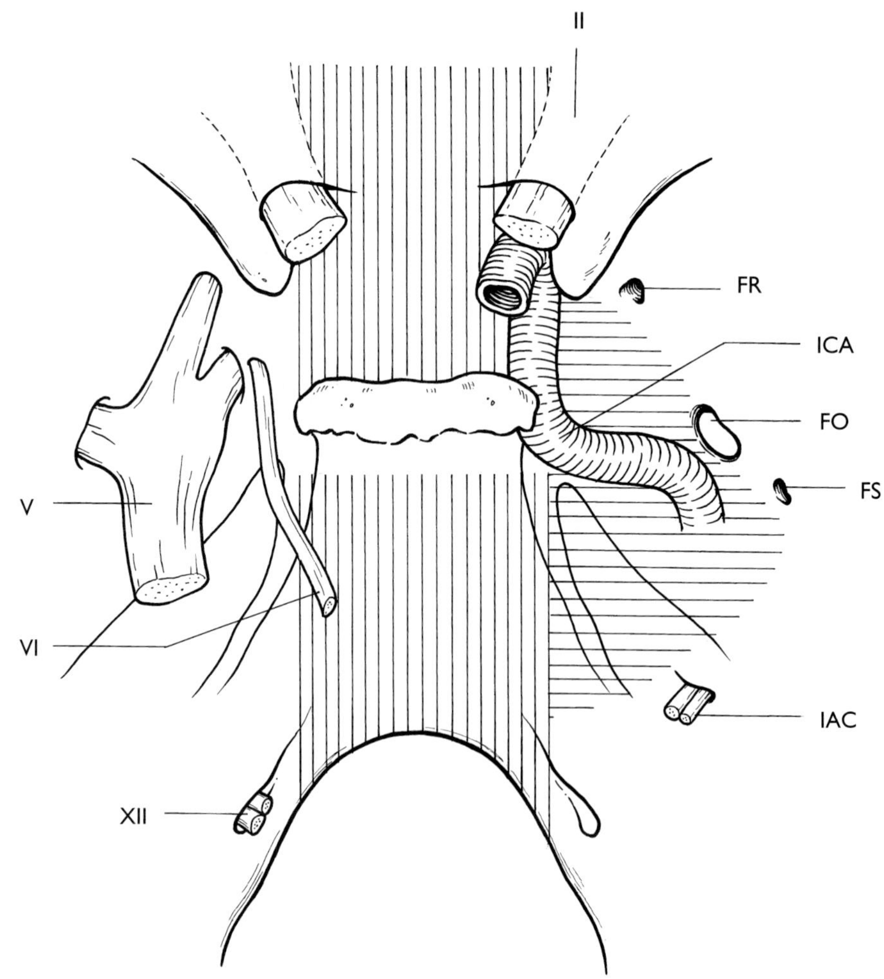

Figure 4-4. Extent of bony exposure of the skull base in the region of the sphenoid and the clivus. The vertical hatching indicates the exposure between the optic nerves, the cavernous ICAs, the 6th nerves, and the hypoglossal nerves obtained by the extended subfrontal approach. Addition of a lateral approach extends the exposure laterally as shown by the horizontal hatching lateral to the ICA. (For explanation of abbreviations, see Appendix 1, p. 373.)

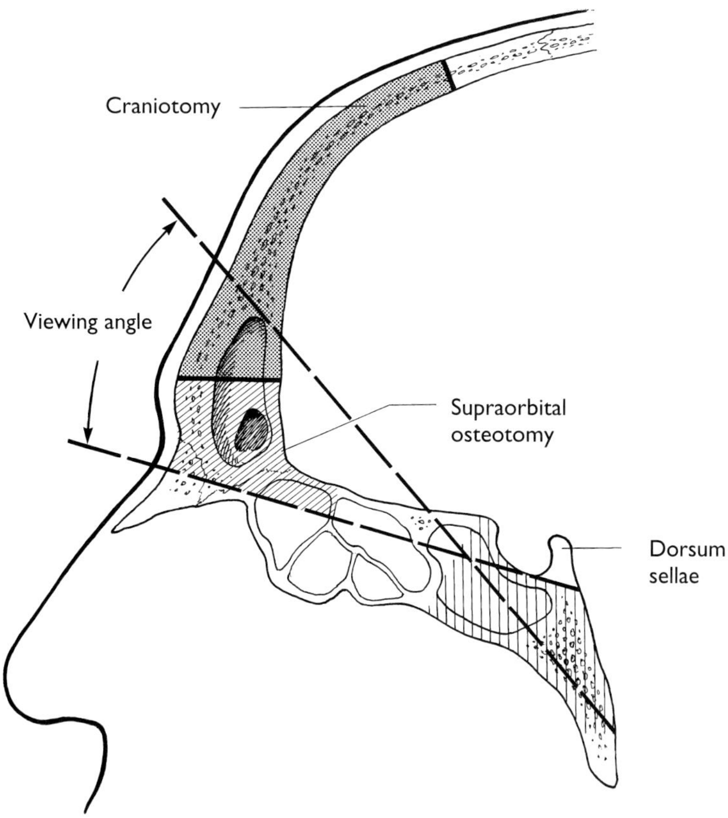

Figure 4-5. Sagittal section through the midline indicating the craniotomy and supraorbital rim removal. The widened view obtained by such bone removal is indicated. The vertical hatch marks indicate the bony exposure of the sphenoid and clivus, but the dorsum sella is hidden from the surgeon's view by the sellar contents.

the nasal mucosa and elevating the entire complex with the frontal dura to be repositioned at the end of the operation. The extradural portions of the optic nerves are decompressed as described before. The sphenoid sinus is widely opened between the optic nerves by drilling off the planum sphenoidale and posterior ethmoidal cells (Fig. 4-6). This provides excellent visualization into the sinus and subsequently the clivus. The soft part of the tumor projecting into the sinus cavity is removed. The microscope is then angled sharply from one side and then the other to inspect the contralateral medial dura of the cavernous sinuses, which overlies the ICA. The medial surfaces of the cavernous sinuses are followed posteriorly to the petrous apex. As much of the surrounding bone as possible is drilled away, keeping in mind the lateral limits of this dissection. Bleeding from the clival and cavernous venous plexus is controlled by packing pieces of rolled surgicel.

Closure consists of exenterating the mucosa of the frontal, ethmoid, and sphenoid sinuses to prevent secondary mucocele formation and packing with autologous fat (Fig. 4-7). If the olfactory nerves have been divided, the dura is closed watertight; however, this is not required if the cribriform plates were left attached to the dura. A long pericranial flap is passed between the optic nerves, above the fat, to cover the clivus (Fig. 4-8). In order for the flap to reach that far posteriorly it is better to route it under the supraorbital rims rather than over them. If the olfactory apparatus was preserved the pericranial flap will have to be button-holed in the middle. If there are doubts about the security of the dural closure, the olfactory apparatus should be sacrificed and priority given to a secure closure with the pericranial flap. The bone reap-

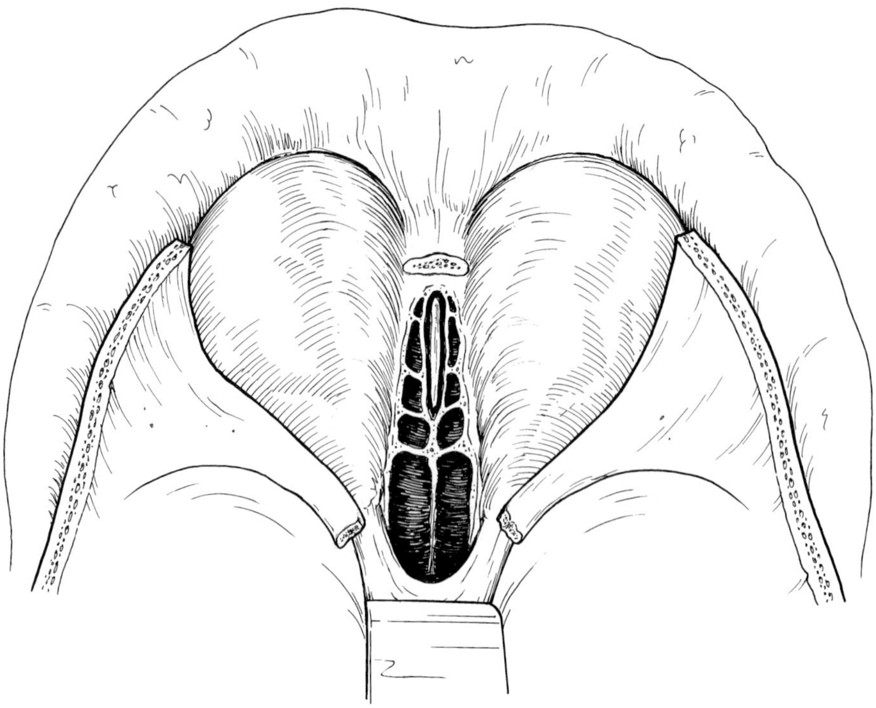

Figure 4-6. Intracranial view after unroofing the orbits and the optic nerves. The sphenoid sinus has been widely opened between the optic nerves. A wide and shallow access to the clivus is thus obtained.

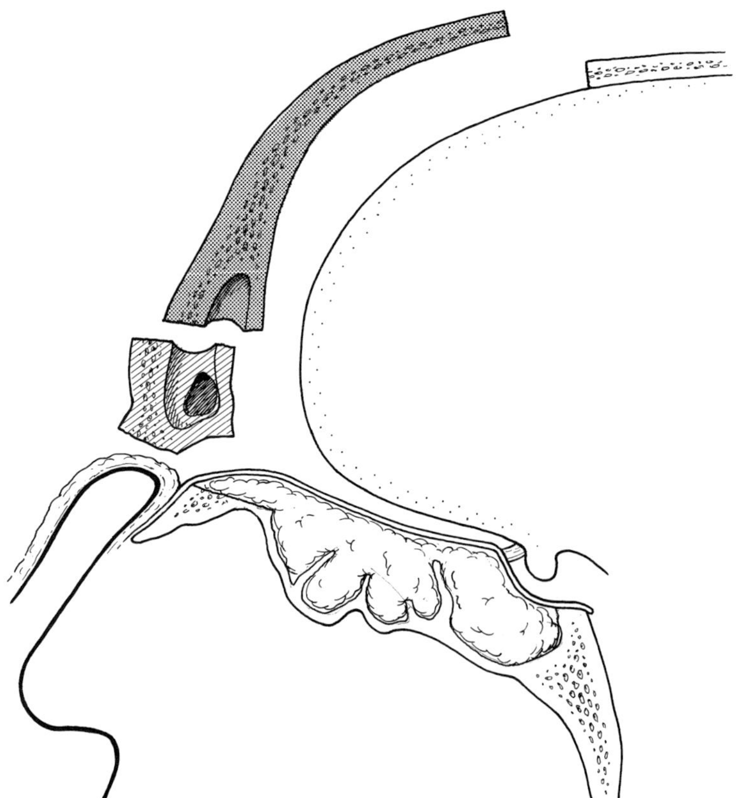

Figure 4-7. Reconstruction is completed by packing fat in the frontal, ethmoidal, and sphenoid sinuses and the tumor cavity. The pericranium is shown passing underneath the supraorbital bar of bone so that it reaches as far back as the clivus.

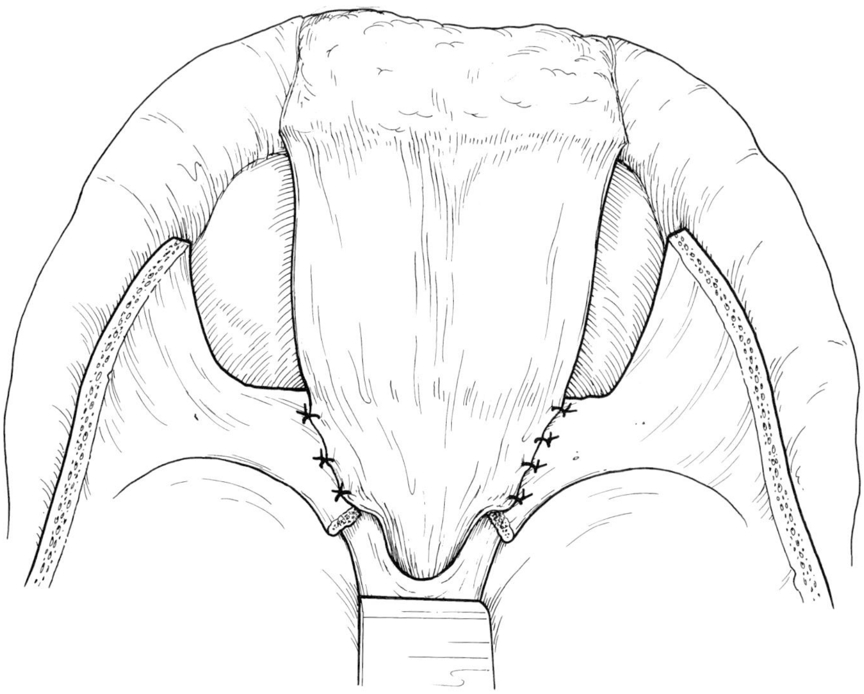

Figure 4-8. Intracranial view of the reconstruction with the pericranium passing between the optic nerves and held with sutures at the edges.

proximation is carried out as described above. Bacitracin-impregnated ½-in. gauze is used to pack the nasal cavity following replacement of the pericranial flap. This serves to aid in hemostasis within the nasal cavity defect, absorb blood and secretions, support soft tissue reconstruction of the anterior cranial fossa floor, and decrease the incidence of tension pneumocephalus.

Postoperative Care

Because of contamination from the paranasal sinuses, which may be frankly infected, broad-spectrum antibiotic coverage consisting of a cephalosporin and metronidazole is continued for 48 hours after the operation or until after the drains and packing are removed (Carran et al., 1991).

Spinal fluid drainage is usually not required after the operation unless the dural repair is felt to be tenuous. If a spinal drain is left, it is regulated by volume rather than by height. The amount of drainage is restricted to 50 to 75 ml per 8 hours and is continued for 5 days or less.

A CT scan is usually performed on the day after the operation to check for brain edema and pneumocephalus, especially if spinal fluid drainage is to be instituted.

Deep venous thrombosis prophylaxis with pneumatic compression stockings and minidose heparin is continued until the patient can ambulate normally.

Complications and Management

Complications and their management (Sen and Sekhar, 1993) are discussed below.

Epidural pneumocephalus, which is commonly seen after such surgery, is seldom under pressure unless there is persistent communication through frontal or ethmoid sinuses that have been incompletely obliterated. A decreased level of consciousness may herald its presence, and if a spinal drain is in place it may further complicate the matter by providing a gradient promoting downward herniation of the brain. Meticulous attention to soft tissue reconstruction of the anterior fossa prevents such occurrence. The spinal drain should be discontinued if the quantity of air increases.

Cerebrospinal fluid fistula may form after inadequate repair of the dural defect. The pericranial flap, which is an excellent barrier of vascularized tissue, must be prepared and inserted carefully. Breakdown of the flap from damage to its vascular supply or pressure necrosis from the bone edges can lead to its failure. The initial treatment for the spinal fluid leak is a spinal drain unless the leak is profuse, which would require re-exploration. In the event of failure of a pericranial flap a temporalis flap with a long piece of pericranium attached to it can be brought in from the side and in rare instances a microvascular free flap may be necessary to reconstruct the barrier.

Despite the routine contamination of the operative field from the paranasal sinuses, the incidence of infection is surprisingly low. This is manifest usually as epidural abscess or meningitis, evident from the edema and erythema of the overlying scalp, changes in the patient's mental status, and the presence of an epidural collection with surrounding enhancement on CT. The infection may also appear in a delayed fashion weeks after the operation. Removal of the bone flap and debridement is necessary with appropriate intravenous antibiotic coverage. Removal of the supraorbital rims is not required because it is a thin piece of bone that gets vascularized quickly.

Brain edema and contusion can occur for several reasons, the most common of which is retraction. Use of the supraorbital osteotomy and other means of brain relaxation such as dehydration and hyperventilation employed judiciously should reduce its incidence. Dissection of the tumor from the brain or injury to cortical drainage veins can also be contributing factors and should be noted on the immediate postoperative CT scans. Steroids and restriction of free water is usually sufficient in limiting this problem. More important, the patient's serum electrolytes must be closely monitored to avoid hyponatremia and anticonvulsant coverage should be maintained so that a seizure does not further complicate the situation.

Results

In a series of 118 malignant skull base tumors, Janecka et al. (1994) reported 63.7 percent disease free at an average follow-up of 30 months whereas 33 percent experienced complications. Catalano et al. (1994) performed a detailed review of the postoperative complications in 73 patients who underwent craniofacial resection for mostly malignant pathology. The incidence of cerebrospinal fluid leakage was 14 percent whereas epidural abscess and osteomyelitis occurred in 22 percent of patients. Sisson et al. (1989) commented on the earlier reports of uniformly dismal outlook in paranasal sinus cancers in the range of 25 to 30 percent survival over 5 years. Because in their report local recurrence was the major cause of death, aggressive treatment of the primary disease was recommended. The nature and biology of the tumor, the possibility of obtaining a healthy margin around the tumor and the response to adjuvant therapy determines the long-term outcome from malignant skull base tumors.

Heffelfinger et al. (1973) reviewed the Mayo Clinic experience with 55 chordomas of the skull base. The average survival from primary therapy was 7.4 years. A more recent report of a series of 60 chordomas and chondrosarcomas (Gay et al., 1994) treated by modern skull base surgery techniques showed a 5-year recurrence-free survival of 76.2 percent. Chordomas had a less favorable control rate than chondrosarcomas. An aggressive initial surgical resection by a single or combined operative approaches seems to play a major role in the long-term outcome. Again, primary treatment rather than treatment for recurrent disease offers a better chance at resection. Thus modern skull base techniques when used appropriately and judiciously can be helpful in the management of these tumors and appear to improve the survival.

References

Blacklock JB, Weber RS, Lee YY, Goepfert H (1989) Transcranial resection of tumors of the paranasal sinuses and nasal cavity. J Neurosurg 71:10–15

Carrau RL, Snyderman CH, Janecka IP et al (1991) Antibiotic prophylaxis in cranial base surgery. Head Neck 13:311–317

Catalano PJ, Biller HF (1993) Extended osteoplastic maxillotomy. Arch Otolaryngol Head Neck Surg 119:394–400

Catalano PJ, Hecht CS, Biller HF et al (1994) Craniofacial resection: an analysis of 73 cases. Arch Otolaryngol Head Neck Surg 120:1203–1208

Cocke EW Jr, Robertson JH, Robertson JT, Crook JP Jr (1990) The extended maxillotomy and subtotal maxillectomy for excision of skull base tumors. Arch Otolaryngol Head Neck Surg 116:92–104

Derome P, Akerman M, Anquez L (1972) Les tumeurs spheno-ethmoidales. Possibilites d'exerese et de reparation chirurgicales. Neurochirurgie, Suppl. 18:1–164

Gay E, Sekhar LN, Rubinstein E et al (1994) Chordomas and chondrosarcomas of the cranial base: results and follow-up of 60 patients. Neurosurgery 36:887–896

Heffelfinger MJ. Dahlin DC, MacCarty CS, Beabout JW (1973) Chordomas and cartilaginous tumors at the skull base. Cancer 32:410–420

Janecka IP, Sen C, Sekhar LN et al (1994) Cranial base surgery: results in 183 patients. Otolaryngol Head Neck Surg 110:539–546

Lanzino G, Sekhar LN, Hirsch WL et al (1993) Chordomas and chondrosarcomas involving the cavernous sinus: review of surgical treatment and outcome in 31 patients. Surg Neurol 40:359–371

Raveh J, Laedrach K, Speiser M et al (1993) The subcranial approach for fronto-orbital and anteroposterior skull base tumors. Arch Otolaryngol Head Neck Surg 119:385–393

Sekhar LN, Janecka IP, Jones NF (1988) Subtemporal infratemporal and basal subfrontal approach to extensive cranial base tumors. Acta Neurochir 92:83–92

Sekhar LN, Nanda A, Sen C et al (1992) The extended frontal approach to tumors of the anterior, middle and posterior skull base. J Neurosurg 76:198–206

Sen C, Sekhar LN (1993) Complications of cranial base surgery. pp. 111–131. In Post K, Friedman E, McCormick P (eds): Postoperative Complications in Intracranial Neurosurgery, Thieme, New York

Sisson GA Sr, Toriumi DM, Atiyah RA (1989) Paranasal sinus malignancy: a comprehensive update. Laryngoscope 99:143–150

Snyderman CH, Janecka IP, Sekhar LN et al (1990) Anterior cranial base reconstruction: role of galeal and pericranial flaps. Laryngoscope 100:607–614

Spetzler RF, Herman JM, Beals S et al (1993) Preservation of olfaction in anterior craniofacial approaches. J Neurosurg 79:48–52

Yamamoto Y, Minakawa H, Yoshida T et al (1993) Role of bone graft in reconstruction of skull base defect: is a bone graft necessary? Skull Base Surg 3:223–229

5

Extended Trans-Sphenoidal Approach to the Pituitary Region and Upper Clivus

Rudolf Fahlbusch
Jürgen Honegger

The first transnasal removal of a pituitary adenoma was reported by Schloffer in 1906. In the following years, Harvey Cushing elaborated the approach and some of his technical principles are still appreciated and in current use. Although Cushing later abandoned the trans-sphenoidal approach, the tradition of trans-sphenoidal surgery was continued by Norman Dott and Oskar Hirsch. Antibiotic and hormonal replacement therapies have widely improved surgical outcome. Re-inauguration and general acceptance of the approach occurred with the advent of microsurgical techniques and radiofluoroscopic control. Introduction of modern imaging techniques such as computed tomography (CT) in the 1970s and magnetic resonance imaging (MRI) in the 1980s have facilitated the decision for the appropriate approach.

The trans-sphenoidal approach has been classically performed for pituitary adenomas within the pituitary fossa. With increasing experience, the approach has been extended. (1) Trans-sphenoidal surgery is now used for pathologies other than pituitary adenomas, (e.g., craniopharyngiomas, chordomas, malignancies, and meningiomas). It is also applied for nontumorous disease such as sphenoidal encephaloceles or post-traumatic cerebrospinal fluid (CSF) leaks. (2) The approach has been extended with respect to the anatomic location of the lesions (Fig. 5-1). Experienced trans-sphenoidal neurosurgeons use the approach for tumors of the clivus. They have learned to deal with tumors invading the cavernous sinus or even arising from the cavernous sinus, but are also aware of the limitations of the approach. In this chapter, we describe modern surgical techniques of the extended trans-sphenoidal approach and emphasize its possibilities and limitations.

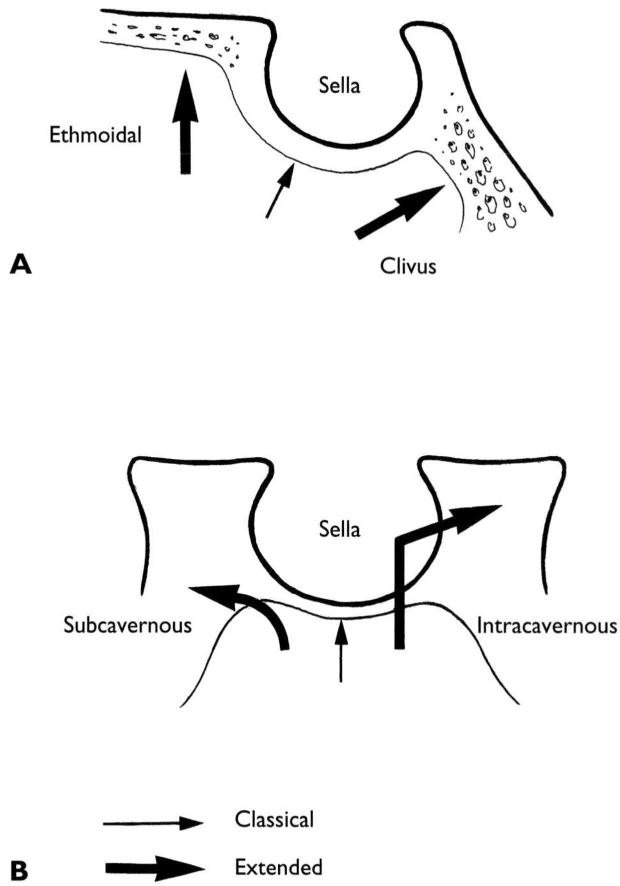

Figure 5-1. Anatomic definition of "classic" and "extended" trans-sphenoidal approach. *(A)* Sagittal view. *(B)* Coronal view.

Indications

The transnasal-transsphenoidal approach is mainly used for extradural lesions in the midline. The posterior ethmoid sinus is the most anterior structure that can be exposed. However, the upper conchae, which hinder opening of the speculum anteriorly, show anatomic variations. The anterior ethmoid is reached by a transethmoidal approach. The sphenoid sinus and the pituitary fossa are classically the main field of surgical exposure. The posterior structures are the upper and middle clivus. The posterior and lower border of the approach are the nasal floor, the choanes, and the epipharynx (Fig. 5-2). The mucosal tunnel can only be extended to this level. The mucosal barrier to the epipharynx is not opened during the trans-sphenoidal approach. The anatomic variability of these structures explains why the lower third of the clivus can be reached in some patients while only the middle of the clivus can be exposed in other patients (Fig. 5-2). For lesions of the lower clivus, the transoral approach is suitable. A combined trans-sphenoidal and transoral approach is used for large lesions in the clival area.

The width of the surgical field is given by the speculum. Direct lateral visualization from the midline is 5 to 10 mm on either side. Lateral resection is performed with curettes. Angulated Fahlbusch curettes (see under Instrumentation and Fig. 5-4) allow tumor removal as far as 20 to 30 mm from the midline.

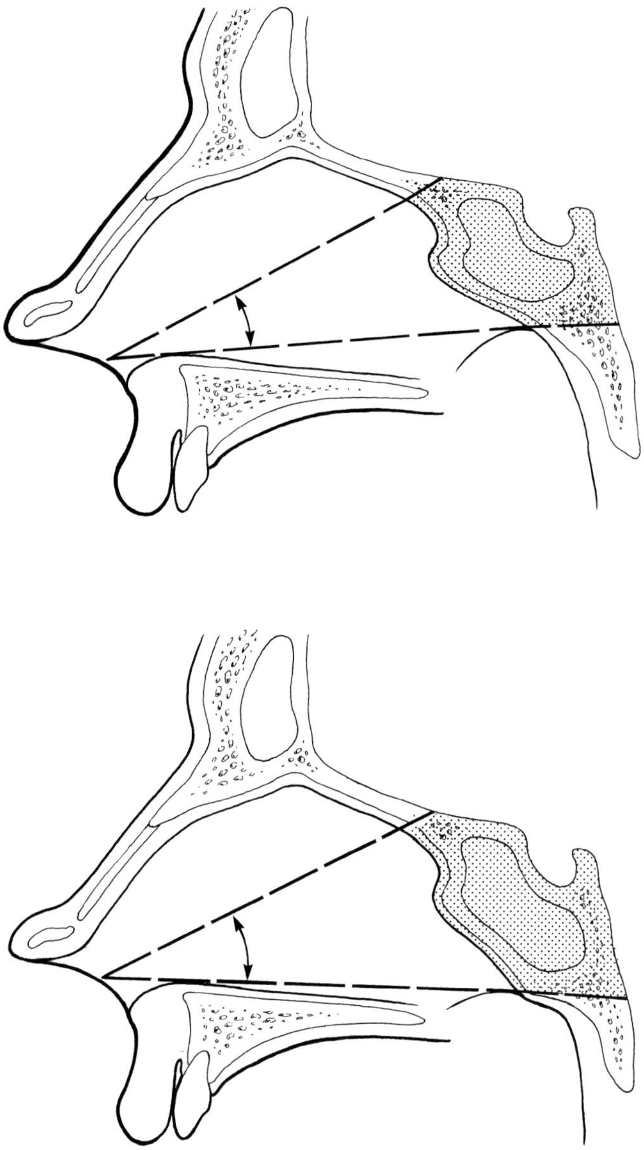

A

B

Figure 5-2. Angle of exposure by the trans-sphenoidal approach depending on anatomic variations: *(A)* High epipharynx. *(B)* Low epipharynx.

A smooth, well-circumscribed upper border of a sellar lesion suggests that the diaphragma sellae is displaced upward and allows trans-sphenoidal removal (Figs. 5-3A & C). An irregular shape indicates an invasive suprasellar extension and precludes trans-sphenoidal removal. Figures 5-3B & D depict other suprasellar extensions that preclude a trans-sphenoidal operation because the suprasellar tumor is unlikely to enter the pituitary fossa during the procedure.

An intradural tumor extension is a contraindication for the approach.

Preoperative Assessment

Neuroradiology

MRI is the technique of choice to depict the extent of the lesion and its relationship to the surrounding structures. MRI demonstrates invasion of the cavernous sinus,

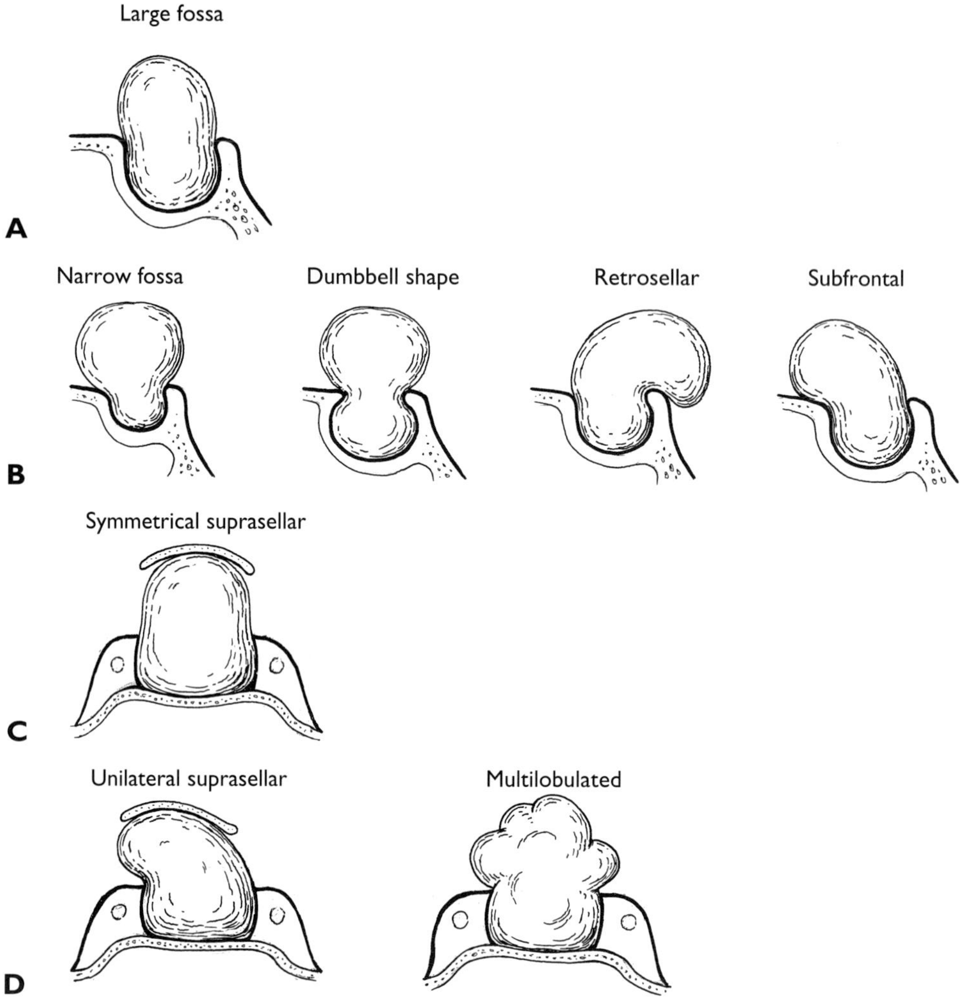

Figure 5-3. Different types of suprasellar tumor extension. *(A & C)* Trans-sphenoidal surgery indicated. *(B & D)* Trans-sphenoidal surgery contraindicated.

sphenoid sinus, and clivus. It shows whether a lesion is located under or above the diaphragm. CT depicts calcifications of a lesion and demonstrates bony destructions of the skull base. In large lesions encroaching upon the cavernous sinus, angiography is performed to demonstrate displacement and narrowing of vessels.

Neuroendocrinology

Neuroendocrine workup is mandatory if the pituitary fossa is involved. It includes dynamic endocrine testing. The insulin tolerance test (ITT) or corticotropin-releasing hormone stimulation or adrenocorticotropic hormone stimulation are used for assessment of the hypothalamo-pituitary-adrenal axis, thyrotropin-releasing hormone stimulation for thyroid axis, and gonadotropin-releasing hormone stimulation for gonadal axis. ITT is the most reliable test for evaluation of growth hormone reserve.

A more than two-fold increase of urine osmolality compared to serum osmolality after an overnight fast indicates undisturbed antidiuretic hormone secretion. In equivocal cases, a water deprivation test proves or excludes diabetes insipidus.

Perioperative hydrocortisone replacement (100 mg intravenously over 24 hours, tapering the dose during the following days) is indispensable in patients with adrenal insufficiency. In slowly growing lesions without urgent ophthalmologic symptoms, a euthyroid state should be attained by replacement therapy before surgery in order to reduce the anesthetic risk.

Ophthalmology

Ophthalmologic workup includes assessment of visual acuity, visual fields, and optomotoric nerve function.

Operative Procedure

Instrumentation

A variety of microsurgical instruments have been specifically designed for the trans-sphenoidal approach. From each type of instrument different variations are available according to the personal preference of the neurosurgeons. The instruments preferred for use in our department are shown in Figure 5-4.

The instrumentation is supplemented by other microsurgical instruments such as microdissectors. Another indispensable instrument is the angulated high-speed diamond drill.

Positioning

We use the supine positioning introduced by Cushing. The patient's head is slightly extended by lowering the head rest of the operating table about 10 to 15 degrees. An x-ray intensifier with lateral view is installed (Fig. 5-5).

Approach

The mucosa of the nasal septum and of the anterior spine is infiltrated with diluted ornipressin solution through the nostrils and the vestibulum oris, and then the draping is arranged leaving an opening for the approach of 4 × 4 cm. The surgeon stands behind the patient's head (Fig. 5-5).

A rhinoseptal approach is routinely used. A sublabial incision is preferred in the case of a large tumor or a small nostril. The versatility to angulate the speculum in relation to the skull base is superior compared to the pernasal approach. We use a 3- to 4-mm horizontal incision above the nasal septum on the inside of the upper lip just a few millimeters from the gingival labial sulcus. With such a short incision, denervation and sensory loss are minimal. The anterior spine and the cartilaginous septum are exposed by blunt dissection of the soft tissue. Then the perichondrium is incised unilaterally. By dissection in the cleavage plane between cartilage and mucosa/perichondrium with a dissector, a mucosal tunnel is created. Exposure of this layer is crucial to prevent tearing of the mucosa. The mucosal tunnel is extended basally to the maxilla. Between cartilage and anterior spine, the mucosa is adherent and must be carefully detached by sharp and blunt dissection. The cartilage is incised basally and can now be deflected to the opposite side. The mucosal tunnel is enlarged by elevation of the mucosa from the anterior spine and the crista nasalis of the opposite side. The anterior spine is removed with a punch or with the diamond drill. At this stage, a small conical speculum (Cushing's type) is inserted, which displaces the cartilage to the opposite side and the microscope is introduced. With a dissector, the border between the bony septum (vomer, lamina perpendicularis ossis ethmoidalis) and the cartilage is separated and the bony septum is exposed in the midline between the blades of the speculum, the approach being bilateral in the depth. The direction is guided by an x-ray intensifier. In the surgical corridor, the bony septum is removed with rongeurs and the mucosal tunnel is extended down to the floor of the sphenoid

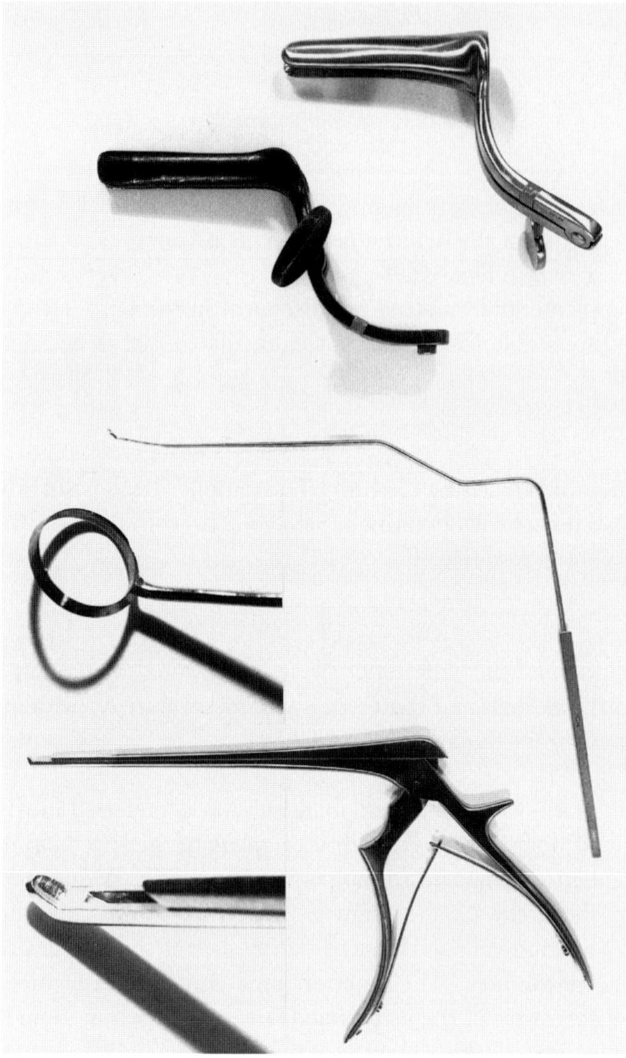

Figure 5-4. *(A–K)* Pituitary instrumentation generally used in our department. *(A)* Hardy nasal bivalve specula, length 80 mm (standard) and 90 mm (acromegalic). *(B)* Conical Cushing's type speculum. *(C)* Fahlbusch curettes. *(D)* Hardy sella punch, 40 degrees up, 1 mm and 2 mm. *(E)* Hardy curettes, bayonet, angled down, 3 mm and 5 mm. *(F)* Fahlbusch scoop, malleable. *(G)* Hardy-Fahlbusch dissector, sharpened inner edge ("pituitary hook"). *(H)* Micropituitary-style scissors, alligator action, semimalleable shaft, straight and curved left and curved right. *(I)* Fahlbusch microscissors with tubular shaft, horizontal cutting, curved or flat. *(J)* Microcup pituitary forceps, semimalleable shaft. *(K)* Pituitary rongeur, straight. *(Figure continues.)*

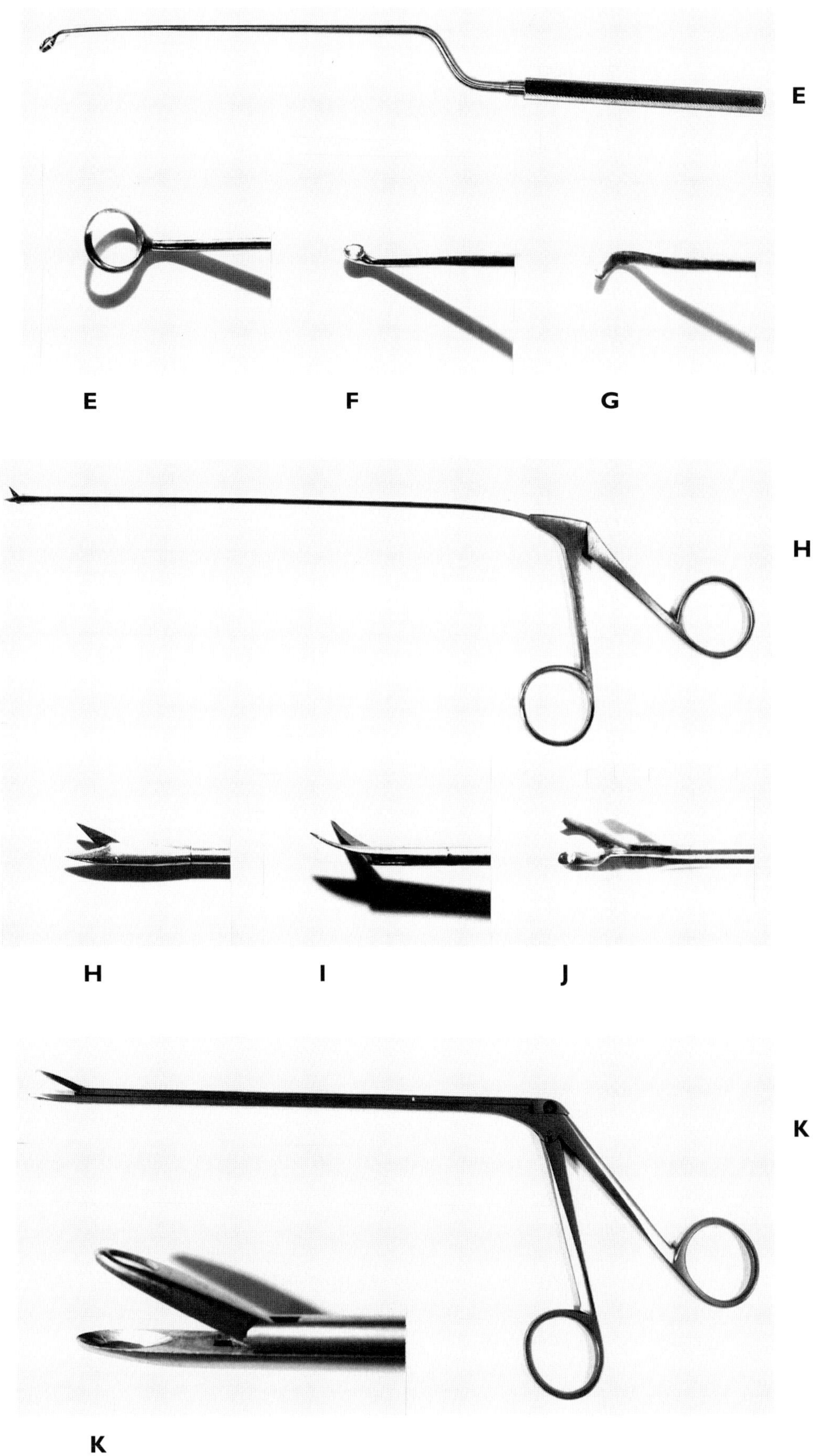

Figure 5-4 (Continued).

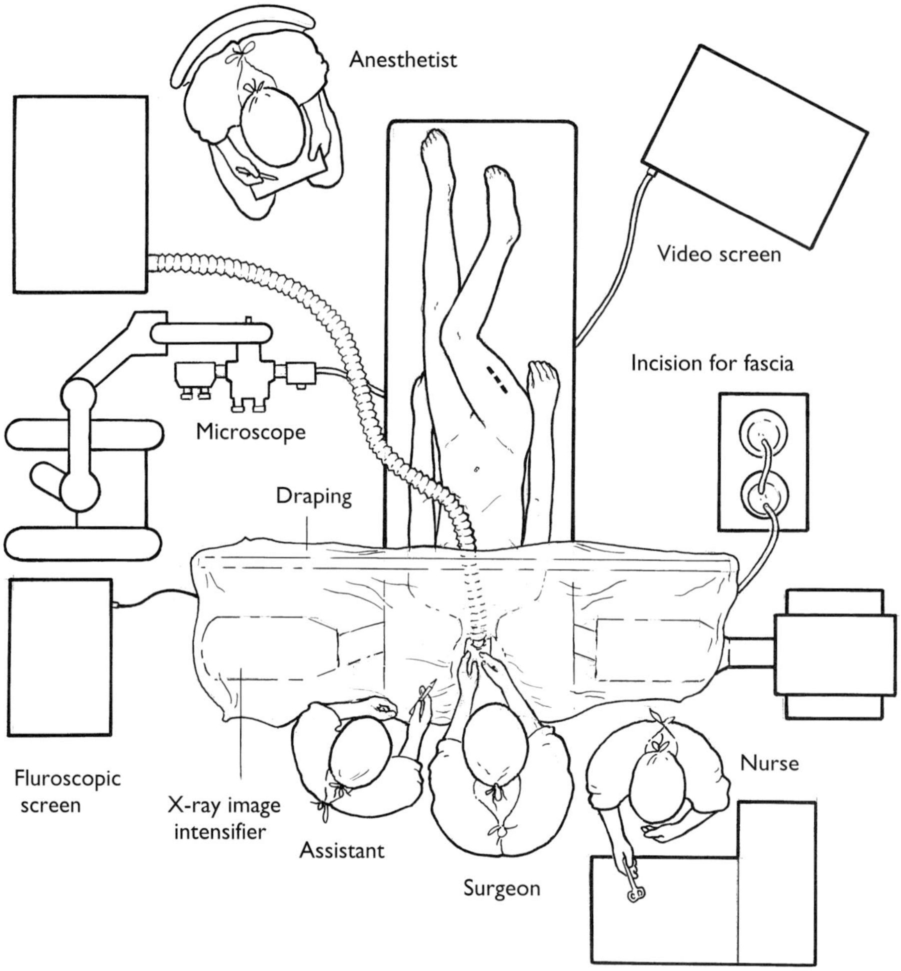

Figure 5-5. Positioning of the patient and arrangement of the equipment in the operating room.

sinus. The sphenoid sinus is opened with a diamond drill and with a punch, followed by insertion of a larger speculum (Hardy's type). Care must be taken to keep the blades just outside the sphenoid floor to prevent fractures of the sphenoid when opening the speculum. With the diamond drill, the sphenoid floor can be removed beyond the blades of the speculum laterally. The sphenoid mucosa is stripped off with forceps, and the sphenoid septum is removed with a rongeur and a diamond drill.

In some instances, the sphenoid is poorly pneumatized. For a wide access to the pituitary fossa, its outline must be fully exposed. Therefore, the sphenoid bone is stepwise removed with the drill. The midline orientation is provided by the insertion of the nasal septum at the sphenoid. MRI shows the course and location of the carotid artery in the sphenoid and helps to avoid vascular injury. The size of the instruments (for example, diameter of the suction tip) is a reliable measure for estimating the possibilities and limitations of lateral exposure. The extent of dorsal exposure to the clivus is supervised by the x-ray image intensifier.

The sellar floor is opened with a diamond drill and a punch. During lateral removal, a firmer attachment of the basal dura to the sellar floor indicates that the border of the cavernous sinus has been reached. In parasellar lesions, removal of bone underneath the cavernous sinus with the drill allows further lateral exposure.

Tumor Removal

Sphenoid Sinus. Tumor can displace or invade the mucosa of the sphenoid sinus. It is removed with forceps or curettes, firm lesions with microscissors. The mucosa is cleared from the sphenoid sinus. Bleeding in the midline can be controlled by bipolar coagulation, and lateral bleeding by angulated bipolar coagulation or by gentle compression with Gelfoam.

Clivus. Trans-sphenoidal surgery is indicated in extradural lesions (Fig. 5-6). Generally, only the upper and middle clivus can be exposed. The approach is contraindicated in intradural lesions penetrating the clivus dura. Two patterns of tumor growth are observed: (1) destruction of the bony structures by a solid mass and (2) diffuse invasion of the bone by tumor.

The former is handled with classical methods of tumor removal. Depending on the consistency, the tumor is removed by curettes or forceps, or by suction. Firm tumors are excised with microscissors or shrunk with coagulation. Often, the exposure is extended to the dura of the clivus, which is the dorsal border of resection. It is often strongly vascularized by the venous plexus, and control of bleeding can be time consuming. Tumor invading and perforating the dura should not be pursued through the defect into the posterior fossa. Visualization of structures (e.g., basilar artery) and control of bleeding is poor behind the level of the dura.

Invaded bone is removed with the drill until a normal bony structure is encountered (Fig. 5-7). Vessels in the bone can often be occluded with the drill. Bone wax on the drill is helpful for difficult and persistent bleeding.

Intrasellar. Having removed the sellar floor, the basal dura is fenestrated. The edges are shrunk by coagulation. A lateral opening can be continued until bleeding from the cavernous sinus occurs, which is controlled by slight compression with Gelfoam or coagulation. If the pituitary gland covers the lesion, the gland is incised in the midline to avoid major damage to the pituitary. The tumor is then removed with curettes. If a capsule is encountered, the content of the capsule is first debulked. Then, the capsule is stepwise dissected externally from the surrounding structures by blunt (and sometimes sharp) dissection with a microdissector or pituitary hook while pulling the capsule to the midline.

Parasellar. Lesions arising from the pituitary fossa may displace the cavernous sinus focally (Fig. 5-8A). They may displace the whole cavernous sinus (Fig. 5-8B). Other lesions show focal or diffuse invasion of the cavernous sinus (Fig. 5-8C).

Parasellar Displacing the Cavernous Sinus. Parasellar lesions can be removed laterally as far as 2 to 3 cm from the midline with curettes (Fig. 5-9). Angulated Fahlbusch curettes allow far lateral manipulation. The smooth wall of the cavernous sinus, palpated with the curette, suggests a noninvasive parasellar extension. After removal of the tumor, the cavernous sinus may shift toward the midline and can often be directly visualized and judged for invasiveness of a lesion.

Parasellar Invading the Cavernous Sinus. We distinguish between local and diffuse invasion of the cavernous sinus by sellar lesions. The surgeon observes perforation or even absence of the medial dural sheet of the cavernous sinus (Fig. 5-10). The cavernous sinus can be entered with curettes between the "trabecular" veins. If the veins are obstructed by tumor, removal can proceed without adverse venous bleeding. The surgeon must be familiar with the anatomy of the cavernous sinus. Curettage is performed carefully to prevent injury of the carotid artery. The lateral border of resec-

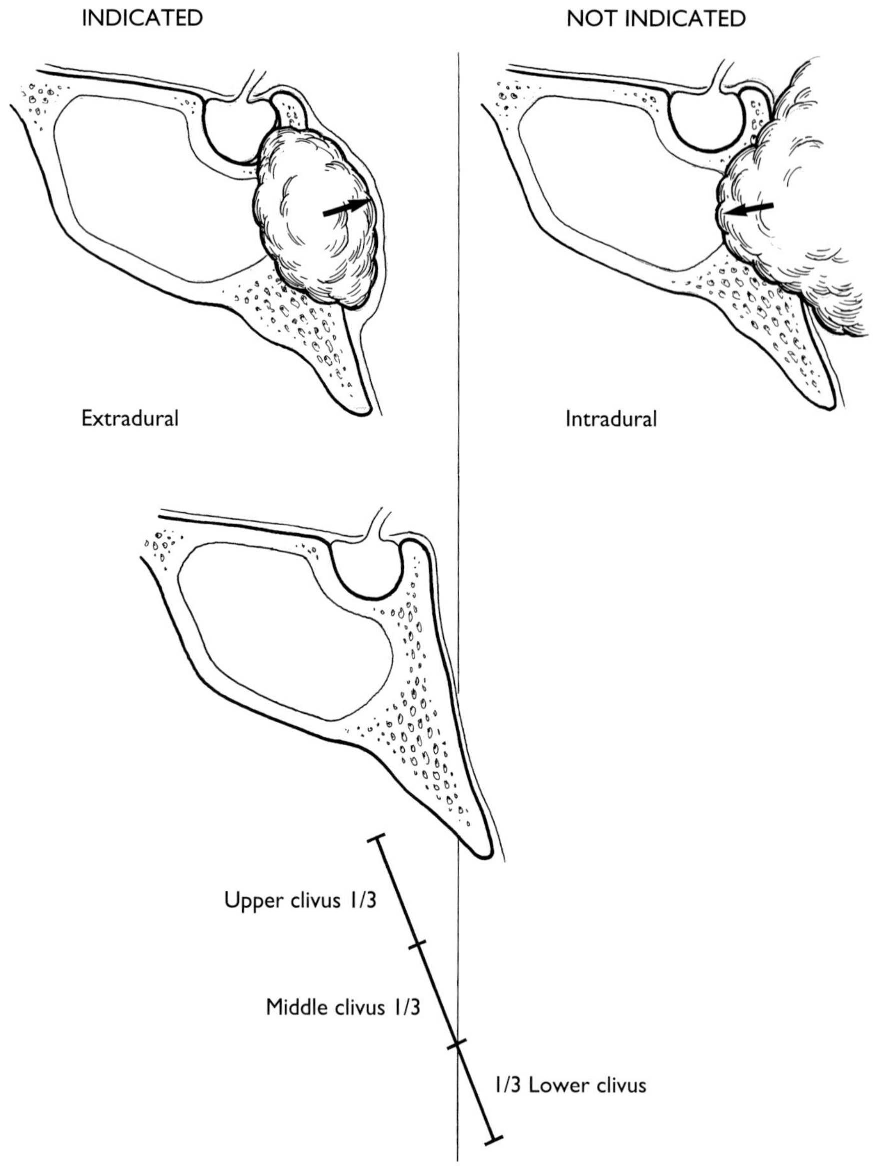

Figure 5-6. Indications and contraindications for trans-sphenoidal surgery in tumors involving the clivus.

tion is the carotid artery. Its pulsations can be palpated with the curette. In cases of major invasiveness, the carotid artery is directly visible. It allows resection around and to some extent lateral to the carotid artery under direct view. Bleeding from the cavernous sinus can be controlled by gentle compression with pieces of Gelfoam (Fig. 5-11).

On the other hand, we have encountered lesions arising from the cavernous sinus that have shown secondary intrasellar extension, such as cavernous sinus meningiomas.

Suprasellar. Once the intrasellar tumor has been removed, the suprasellar portion can enter the empty pituitary fossa. In some instances, descent of suprasellar tumor is only accomplished by an increase of the intracranial pressure using positive end-expiratory pressure ventilation or bilateral jugular vein compression (Fig. 5-12).

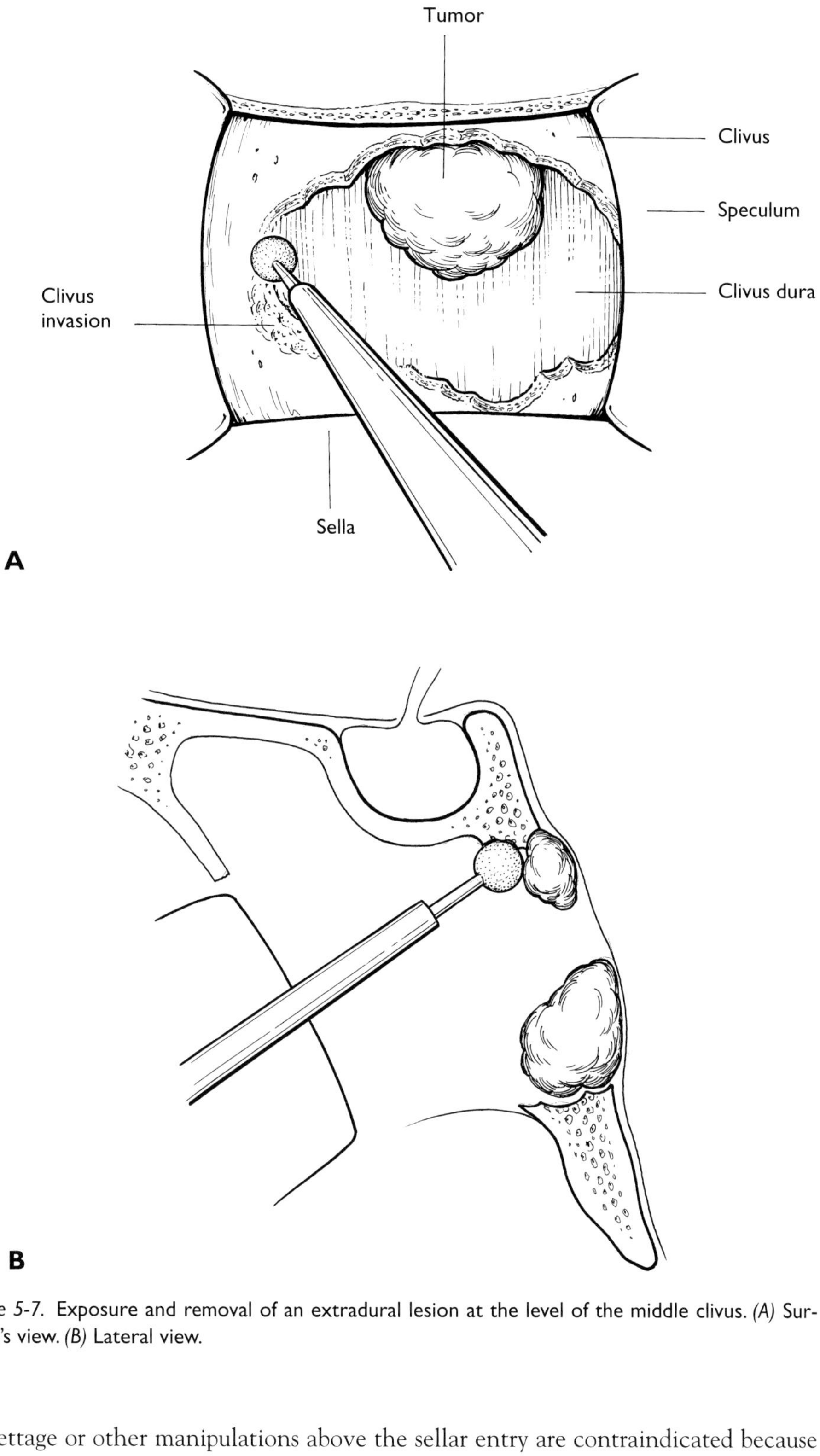

Figure 5-7. Exposure and removal of an extradural lesion at the level of the middle clivus. *(A)* Surgeon's view. *(B)* Lateral view.

Curettage or other manipulations above the sellar entry are contraindicated because of the risk of damage to the optic pathways or of producing uncontrollable bleeding.

Closure

The surgical field is closed with fascia lata (Fig. 5-13). For closure of the pituitary fossa, one square piece of fascia is placed on the edges of the basal dura. A larger piece of fascia widely covers the opening from the planum sphenoidale to the clivus.

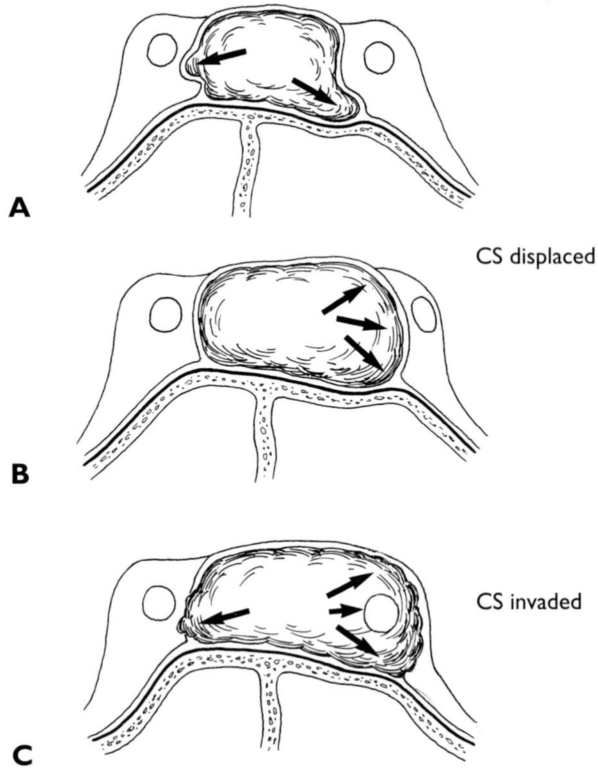

Figure 5-8. Types of cavernous sinus (CS) involvement. *(A)* Local displacement. *(B)* General displacement. *(C)* Focal or diffuse invasion.

Fibrin glue is used as sealant. If a large CSF leak has been encountered, the sphenoid sinus is additionally packed with fat or muscle from the thigh. Exposed dura at the clivus is closed in a similar manner. Once an intraoperative CSF fistula is encountered, a lumbar CSF drainage is inserted in the operating room and 20 ml CSF are withdrawn three times daily over a 3- to 4-day period to lower the intracranial pressure and to prevent a postoperative CSF leak.

Pathologies

Pituitary Adenoma

Pituitary adenomas surpass the frequency of other pathologies in the pituitary and clivus area (Table 5-1). They arise from the anterior pituitary lobe.

Small nonfunctioning pituitary adenomas that are confined to the pituitary fossa and subdiaphragmatic space are operated on if they compromise vision or cause pituitary deficiency. Large adenomas should be removed surgically to prevent progression and deteriorating symptoms. For parasellar adenomas invading the cavernous sinus, a trans-sphenoidal approach is appropriate. However, a temporal extension or parasellar supraclinoidal extension necessitates transcranial surgery. Suprasellar adenomas are removed transcranially in the case of a major retrosellar hump, subfrontal extension, small pituitary fossa, or a narrow sella entry (Fig. 5-4B & D). A multilobulated or asymmetric suprasellar portion suggests perforation of the diaphragm and also requires transcranial surgery. In nonfunctioning adenomas, a transcranial approach is more often required than in hormone-secreting adenomas. Often, they are not diagnosed until they are large in size.

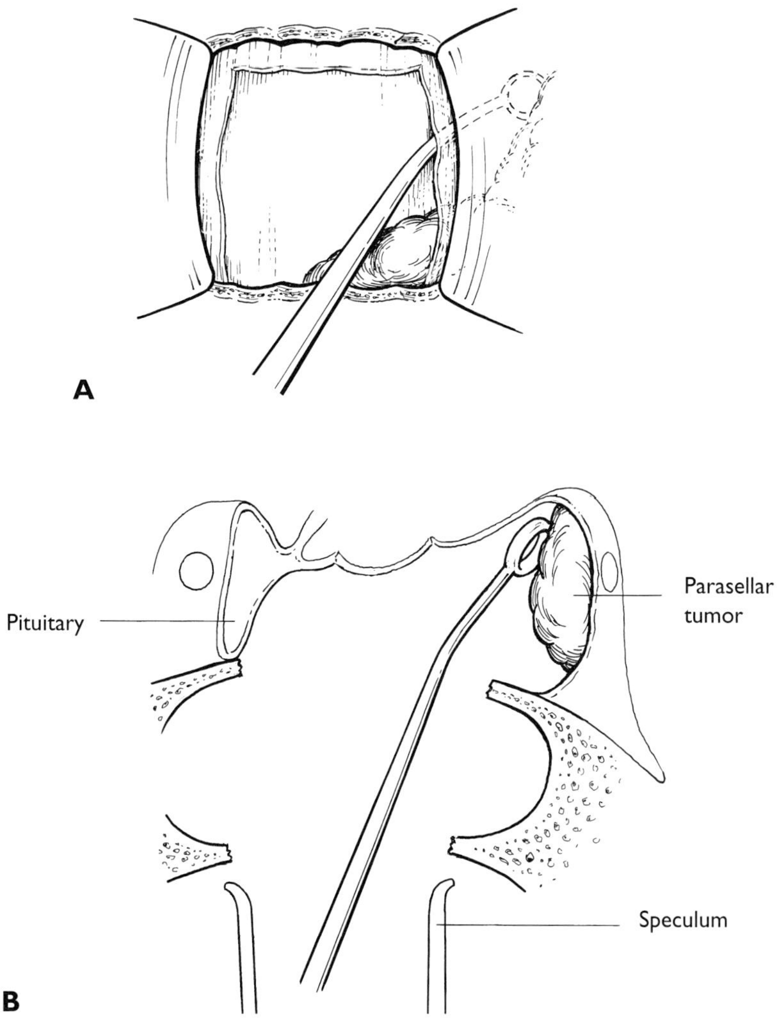

Figure 5-9. Removal of parasellar tumors displacing the cavernous sinus. *(A)* Surgeon's view. *(B)* Coronal view.

Because of the benign nature of pituitary adenomas and the high control rate of residual tumor by radiotherapy, the surgical management is less aggressive than in other lesions (e.g., craniopharyngiomas).

Prolactinomas are operated on if they are nonresponsive to dopamine agonist therapy or if dopamine agonists are not tolerated. Surgery is also considered in mesoadenomas (5 to 10 mm) and in macroadenomas (> 10 mm) if the patient desires pregnancy. Pretreatment with long-acting bromocriptine (Parlodel LAR 100 mg) for 1 to 3 months is an adjunct to surgical therapy. Suprasellar or parasellar adenomas may then enter the fossa and become accessible by the trans-sphenoidal approach.

In Cushing's disease and in acromegaly, hormone excess clearly impairs life expectancy. Cushing's disease is usually associated with microadenomas. Pretreatment of hypercortisolism with ketoconazole or metyrapone improves the patient's general condition before surgery and is done in severe cases. Trans-sphenoidal exploration is the initial therapy of choice. In acromegaly, the trans-sphenoidal approach is suitable in the vast majority of cases. About 5 percent of our patients required a combined transcranial and trans-sphenoidal operation. Pretreatment with the somatostatin-analog octreotide 3 × 100 μg daily for 2 to 3 months is increasingly

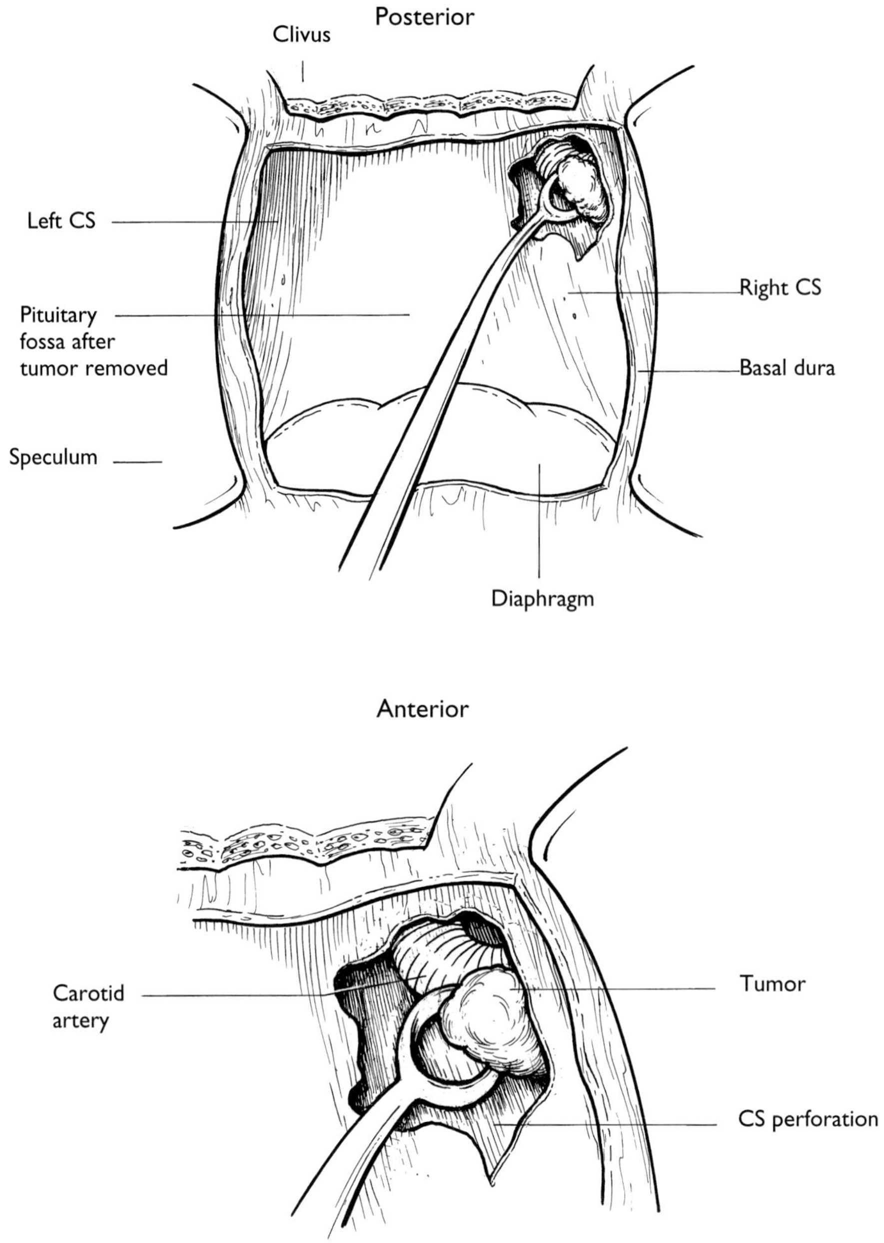

A

B

Figure 5-10. Removal of tumor from within the cavernous sinus. *(A)* Surgeon's view. *(B)* Magnification of the invaded cavernous sinus area.

recommended by experienced neurosurgeons. It is felt that pretreatment softens the adenoma and facilitates its removal. It also lowers growth hormone levels and improves the patient's condition. However, tumor shrinkage is only achieved in a minority of cases by pretreatment.

Craniopharyngioma

Craniopharyngiomas arise in the hypothalamo-pituitary region. Trans-sphenoidal resection is indicated in craniopharyngiomas arising from the pituitary fossa with subdiaphragmatic–extra-arachnoidal location. This type of craniopharyngioma is generally confined to the intrasellar and suprasellar/extra-arachnoidal compartment and shows no invasion of the cavernous sinus and clivus.

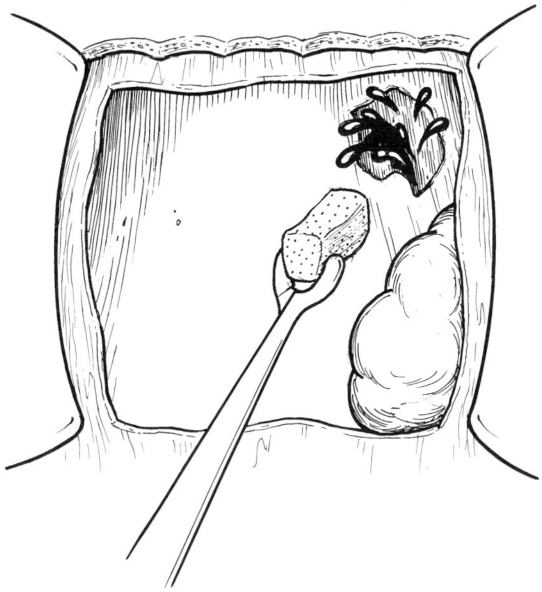

A

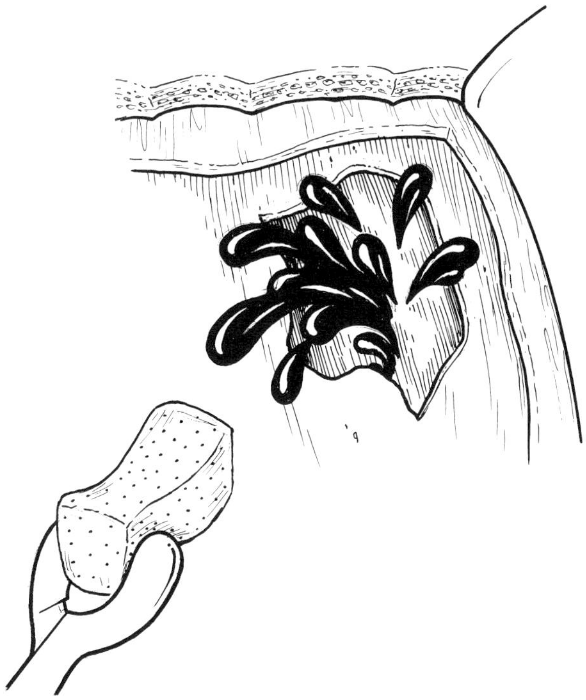

B

Figure 5-11. Control of bleeding from the cavernous sinus by Gelfoam. *(A)* Surgeon's view. *(B)* Magnification of the cavernous sinus area.

Removal commences with intracapsular debulking. Some characteristics render trans-sphenoidal removal of craniopharyngiomas difficult: (1) The pituitary gland is displaced anteriorly in 50 percent of cases. The pituitary gland must first be divided to visualize the craniopharyngioma. (2) The capsule firmly adheres to the surrounding structures. It is detached by blunt or sharp external dissection. (3) Another problem is the attachment of the capsule to the pituitary stalk. It is excised with microscissors and the stalk is usually preserved. (4) A large CSF leak is frequently encountered after complete excision because excision of the diaphragm with the

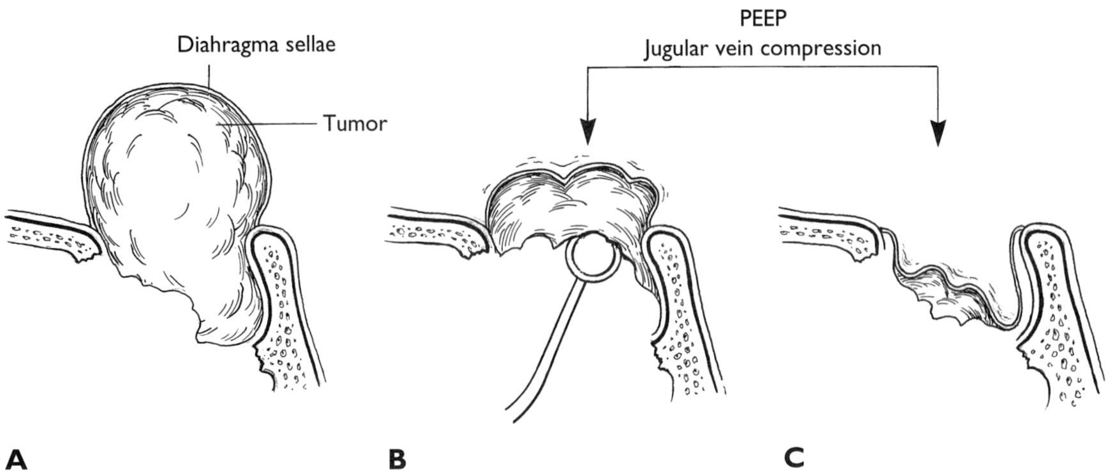

Figure 5-12. **(A–C)** Removal of a suprasellar tumor.

adherent capsule is sometimes required for radical removal. In other cases, the craniopharyngioma is only covered by an arachnoid layer. Careful closure of the CSF leak is essential.

Ectopic nasopharyngeal craniopharyngiomas are extremely rare.

Chordoma

Chordomas are locally invasive lesions arising from notochord remnants. Clival chordomas characteristically bulge the clival dura toward the brain stem. The pituitary fossa is often spared. Tumor consistency allows removal with curettes. Invaded bone is removed with the diamond drill. The dorsal border of resection is the clival dura. Extension of chordomas to the lower clivus may require a combined trans-sphenoidal and transoral approach. The clinically prevailing symptom of 6th nerve palsy is likely to regress after surgery. An exemplary case of a chordoma before and after removal is demonstrated in Figure 5-14. Chordomas are prone to recur. Re-operations are performed if patients present with new symptoms, and many patients

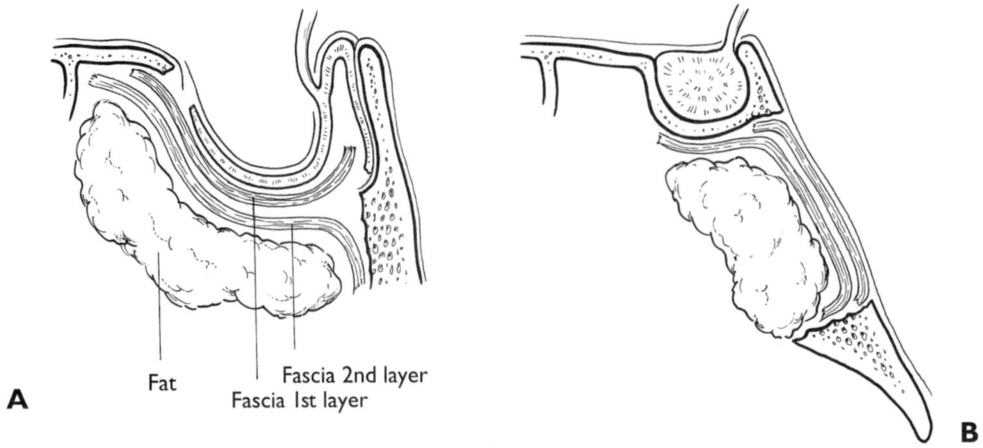

Figure 5-13. Closure of the surgical defect. The use of fat is optional. **(A)** Closure of the pituitary fossa. **(B)** Closure of a clivus defect.

Table 5-1. Trans-Sphenoidal Operations: Erlangen December 1982–June 1994

Pituitary adenomas		1,592
Acromegaly	424	
Prolactinomas	371	
Nonfunctioning adenomas	650	
Cushing's disease	242	
Nelson tumors	25	
TSH-omas	14	
Craniopharyngiomas		45
Rathke's cysts		9
Colloid cysts		9
Meningiomas		14
Malignomas		15
Chordomas		13
Chondromas		2
Inflammatory lesions		6
Epidermoid		3
Arachnoid cysts		3
Encephaloceles		3
Other lesions		4
Total		1,718

A

B

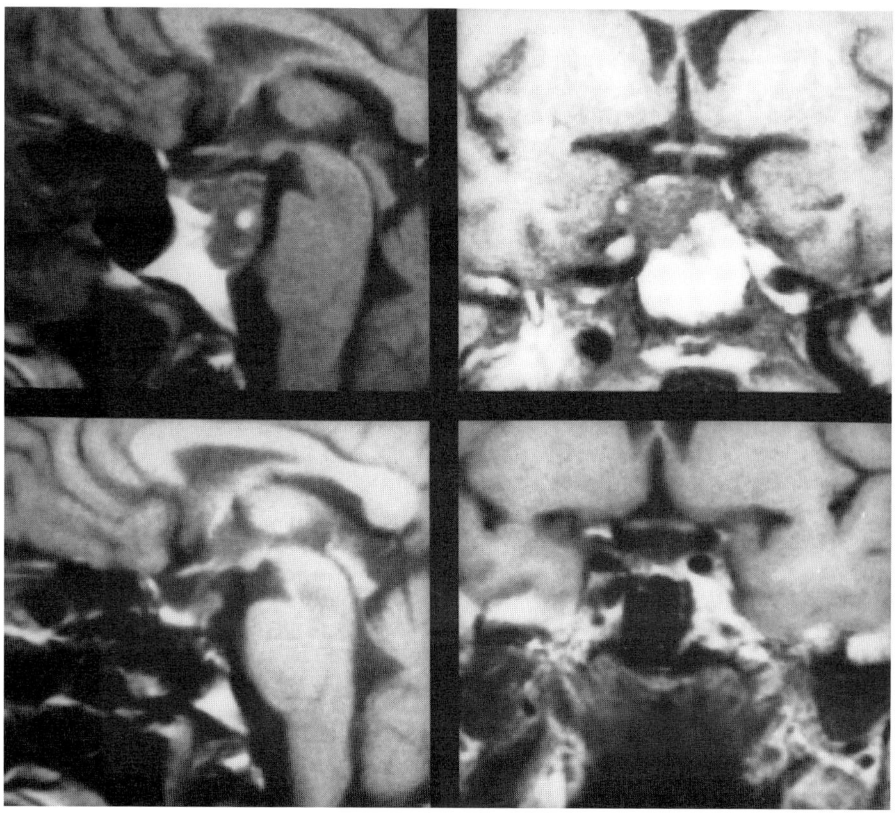

Figure 5-14. MRI of a chordoma. *(A)* Before surgery. *(B)* After trans-sphenoidal removal.

undergo several surgical procedures. Trans-sphenoidal procedures are restricted to chordomas in the midline with extradural location.

Meningioma

Cavernous sinus meningiomas frequently extend into the pituitary fossa and invade the sphenoid bone. If patients harboring such lesions present with incomplete oculomotor palsy or trigeminal pain, a trans-sphenoidal approach allows decompression of the cavernous sinus with relief of symptoms. A radical transcranial resection carries a high risk of an additional neurologic deficit. It is used in patients with severe cavernous sinus syndrome.

Preoperative MRI and angiography is mandatory to minimize the risk of vascular injury. The thickened floor of the fossa and the invaded sphenoid bone adjacent to the cavernous sinus are drilled away for bony decompression. Next, the basal dura is opened. The intrasellar and parasellar portion medial to the carotid artery is resected.

Malignancy

It is necessary to distinguish three types of malignancies:

1. Primary malignancies usually arising from the sphenoid sinus mucosa (e.g., adenocarcinoma).
2. Metastatic deposits with predilection for the pituitary gland.
3. Malignomas with secondary extension to the pituitary and clivus region (e.g., esthesioneuroblastomas).

Malignancies are characterized by destruction of the bony structures. In malignancy, a higher blood loss should be anticipated due to higher vascularity and invasion of vascular structures such as the cavernous sinus. In malignancies involving the clivus, penetration of the clivus dura is unusual, therefore allowing removal by the trans-sphenoidal route.

Complications

The risk of postoperative CSF liquorrhea requiring re-exploration and sealing of the leak is about 1 percent in large series of pituitary adenomas. The incidence of meningitis is approximately 0.5 percent. In more recent series, the risk of postoperative bleeding in the operative field is below 0.5 percent. Another infrequent complication is a transient optomotor nerve palsy. We have never observed a permanent deficit. Patients with normal preoperative vision are not at risk of a postoperative deficit. Deterioration of a pre-existing chiasmal syndrome is rarely observed. It can be caused by rebleeding, or by adherence of suprasellar tumor to the chiasm. It is important to avoid undue manipulation above the sellar entry.

Complications from the nasal approach such as sinusitis, mucocele formation, epistaxis, and septum hematoma are sometimes observed. A postoperative nasoseptal perforation is usually asymptomatic. However, permanent troublesome problems (e.g., septum deviation, saddle nose deformity, nasal synechia) are rare.

Only in large tumors, a certain risk of postoperative pituitary deficiency is observed. The risk of pituitary failure is much higher after transcranial procedures. Craniopharyngiomas are an exception. Due to their frequent origin at the pituitary stalk, a high risk of postoperative diabetes insipidus is also found after trans-sphenoidal removal.

Devastating injury to the carotid artery is an extremely rare complication.

Table 5-2. Complications of Trans-sphenoidal Surgery for Lesions Involving the Clivus

	Pituitary Adenomas (n = 71)	Other Lesions (n = 44)
Mortality	1	0
Rhinoliquorrhea	1	0
Meningitis	0	0
Epistaxis	1	0
Subarachnoid hemorrhage	1	0
Optomotor deficit		
Transitory	0	0
Permanent	0	0
Brain stem injury	0	1

In large series, the mortality rate of the trans-sphenoidal approach ranges from 0.3 to 1.4 percent.

Results

Between December 1982 and June 1994, 1,718 transsphenoidal operations were performed in our department (Table 5-1). The majority of operations (n = 1,592) were done in patients harboring pituitary adenomas.

In our department, the mortality rate of trans-sphenoidal surgery for pituitary adenomas has been 0.19 percent. Mortality increases with the size of the adenomas. No operative death occurred in other lesions. The clivus was involved in 115 lesions. The mortality in lesions involving the clivus was 0.9 percent (Table 5-2).

Suggested Readings

Buchfelder M, Fahlbusch R (1992) Risiken und Komplikationen bei Operationen von Prozessen im Sellabereich. Nervenheilkunde 11:105–111

Buchfelder M, Fahlbusch R, Huk WJ, Thierauf P (1987) Intrasphenoidal encephaloceles—a clinical entity. Acta Neurochir (Wien) 89:10–15

Fahlbusch R, Buchfelder M (1993) The transsphenoidal approach to invasive sellar and clival lesions. pp. 337–349. In Sekhar LN, Janecka IP (eds): Surgery of Cranial Base Tumors. Lippincott-Raven Press, Philadelphia

Hardy J (1969) Transsphenoidal microsurgery of the normal and pathological pituitary. Clin Neurosurg 16:185–217

Hardy J, Vezina JL (1976) Transsphenoidal neurosurgery of intracranial neoplasm. pp. 261–274. In Thompson RA, Green JR (eds): Advances in Neurology. Lippincott-Raven, Philadelphia

Honegger J, Buchfelder M, Fahlbusch R, et al (1992) Transsphenoidal microsurgery for craniopharyngioma. Surg Neurol 37:189–196

Honegger J, Fahlbusch R, Buchfelder M et al (1993) The role of transsphenoidal microsurgery in the management of sellar and parasellar meningioma. Surg Neur 39:18–24

Laws ER, Kern EB (1976) Complications of trans-sphenoidal surgery. Clin Neurosurg 23:401–416

6

Alternative Endonasal and Paranasal Approaches

Michael Torrens
Savvas Kazanas

The approaches described in this chapter all share the attribute that they transgress the nasal mucosa. This, from our experience of 25 years, has created no particular problem. If a submucosal or trans-septal route has advantages they are not particularly in the avoidance of infective complications. The historical evolution of some of these approaches, particularly those related to the pituitary, has been described by Welbourn (1986).

The approaches included below are:

- Endonasal trans-sphenoidal microscopic
- Endonasal endoscopic
    - Trans-sphenoidal
    - Other sinus surgery
- Paranasal
    - Transethmoidal
    - Lateral rhinotomy

Endonasal Trans-Sphenoidal Microscopic Approach

This represents a simple and rapid alternative to the trans-septal approach. As such it requires only a brief description.

Indications

Pituitary tumors confined to the fossa can be accessed but significant extensions may require a larger exposure. Clival and other lesions can easily be biopsied under direct vision but removal may require an extended approach. Cerebrospinal fluid (CSF) leaks known to be from the sphenoid can be closed, but those involving the ethmoid are better approached transethmoidally.

Contraindications include a very small nostril or grossly distorted internal anatomy such as may occur after trauma.

Positioning

The position described in Chapter 5 may be used but we prefer a less hyperextended approach. The patient is supine with the head slightly extended and rotated 15 degrees to the side of the surgical approach, usually the right for a right-handed surgeon. The surgeon stands or sits by the right shoulder. The use of an image intensifier is recommended as the detail of the intranasal anatomy is not as clear as with a central septal approach. The nasal cavity is packed with gauze soaked in a combined vasoconstrictor-antiseptic solution.

Instrumentation

It is necessary to use a pituitary speculum with narrow (13-mm) blades (e.g., Fehling NBN 6) in order to pass through the nostril. Otherwise the equipment is the same as for any trans-sphenoidal operation. Generally instruments of small size are preferable.

Surgical Technique

After removal of the intranasal pack the speculum is inserted through the nostril up to the anterior wall of the sphenoid. While still closed the tip of the speculum is deviated to the contralateral side to dislocate the back of the nasal septum. The blades are then opened. The skin of a small nostril may tear at the lateral corner but this is easily repaired with one stitch at the end of the procedure.

The operating microscope is introduced and the anterior wall of the sphenoid is opened. The remainder of the operation proceeds in a traditional way.

After packing of the sphenoid sinus (when necessary) the speculum is removed. The septum is straightened and kept in position by a nasal pack on the opposite side. The ipsilateral nasal cavity is then packed. The packs remain in place for at least 48 hours.

The advantages are the speed, simplicity, and the relatively little disturbance of nasal anatomy. The disadvantages are that the size of the access is reduced to about 60 percent of that created in a trans-septal approach and the direction of access is from one side, which may disorient the inexperienced surgeon. The complications are no different from other approaches.

Endonasal Endoscopic Approaches

For those wishing to pursue the goal of minimally invasive surgery the logical next step after the endonasal microscopic approach to the pituitary is to perform the same procedure endoscopically. This has recently been described (Torrens, 1995) but it is still in an early stage of development and cannot yet be recommended as a routine procedure. It is included for the sake of interest and in the hope that it will stimulate others. However, nasal endoscopy has already proven its usefulness in other situations.

Indications
Biopsy
Recurrent sinusitis
Orbital complications of acute sinusitis
Nasal polyps
Mucoceles
Dacrocystorhinostomy
Orbital decompression
Decompression of optic nerve
Repair of CSF leaks
Traumatic hemorrhage
Removal of foreign bodies
Laser ablation of epipharyngeal tumor
Intrasinus pathology
Vidian neurectomy
Pituitary tumors

Conditions that require en bloc removal are inappropriate for endoscopy, except as part of an assessment.

Positioning

The positioning is as described above. Additional space around the head is needed as an assistant will need to hold and move the endoscope. An image intensifier is useful for assisting orientation especially in the learning phase. The nose should be packed as described above.

Instrumentation

Pituitary operations
Rigid endoscopes, 2.5 and 4.0 mm diameter, 0 degrees and 2.5 mm 90 degrees (the sheath is unnecessary)
Camera and high-definition television (HDTV) monitor
Pituitary microinstruments
Long, insulated bipolar forceps
Landolt bipolar coagulator
Endoscopic bipolar electrode
Neodymium (Nd) YAG laser if available
Bayonet microchisel
Elongated small-caliber ultrasonic aspirator

(Continues)

Endoscopic sinus surgery
Rigid endoscopes 4.00 mm (0, 25, and 75 degrees) and 2.7 mm (25 degrees)
Cottle's elevator
Turbinate scissors
Blakesley-Weil forceps (straight, 45 and 90 degrees) thin and broad
Double-spoon angled forceps
Suction tubes, curved and straight
Bipolar forceps, angled and straight
Sinus punch forceps (upward, straight, retrograde)
Ostrom reverse cutting forceps
Bent spoon
Sickle knife

Pituitary Operations

If the septum of the sphenoid sinus is asymmetric, the side of the larger cavity should be chosen. A dual port approach (with the endoscope through one nostril and an instrument channel through the other) is feasible but has not been found to be an advantage. It is simple to pass the necessary instruments freehand alongside the endoscope on one side only (Figs. 6-1 and 6-2).

The nostril and atrium are opened with a simple Cottle nasal speculum. The 4-mm endoscope is inserted and the rostrum of the sphenoid identified. Unless the ostium of the sphenoid sinus is large it will be confined to the sphenoethmoidal recess. It may be possible to enlarge it but usually it is easier to open the anterior wall of the sinus with a microchisel and then enlarge the opening with Kerrison punches. The opening should be about 15 mm in diameter. The septum of the sphenoid sinus can be perforated with a chisel and removed with rongeurs as appropriate.

The image intensifier may be useful for defining the limits of the pituitary fossa, especially when it is small. The anterior wall of the fossa is opened with a

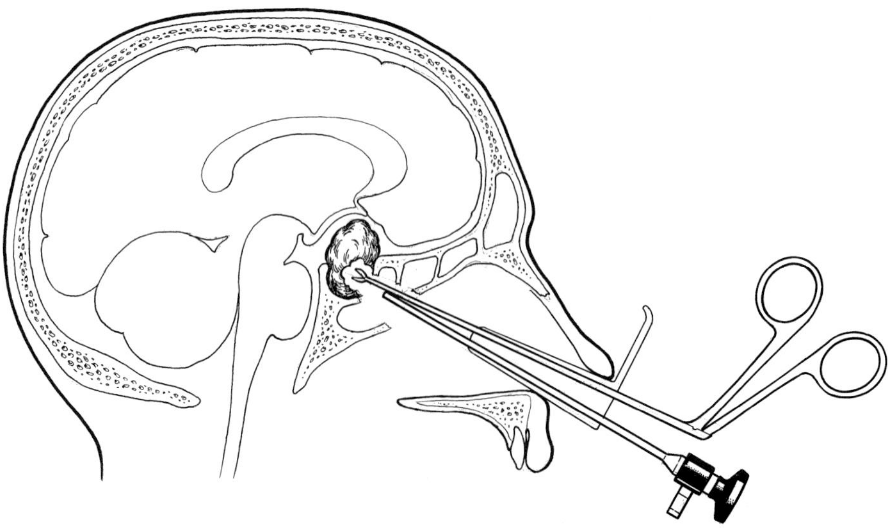

Figure 6-1. Edoscopic access to the pituitary.

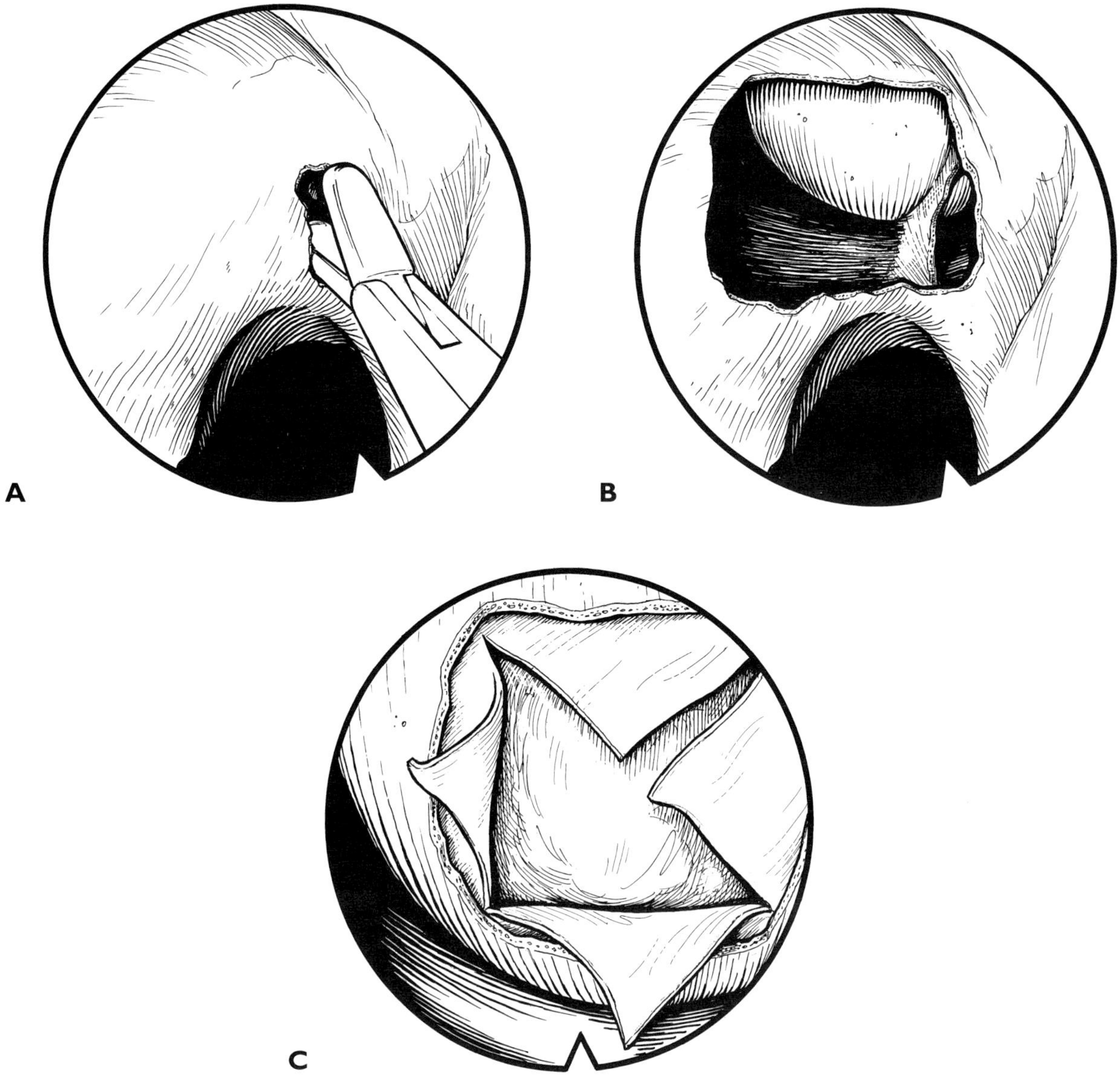

Figure 6-2. Endoscopic drawings of the trans-sphenoidal approach to the pituitary fossa. *(A)* Opening the anterior wall of the sphenoid sinus above the choana on the right side. *(B)* View into the sphenoid sinus showing an enlarged pituitary fossa. Part of the sphenoid sinus septum has been removed. *(C)* The anterior wall of the pituitary fossa has been opened and a cruciate incision made in the dura.

microchisel and micropunches (Hardy 1 mm, Codman). The dura of the pituitary fossa is best incised with the Nd YAG laser using a fiber with a conical tip. Bleeding from transverse sinuses within the dura can be controlled with the Landolt bipolar coagulator (Aesculap).

Removal of the pituitary tumor is technically the same as in a microscopic operation. It is important to keep the distal lens of the endoscope free from obscuration by blood, first by appropriate suction and second by withdrawing it a little if obscuration is imminent. Once the lens has blood on it, it must be completely removed for cleaning, which wastes time.

To visualize "around the corner" laterally or superiorly in the pituitary fossa it is useful to have a 2.5-mm, 90-degree endoscope. Pass this into position under the visual control of the 0-degree endoscope, fix its position, and then transfer the camera from one to the other. Orientation is a matter of experience and "in vitro" practice is useful.

The technique for closure is also the same as in the microscopic operation.

Endoscopic Sinus Surgery (Fig. 6-3)

Total Sphenoethmoidectomy and Related Procedures. Whether under local or general anesthesia the uncinate process, the anterolateral wall of the middle turbinate, and the bulla ethmoidalis are infiltrated with Xylocaine 2 percent—adrenaline 1/80,000 solution.

Using a curved sickle knife and a Blakesley-Weil forceps the uncinate process (see Fig. 2-7) is transected by an incision parallel to the lamina papyracea and resected. The infundibulum is now open. By gently pushing with a thin Blakesley-Weil forceps the medial part of the anterior wall of the bulla ethmoidalis is entered and the open-

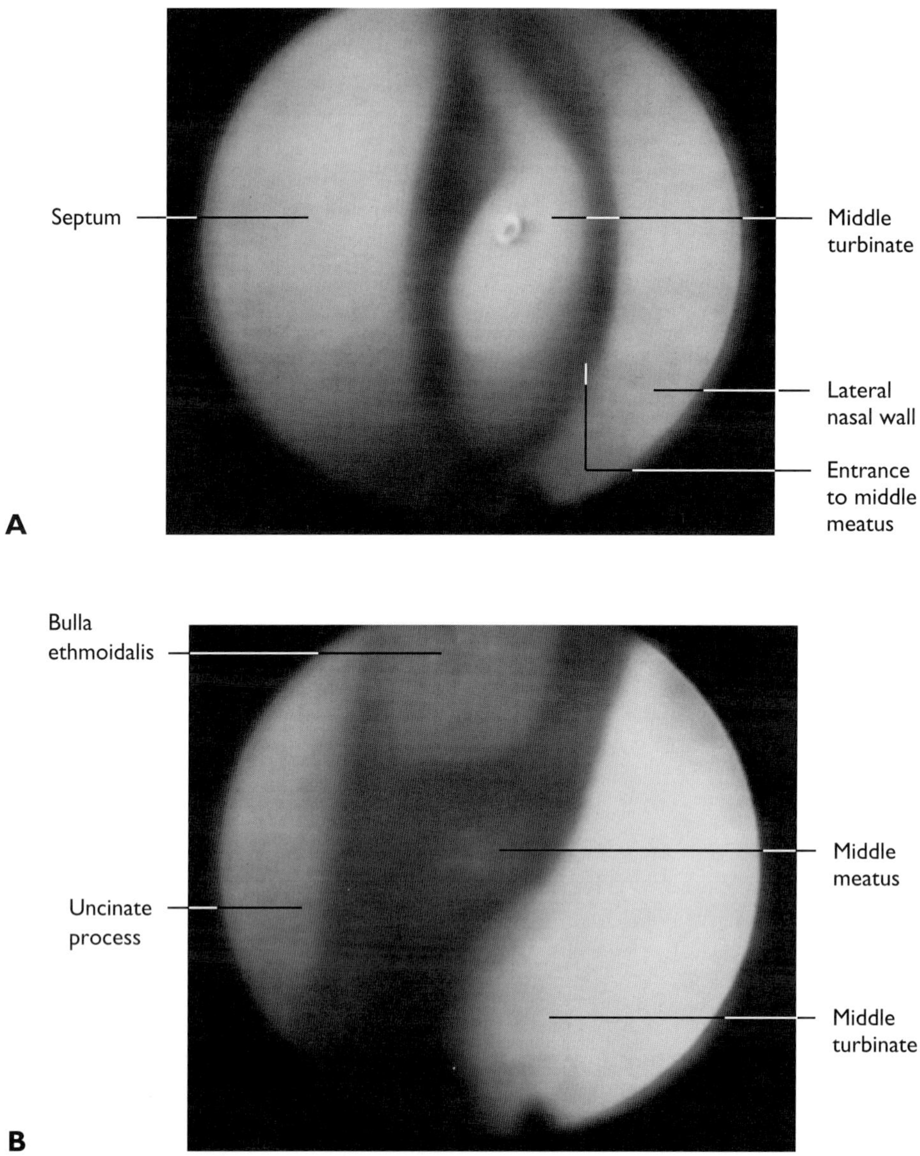

Figure 6-3. Photographs of nasal endoscopy. *(A)* Approaching the left middle meatus. *(B)* Inside the right middle meatus at the region of the infundibulum. *(Figure continues.)*

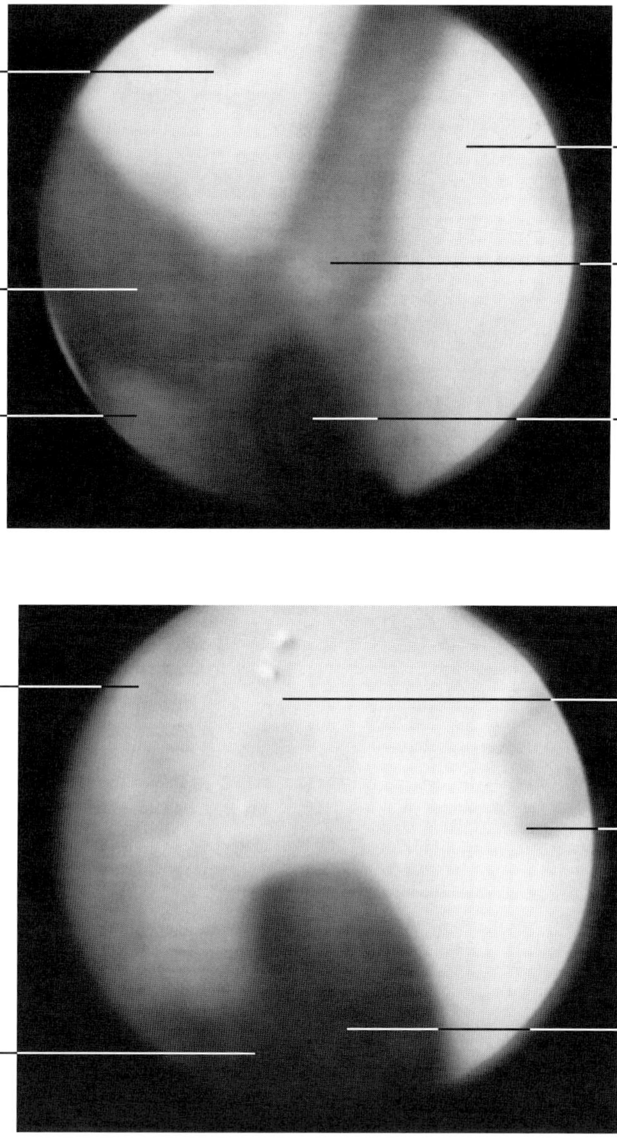

Figure 6-3 (Continued). (C) The posterior end of the right middle meatus. *(D)* The anterior wall of the right sphenoid sinus above the choana.

ing is enlarged until the ground or basal lamella can be identified. This is the wall of bone between the anterior and posterior ethmoidal cells and is the thickest structure that will be encountered.

At the junction between the anterior wall of the bulla ethmoidalis and the ethmoidal roof (just behind the frontal recess) the anterior ethmoidal artery usually runs in a thin, occasionally dehiscent, bony canal across the ethmoids. It is important not to interfere with this area if it is not necessary.

The thick ground lamella can be indented with the same instruments as the bulla, as far medially (to avoid any trauma to the optic nerve that may run adjacent to the posterior ethmoids) and inferiorly (to avoid inadvertent penetration of the skull base) as is possible. With exactly the same direction of excision (medial and inferior) the posterior ethmoids are resected, bearing in mind that the path through the posterior ethmoid does not lead to the anterior wall of the sphenoidal sinus in the region of its natural ostium, but farther superiorly and laterally. There are cases of pneumatization in which the cells of the posterior ethmoid extend lateral to the sphenoid and may even extend above it (Onodi cells; Stammberger, 1991).

The anterior wall of the sphenoid sinus is the posterior wall of the sphenoethmoidal recess and to identify this area an endoscope light in the nasal cavity or any curved instrument advanced into the sphenoethmoidal recess can be very useful for orientation. The sphenoid sinus is entered, again as far medially (to avoid the internal carotid artery and optic nerve) and inferiorly (below the skull base or pathology of the pituitary fossa) as is possible.

For opening the frontal recess the cranial extensions of the uncinate process and perhaps the junction between middle turbinate and lateral nasal wall, including the agger nasi, must be removed. The ostium of the frontal sinus is sometimes very difficult to identify, because there are various anatomic variations. In this area, more often than in any other, it is possible to cause a CSF leak if there is any force applied to the bony walls. The ostium of the frontal sinus must be able to drain easily and it is better to avoid it completely if possible because of the probability of causing adhesions and stenosis.

A middle meatal antrostomy is the enlargement of the normal ostium of the maxillary sinus. This opening can be performed by small curettes, the Ostrom reverse cutting forceps, or Blakesley-Weil forceps. The limits of a total opening are the lacrimal bone anteriorly, the root of the inferior meatus inferiorly, the perpendicular plate of the palatine bone posteriorly, and the horizontal level of the bulla ethmoidalis superiorly.

For all these procedures the use of a 0-degree endoscope is preferable in order to have the better orientation provided by a direct view. To open the frontal recess a 25-degree endoscope is better. Also very important is the study of CT scans preoperatively and their presence in the theater for use during the operation.

By this basic technique a number of procedures can be performed very precisely, with less damage, without external scar, and with less morbidity and fewer complications. Such complications are fewer in number and severity in experienced hands. They include orbital hematoma, loss of vision, nasolacrimal duct stenosis, CSF rhinorrhea, meningitis, pneumocephalus, mucocele, nasal synechiae, and wound infection (Vleming et al., 1992).

Endoscopic Management of CSF Leaks (Mattox and Kennedy, 1990). By endoscopy or, if not so visible, by intrathecal injection of fluorescein together with endoscopy, the precise site of the leak is identified. If there is a significantly large defect the surrounding dura is elevated. A graft such as temporalis muscle and fascia, abdominal fat, or lyophilized cartilage is inserted to support the intracranial side and fibrin glue or microfibrillar collagen used to secure the seal.

The sinus mucosa is carefully elevated from the surrounding bone for at least 5 mm in all directions. A free mucoperiosteal flap from the septum (contralateral side) is placed over the defect and its edges tucked under the mucosal edges around the defect. Fibrin glue or collagen is again used to hold the flap. Gelfoam is laid over this. Firm packing of the nose is performed and this is left in place for the next 5 to 7 days.

Endoscopic Transnasal Orbital Decompression (Kennedy et al., 1990). With the patient in the supine position under general anesthesia a total ethmoidectomy is performed as described above. The medial orbital wall and the skull base are skeletonized. The orbital apex and if possible the optic canal are identified posteriorly. The anterior ethmoid artery is identified and the frontal recess is opened. A full middle meatal antrostomy is performed. Its limits are the posterior margin of the nasolacrimal duct anteriorly, the root of the inferior turbinate inferiorly, and the posterior limit of the maxillary sinus posteriorly. The infraorbital nerve is identified within the sinus and defines the lateral limit for the removal of the orbital floor. After this, the medial orbital wall and the medial orbital floor are removed with an angled spoon, fine Blakesley forceps, and 70- or 110-degree Giraffe forceps under direct endoscopic control. These walls are removed to the orbital apex posteriorly, leaving a small rim of bone anterior to the optic nerve. Anteriorly, the medial orbital wall in the region of the frontal recess is preserved. After completing the resection of the bony orbital walls, the periorbitum is incised with a sickle knife in linear strokes from posterior to anterior in all the exposed area. This allows herniation of orbital fat into the opened sinuses. At the end of the operation a Mecorel sponge in a rubber finger cot is coated with antibiotic ointment and placed lateral to the middle turbinate. This sponge should be removed the next day.

This operation combined with a lateral orbitotomy gives excellent optical results and an external ethmoidectomy or Caldwell-Luc antrostomy is avoided.

The performance of a sphenoethmoidectomy with extension of the medial orbital decompression posteriorly to access and remove the medial wall of the optic foramen and canal provides an endoscopic optic nerve decompression in cases of traumatic optic neuropathy (Stammberger, 1994).

Paranasal Approaches

There are a large number of technical variations to this approach, which can extend from the brow-frontal sinus to the upper lip–maxillary sinus. It is similar to the face-splitting incision described in Chapter 9. Bilateral access without facial scarring can be obtained by the facial degloving approach (Ch. 7). The central facial minitranslocation described by Janecka (Ch. 8) provides similar but more extensive exposure, as do the Le Fort 1 maxillotomies described in Chapters 10 and 11.

Two variations of the paranasal route are described here, a simple transethmoidal approach and a more extended lateral rhinotomy. The extent of access as related to the anatomy of the lateral nasal wall is shown in Figure 6-4.

Transethmoidal Operations

Indications
Optic nerve decompression
Medial orbital lesions posterior to globe
Medial orbital decompression
Pituitary and upper clival tumors
Unilateral frontoethmoidal pathology
Sphenoethmoidal or frontal CSF leaks

Surgical Technique. The transethmoidal approach (Fig. 6-5) also known as external frontoethmoidectomy or Lynch's operation (Lynch, 1921) has a number of variations and extensions. The basic technique to be described here involves an approach via the lamina papyracea of the medial orbital wall.

A "C"-shaped incision 3 cm long is made centered 8- to 10-mm medial to the internal canthus (Fig. 6-5A). This is continued down to and through the periosteum.

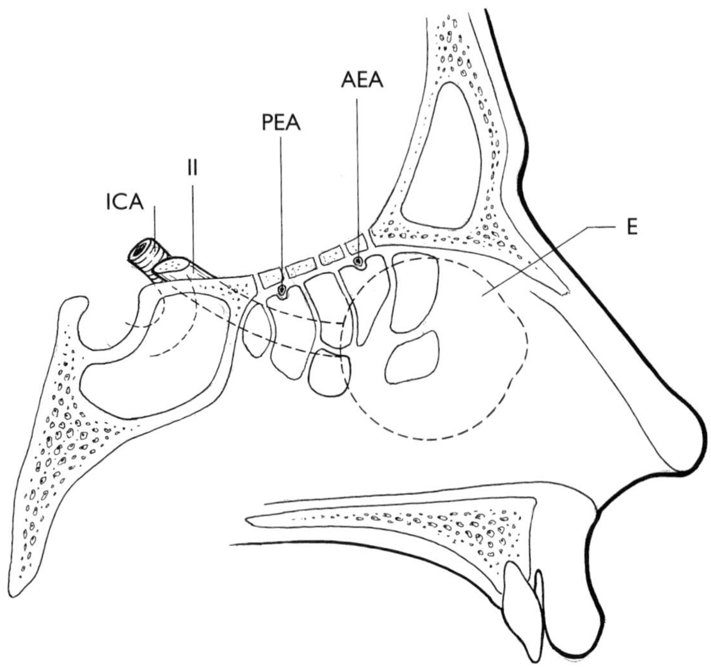

A

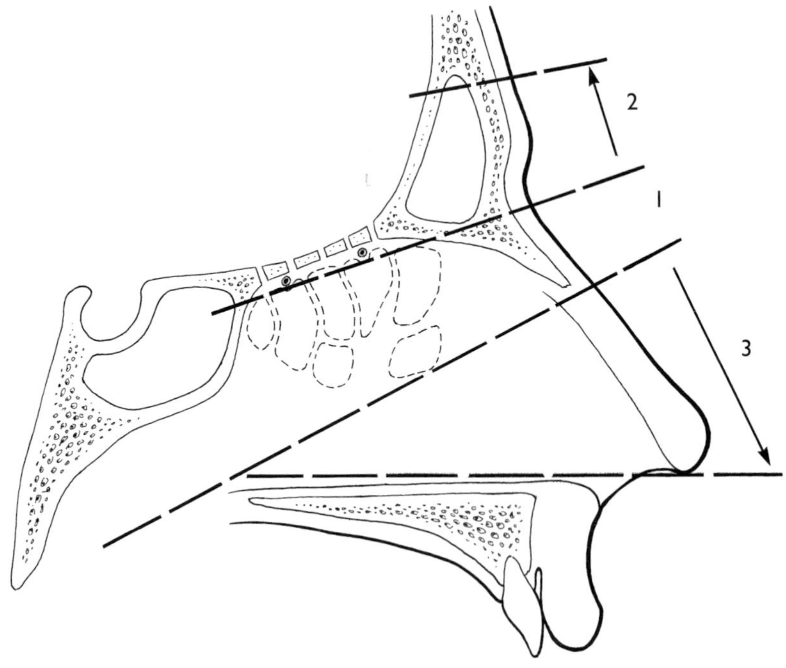

B

Figure 6-4. Anatomy of the lateral wall of the nasal cavity in relation to surgical access by ethmoidectomy. *(A)* The location of the ethmoidal sinuses, optic nerve, and carotid and ethmoidal arteries. *(B)* 1, Access by the route through the lamina papyracea. 2, Extension upward allows access to the frontal sinus and anterocentral base. 3, Extension downward allows more space for instrumental access and better visualization upward but does not improve the extent of exposure downward to the clivus. (For explanations of abbreviations, see Appendix 1, p. 373.)

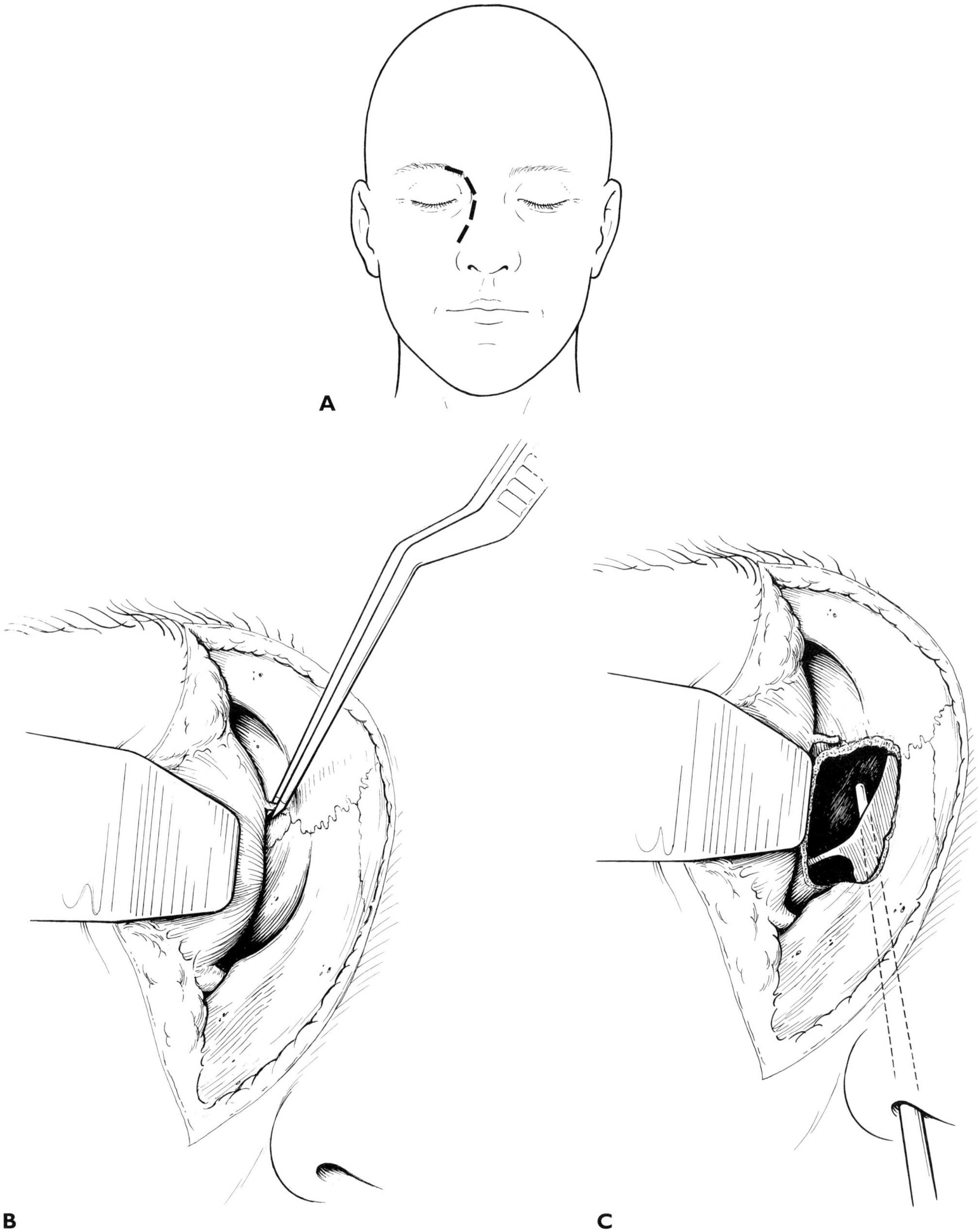

Figure 6-5. The transethmoidal approach via the lamina papyracea. *(A)* Incision 1-cm medial to the medial edge of the orbit. *(B)* Subperiosteal dissection exposing the medial orbital wall. The contents of the nasolacrimal fossa are protected. The anterior ethmoidal artery is coagulated with bipolar forceps. *(C)* The medial wall of the orbit has been excised. The ethmoid cells are removed with rongeurs keeping below the level of the anterior ethmoidal artery. An instrument passed through the nose helps to identify the sphenoethmoidal recess. *(Figure continues.)*

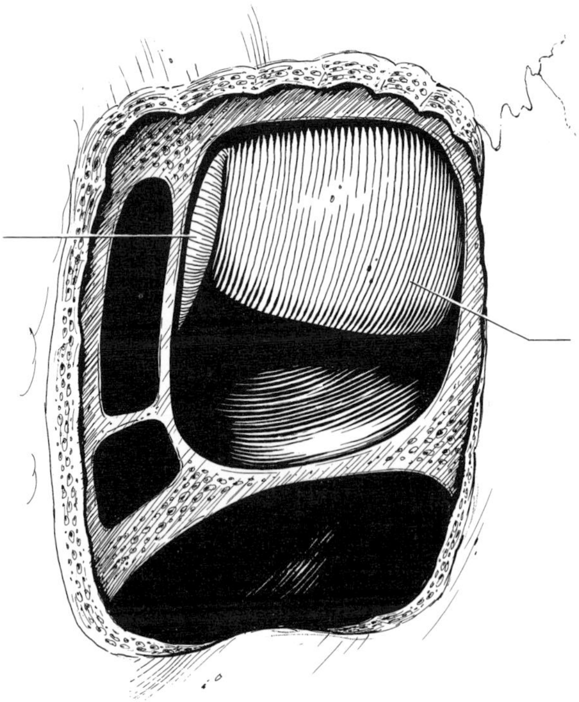

D

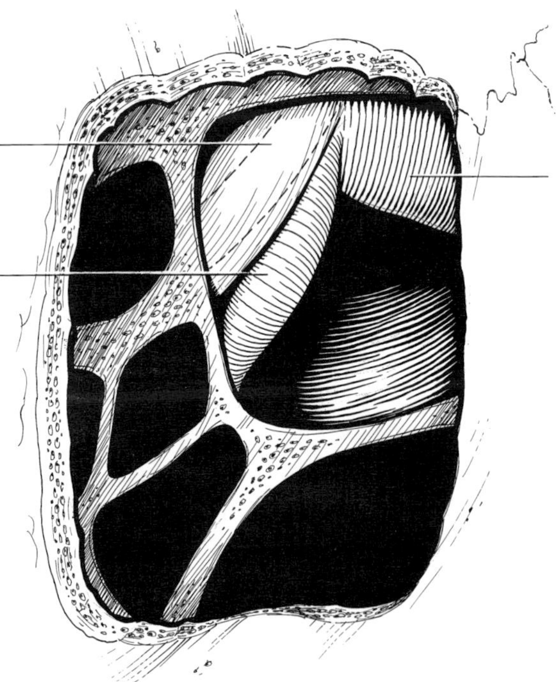

E

Figure 6-5 (Continued). (D) Opening of the right side of the sphenoidal sinus reveals an enlarged pituitary fossa. A prominent area over the carotid artery may or may not be present. Direction of the microscope toward the left will allow the removal of the sphenoid septum and full opening of the left side of the sinus. The view to the left is usually better than the view to the right. *(E)* In a case requiring optic nerve decompression, the microscope has been directed to the right and the medial wall of the orbit removed back to the apex. The prominence of the optic nerve is seen in the lateral wall of the sphenoid sinus. This is unroofed with a diamond drill and followed forward to the orbital foramen.

Hemostasis of small arteries is performed with bipolar diathermy. Subperiosteal dissection laterally is continued into the orbit to expose the whole medial wall. The structures in the lacrimal fossa are lifted out without damaging the lacrimal duct. One foot of the attachment of the medial canthus should be preserved to avoid later telecanthus. Otherwise the periosteum seems to reattach without problems.

A retractor is inserted to retain the periorbitum without undue pressure. The anterior ethmoidal artery should be identified and coagulated but not cut (Fig. 6-5B). This is a marker of the level of the cribriform plate (see Ch. 2). If the subsequent ethmoidectomy is kept below this level there is less chance of damage to the cribriform area with consequent CSF leak.

The thin bone of the lamina papyracea is removed, anteriorly until it beomes too thick to cut easily with a punch and posteriorly as far as necessary for the particular procedure. If appropriate, a small flap of bone is taken from the medial orbital wall to use in later reconstruction. The posterior ethmoidal artery will require diathermy and section in approaches to the optic nerve.

The ethmoidal cells are removed with rongeurs until the sphenoethmoidal recess is reached (Fig. 6-5C). It is helpful to have an instrument that has been passed intranasally to identify when the nasal cavity (sphenoethmoidal recess) has been reached. The sphenoid sinus is then opened with a microchisel and punches. This is easier than searching for the ostium. With such a lateral approach it is essential to know, from MRI and CT scans, the anatomy of the posterior ethmoidal and sphenoid area in relation to the carotid artery and optic nerve.

Once the sphenoid sinus has been opened (Fig. 6-5D & E), any operation on the pituitary proceeds as described earlier. The advantage of the approach is a significantly shorter route of access and consequent ease of instrument manipulation. The disadvantage is the facial scar. Some surgeons also consider that the higher angle of approach is a disadvantage because it reduces the view upward into the pituitary fossa. In fact the difference in view angle is relatively small and is irrelevant if endoscopy is employed to "look around the corner" upward.

Extradural tumors involving the clivus can often be managed by this approach. Even larger lesions of the upper and middle third can be excised with only modest inferior and medial extensions to the approach (Samii, 1995). A view to the contralateral petrous apex area is obtained and the contralateral posteromedial orbit can also be explored.

Much of the ipsilateral medial orbital wall is removed in this approach. For orbital decompression or access to the posteromedial orbit the bone removal must be more extensive.

To decompress the optic nerve (Joseph et al., 1990; Levin et al., 1994) the lamina papyracea is removed as described above. A microdrill with a small cutting burr is employed to thin the medial wall of the optic foramen continuing posteriorly along the optic canal in the medial wall of the sphenoid sinus. A small curette or elevator is then used to break the thin shell of bone away from the nerve. Alternatively the nerve may be identified in the lateral wall of the sphenoid sinus (Fig. 6-5E) and followed forward. Joseph et al. (1990) discuss the fact that the results of extracranial, transethmoidal decompression are better than those after decompression by craniotomy and consider that this may be due to the concomitant orbital decompression. Levin et al. (1994) obtained improvement of vision in 71 percent of 31 cases operated within 6 days. In a larger series of 70 operated eyes, Fujitani et al. (1986) obtained a success rate of 48 percent but emphasized that this success can be achieved as late as 3 weeks after injury.

In cases with more extensive frontobasal trauma Raveh et al. (1988) recommend a one-stage repair and craniofacial reconstruction by a modified transethmoidal route.

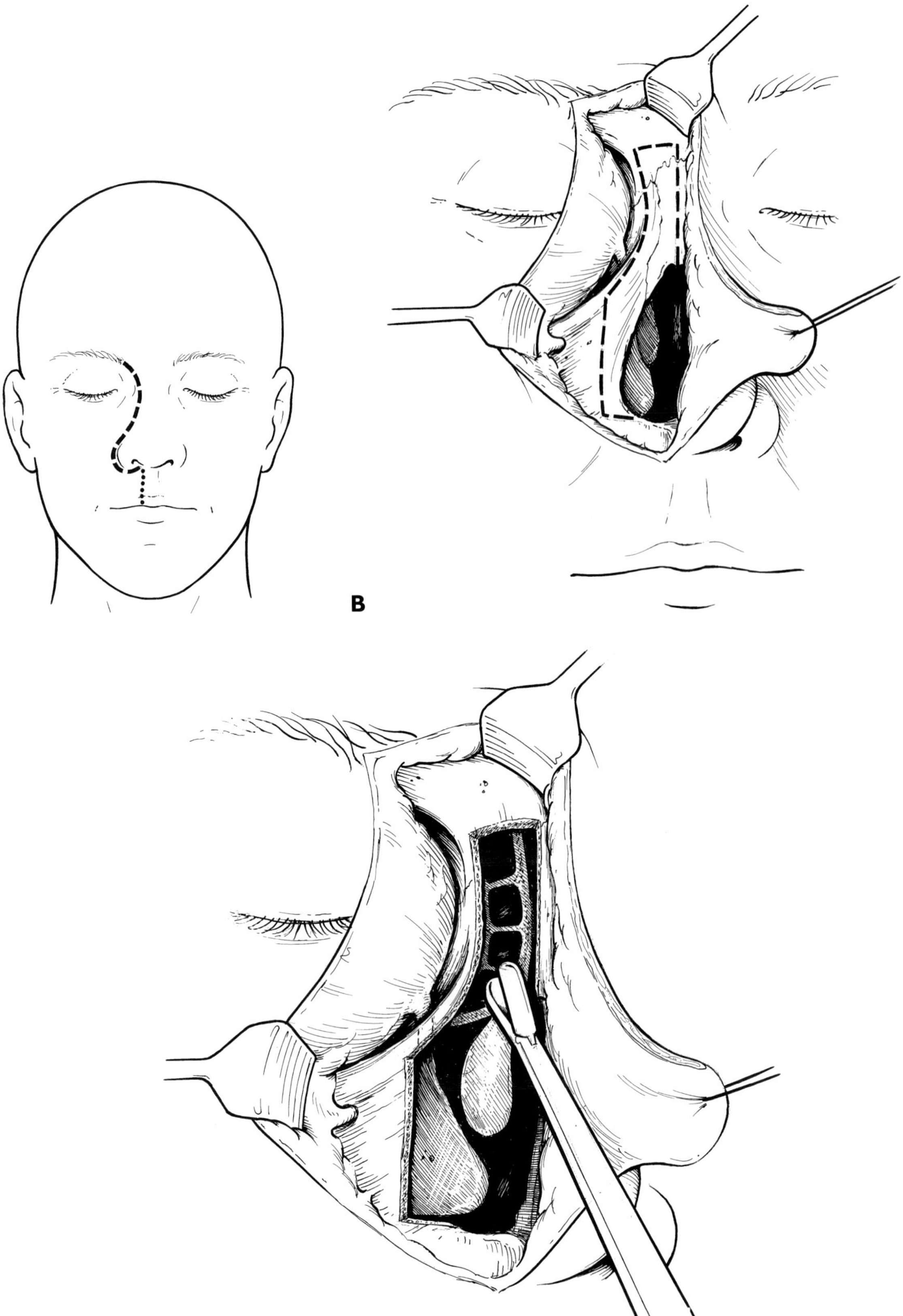
A

B

C

Figure 6-6. The lateral rhinotomy approach. *(A)* The paranasal incision can be extended downward through the upper lip (dashed line) to allow a more extensive transmaxillary approach. *(B)* The nostril with its cartilages is retracted medially and subperiosteal dissection proceeds to the nasion, medial orbit, and infraorbital foramen. The broken line indicates the extent of the osteotomy. *(C)* Following osteotomy the ethmoid cells are removed. The lateral wall of the nasal cavity including the middle turbinate may be preserved if desired, being retracted medially or laterally as required. The nasolacrimal duct (dashed line) is protected. *(Figure continues.)*

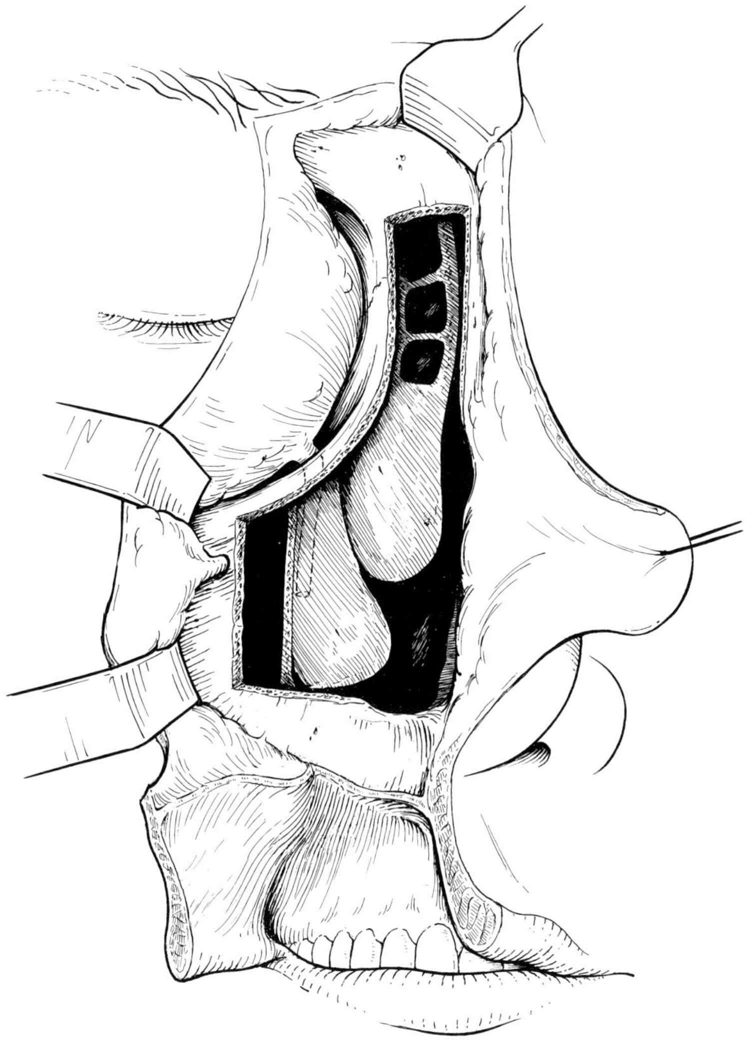

D

Figure 6-6 (Continued). (D) An extended transethmoidomaxillary approach. The middle turbinate can be removed. The inferior turbinate can be retracted laterally, thus preserving the nasolacrimal duct (dashed line). Further extension of the approach can be made upward by including the nasolacrimal fossa in the osteotomy and removing the lamina papyracea as in Figure 6-5. In such cases a reconstruction of the nasolacrimal duct will be required.

By this means transfrontal craniotomy is avoided. They report 395 procedures with a low rate of complications.

Modifications of the approach include frontonasal osteotomy, allowing access to the frontal sinus, and performance of the ethmoidectomy without violating the medial orbital wall, as illustrated in Figure 6-6.

Lateral Rhinotomy (Moure, 1922; Mertz et al., 1983; Lund, 1992)

Indications. Indications for lateral rhinotomy include procedures as discussed above requiring a lower or more extended approach, or both.

Surgical Technique. The surgical technique (Fig. 6-6) is as follows. Under general anesthesia and with the patient in reverse Trendelenburg position, local anesthetic (Xylocaine 1 percent–adrenaline) is injected in the incisional area. Tarsorrhaphy may be performed to protect the eye.

A paralateronasal incision is performed, from the medial extremity of the eyebrow, around the medial canthus, down the nasomaxillary groove, and, after following the ala round, finishing at the base of the columella (Fig. 6-6A). When necessary this can be extended down through the lip, greatly increasing the potential access.

The skin and periosteum are elevated together. Medially the exposure extends over the nasal bone and frontonasal process. Laterally exposed, from below upward, are the canine fossa, the infraorbital foramen, and the lacrimal sac (displaced laterally). The medial canthal ligament is detached from the lacrimal crests and the orbital periosteum freed from the medial orbital wall (lamina papyracea). The anterior ethmoidal vessels are cauterized and divided. Superiorly, the elevation ends after exposing the frontonasal suture and a portion of frontal bone.

After careful hemostasis a section of the bone can be removed by three osteotomies (Fig. 6-6B) performed with a microdrill or, preferably, its saw attachment. A vertical osteotomy is made from the lateral pyriform fossa up to the orbital rim continuing just medial to the lacrimal fossa and orbit up to the root of the nose. A second osteotomy (parallel to the first) separates the two nasal bones and a third horizontal osteotomy unites the upper parts of the first two. This plate of bone is removed by elevating it with a chisel. Later it must be replaced and fixed by wire sutures passed through holes in the nasal bones or low-profile microplates.

The ethmoidectomy (Fig. 6-6C) is as extensive as required. The middle turbinate and thus the lateral nasal wall may be preserved and retracted medially or laterally as required. Alternatively, a complete clearance with removal or contralateral dislocation of the nasal septum may be performed.

The performance of a medial maxillectomy (Fig. 6-6D), after extending the incision through the lip, greatly increases the width of the exposure. Combined with clearance of the pterygopalatine fossa and drilling of the pterygoid plates, this can produce an excellent exposure of the clivus and petrous apex region without the need for mobilization of the maxilla. Preservation of the inferior turbinate protects the nasolacrimal duct.

Variations of the exposure have been described that preserve the vascular supply to the osteotomized bone fragment. The bone may be left attached to the lateral skin flap by avoiding the subperiosteal elevation over the nasal bone and medial orbital wall. The medial orbit is then osteotomized with a chisel from below and the nasal bone opened like a door on the lateral periosteal hinge. Swearingen et al. (1995) describe a bilateral osteotomy of the nasal bones with the rotation of a nasal pedicle to the contralateral side. Removal of the septum, middle turbinate, and, if necessary, a medial maxillectomy provides a wider exposure of the clivus.

References

Fujitani T, Inoue K, Takahashi T (1986) Indirect traumatic optic neuropathy—visual outcome of operative and nonoperative cases. Jpn J Ophthalmol 30:125–134

Joseph MP, Lessell S, Rizzo J, Momose KJ (1990) Extracranial optic nerve decompression for traumatic optic neuropathy. Arch Ophthalmol 108:1091–1093

Kennedy DW, Goodstein ML, Miller NR, Zinreich SJ (1990) Endoscopic transnasal orbital decompression. Arch Otolaryngol Head Neck Surg 116:275–282

Levin LA, Joseph MP, Rizzo JF, Lessell S (1994) Optic canal decompression in indirect optic nerve trauma. Ophthalmology 101:566–569

Lund VJ (1992) Lateral Rhinotomy in Operative Surgery, Head and Neck. Part 2. Butterworth-Heinemann, London

Lynch RC (1921) The technique of a radical frontal sinus operation which has given me the best results. Laryngoscope 31:1–5

Mattox DE, Kennedy DW (1990) Endoscopic management of cerebrospinal fluid leaks and cephalocoeles. Laryngoscope 100:857–862
Mertz JS, Pearson BW, Kern EB (1983) Lateral rhinotomy: indications, technique and review of 226 patients. Arch Otolaryngol 109:235–239
Moure EJ (1922) Techniques chirurgicales oto-rhino-laryngologiques. Libraire Oc Douin, Paris
Raveh J, Vuillemin T, Sutter F (1988) Subcranial management of 395 combined frontobasal-midface fractures. Arch Otolaryngol Head Neck Surg 114:1114–1122
Samii M (1995) Editorial comment in Swearingen B, Joseph M, Cheyney M, Osemann RG (1995) A modified transfacial approach to the clivus. Neurosurgery 36:101–105
Stammberger H (1991) Functional Endoscopic Sinus Surgery. Marcel Decker, Philadelphia
Stammberger H (1994) Endoscopic Optic Canal Decompression. Seventh Panhellenic ENT Congress, Heraklion, Crete
Swearingen B, Joseph M, Cheyney M, Ojemann RG (1995) A modified transfacial approach to the clivus. Neurosurgery 36:101–105
Torrens MJ (1995) Endoscopic neurosurgery. Neurosurg Q 5:18–33
Vleming M, Middelweerd RJ, de Vries N (1992) Complications of endoscopic sinus surgery. Arch Otolaryngol Head Neck Surg 118:617–623
Welbourn RB (1986) The evolution of transsphenoidal pituitary microsurgery. Surgery 100:1185–1190

7

Transfacial Approach to the Skull Base with the Degloving Procedure

Kazuhiko Kyoshima
Kiyoshi Matsuo

The approaches to the central skull base may be broadly classified into anterior and lateral routes. There are some specific indications for an anterior approach. Its principal advantage is that the major vessels and cranial nerves are not encountered early during the approach.

Various techniques of facial degloving procedure have been described and successfully used. (Casson et al., 1974; Koch and Price, 1990; Mattox, 1989; Price, 1986; Uttley et al., 1989). This chapter describes a transfacial approach that is combined with the midface degloving procedure, and with nasomaxillary and Le Fort 1 osteotomies.

Surgical Technique

The operation is carried out under general anesthesia with orotracheal intubation. Preoperative tracheotomy is usually not necessary. With the patient in a supine position, the head is fixed (in a skull fixation system) with chin-up tilt of about 15 degrees. The surgeon may work from the lateral or frontal side.

Midface Degloving Procedure

The medial palpebral ligament is first dissected and wired after making a small skin incision near the medial angle of the eye on each side. These wires are connected to each other under the nasal skin at the end of surgery.

Bilateral circumferential mucosal incisions are made in the nares (Fig. 7-1A). These are started with a transfixion incision in the membranous septum between the cartilaginous septum and the medial crura of the lower lateral cartilages (Fig. 7-1B).

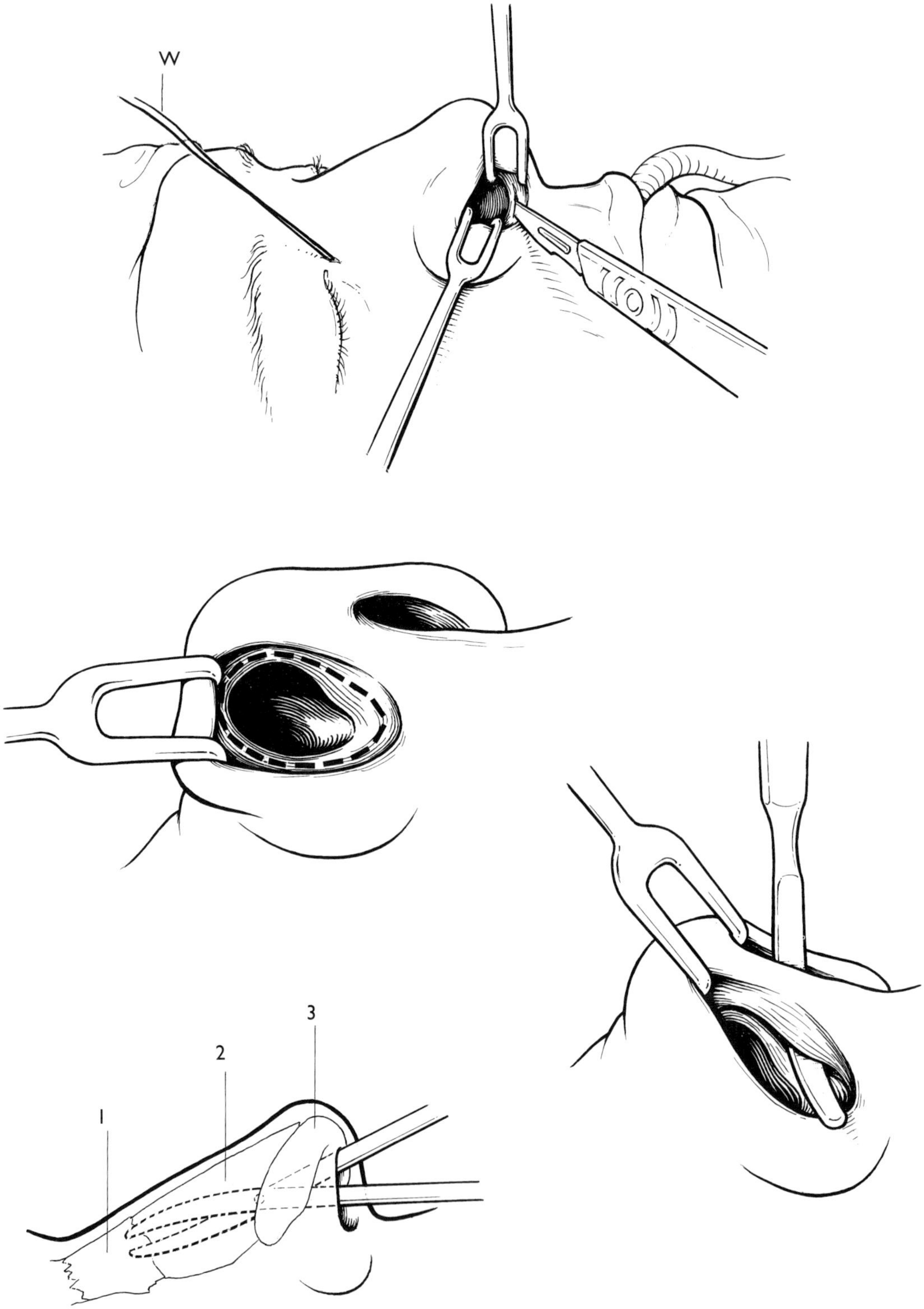

A

B

C

Figure 7-1. Midface degloving procedure. *(A)* Intranasal incision. Circumferential mucosal incisions are made in the nares. *(B)* Transfixion incision. A transfixion incision is connected bilaterally with intercartilaginous, pyriform, and nasal floor incisions. *(C)* Intercartilaginous incision. The soft tissues of the nasal dorsum are separated from the upper lateral cartilage and nasal bone through an intercartilaginous incision in the subperiosteal plane. 1, nasal bone; 2, upper lateral cartilage; 3, lower lateral cartilage (lateral crus); W, wiring of medial palpebral ligament.

This incision is continued across the floor of the nose at the margin of the pyriform aperture. The upper end of the transfixion incision is carried across the dome of the nose between the upper lateral cartilages and the lower lateral cartilages (intercartilaginous incision). This incision is then extended laterally and inferiorly to reach the incision in the floor of the nose. The soft tissues of the nasal dorsum are separated from the upper lateral cartilages and nasal bones through the intercartilaginous incisions bilaterally in a subperiosteal plane (Fig. 7-1C). All fibrous attachments between the septum and the skin of the nasal tip area are divided. Thus, the nasal tip including its lower lateral cartilage skeleton is separated. Extension of the incision circumferentially within the nasal vestibule at the skin–mucosal junction completes the release of the nasal soft tissue at the pyriform aperture. The soft tissues of the nasal dorsum are widely elevated in the subperiosteal plane.

A sublabial incision is made 4 to 5 mm above the labiogingival sulcus. The incision extends much more laterally than the conventional incision for trans-sphenoidal surgery. It may extend up to or beyond the first molar on both sides (Fig. 7-2). The skin and soft tissue of the face (superior to the upper lip) is then dissected in the subperiosteal plane, sparing each infraorbital nerve. Facial soft tissues including lip, cheeks, nasal tip and alae, columella, and nasal skin are then reflected superiorly (Fig. 7-3). The elevation is wide and can be as high as the infraorbital rim and the glabella.

Osteotomies of Facial Bone

Nasomaxillary Osteotomy. A nasomaxillary osteotomy is first done as shown in Figure 7-4 after marking the site of the projected Le Fort 1 osteotomy. An osteotomy is made in the maxillary bone medial to the inferior orbital foramen. The mucosa under the nasal bone is separated from it and an osteotomy of the nasal bone is per-

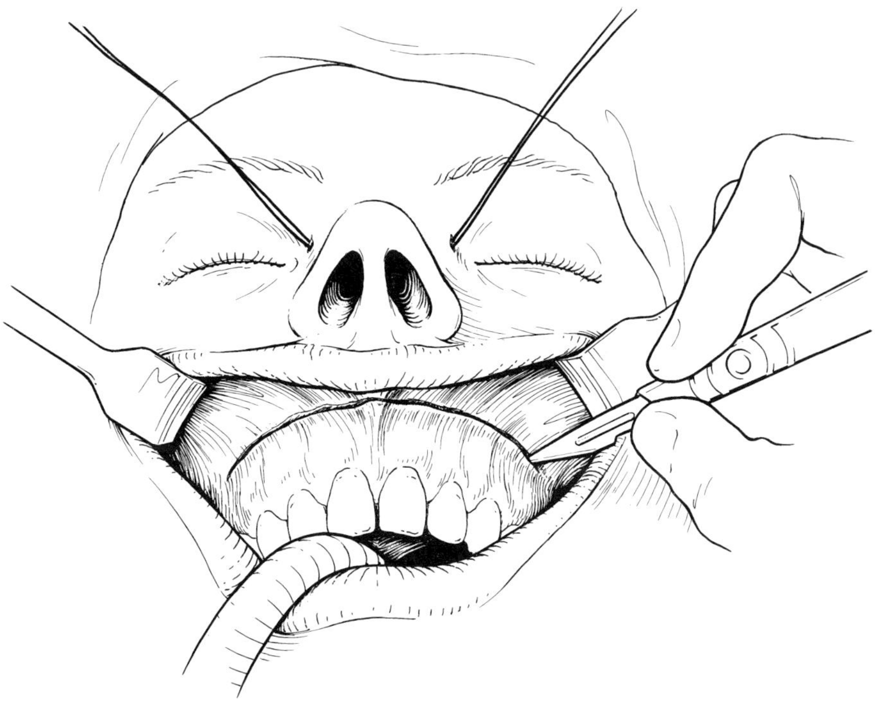

Figure 7-2. Sublabial incision. The incision extends to the first molar tooth on each side. Labial mucosa remains on the gingival side to facilitate closure.

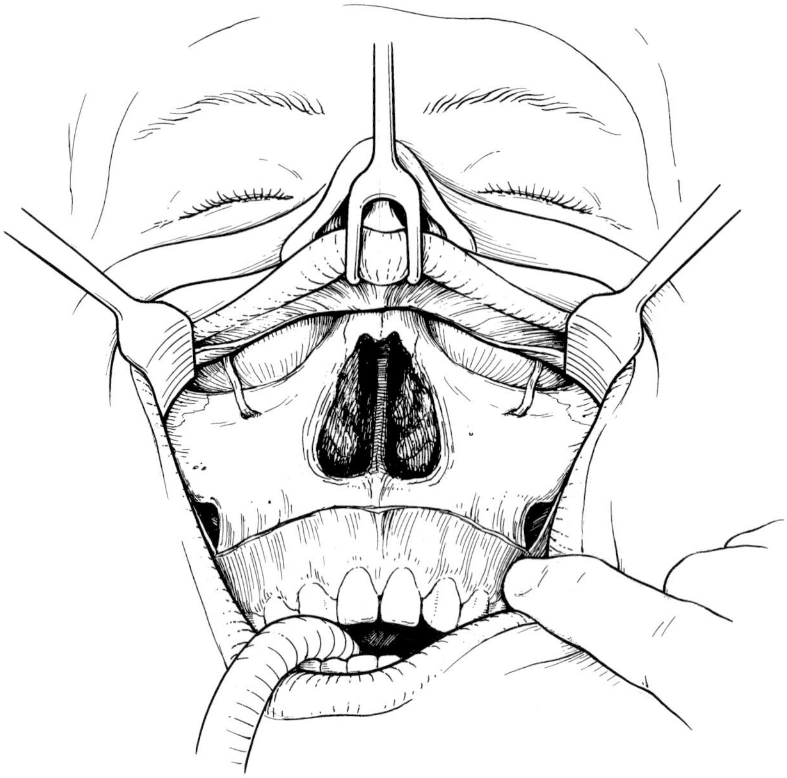

Figure 7-3. Elevation of midfacial soft tissues. The midfacial soft tissues are reflected. The infraorbital nerves, orbital rims, and glabella are seen.

formed near the frontonasal suture transversely, while taking care to preserve the nasolacrimal duct on both sides. The nasomaxillary bone fragment is then removed.

Le Fort 1 Osteotomy with Pediculated Cartilaginous Septum. Le Fort 1 osteotomy with the cartilaginous septum is carried out with a power-driven bone saw, chisels, and hammer.

The nasal cavity is opened by dissecting the attachment of the nasal septum at the nasal dorsum. The nasal septum is cut in full thickness with scissors between the cartilaginous septum and the perpendicular plate of the ethmoidal bone (Fig. 7-5), and the cartilaginous septum is freed from the vomer (Fig. 7-6). A sagittal mucosal incision is made in the lateral wall of the pyriform aperture near the lateral margin of the nasal floor preserving the greater palatine artery on both sides. After horizontal osteotomy of maxilla, the lateral wall of the pyriform aperture is cut from anterior to posterior along the sagittal mucosal incision. Thus, the cartilaginous septum with mucosa continuing onto the maxilla is obtained.

The maxillary segment is separated from the pterygoid plates with a curved chisel. The maxilla, with pediculated cartilaginous septum attached, can then be down-fractured to gain mobility and full posterior exposure (Fig. 7-7). Turbinectomy of the inferior and middle nasal conchae provides more lateral exposure.

Access to Central Skull Base

The mucosa of the bony septum is divided on each side. Access to the central skull base is obtained by removal of the bony septum and by retracting the mucosa laterally. The pediculated cartilaginous septum is also retracted laterally during proce-

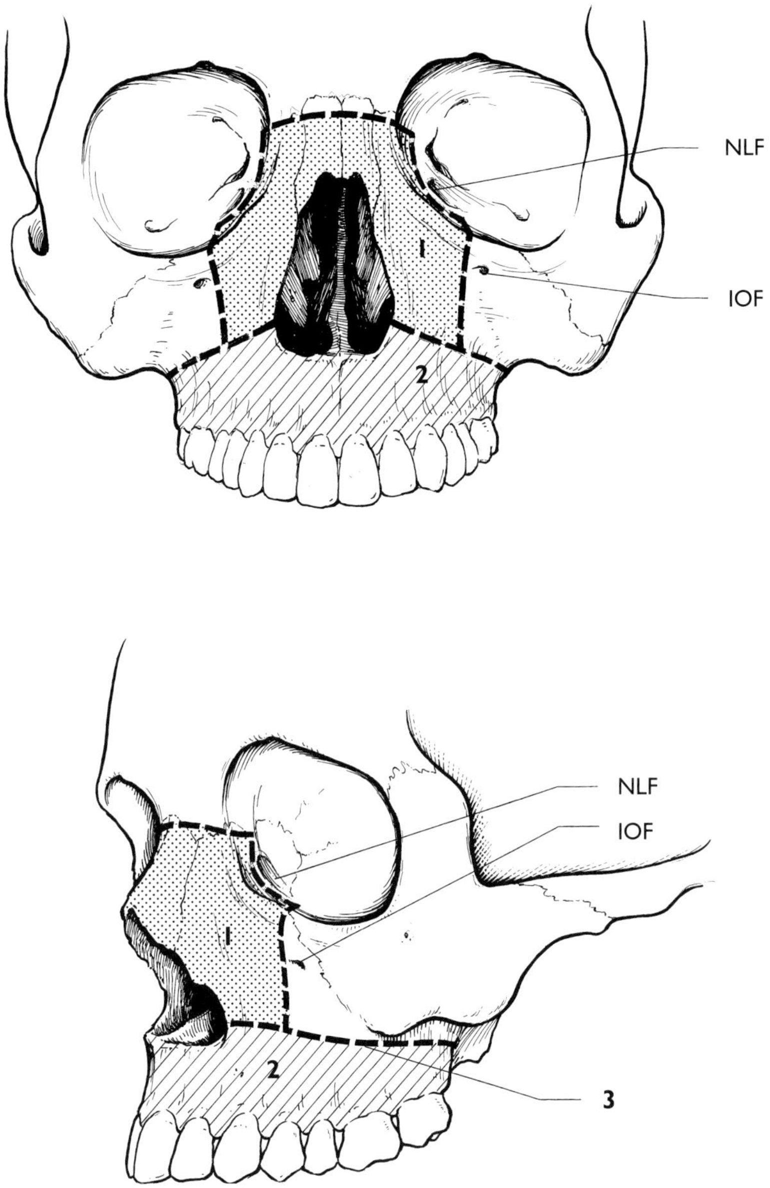

Figure 7-4. Osteotomies of facial bone. 1, nasomaxillary osteotomy; 2, Le Fort 1 osteotomy; 3, horizontal osteotomy of maxilla; IOF, infraorbital foramen; NLF, nasolacrimal fossa.

dures. The nasomaxillary osteotomy provides access to the lower clivus and upper cervical spine under the mucosa of the posterior pharyngeal wall. The downward displacement of the maxilla provides a wider exposure of posterior aspect of the upper nasopharynx and central skull base area and a good view laterally. An exposure by a selective trans-sphenoidal approach is limited by the lateral wall of the pyriform aperture. Thus, by the combination of the nasomaxillary and Le Fort 1 osteotomies, the central skull base is accessible from the frontal base to the C2 level of the cervical spine. The lower clivus and cervical portion are exposed by dissection under the pharyngeal mucosa (Fig. 7-8).

Reconstruction and Wound Closure

The dead space after removal of the tumor and clival bone is filled with autogenous material such as abdominal fat and fascia lata strengthened by fibrin glue. The

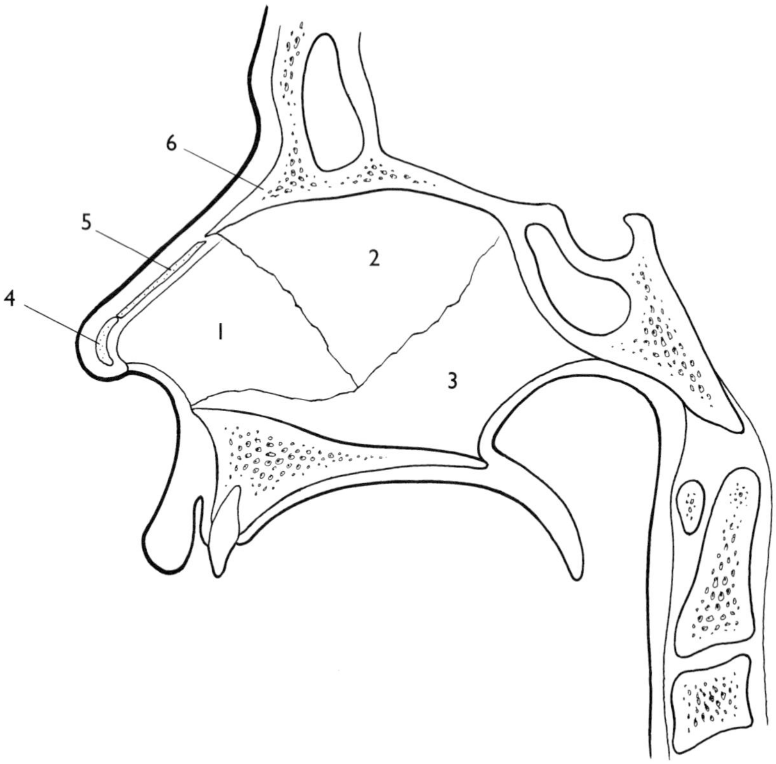

Figure 7-5. Midfacial sagittal section. 1, cartilaginous septum; 2, perpendicular plate of ethmoidal bone; 3, vomer; 4, lower lateral cartilage; 5, upper lateral cartilage; 6, nasal bone.

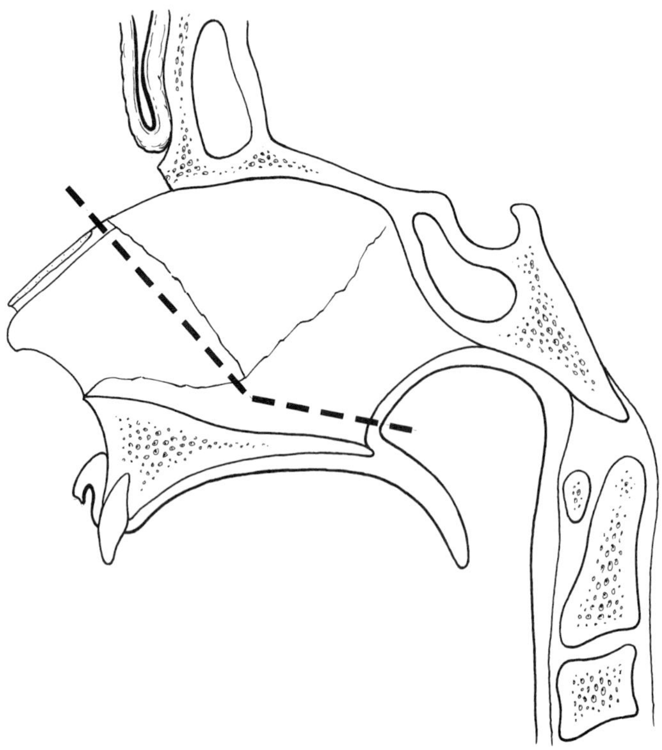

Figure 7-6. Dissection of the nasal septum. The cartilaginous septum is cut and freed from the bony septum in full thickness (dashed line). The septal mucosa of the choanae is also dissected. The nasal bone is removed and nasal skin including lower lateral cartilages is reflected superiorly.

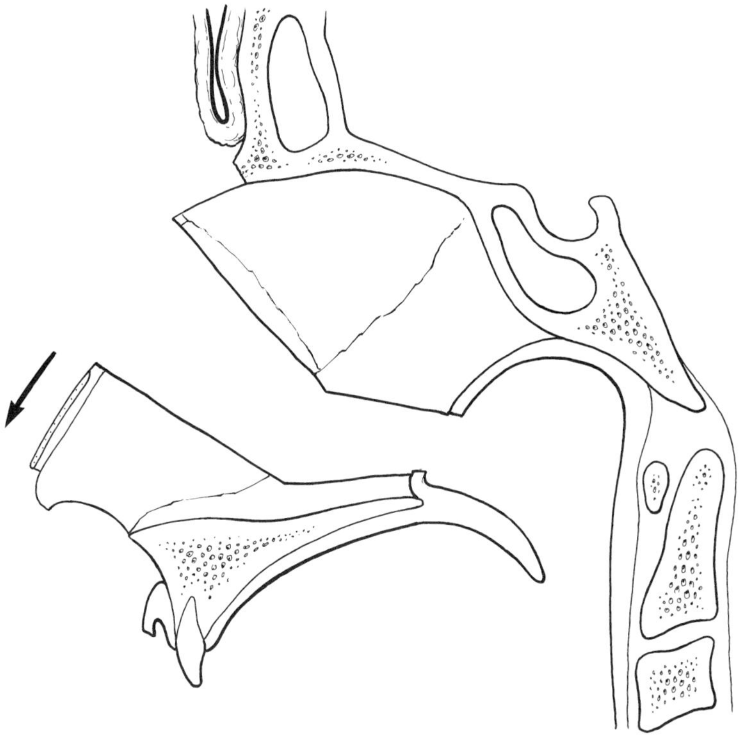

Figure 7-7. Down-fracture of maxilla with pediculated cartilaginous septum.

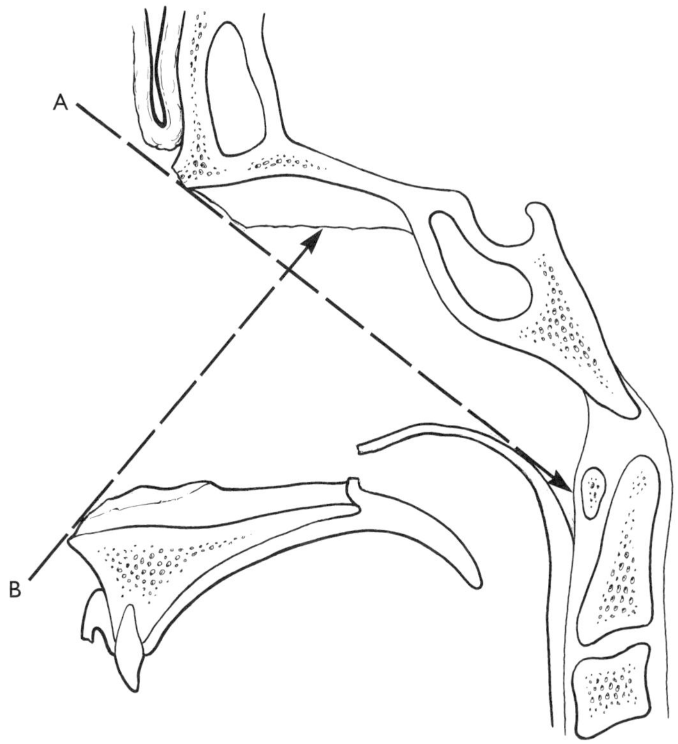

Figure 7-8. Access to central skull base by transfacial degloving approach. Arrow A shows access to lower clivus and upper cervical spine under the mucosa and muscle of the pharyngeal wall. Arrow B shows access to the frontal base. The cartilaginous septum is retracted laterally.

mucosa of the bony septum is closed without tension and complete separation from the nasal cavity is obtained. There remains a defect of the bony septum (Fig. 7-9). The facial bone is stabilized with miniplates. The cavity is packed with antibiotic-soaked petroleum gauze that is brought out through the nares. The upper lateral cartilages and the cartilaginous septum are sutured reconstructing the nasal dorsum. Sublabial and intranasal incisions are finally closed.

Limitation and Extension of the Operative Field

The procedure may not provide a sufficient lateral exposure because it is limited by the pterygoid plates. In combination with other approaches a wider exposure can be obtained.

The transmaxillary approach is easily combined with this technique, for tumors of the posterior sphenoid and clivus that have lateral extensions.

Additional transverse incisions of the mucosa at the choanae also provide a more lateral exposure, and a longitudinal incision of the pharyngeal mucosa downward, including the septal mucosa of the choanae, gains a more inferior exposure. In such a situation the mucosa of the bony septum may be used for closure of the pharyngeal mucosa in cases where there is a defect in it.

If a tumor extends intradurally, opening the dura facilitates its exposure. A bifrontal craniotomy and frontobasal interhemispheric approach can also be combined with this approach wherever necessary.

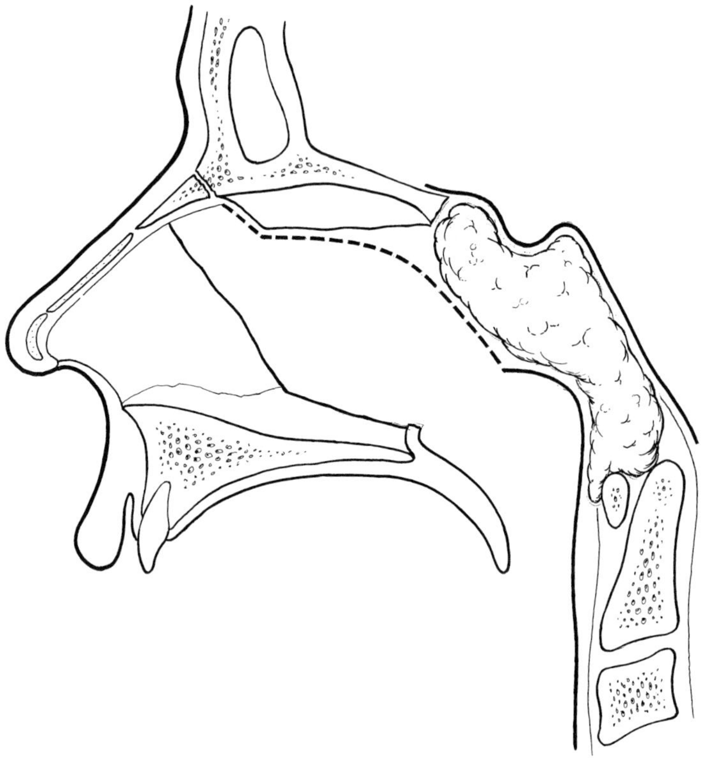

Figure 7-9. Closure of posterior nasopharynx. The mucosa of the bony septum is closed (dashed line) after filling the dead space with fat. The resulting defect of the bony nasal septum is seen. The cartilaginous septum is preserved.

The pterygoid plates are the main obstructing factor in expanding the lateral exposure in the depth. Drilling of the pterygoid plate provides a more wider operative field to the lateral side. The pterygoid plate can be fractured outward or drilled off.

Advantages

The procedures are technically relatively simple. This technique does not involve any external incisions over the face and hence the cosmetic result is excellent. There are no significant problems related to malocclusion. In our experience the postoperative discomfort is slight and settles quickly. Maintaining a vascularized mucosa fed by the greater palatine arteries limits the postoperative resorption of the cartilaginous septum and thus deformity of nasal dorsum.

Nasomaxillary osteotomy provides access to the lower clivus and upper cervical region, and Le Fort 1 osteotomy with down-fracture affords a direct line of vision to the clivus and the mucosa of the posterior pharyngeal wall. Thus, the combined technique provides sufficient access from the frontal base down to approximately C2 and also wide working space especially longitudinally. It allows good access to epidural lesions located in the midline, between the carotid arteries, with a minimal risk of damage to neurovascular structures. The risk of wound breakdown and infection is also small.

The exposure obtained is larger than that obtained by the combination of trans-oral and trans-sphenoidal approaches and can be expanded in superior, lateral, and inferior directions by combining other approaches.

References

Casson PR, Bananno PC, Converse JM (1974) The midface degloving procedure. Plast Reconstr Surg 63:102–103

Koch WM, Price JC (1990) Midface degloving approach to tumors involving the skull base. pp. 302–305. In Wilkins RH, Rengachary SS (eds.): Neurosurgery Update I. Diagnosis, Operative Technique, and Neuro-Oncology. McGraw-Hill, New York

Mattox D (1989) Midfacial degloving for exposure of the clivus. pp. 371–376. In Long DM (ed): Atlas of Operative Neurosurgical Technique. Vol 1. Cranial Operations. Williams & Wilkins, Baltimore

Price JC (1986) The midfacial degloving approach to the central skull-base. Ear Nose Throat J 65:174–180

Uttley D, Moore A, Archer DJ (1989) Surgical management of midline skull-base tumors: a new approach. J Neurosurg 71:705–710

8

Facial Translocation Approach to the Skull Base

Ivo P. Janecka

Surgical approaches to the skull base are designed to permit the operative manipulation of cranial base anatomy and pathology. Detailed knowledge of normal anatomy as well as developmental variations permit the distinction of pathologic processes during surgery, which is one of the principles of surgical oncology. A number of objectives must be reached in order to fulfill the goal of surgical therapy: control of a neoplastic process or repair of congenital/traumatic deformity.

The intimate relationship of the skull base to the cranial as well as facial structures requires tissue displacement of one or both of these compartments to reach the desired section of the skull base. It is important to consider the effects of surgery on the normal but surgically manipulated tissues in order to select the most optimal approach. Any operative tissue displacement produces alterations in the anatomy and physiology of affected structures. Such changes have variable consequences depending on whether they occur in the neurocranium or the facial viscerocranium. For example, facial swelling is usually self-limiting with minimal long-term consequences for the patient. Similar edema, however, may be very deleterious when it involves the neurocranium.

The current underlying principle of skull base approaches is to minimize brain retraction while maximizing skull base visualization. This concept facilitates three-dimensional tumor resection, tumor margin verification, and functional reconstruction with appropriate aesthetic concerns.

In general, surgical treatment of lesions located anterior to the neuraxis should be done through an anterior approach. This requires selection of a transfacial approach because of the anteroinferior anatomic relationship of the facial viscerocranium to the cranial base.

This chapter is adapted with permission from Janecka (1993) and Janecka (1996).

The advantages of transfacial approaches include the following:

1. Facial anatomy has developed through the embryonic fusion of nasofrontal, maxillary, and mandibular processes. Normally, the fusion takes place in the midline or in the paramedian region, thus logically presenting optimal lines of "separation" of facial units for a surgical approach, permitting the least traumatic displacement.
2. The primary blood supply to the "facial units" is through the external carotid system, which also has a lateral-to-medial direction of flow, thus ensuring viability of displaced surgical units.
3. The midface contains multiple "hollow" anatomic spaces (oronasal cavity, nasopharynx, paranasal sinuses), which facilitate the relative ease of surgical access to the central skull base.
4. Displacement of facial units for an approach to the central cranial base offers much greater tolerance to postoperative surgical swelling, as opposed to similar displacement of the contents of the neurocranium.
5. Re-establishment of the normal anatomy, following repositioning of the facial units during the reconstructive phase of surgery, has a high degree of functional as well as aesthetic achievement.

However, transfacial approaches also have certain disadvantages, such as:

1. Contamination of the surgical wound with oropharyngeal bacterial flora.
2. The need for facial incisions with subsequent scar development.
3. Emotional considerations for the patient related to "surgical facial disassembly."
4. The potential need for supplementary airway management (postoperative endotracheal intubation, temporary tracheostomy).

In the past, several surgeons worked on achieving additional exposure of the craniofacial region for oncologic reasons, including Barbosa (1961) for lateral exposure of the maxilla and Altemir (1986) for the nasomaxillary area.

Patient Selection

To be considered for transfacial surgery, the patient must have a pathologic entity located at the anterolateral cranial base or the craniovertebral junction, judged to be best treated with surgery. This would include benign and malignant tumors as well as congenital and post-traumatic deformities.

Also necessary is adequate imaging to define the extent of the pathologic process as well as to show the key neighboring anatomic structures and the potential for their preservation. This may include computed tomography (CT), magnetic resonance imaging (MRI) (static and dynamic), and four-vessel angiography. Numerous questions need to be answered by the imaging studies: the true extent of the lesion, its relationship to the key anatomic structures (e.g., vessels, dura, brain stem, cranial nerves), and the potential expendability of such structures during surgical resection.

A patient would not be considered for this type of surgery if the lesion (e.g., lymphoma, most metastatic lesions) is best treated by nonsurgical modalities, or if there is an active infection in the oronasopharynx.

The timing of surgery is guided by the nature of the pathologic process and the urgency for its treatment, as well as the patient's overall medical status. In general, malignant processes are treated expeditiously. Benign tumors and congenital deformities are treated electively.

A preoperative biopsy for tissue diagnosis will differentiate the neoplasms into surgical and nonsurgical categories. Those patients with malignant tumors for which transfacial surgery is not recommended are usually offered radiotherapy, chemotherapy, or both. External beam radiotherapy may be supplemented with brachytherapy. Some benign lesions may be followed with scans to assess their growth potential, if the surgical treatment has a high likelihood of worsening the patient's deficit.

Transfacial approaches create potential risks to the function and aesthetics of the following structures: skin, dentition, maxillofacial skeleton, mucosal lining of the upper airway, paranasal sinuses, eustachian tubes, superior pharyngeal constrictor muscles, soft and hard palate, and tongue. From the neurovascular point of view, the locations of the upper cervical and petrous segments of the internal carotid arteries as well as cranial nerves V_3 (especially the lingual nerve), XII, and V_2 (and the vidian nerve) must be recognized. Furthermore, the vertebral arteries are at potential risk, especially in congenital anomalies of the craniovertebral junction with an associated asymmetry. If they are exposed during surgery, these vessels should be covered with vascularized tissue to prevent the likelihood of subsequent vessel rupture.

The potential postoperative risks are related to the quality of wound healing, involving the dura as well as the wall of the oropharynx. Cerebrospinal fluid (CSF) leakage and breakdown of the wound closure are highly undesirable and require intensive treatment.

Preoperative Planning

All patients are given a broad-spectrum antibiotic (a third-generation cephalosporin such as Rocephin), which is started within 1 hour prior to surgery and continued for approximately 48 hours postoperatively or until the spinal drain is removed. Most patients are not given an anticonvulsant except when a basal subfrontal approach is added to the procedure. Preoperative oral irrigation with a clindamycin solution may be used to reduce microbial flora.

Surgical Technique

Anesthetic Technique

Anesthesia is usually induced with pentobarbital and maintained with enflurane. Oral endotracheal intubation is usually satisfactory (a contoured Rey tube is preferred). In rare cases, preliminary tracheostomy is performed. Neurophysiologic monitoring includes monitoring of cranial nerve XII (by tongue electromyography) as well as monitoring of brain stem evoked potentials. All patients have arterial as well as central venous pressure lines. Elective hypotension is not used. All patients have a precordial stethoscope to alert the anesthesiology team to venous air embolism. When dural transgression is anticipated, a spinal drain is inserted.

Patient Positioning

Most patients are positioned supine on the operating table with the head resting in a headrest. Occasionally, rigid head fixation is used. An alternative position is a right lateral position (for right-handed surgeons) for a limited midline lesion that is approached transorally. The advantage of this position is gravity-dependent drainage away from the immediate surgical field.

Draping

Complete preparation of the face and neck is performed with Betadine, and the oropharynx is irrigated with diluted Betadine solution. This area is then draped. In addition, the lateral thigh is prepared and draped as a fascia lata donor site.

Operative Technique

Modular craniofacial disassembly is the principle of the facial translocation approach to the skull base (Fig. 8-1). It is based on creation of composite facial units that are designed along key neurovascular anatomy and aesthetic lines. The individual units merge into larger composites without compromising their function. It is possible to attach eponyms to the technical variations of facial translocation for ease of communication and comparison. Thus, we can recognize "mini," "standard," "expanded" (vertically, medially, posteriorly), "bilateral," etc. facial translocation procedures. Complementary craniotomies or craniectomies are added to these approaches as necessary to assist with three-dimensional tumor resection.

Mini facial translocation—central is designed to reach the medial orbit, sphenoid and ethmoid sinus, and inferior clivus. The port of entry is through the displaced ipsilateral nasal bone and the nasal process of the maxilla (with an attached medial canthal ligament, the lacrimal duct, and skin). The skin incision is made along the lateral aspect of the nose and the inferior aspect of the eyebrow with triangular design at the level of the medial canthal ligament. Osteotomies create a rectangular pattern with the lateral extent being just medial to the infraorbital nerve. Rigid fixation is accomplished with microplating (Fig. 8-2).

Mini facial translocation—lateral opens the infratemporal fossa. The incisions run from the inner canthus horizontally to the preauricular area and then vertically in front of the ear. The head of the mandible is either displaced or resected following a temporary removal of zygomatic arch and malar eminence (Fig. 8-3).

Standard facial translocation achieves surgical access to anterolateral skull base. It was originally described by Janecka et al. (1990). The ipsilateral facial skin (including the lower eyelid) is displaced laterally and inferiorly with the underlying maxilla (with or without the hard palate). The nasal incision may extend inferiorly to include an upper lip split. Superior incision continues from the nose to the inferior fornix of the lower eyelid, through the lateral canthus horizontally to the preauricu-

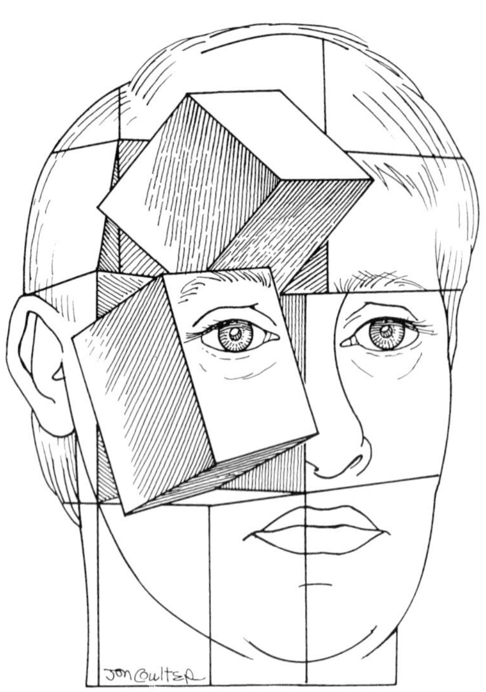

Figure 8-1. Modular craniofacial disassembly.

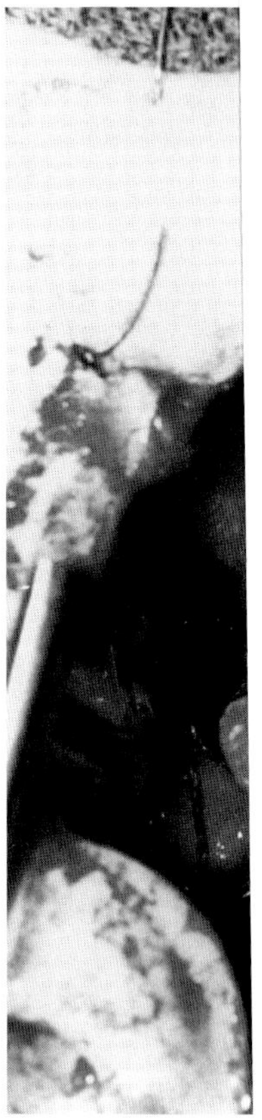
E

Figure 8-2 (Continued). (E)
(F) Replacement of compos

lar area. In some cases (more anterior tumors) it is possible to conclude this incision about 1.5 cm beyond the lateral canthus after identifying and preserving the most anterior frontal branch of the facial nerve. This point then serves as the point of rotation of displaced tissue, which gives sufficient surgical space for access to some paracentral tumors. When the entire extent of the horizontal temple incision is needed, the frontal branches of the facial nerve are identified with a nerve stimulator, placed in silicone tubings, and transected. During reconstruction these transected tubings are reconnected and the continuity of the facial nerve branches is re-established. Osteotomies correlate to Le Fort 1 and 2 or the midpalatal lines when the entire maxilla is being displaced. The infra-orbital nerve is electively sectioned along the floor of the orbit, tagged, and repaired at the end of the procedure. Rigid fixation is achieved with mini- and microplates. With this technique of facial translocation, good exposure of the anterolateral skull base is achieved, especially when the infratemporal fossa is involved as well (Fig. 8-4).

Extended facial translocation—medial incorporates the standard translocation unit plus the nose and the medial one-half of the opposite face (up to the infraorbital nerve). It can be rotated at the Le Fort 1 level or include the ipsilateral palate and upper lip split. The skin incisions are similar to the standard technique except the paranasal incision is made on the contralateral side. The surgical exposure includes the ipsilateral infratemporal fossa and central and paracentral skull base bilaterally. The entire clivus is accessible as are the optic nerves, both precavernous internal carotid arteries, and the nasopharynx. The wide communication with the infratemporal fossa allows the placement of the temporalis muscle flap for vascularized reconstruction of the skull base defect. Bony fixation of craniofacial osteotomies is done with miniplates and a lag screw for the palate. The occlusal plane is re-established with the help of an orthognathic split. In addition a palatal split is attached to the maxillary dentition for additional stability and protection of the palatal incision. Temporary silicone intranasal stents are inserted as are bilateral lacrimal stents (Fig. 8-5).

Extended facial translocation—medial and inferior includes the above procedure with an inferior extension via a mandibular split (Fig. 8-6). The lower lip incision is performed in a zigzag fashion to conform to the tension lines of the skin with an extension horizontally into the upper neck. Mandibular osteotomy is performed just medial to the mental foramen. Usually an interdental space is found wide enough to permit placement of a reciprocating saw for the osteotomy. This is performed in a step fashion, which then permits more stable reconstructive reapproximation of the bone. Prior to the osteotomy it is wise to select an appropriate miniplate for eventual fixation, contour it to the mandible, and create drill holes. This assists in the postoperative re-establishment of a normal occlusion. This extended translocation procedure adds a significant inferior cranial as well as upper cervical surgical access.

Extended facial translocation—posterior incorporates the ear, temporal bone, and posterior fossa into its surgical access. The horizontal temple incision of the standard translocation is extended posteriorly just above the external ear and curves inferiorly over the occipital bone to the neck. This provides access to the anterior as well as posterior aspect of the temporal bone with control of the key neurovascular structures (Fig. 8-7).

Bilateral facial translocation combines complete right and left basic translocation units with or without palatal split. The exposure incorporates both infratemporal fossae, and the central and the entire paracentral skull base. Both distal cervical internal carotid arteries (ICAs) are in view as is the full clivus. The palatal split permits a reach to the level of C2-C3. If further inferior extension is needed, a mandibular split can be added so a vertical reach to C3-C4 is accomplished. A sin-

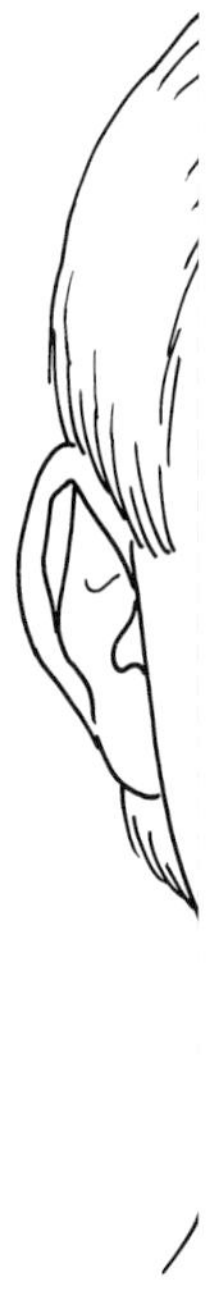

A

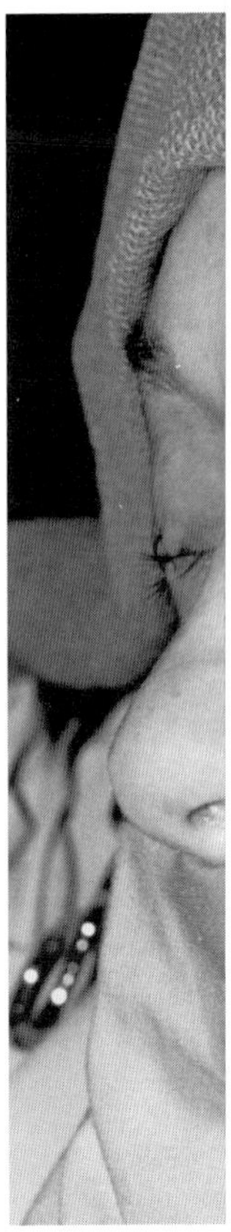

C

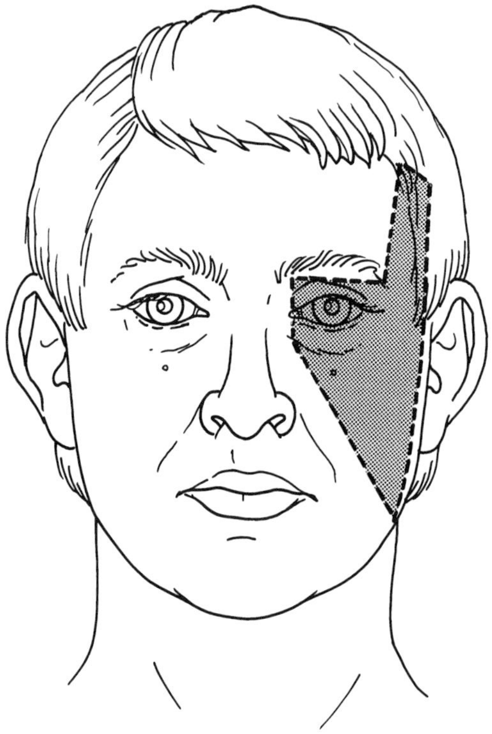

A

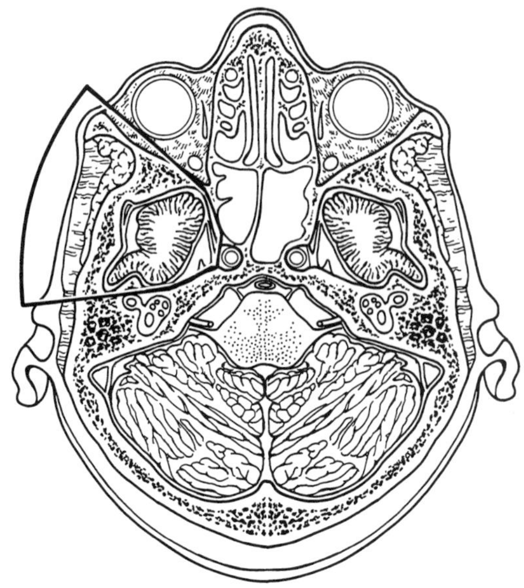

B

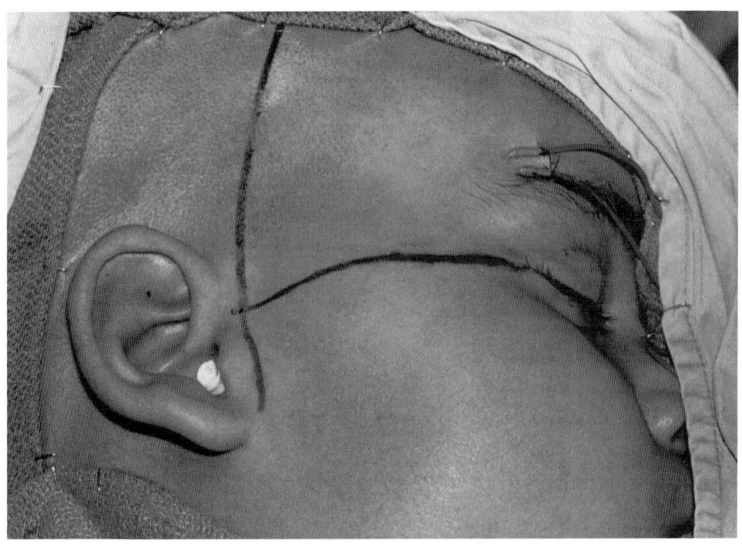

C

Figure 8-3. *(A)* Schema of mini facial translocation—lateral. *(B)* Outline of surgical field. *(C)* Clinical example—skin incisions. *(Figure continues.)*

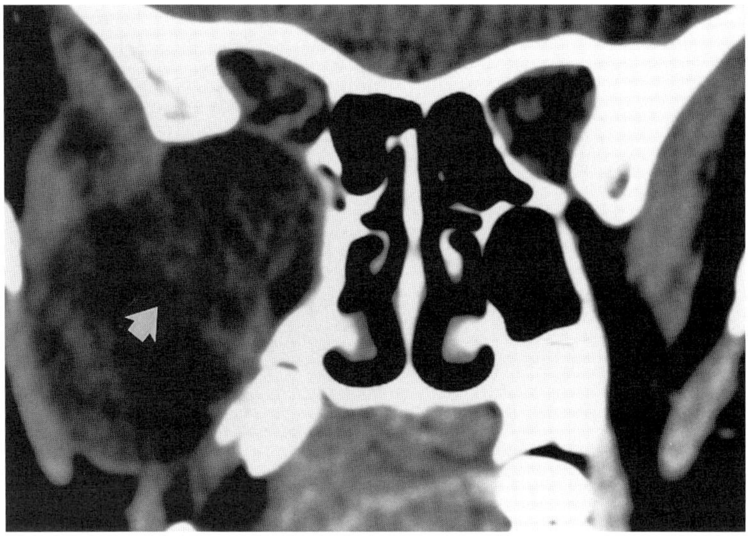

D

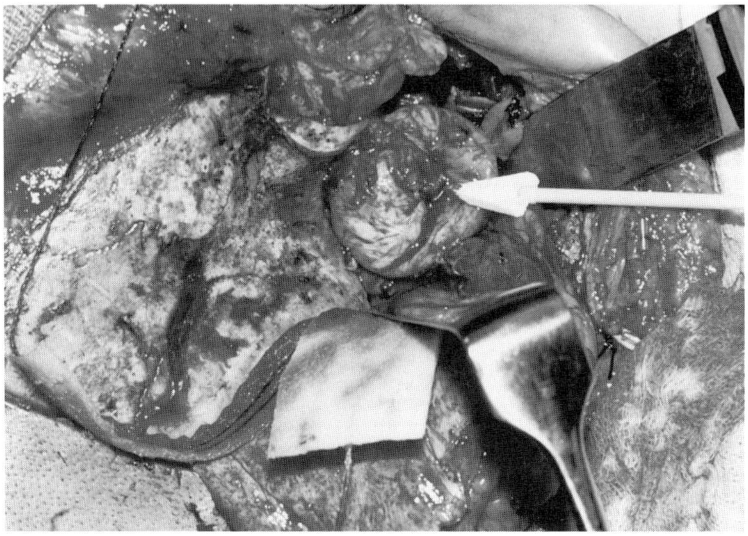

E

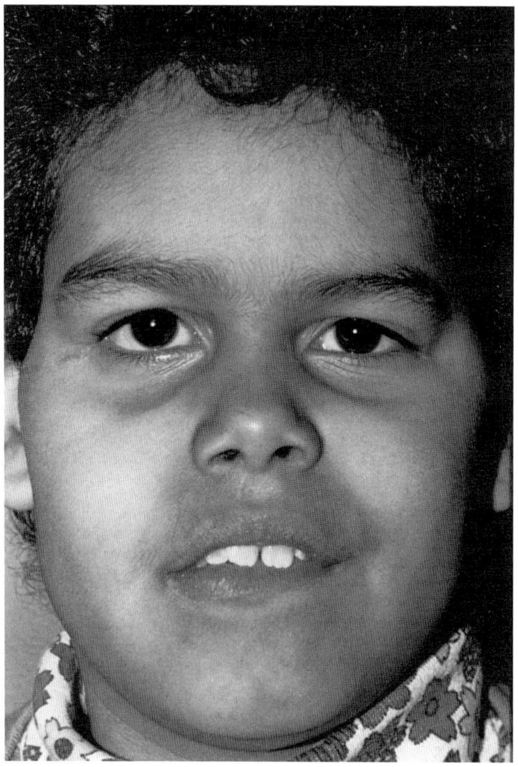

F

Figure 8-3 (Continued). (D) Coronal CT demonstrating cystic mass (encephalocele; arrow) in the right infratemporal fossa with extension to the orbital fissure. *(E)* Surgical view of right temporal and infratemporal fossa with arrow pointing to the cystic mass exiting from right middle fossa. *(F)* Patient's postoperative appearance at 6 months.

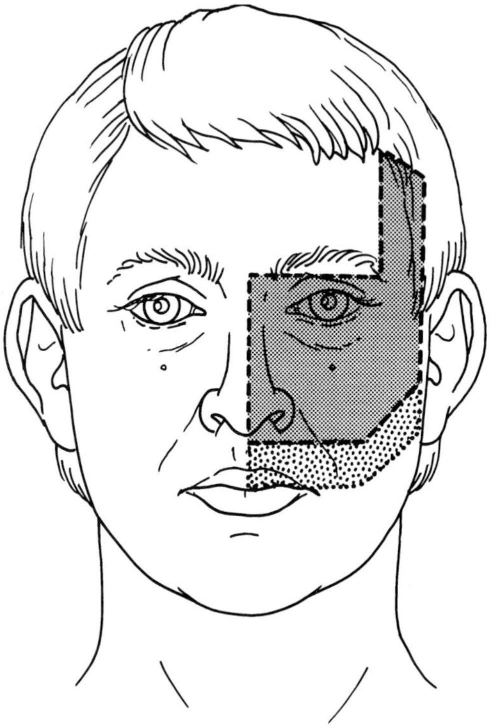

A

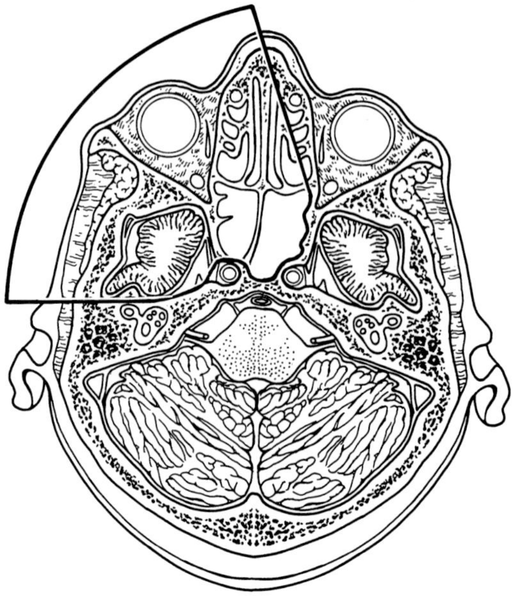

B

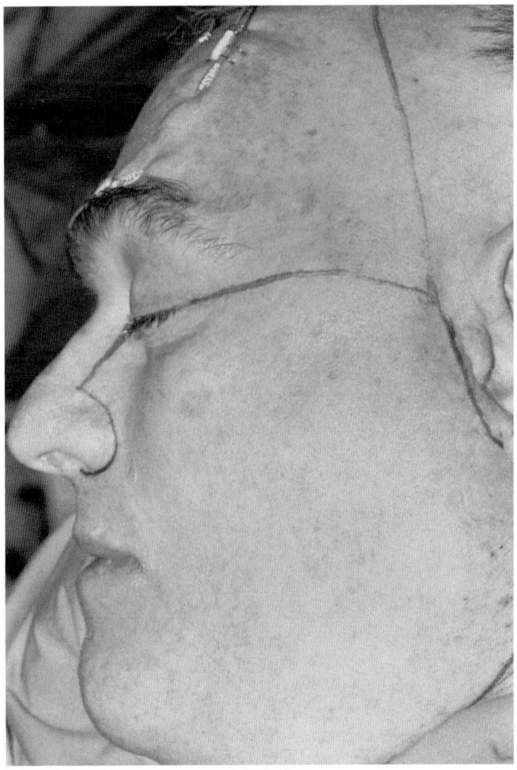

C_1

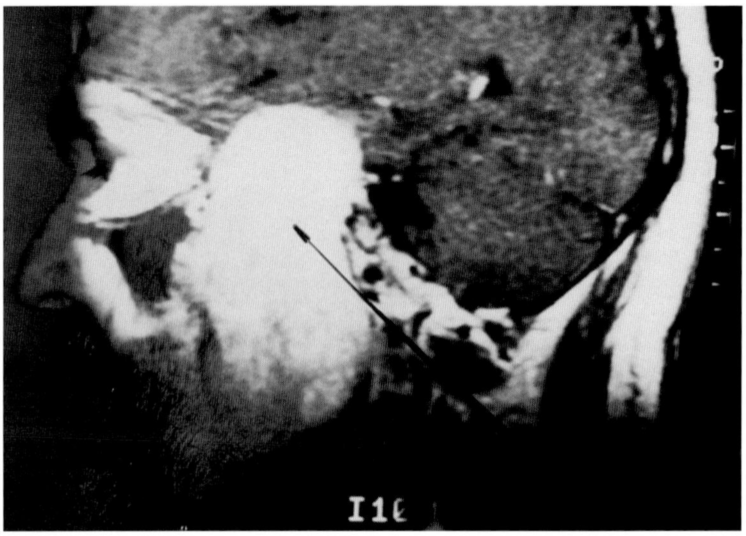

C_2

Figure 8-4. *(A)* Schema of standard facial translocation with palatal extension (dotted). *(B)* Outline of surgical field. *(C_1)* Clinical example (translocation without palatal split)—skin incisions. *(C_2)* Composite slide of patient's lateral photograph and lateral MRI demonstrating (pointer) a transcranial neurofibroma. *(Figure continues.)*

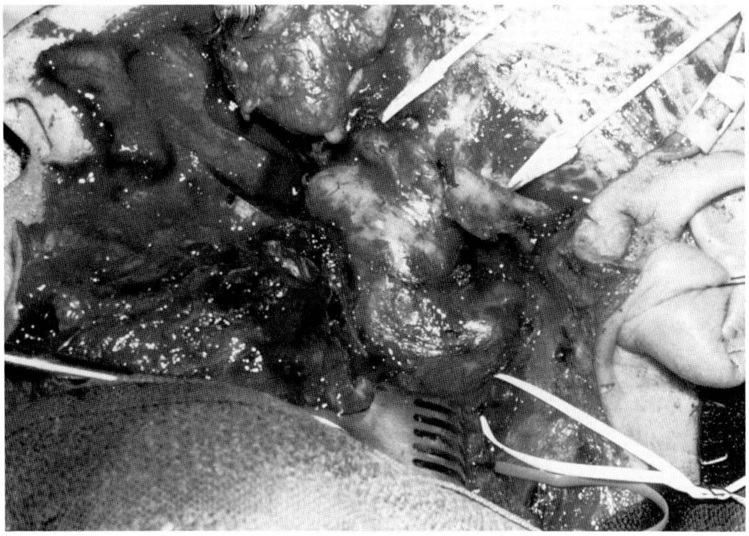

C3

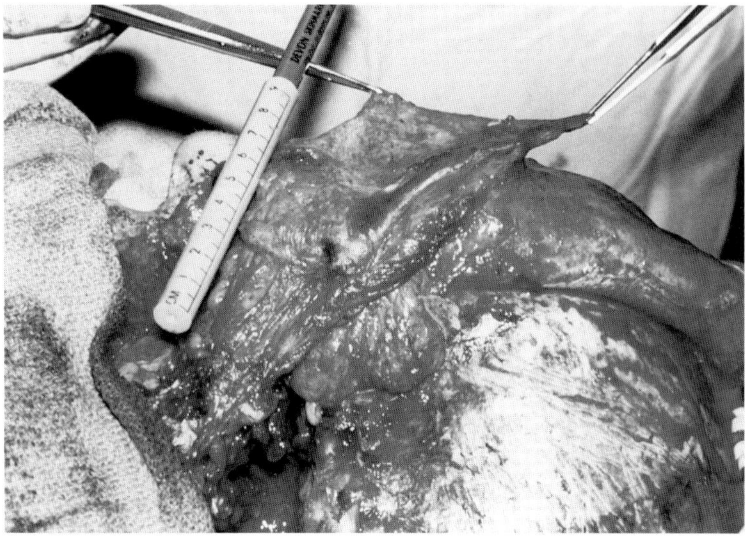

C4

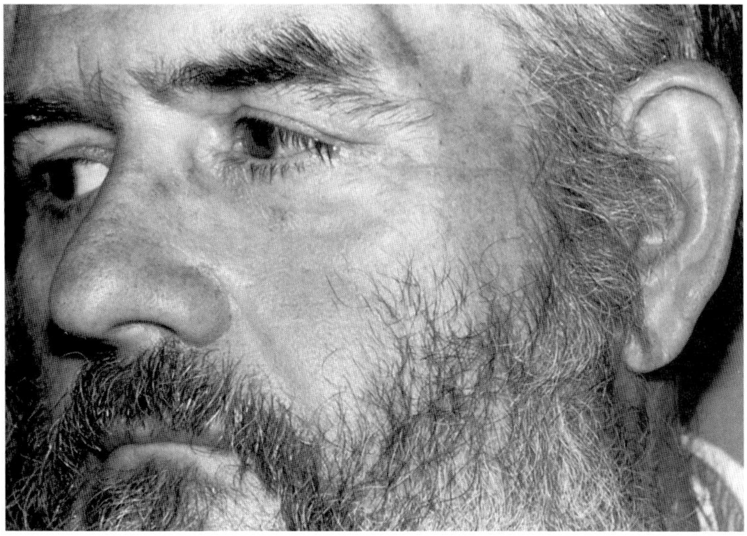

C5

Figure 8-4 (Continued). *(C_3)* Surgical view of left temporal and infratemporal fossae with exposure of the tumor (arrows). *(C_4)* Medial rotation of left temporalis muscle used for reconstruction. *(C_5)* Patient's appearance 1 year postoperatively. *(Figure continues.)*

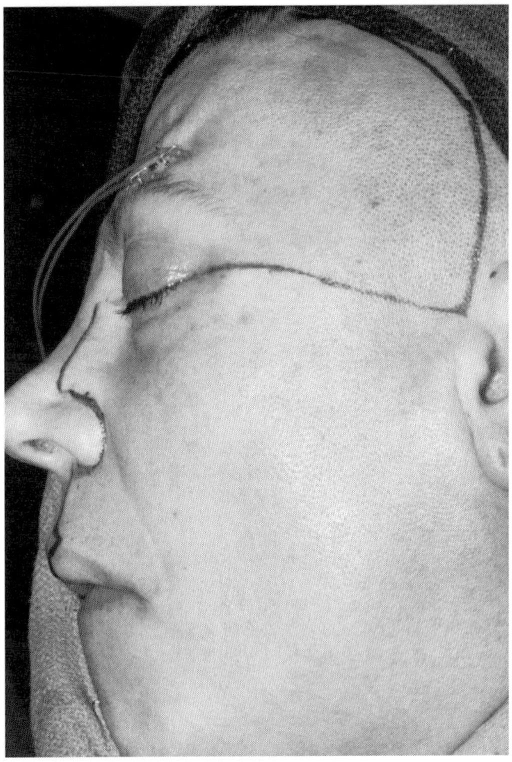

D₁

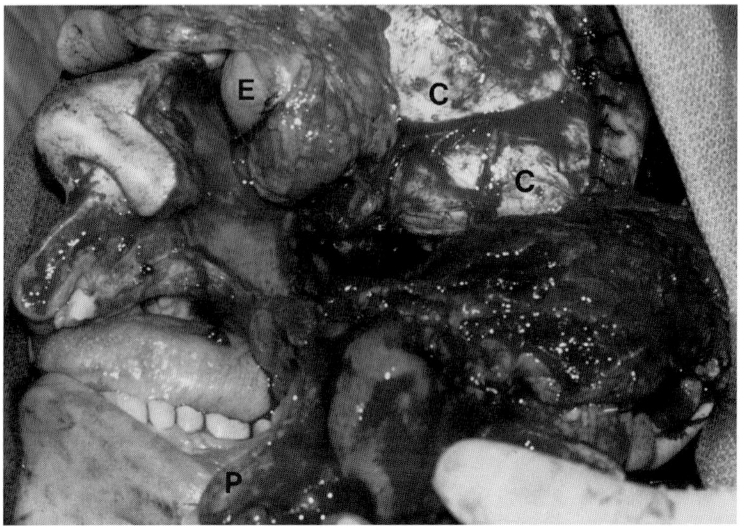

D₂

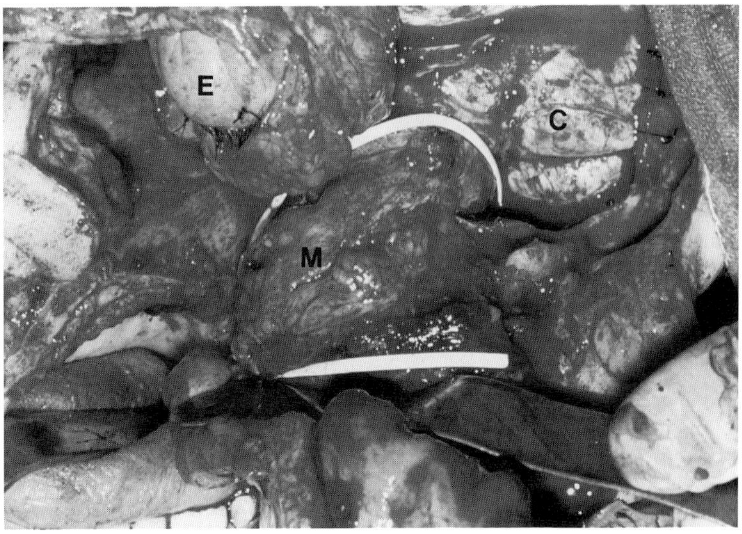

D₃

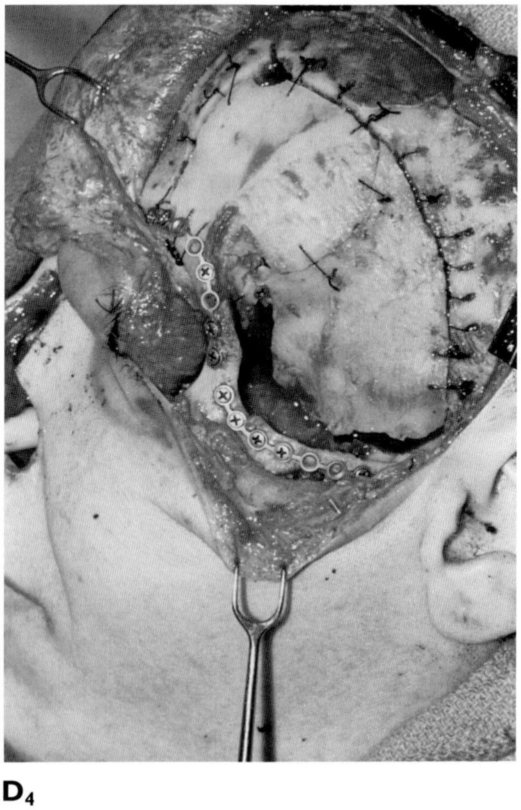

D₄

Figure 8-4 (Continued). (D_1) Clinical example (translocation with palatal split)—skin incisions. *(D_2)* Surgical view; frontotemporal craniotomy (C); eye (E); translocated left palate (P). *(D_3)* Transferred left temporalis muscle (M) into the surgical defect; eye (E); craniotomy (C). *(D_4)* Bony fixation; facial skeleton (miniplates); craniotomy (sutures). *(Figure continues.)*

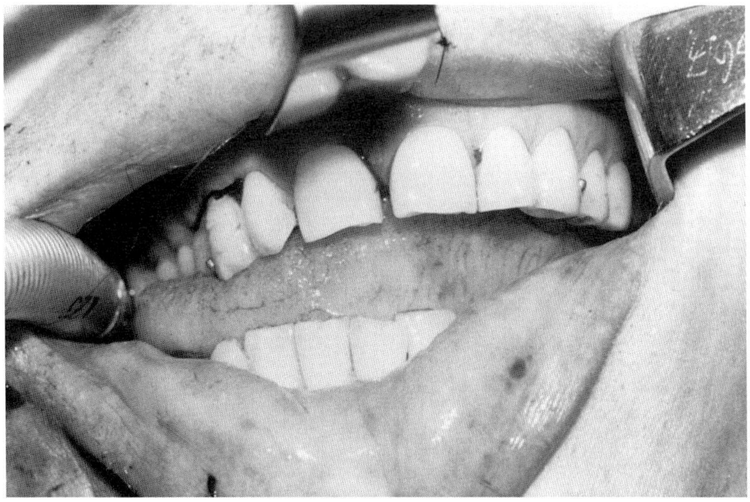

D_5

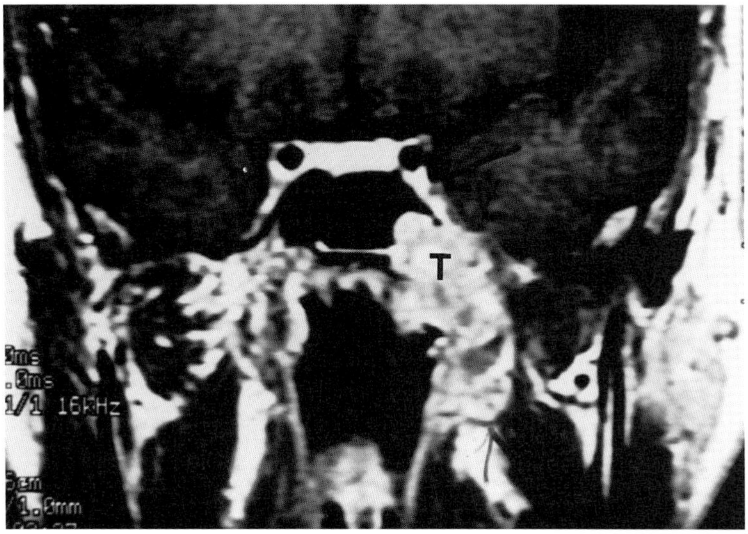

D_6

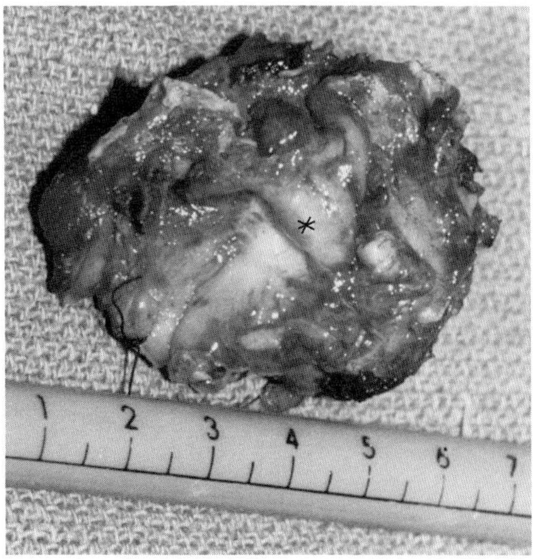

D_7

Figure 8-4 (Continued). (D_5) Re-established occlusion at the end of surgery. *(D_6)* Coronal MRI demonstrating patient's tumor (T) in left nasopharynx and middle fossa. *(D_7)* Surgical specimen includes left lateral and posterior nasopharynx, foramen lacerum, and contents of infratemporal fossa; left eustachian tube (*). *(Figure continues.)*

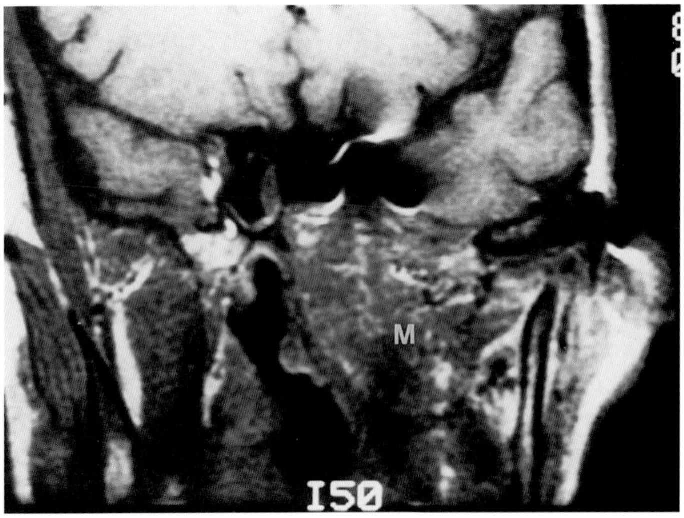

D₈

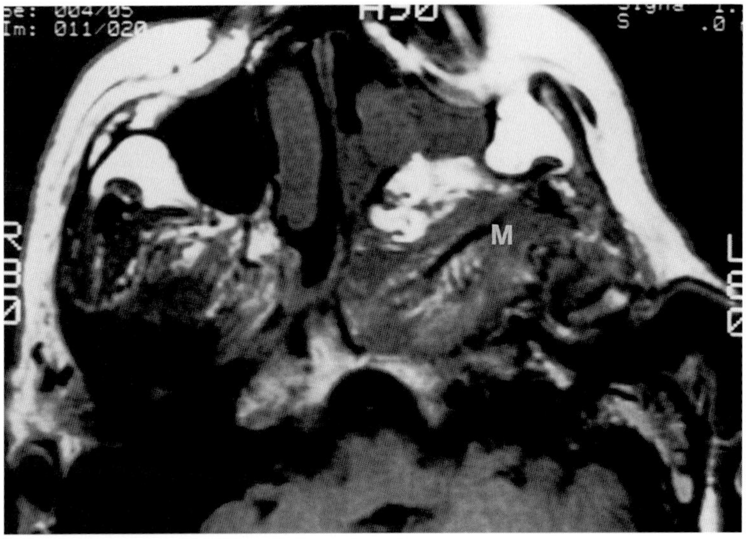

D₉

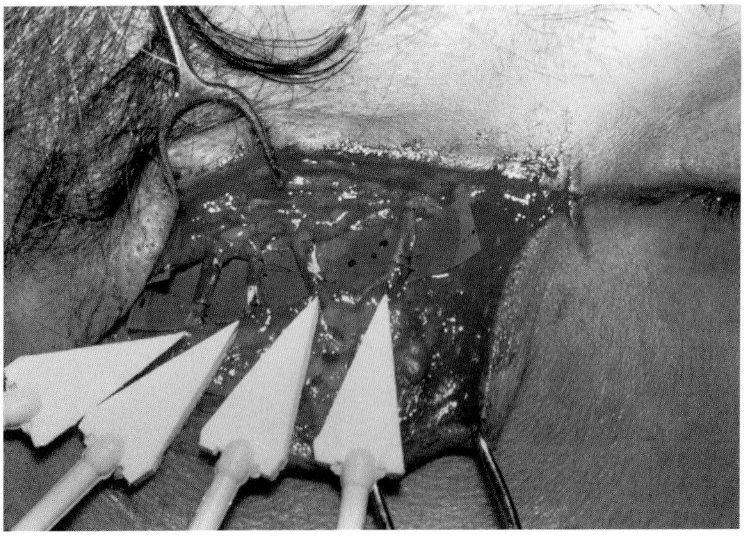

E₁

Figure 8-4 (Continued). *(D_8)* Coronal MRI demonstrating the temporalis muscle (M) transferred into the surgical defect. *(D_9)* Axial MRI demonstrating the transferred temporalis muscle (M); the central signal void in the muscle represents its tendon. *(E_1)* Clinical example—isolation and placement of silicone tubings around frontalis branches of left facial nerve above the zygomatic arch (arrows). *(Figure continues.)*

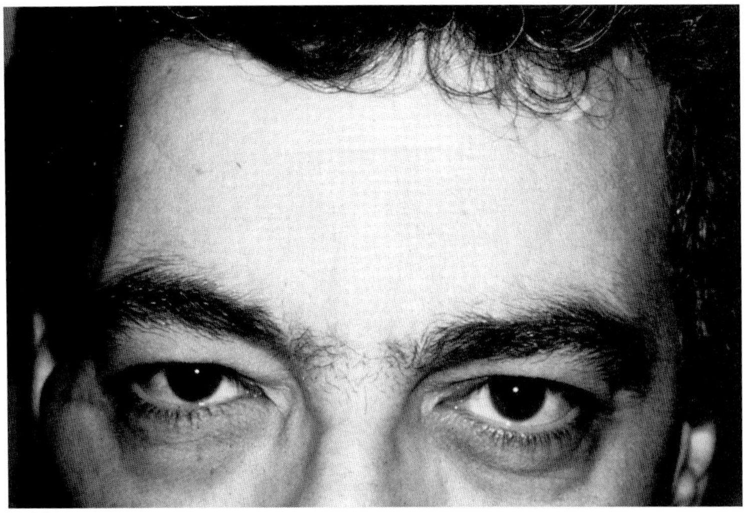

E_2

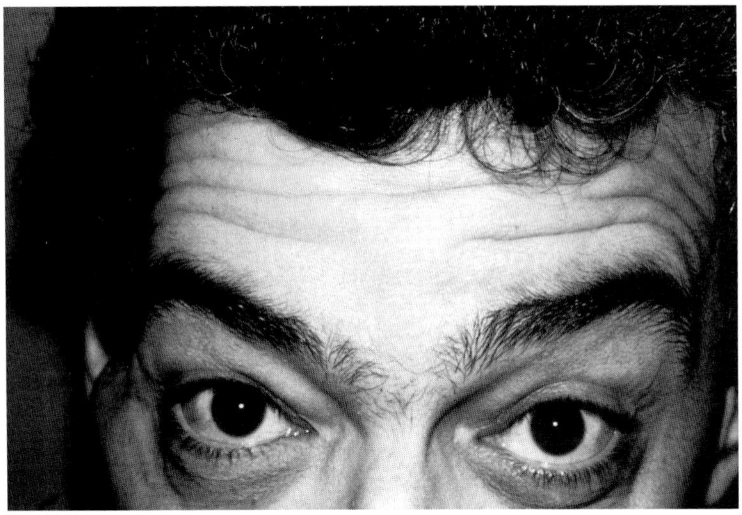

E_3

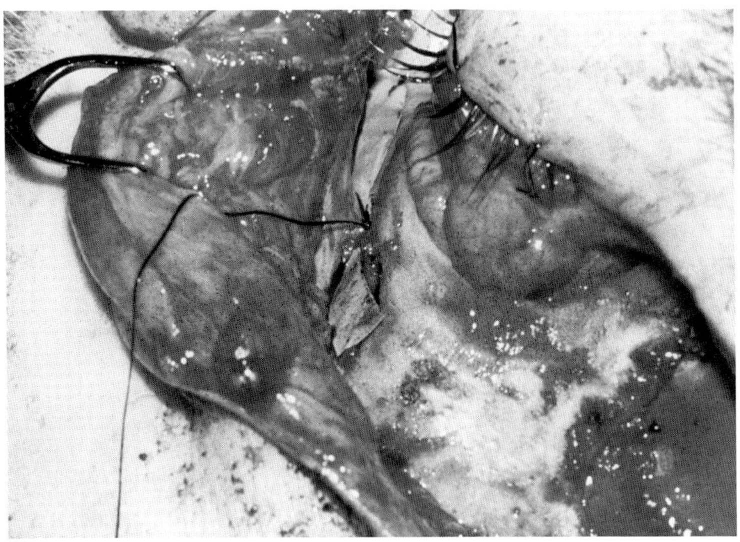

F

Figure 8-4 (Continued). *(E_2)* Patient's postoperative (1 year) forehead appearance in repose. *(E_3)* Forehead movement at 1 year following repair of frontalis branches of the left facial nerve. *(F)* Repair of left infraorbital nerve at the completion of facial translocation. *(Figure continues.)*

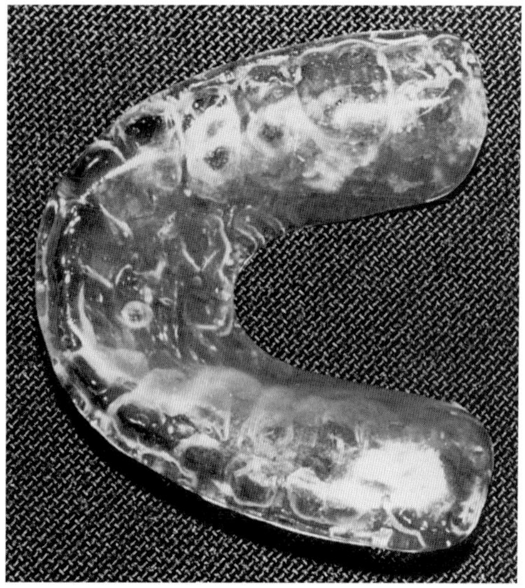

G₁

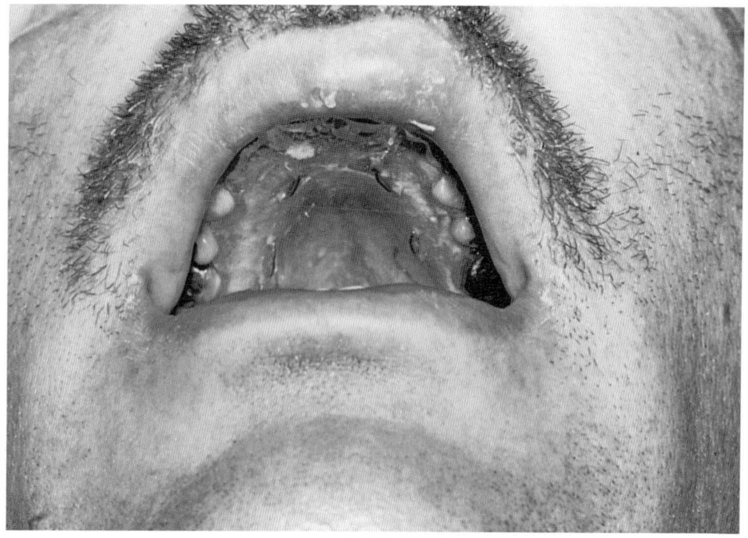

G₂

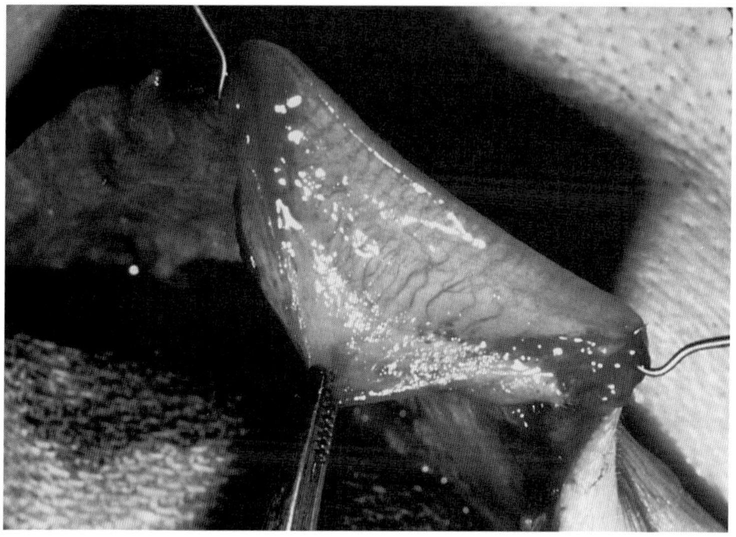

H₁

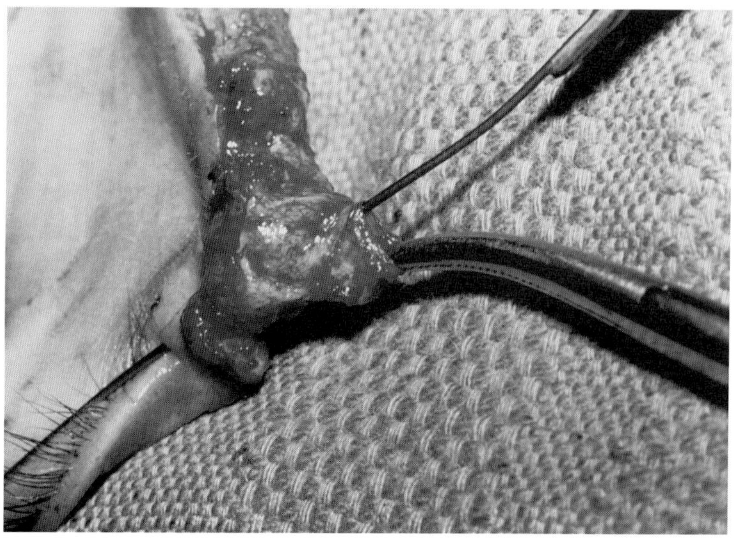

H₂

Figure 8-4 (Continued). *(G_1)* Occlusal splint used intraoperatively to re-establish patient's occlusion following palatal split. *(G_2)* Another type of occlusal split with palatal extension. *(H_1)* Lower lid fornix demonstrating level of transection. *(H_2)* Left lower lid with a probe in the lacrimal drainage system; probe is seen entering inferior canaliculus and exiting via nasolacrimal duct (held by a clamp). *(Figure continues.)*

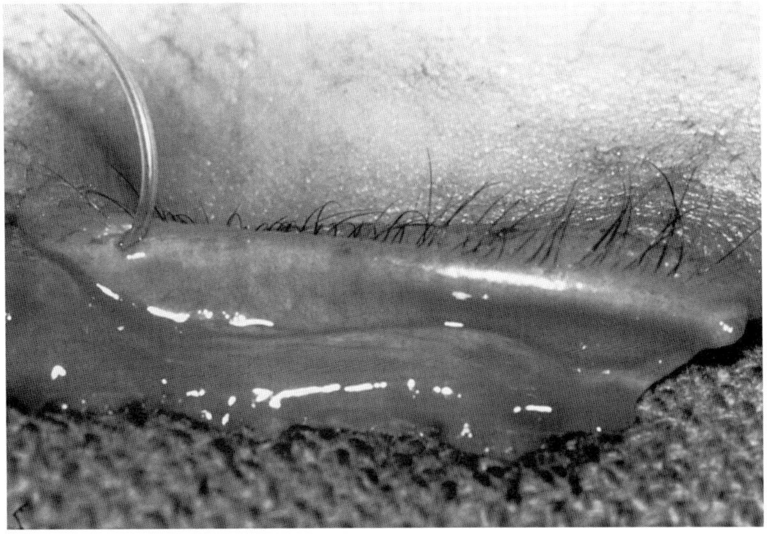

H_3

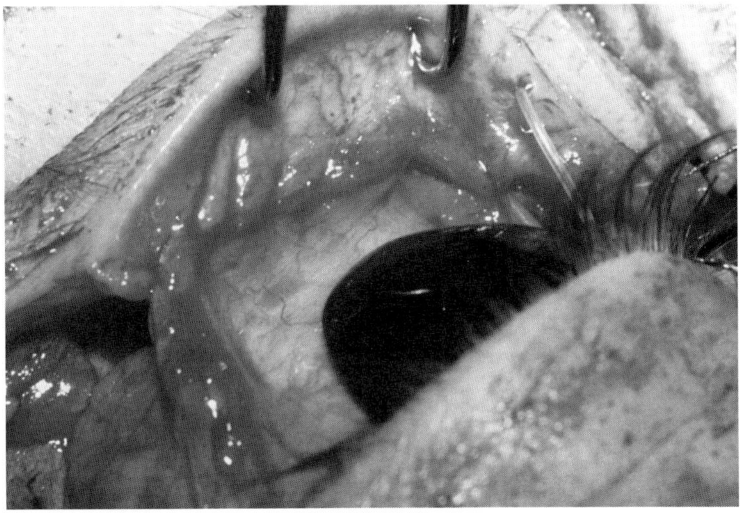

H_4

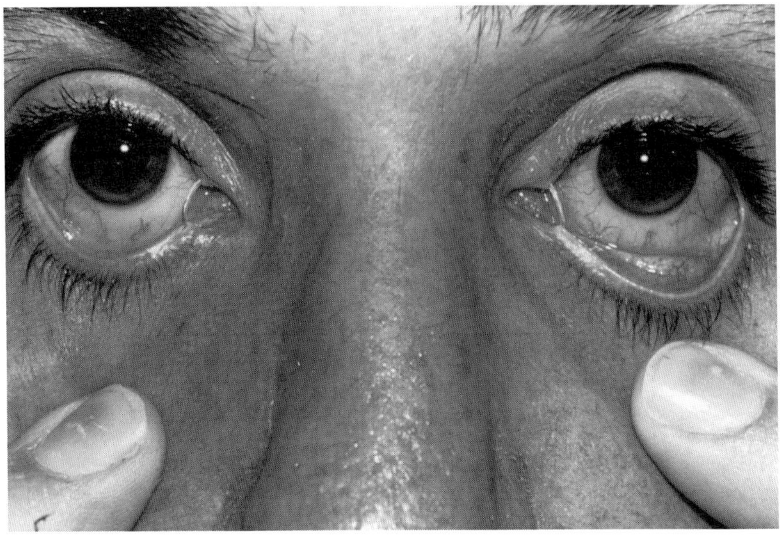

H_5

Figure 8-4 (Continued). *(H_3)* Close-up of right lower lid with a lacrimal stent in the inferior canaliculus. *(H_4)* Suturing of conjunctiva of the left inferior fornix; lacrimal stent is seen between superior and inferior canaliculus; dark lens protects the cornea. *(H_5)* Patient's appearance 3 months postoperatively following extended facial translocation (medial); lacrimal stents are visible in both eyes between superior and inferior canaliculi.

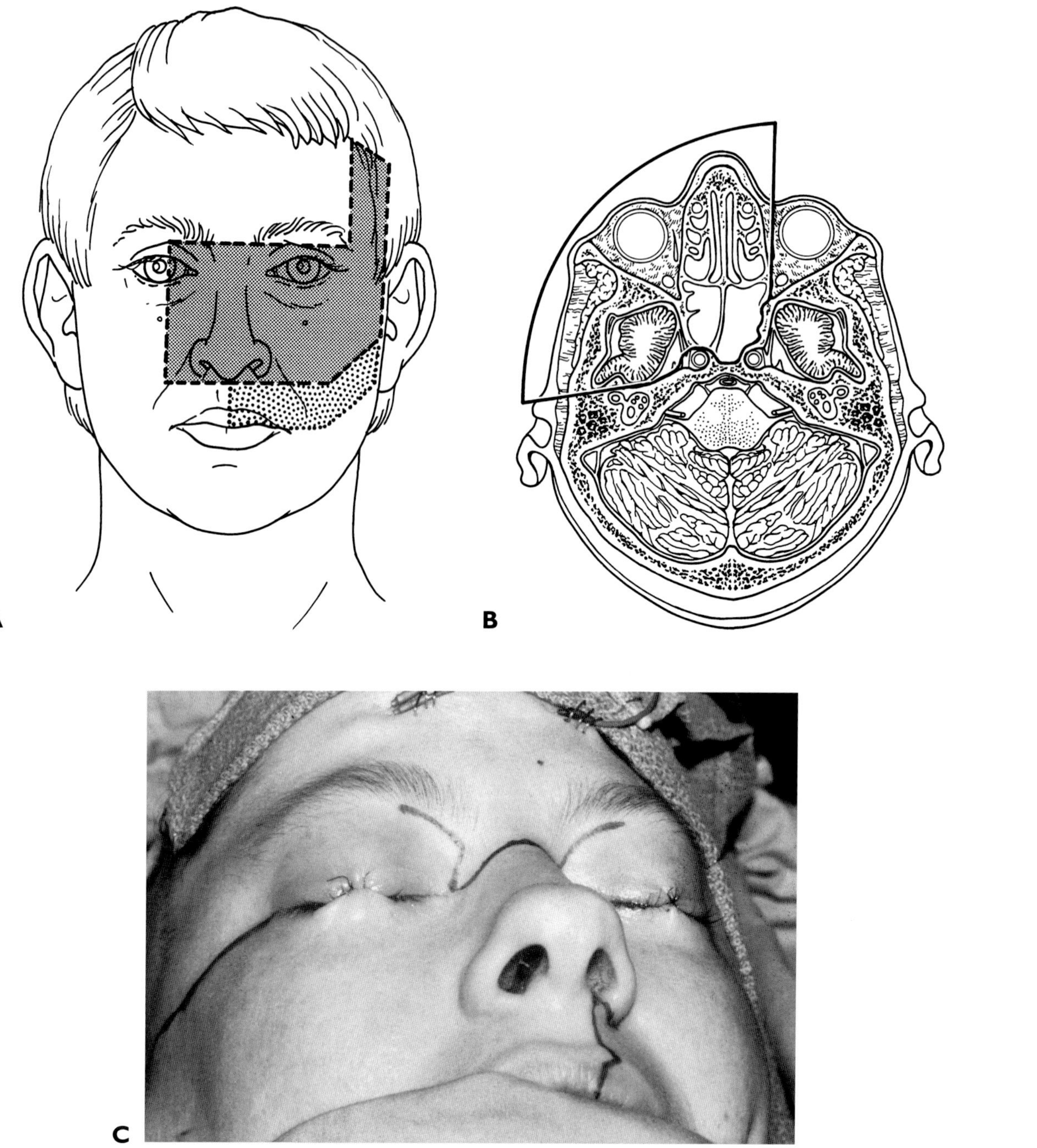

A B C

Figure 8-5. *(A)* Schema of extended facial translocation—medial with palatal extension (dotted). *(B)* Outline of surgical field. *(C)* Clinical example—outline of skin incisions. *(Figure continues.)*

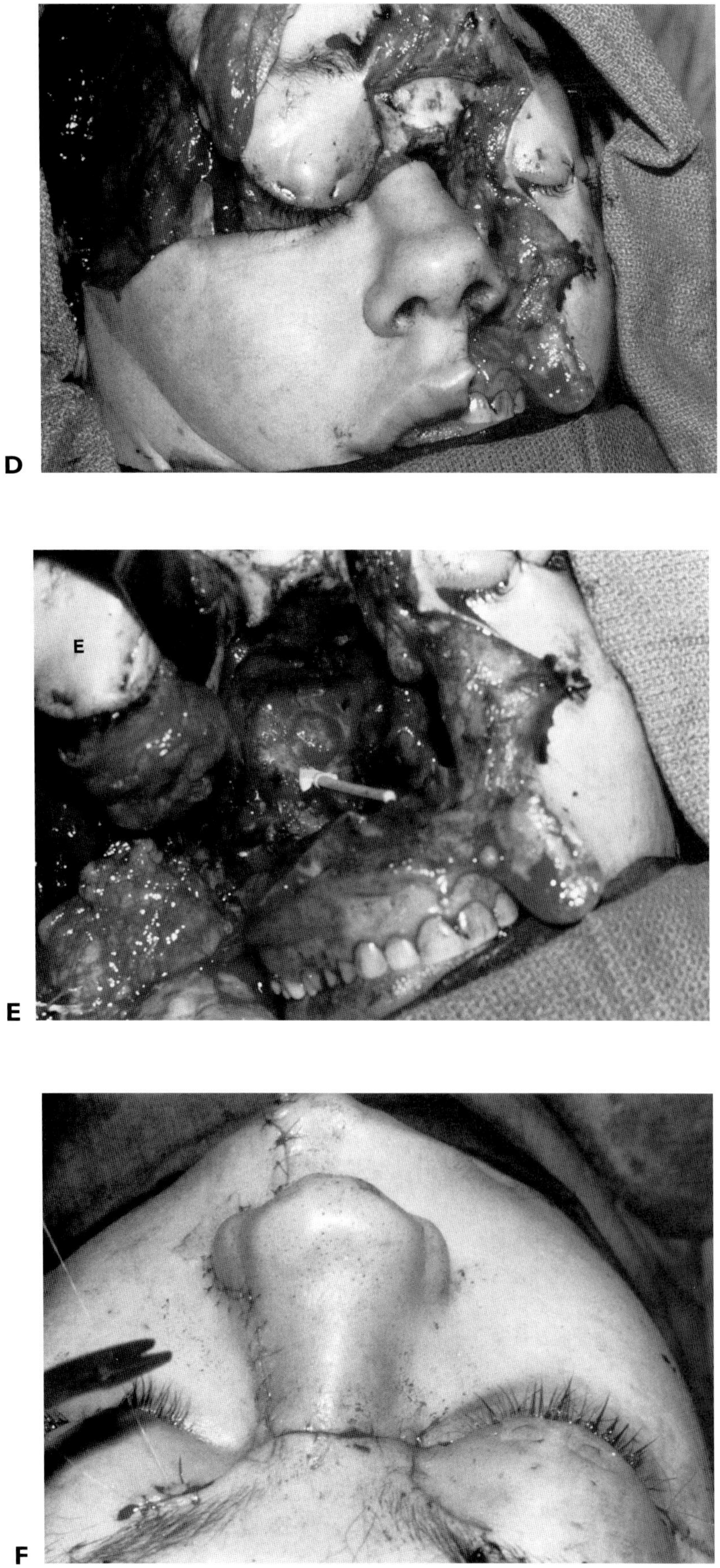

Figure 8-5 (Continued). *(D)* Incisions performed. *(E)* Close-up of surgical view following resection of fibrous dysplasia; arrow is at the clival dura; right eye (E). *(F)* Surgical closure; superior view. *(Figure continues.)*

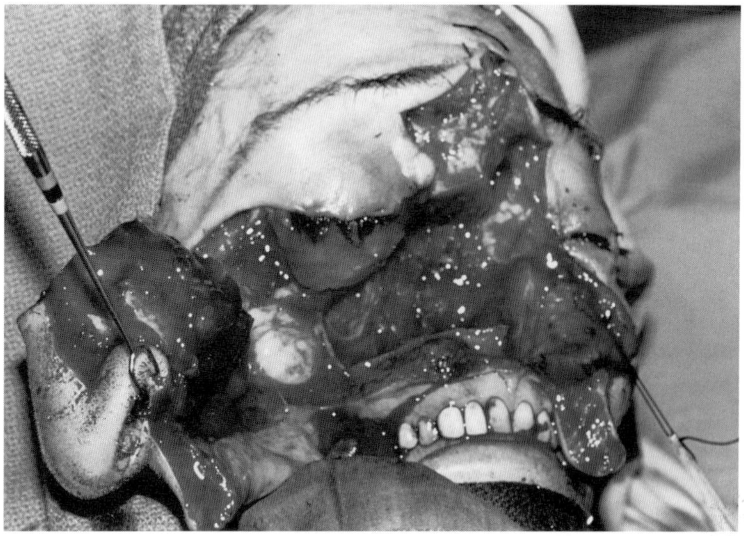

G

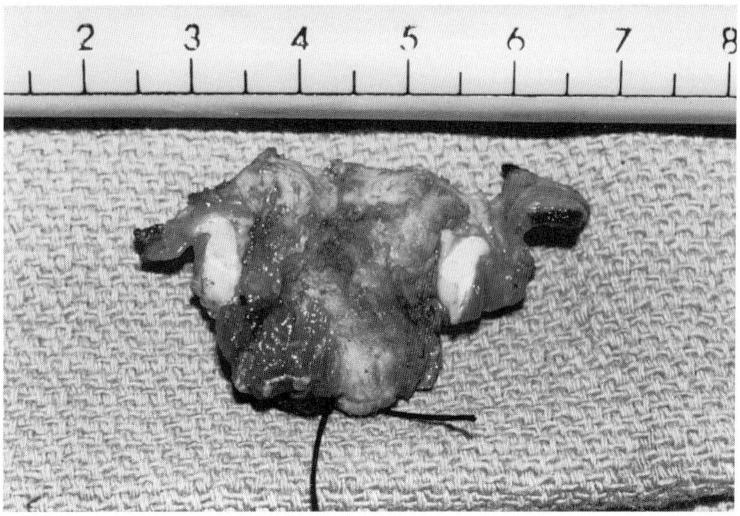

H

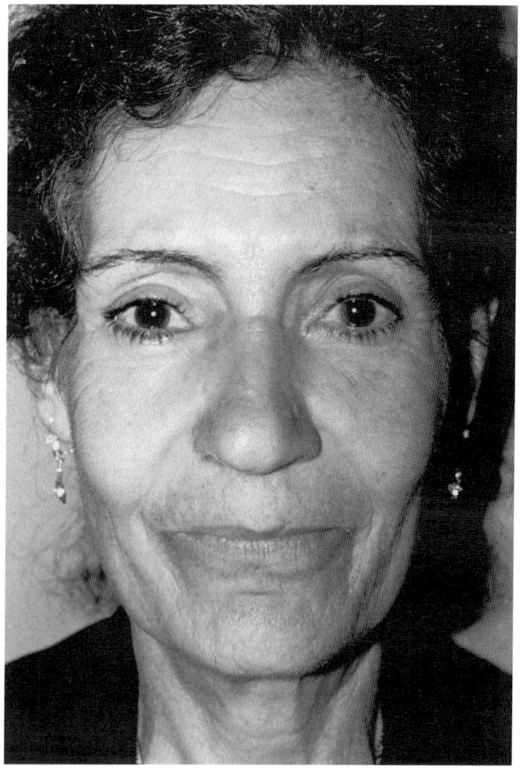

I

Figure 8-5 (Continued). *(G)* Surgical exposure of another patient (nasopharyngeal cancer). *(H)* Surgical specimen including both lateral walls and the posterior wall of nasopharynx; eustachian tube cartilages are prominently white at 3 and 9 o'clock. *(I)* Patient's appearance 1 year postoperatively.

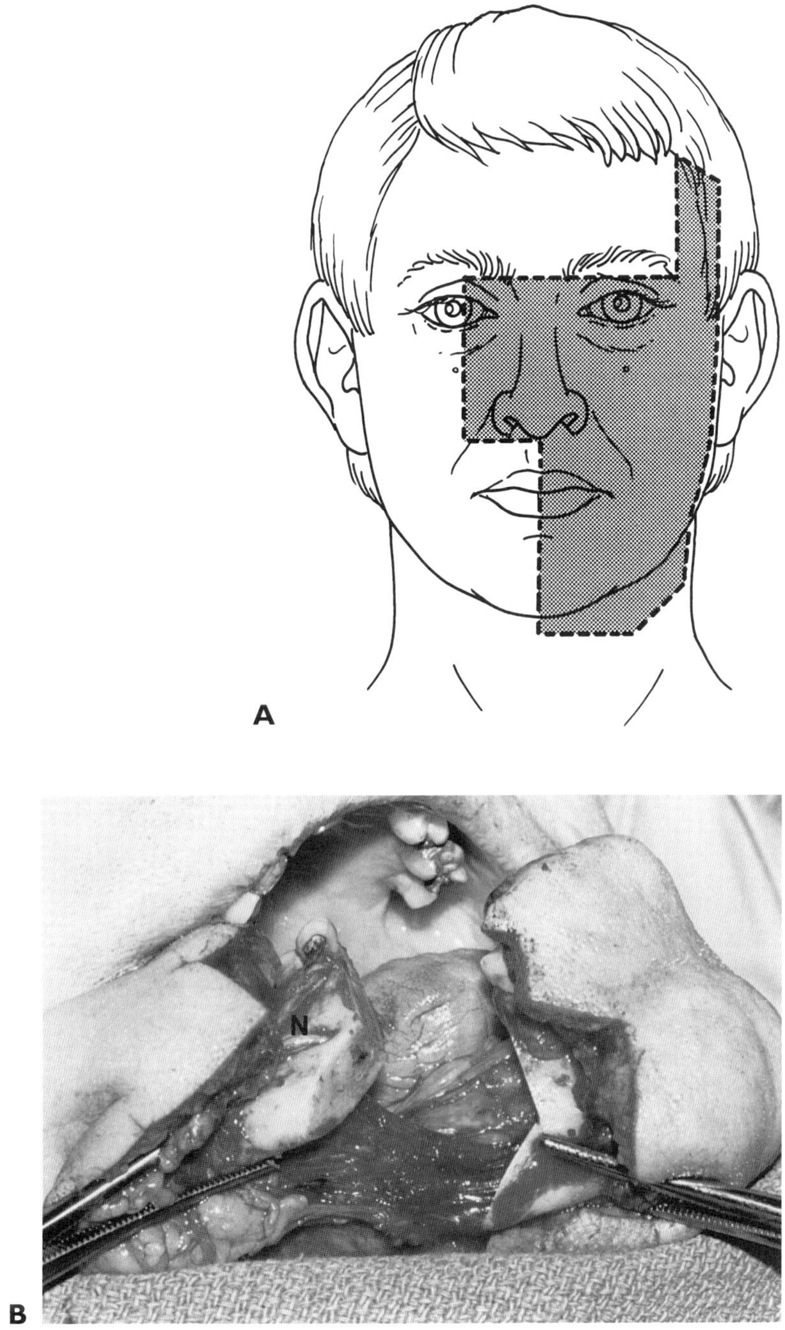

Figure 8-6. *(A)* Schema of extended facial translocation—medial and inferior. *(B)* Clinical example of right parasymphyseal mandibular split used in inferior extension of facial translocation; right mental nerve (N).

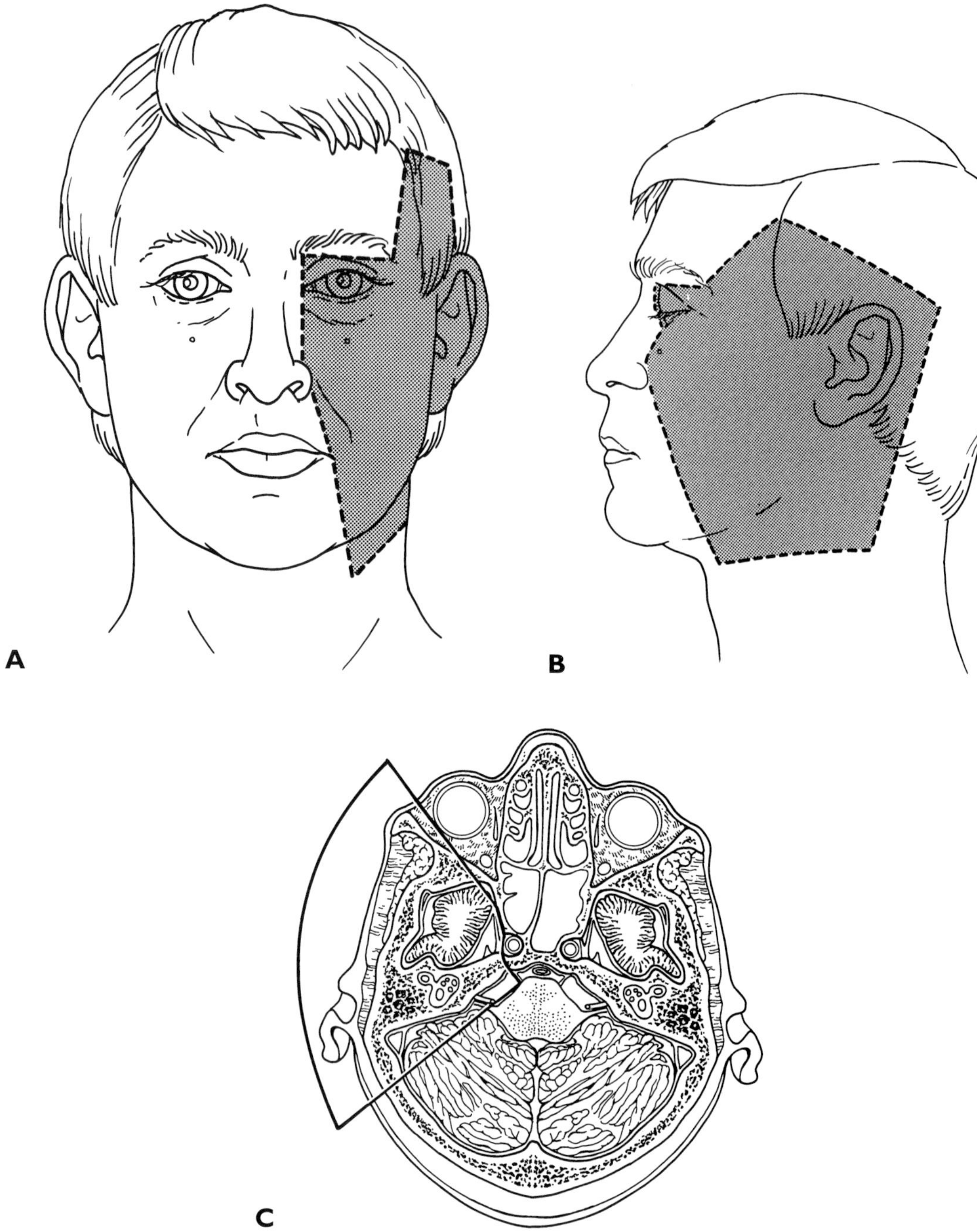

Figure 8-7. *(A)* Schema of extended facial translocation—posterior. *(B)* Side view. *(C)* Outline of surgical field. *(Figure continues.)*

gle temporalis muscle flap is sufficient for the coverage of the surgical defect at the skull base (Fig. 8-8).

Closure Techniques

Following extirpation of the lesion at the cranial base, the dura is repaired or examined for intactness. If a suture repair is performed, fibrin glue is also used to reinforce the dural closure. A separate segment of fascia lata or pericranium may be applied directly to this suture line.

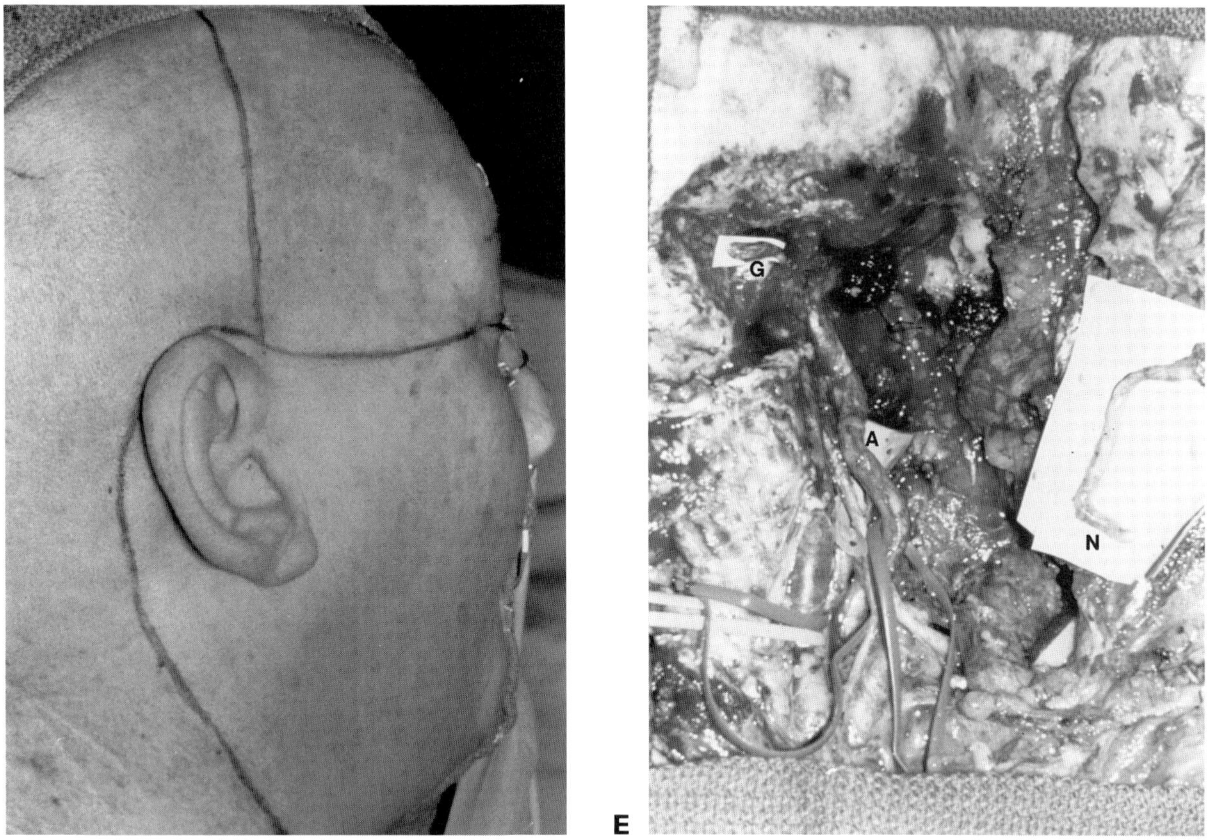

Figure 8-7 (Continued). (D) Clinical example—skin incisions. *(E)* Surgical view following resection of mucoepidermoid carcinoma; internal carotid artery: (A) decompressed to the precavernous segment; facial nerve at geniculate ganglion (G) prior to nerve grafting; nerve graft (N).

Following large resection with dural or vessel exposure, an ipsilateral temporalis muscle flap is transferred into the wound from the temporal fossa and laid into the central and paracentral skull base. The attached deep temporalis fascia permits circumferential suturing of this muscle-fascia unit to the surrounding soft and bony tissues under moderate tension, thus preventing postoperative gravity-dependent displacement of the temporalis muscle. (The temporal fossa donor defect may be filled with an abdominal fat graft or later with an implant.) The remnant of nasopharyngeal mucosa with the underlining pharyngeal constrictor muscle may then be placed over this temporalis muscle. If pharyngeal mucosa is not available, it is reasonable to leave the temporalis muscle exposed to the nasopharynx. Usually within several weeks, mucosal coverage develops from the periphery of the nasopharynx. It is important, however, to suture the periphery of the muscle to the surrounding structures to ensure support and to seal the surgical site.

The compound vascularized facial segments are repositioned. The dental occlusal plane is re-established with a prefabricated occlusal splint fashioned preoperatively from the patient's dental models. The lateral orbital and central nasal osteotomies are stabilized with miniplates. Large orbital defects are reconstructed with titanium mesh (Fig. 8-9). A horizontal lag screw is placed at the region of the nasal spine (above the roots of the central incisor teeth) for anterior palatal stabilization.

Specialized Instrumentation for Facial Osteotomies

A Zimmer Micro 100 reciprocating saw is used. It offers 1-mm-thick blades in short and long versions, ideal for facial osteotomies. For drilling, the Midas Rex system is

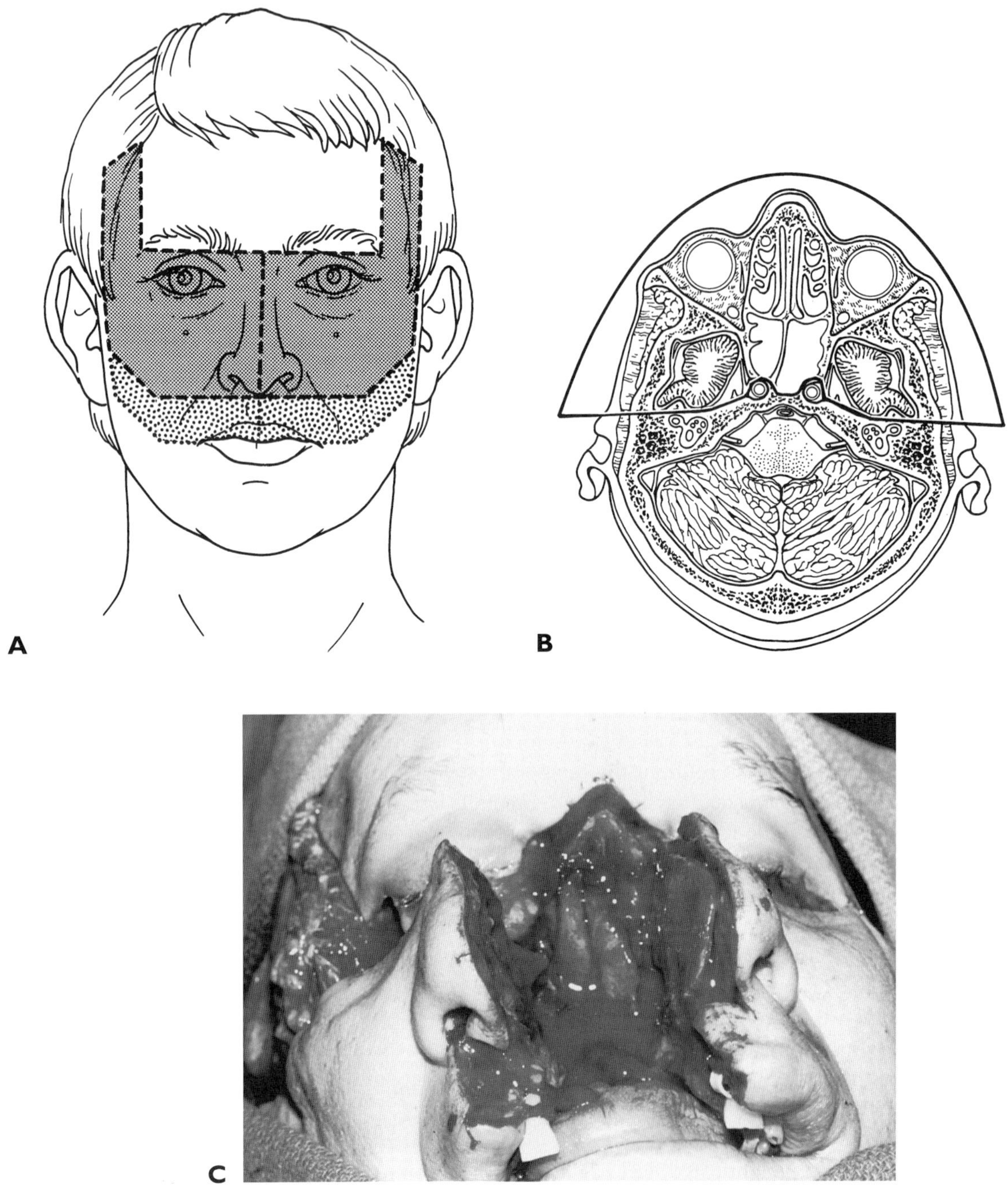

Figure 8-8. *(A)* Schema of bilateral facial translocation; dotted area includes palatal split. *(B)* Outline of surgical field in an axial plane. *(C)* Clinical example—facial/palatal split. *(Figure continues.)*

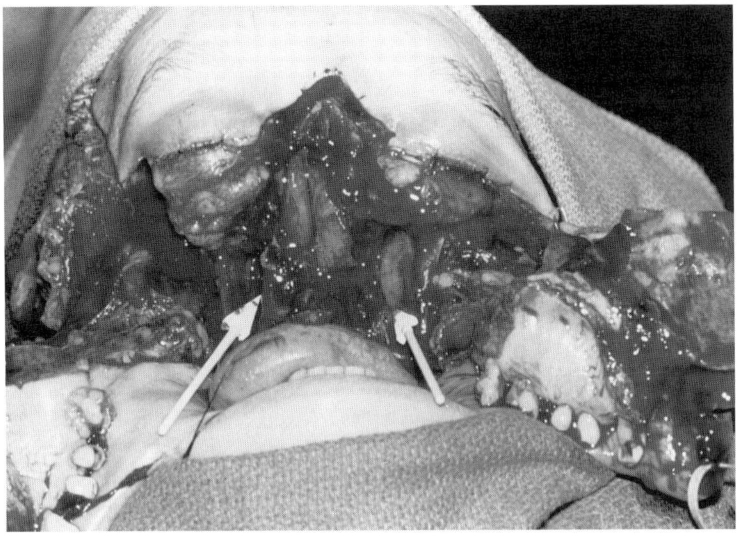

D

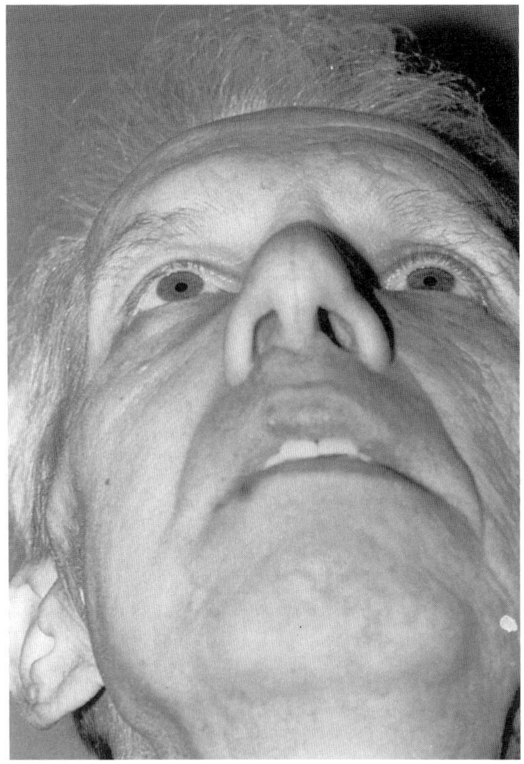

E

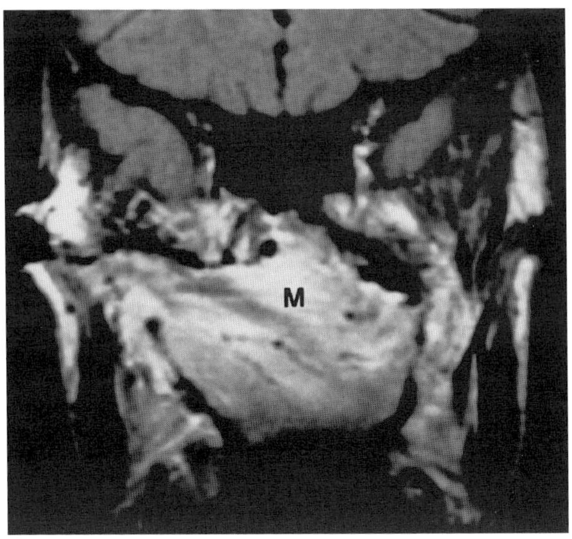

F

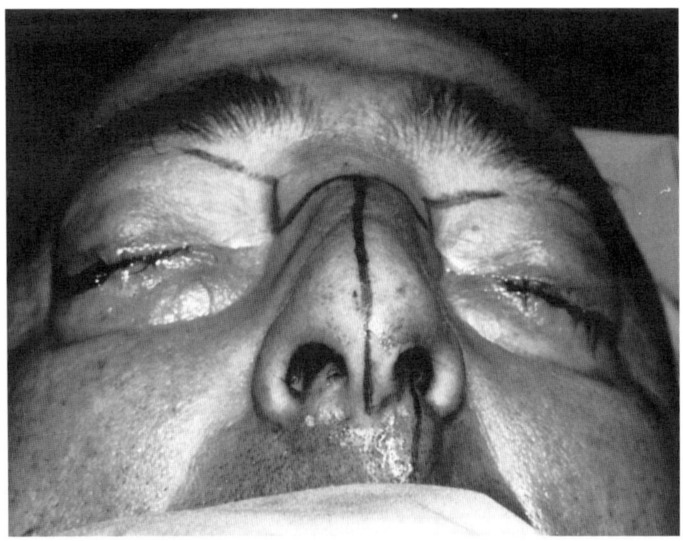

G

Figure 8-8 (Continued). (D) Extent of surgical exposure; arrows delineate nasopharyngeal cancer; displaced facial segments (with palatal halves with dentition) are lateral. *(E)* Postoperative result at 1 year. *(F)* Coronal postoperative MRI demonstrating transferred right temporalis muscle (M) into the surgical defect; notice the extent of the reach across the midline. *(G)* Another patient—skin incisions. *(Figure continues.)*

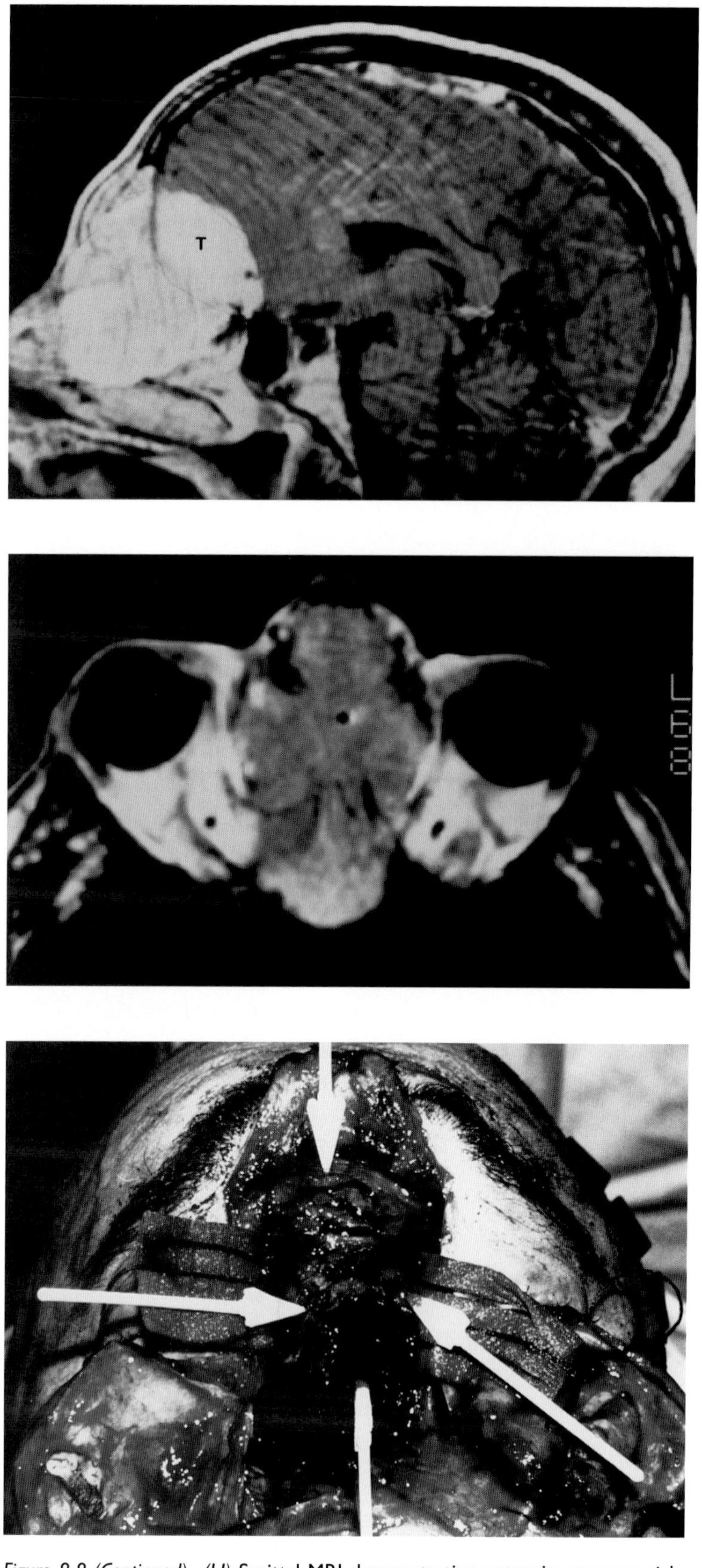

H

I

J

Figure 8-8 (Continued). (H) Sagittal MRI demonstrating extensive transcranial meningioma (T) with signs of an increased intracranial pressure. *(I)* Axial MRI showing tumor encroaching on both orbits. *(J)* Surgical exposure; arrows outline meningioma. *(Figure continues.)*

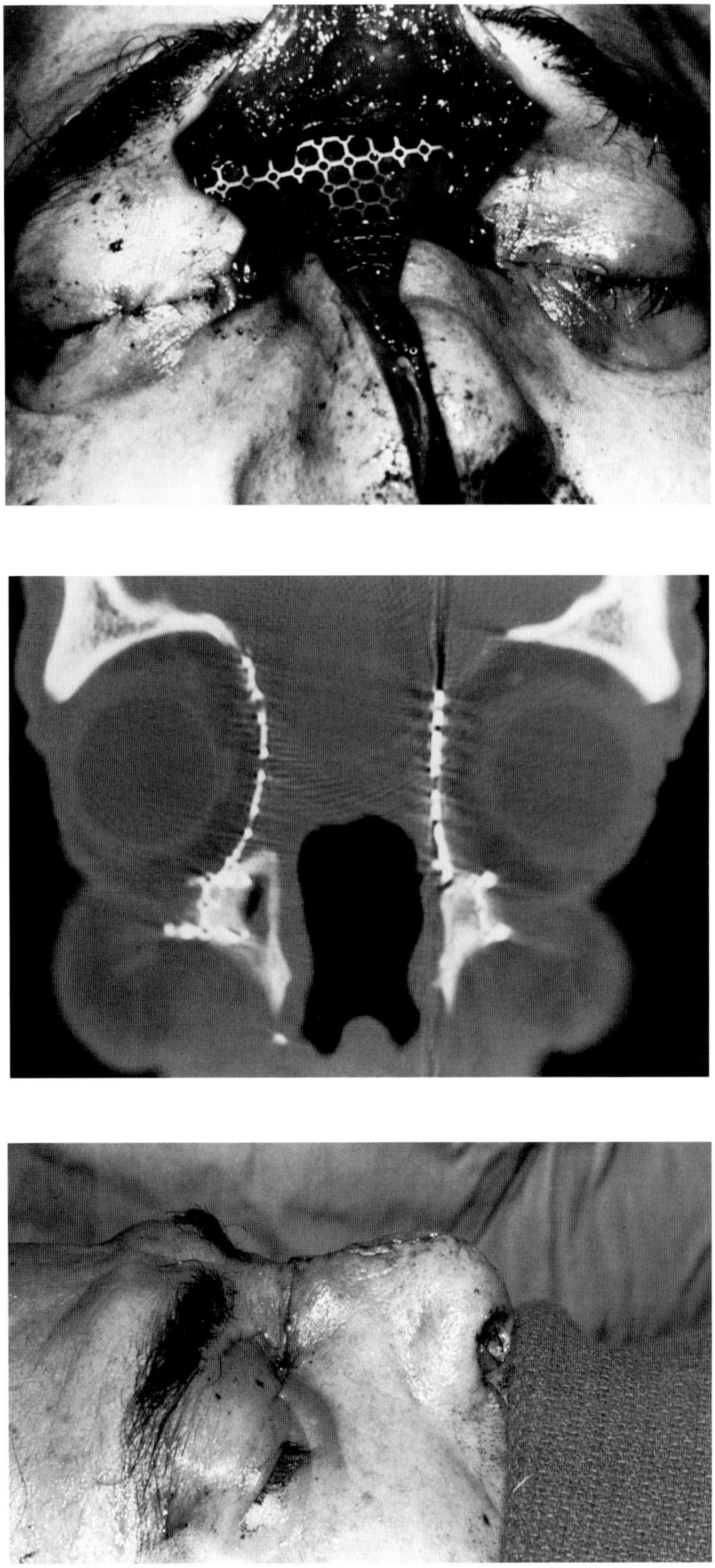

K

L

M

Figure 8-8 (Continued). *(K)* Bony defect was reconstructed with metal mesh. *(L)* Coronal CT demonstrating reconstruction of both medial orbital walls with metal mesh. *(M)* Lateral view of wound closure and reconstruction of nasal projection.

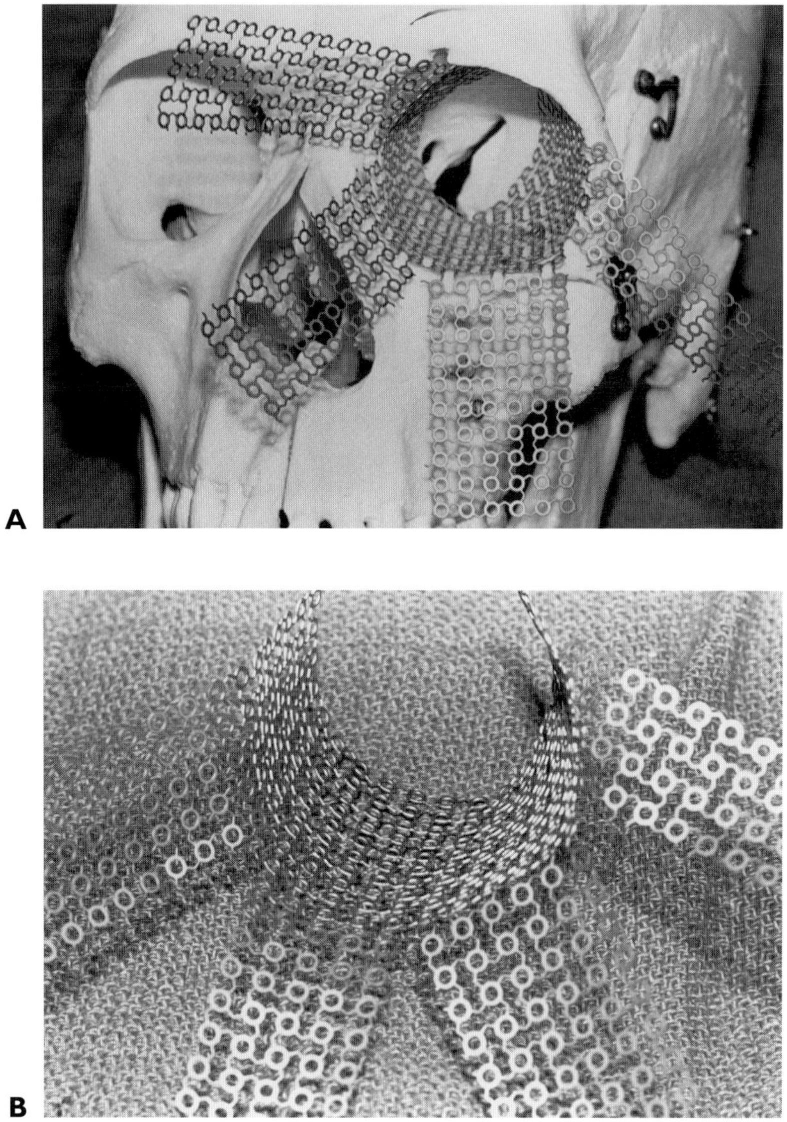

Figure 8-9. *(A)* Intraoperative formation of orbital reconstructive plate on skull model. *(B)* Close-up view of contoured orbital mesh (Leibinger; dynamic mesh). *(Figure continues.)*

used, with straight or angulated hand pieces. It comes with appropriate long attachments suitable for deep central skull base surgery. Cutting as well as diamond burrs are used with suction irrigation. For adequate microsurgical visualization, the Zeiss microscope on a Contraves stand is very useful. Bipolar cautery is essential. Bone plating systems are available from several manufacturers. I have used sets from Leibinger, Synthes, and Howmedica.

Postoperative Management

Most patients are extubated at the completion of skull base surgery. Elective temporary tracheostomy is performed in patients with palatal transections. All suction drains maintain vacuum through a closed bulb system or a wall unit. External dressing is seldom used. Arterial and central venous pressure lines remain in during the immediate postoperative period as does the Foley catheter. Both lower extremities

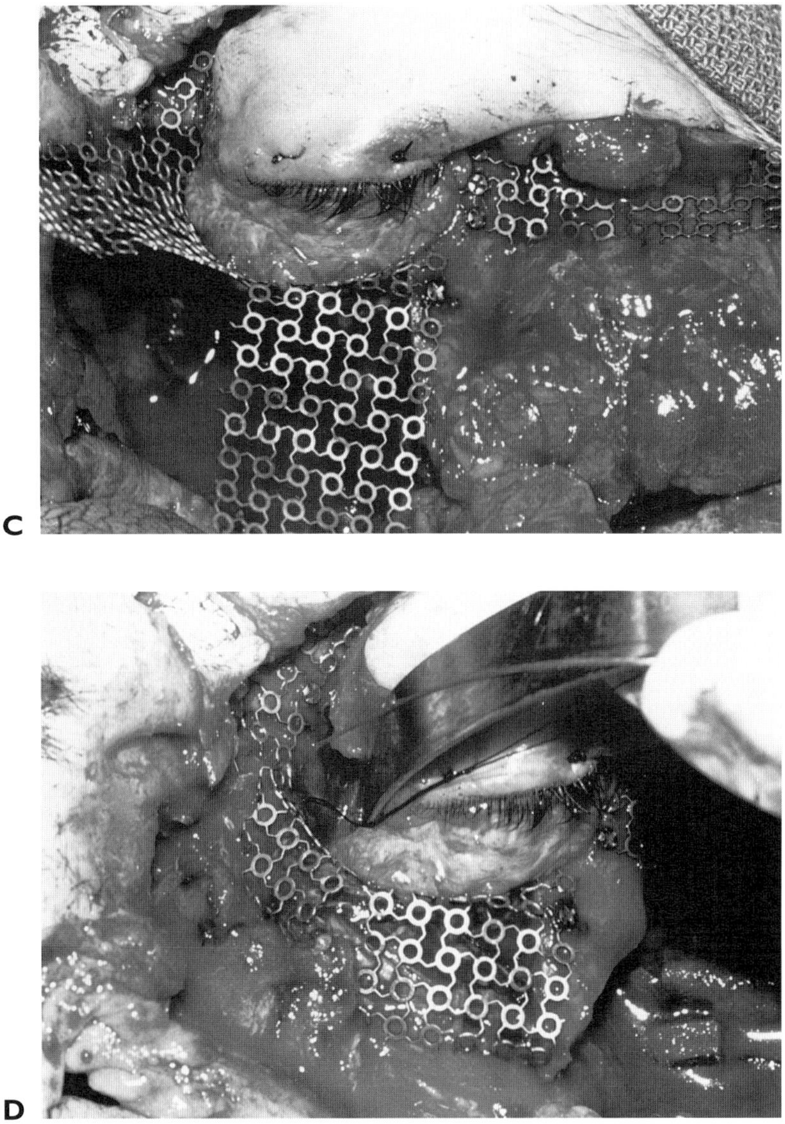

Figure 8-9 (Continued). (C) Inserted contoured mesh into left orbit with lateral screw fixation. *(D)* Inserted mesh with medial screw fixation in left orbit.

are covered with intermittent air compression stockings to maintain venous circulation. Once ambulation is resumed, they are discontinued. Nasogastric tube is connected to a low suction until bowel activity resumes. Tube feeding is started and continued until oral intake is resumed. Antibiotic coverage is usually discontinued after 48 to 72 hours. If spinal drain is in place, 50 to 75 cc are removed every shift for 2 to 4 days. A CT scan is done within the first 24 to 48 hours to ascertain the immediate postsurgical changes (looking for collections of blood, CSF, or air). General systemic as well as neurologic examinations are continued throughout the postoperative period.

Complications

Complications at the skull base may be quite hazardous. The major complications tend to fall into three categories: bleeding, infection, and wound healing problems.

The sometimes bothersome venous bleeding at the skull base is usually controlled intraoperatively with bone wax or Gelfoam. Arterial bleeding may be encountered from the vertebral as well as the carotid arteries. Repair should be attempted following application of temporary vascular clips.

Infection is often the result of the presence of nonvascularized tissue, postsurgical "dead space" or both. The transfer of the temporalis muscle provides vascularized reconstruction of the surgical defect. Postoperative CSF leakage with the threat of meningitis is also possible and should be treated aggressively with spinal drainage, reoperation, or both. Beta-2-transferrin electrophoresis of suspected fluid is currently the most accurate test to document CSF leakage.

Wound healing problems are more frequent in patients who have had previous surgery and/or radiotherapy. They include minor or major tissue necrosis. When it develops the extent of local wound care is dependent on the size and location of the necrosis. When it overlies an essential structure, surgical debridement and vascularized tissue transfer are indicated.

Certain surgical steps lessen the potential for complications. First and foremost is the assurance of displaced tissue viability. This requires detailed knowledge of the vascular anatomy and judicial use of electrocoagulation. The use of vascularized muscle transfer (temporalis or microvascular flap) to provide vascularized coverage of the surgical site is the second essential element in lessening the risk of postoperative complications. This step also increases the chances for a seal of the CSF-containing space. When pharyngeal or palatal incisions or both are also used for exposure, a layered closure with mattress sutures should be performed.

References

Altemir FH (1986) Transfacial access to the retromaxillary area. J Maxillofac Surg 14:119–182

Barbosa J (1961) Surgery of extensive cancer of paranasal sinuses. Arch Otolaryngol 73:129

Janecka IP (1993) Transfacial approaches to the skull and upper cervical spine. In: Neurological Operative Atlas. Vol. 3. No. 3. Williams & Wilkins, Baltimore

Janecka IP (1996) Transfacial approaches to the skull base. In Myers CN (ed): Operative Otolaryngology. WB Saunders, Philadelphia

Janecka IP, Sen Ch, Sekhar LN, Arriaga M (1990) Facial translocation: a new approach to the cranial base. Otolaryngol Head Neck Surg 103:413–419

9

Surgical Approaches to the Orbit

Spiros A. Lazarou

Orbital decompression in Grave's disease, tumor extirpation, and trauma make up the vast majority of indications for orbital surgery. In this chapter the osteotomies necessary to access and extirpate tumors as well as the variety of approaches for orbital decompression are reviewed.

Tumors affecting the orbit may originate intraorbitally, from the bone of the orbit itself, or extraorbitally (Table 9-1). The precise choice of approach, therefore, will depend on the size, location, and nature of the pathology as well as the experience and preferences of the surgeon (Fig. 9-1).

Most small benign soft tissue intraorbital tumors in the anterior half of the orbit may be approached anteriorly without the need for osteotomy. Often a medial or lateral rectus muscle may need to be disinserted from the globe to approach the tumor. Most other tumors will need an osteotomy of some kind.

Anterior superior benign soft tissue tumors may require a superior rim osteotomy for easier access. Benign soft tissue intraorbital lesions that do not reach the apex and are in the lateral half of the orbit may be approached extracranially through a lateral orbitotomy. Lesions approaching the apex, large benign tumors, tumors of intracranial origin, tumors of bony origin, and all skull base malignancies of extraorbital origin require a more extensive transcranial or transfacial approach. Tumors of intracranial origin may require frontal or frontotemporal craniotomy followed by the removal of superior and lateral rims and orbital walls along with the zygoma and zygomatic arch as needed depending on the location of the lesion. Tumors of centromedial origin require a face-splitting approach with removal of the medial orbit necessitating reconstruction of medial canthi and possibly the lacrimal system. Tumors of inferior origin may require partial or total removal of the zygoma, maxilla, or both as well. Malignancies of intraorbital origin require exenteration. Aggressive, extensive malignancies in, or invading, the orbit may require total en bloc orbitectomy. This chapter, being oriented toward skull base surgery, concentrates mainly on those procedures involving an osteotomy.

The orbit itself is a cavity surrounded by cavities. These include the anterior and middle fossae; the infratemporal fossae; the nose, nasopharynx, and nasolacrimal duct canal; and the maxillary, frontal, and ethmoid sinuses. Tumors may invade the orbit by direct bony extension or via foramina, for example, meningiomas from the middle cranial fossa.

Table 9-1. Tumor Origination

Tumors of intraorbital origin
Benign
Schwannoma
Glioma
Meningioma
Vascular lesions
Hemangioma
Arteriovenous malformation (AVM)
Lymphangioma
Neurofibroma
Malignant
Rhabdomyosarcoma
Gliomas
Hemangioendotheliomas
Hemangiopericytoma
Melanoma
Retinoblastoma
Medulloepithelioma
Neurofibrosarcoma
Lacrimal adenocarcinoma
Tumors of osseous and cartilaginous origin
Benign
Osteoma
Osteoid osteoma
Osteoblastoma
Chondroma
Hemangioendothelioma
Malignant
Osteosarcoma
Chondrosarcoma
Myeloma
Chordoma
Ewing's sarcoma
Pseudotumors of bone
Aneurysmal bone cyst
Fibrous dysplasia
Brown tumor
Giant cell reparative granuloma
Eosinophilic granuloma
Ossifying fibroma
Hand-Schüller-Christian disease
Tolosa-Hunt syndrome
Tumors of extraorbital origin
Benign
Neurofibroma
Meningioma
Pituitary adenoma
Neurinoma
Inverting papilloma
Fibroma (and related tumors)

(Continues)

Table 9-1. *(Continued)*

Malignant
Squamous cell cancer
Adenocarcinoma
Mucoepidermoid cancer
Adenoid cystic cancer
Melanoma
Basal cell cancer
Sebaceous cell cancer
Eccrine sweat gland cancer
Esthesioneuroblastoma
Glioblastoma
Fibrosarcoma
Fibrous histiocytoma
Lymphoma
Neurilemmoma
Liposarcoma
Fibrous histiocytoma
Meningioma
Hemangiopericytoma
Merkel's tumor
Metastatic tumors

Investigations

The history and physical examination determine the special investigations. Important signs and symptoms include visual impairment, impairment of eye movement, displacement of the eye, and malfunction of the lacrimal drainage system. Adjacent systems and structures must also be assessed such as airway passages and in particular cranial nerves V and VII.

Computed tomography (CT) with and without contrast is helpful when there is the possibility of bone involvement by invasion or mass effect. Most tumors can be defined and density differentiation can further enhance soft tissue delineation. Magnetic resonance imaging (MRI) is the definitive investigation for the orbit and can give precise soft tissue information. It is especially useful in studying optic nerve masses. Angiography may be performed if a vascular tumor is suspected. MR angiography is also an option. Occasionally orbital venography is useful. Special investigations to assess the lacrimal system may also be done. These include simple office examinations such as lacrimal irrigation, fluorescein dye test, saccharine taste test, and in unusual circumstances dacrocystography with radiopaque dyes.

Operative Procedures

Anterior Approaches

For the sake of completeness a few comments will be made on the anterior approaches that do not involve the skull base (Fig. 9-2). The orbit may be viewed as a four-sided cavity for surgical purposes. Therefore, anterior approaches to the orbit may be classified as medial, lateral, superior, inferior, or some combination thereof.

Medial. The orbit may be approached through a "C" incision centered 1 cm medial to the medial canthus for small tumors in the medial quadrant of the orbit that do

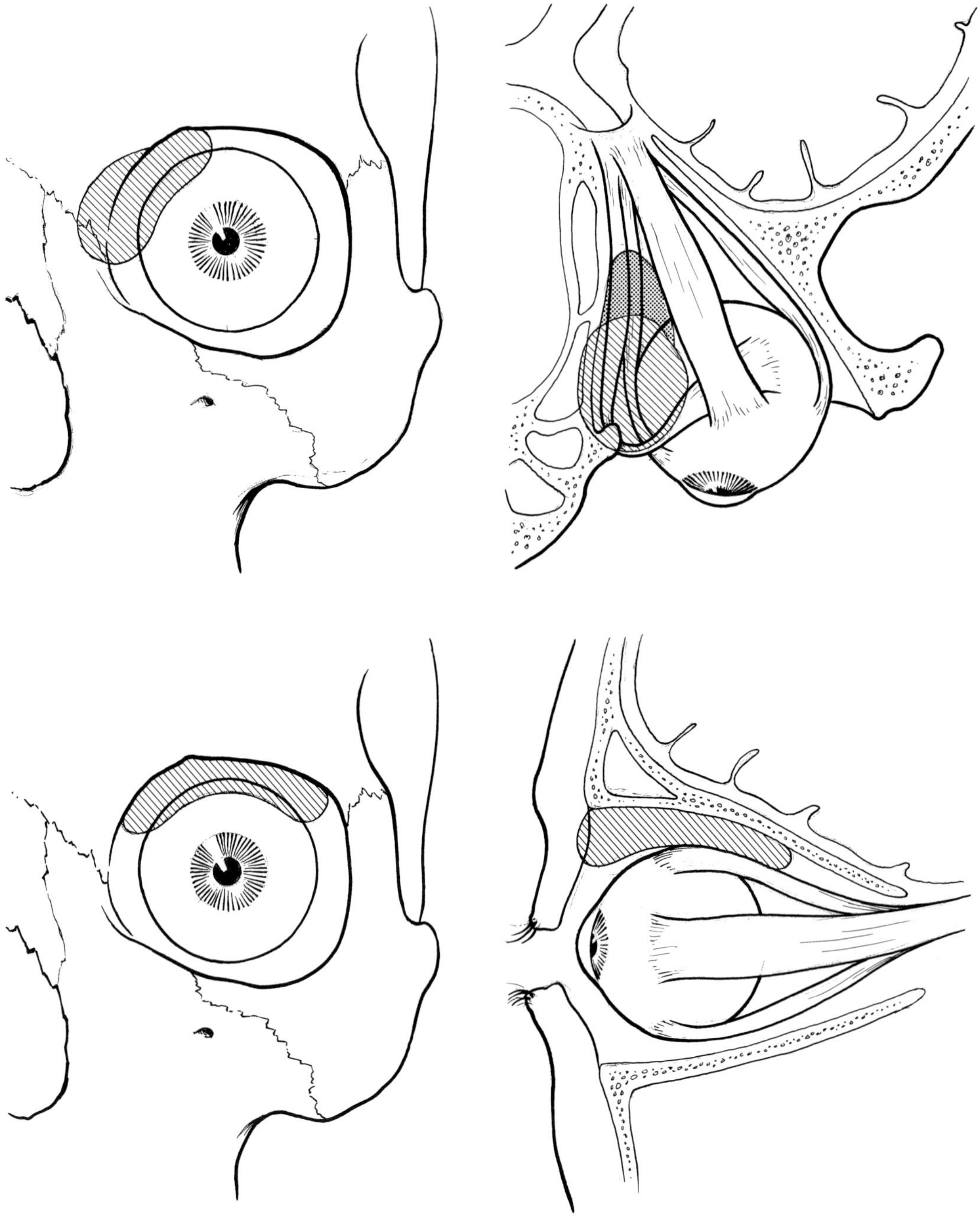

A

B

Figure 9-1. *(A)* The shaded area illustrates pathology approachable by a medial incision. The darker shaded area posteriorly may be difficult to reach by a simple medial incision. The experience and expertise of the individual surgeon will determine whether another approach is required. *(B)* The shaded area illustrates pathology best reached through a superior approach. *(Figure continues.)*

not reach the optic canal. Anatomically, one is limited inferiorly by the lacrimal system and medial canthi which, if detached, will need to be reconstructed. Often the medial rectus muscle needs to be detached from the globe for access as in the medial conjunctival incision. It is wise to place a limbal suture to allow globe rotation.

Inferior. Inferior approaches to the orbit may be accomplished through a variety of incisions. These include conjunctival, subciliary, and lower lid incisions. The antral

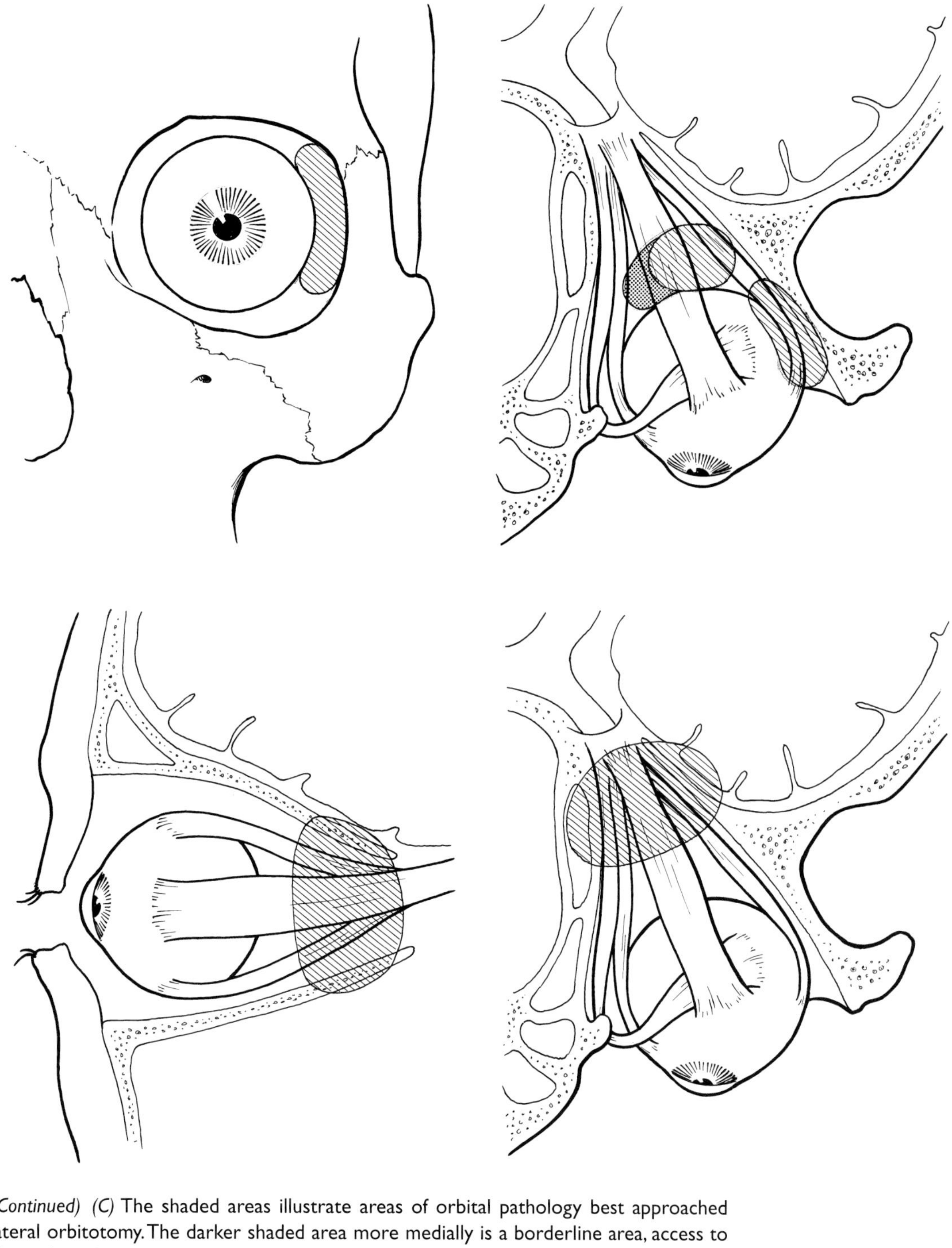

C

D

Figure 9-1 (Continued) (C) The shaded areas illustrate areas of orbital pathology best approached through a lateral orbitotomy. The darker shaded area more medially is a borderline area, access to which will depend on the experience of the surgeon. *(D)* The shaded area indicates orbital pathology best approached transcranially.

approach, intraorally, is of historic interest only. A subconjunctival incision may be used with or without a lateral canthal extension for increased access. I believe the extension directly from the corner of the lateral canthus leaves an aesthetically displeasing result. Therefore, the lateral extension is started 1 mm anterior to this (Fig. 9-2). Upon reaching the subciliary level, 1 or 2 mm below the lashes, one should continue laterally a few more millimeters as in a blepharoplasty and then diagonally downward into the crow's feet. A subciliary incision is placed 1 or 2 mm

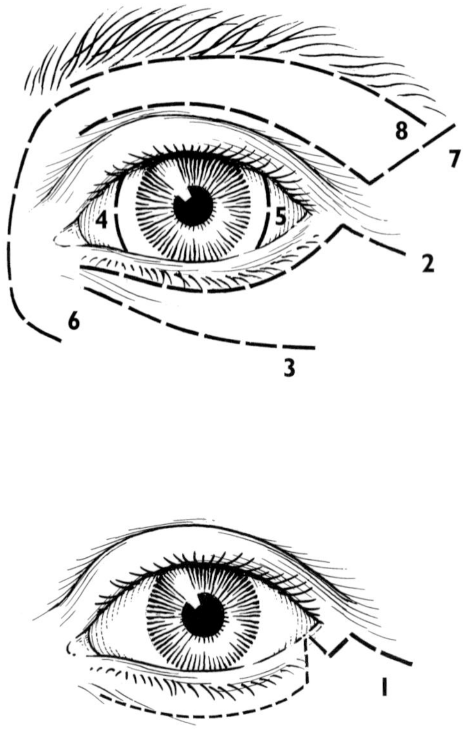

Figure 9-2. Anterior approaches. 1, Conjunctival with lateral extension. 2, Subciliary. 3, Infraorbital. 4, Medial globe. 5, Lateral globe. 6, Medial. 7, Upper lid. 8, Supraorbital.

below the lash. A lower lid incision is the most direct approach to the inferior orbital rim.

Lateral. A lateral conjunctival incision for small anterior tumors may be used in the lateral quadrant. The lateral rectus often needs to be detached from the globe.

Superior. An upper lid incision may be used as in a blepharoplasty, in which case repair of the levator muscle is required. A supraorbital rim incision may be used for an anterior tumor such as a neurofibroma, superior orbital schwannoma, dermoid cysts, or mucoceles. One can make this incision the full length of the supraorbital rim. If staying extraperiosteally then the incision is only through the skin and careful dissection follows. Injury to the superior orbital nerve (SON) should be avoided; the whereabouts of this nerve can be located by palpating the supraorbital notch. If the dissection is to be subperiosteal then the nerve must be dissected free of the notch.

Certain tumors may require the overhanging supraorbital rim to be osteotomized temporarily (Fig. 9-3). The SON must be dissected free of its notch in this case. Occasionally the nerve is encased in bone and this needs to be osteotomized with a chisel. The incision is made directly onto the ridge below the eyebrow. Subperiosteal dissection is continued when certain preservation of the SON is obtained. Clean entrances into the frontal sinus need no special reconstruction.

Lateral Orbitotomy Approach

A large number of benign intraorbital soft tissue tumors may be accessed through a lateral orbitotomy (Fig. 9-4). A lazy "S" incision over the lateral third of the eyebrow proceeding along the lateral rim and curving along the zygomatic arch may be performed (Fig. 9-4A) giving direct access to the lateral orbit. Lateral extension of the

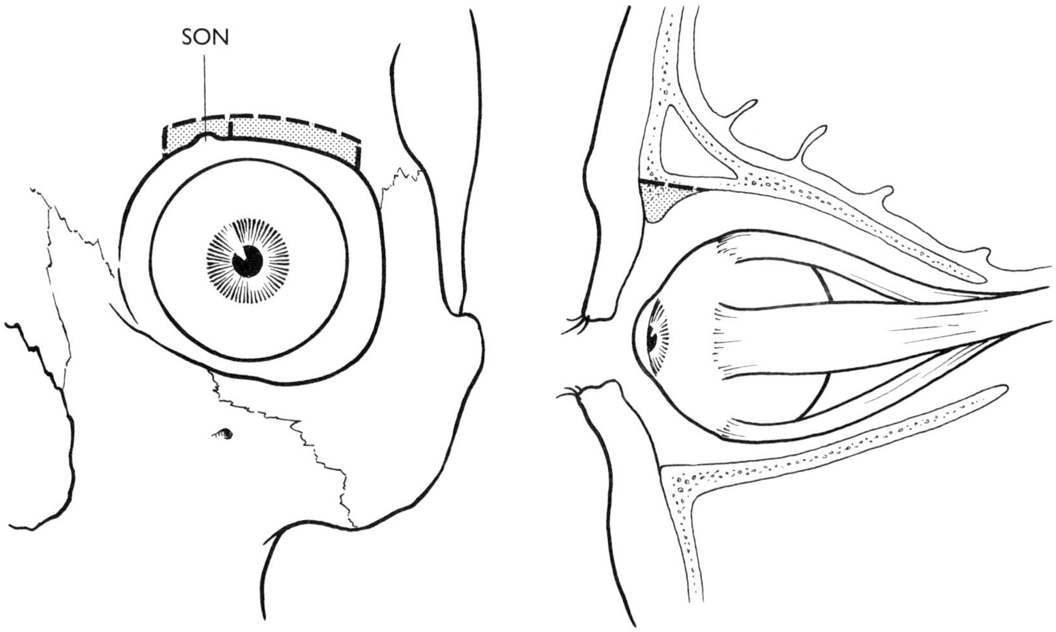

Figure 9-3. Osteotomy of the superior orbital ridge. There may be up to 1 cm of orbital contents behind the rim. The medial extension of the orbitotomy may vary. The supraorbital nerve (SON) must be dissected out of its notch if the osteotomy is to include this area.

incision is limited by the frontal branch of the facial nerve, which crosses the zygomatic arch 2 to 3 cm behind the lateral orbital rim. The incision is carried directly down to the bone (Fig. 9-4B). Subperiosteal dissection includes elevating and retracting the temporalis muscle until there is adequate visualization of the lateral wall. Subperiosteal dissection then continues around the rim intraorbitally (Fig. 9-4C). The zygomaticotemporal and zygomaticofacial nerves branch off the maxillary division of the trigeminal nerve and exit along the lateral wall. These, along with their accompanying artery, will need to be cauterized. The extent of the osteotomy (Fig. 9-4D) is decided and the bone removed. The osteotomy may be extended from just above the frontozygomatic suture area down to the zygoma and may include a variable part of the lateral orbital wall. The globe must be protected during the osteotomy with a ribbon retractor, and the temporalis muscle is retracted posteriorly. A reciprocating saw is used along with irrigation. The periorbitum is incised (Fig. 9-4E) and the dissection continues as required to remove the tumor.

An alternative approach involves the use of the bicoronal incision. With this one is able to access all but the inferior orbit through a combined intra- and extracranial approach if extension should prove necessary. There are benefits to this approach even if it is used only for extracranial access as with the lateral orbitotomy. This includes wider area of exposure without severe traction to tissues, avoidance of injury to the frontal branch of facial nerve, avoidance of visible scar, wider osteotomy, and visibility of the other side for comparison during reconstruction. One is also better prepared for unexpected findings. A bicoronal incision, in and of itself, does not prolong hospitalization.

Transcranial Approaches

For tumors requiring extra- and intracranial approach a bicoronal incision is used. This is preferable to a hemicoronal incision when that option is a possibility because if more exposure is required it is difficult to achieve without compromising aesthetic

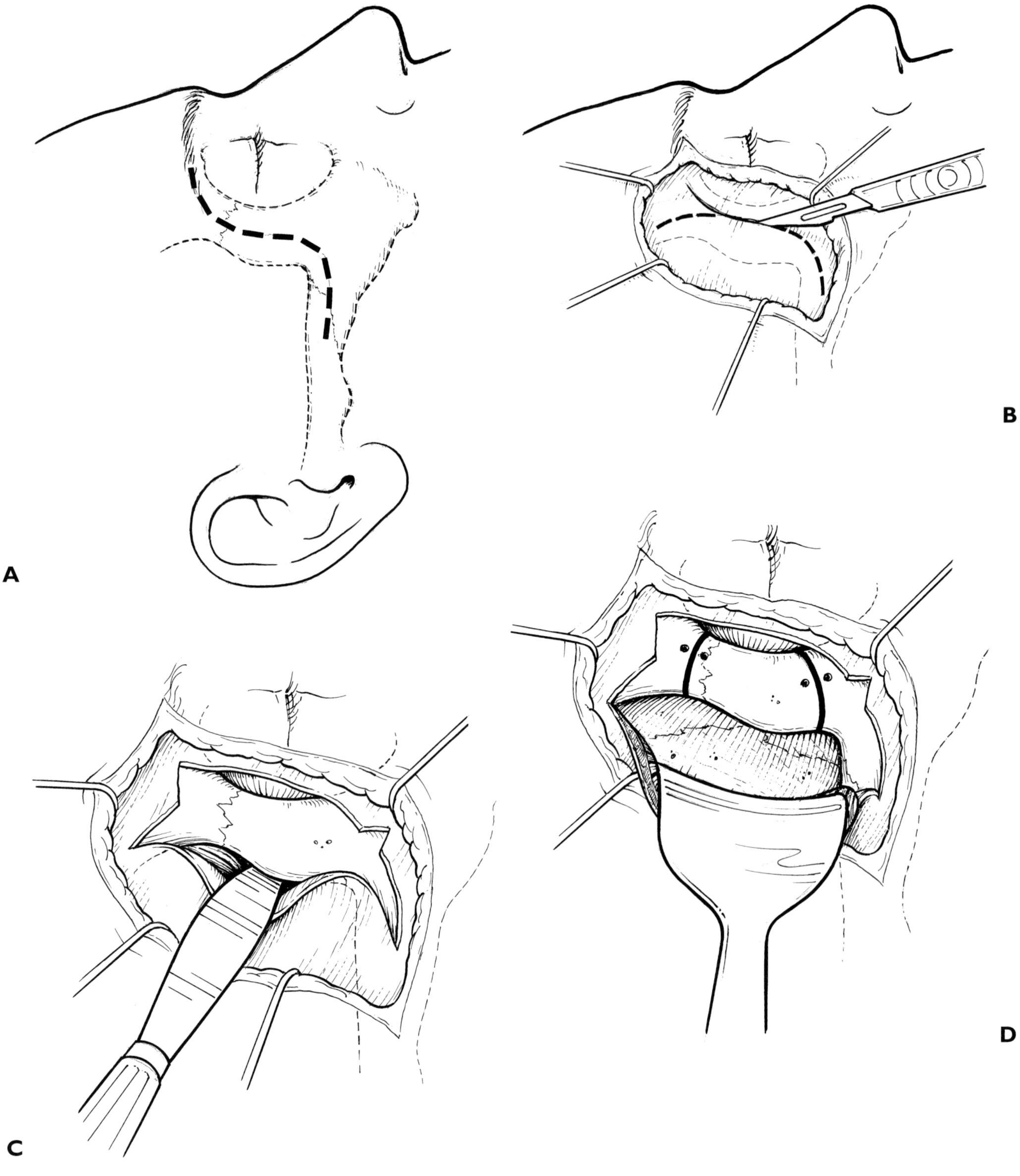

Figure 9-4. Lateral orbitotomy. *(A)* The incision should begin at the lateral third of the eyebrow, just above it and not in it. After following the frontal process of the zygoma it should continue no more than 3 cm along the superior margin of the zygomatic arch to avoid injury to the frontalis branches of the facial nerve. *(B)* After blunt dissection superficial to the temporalis fascia to elevate the skin, the periosteum and temporalis fascia is incised as shown with relaxing incisions as needed. *(C)* Subperiosteal dissection is performed around the rim into the orbit and the temporalis muscle is retracted posteriorly. *(D)* The osteotomy is performed with holes placed for reattachment. *(Figure continues.)*

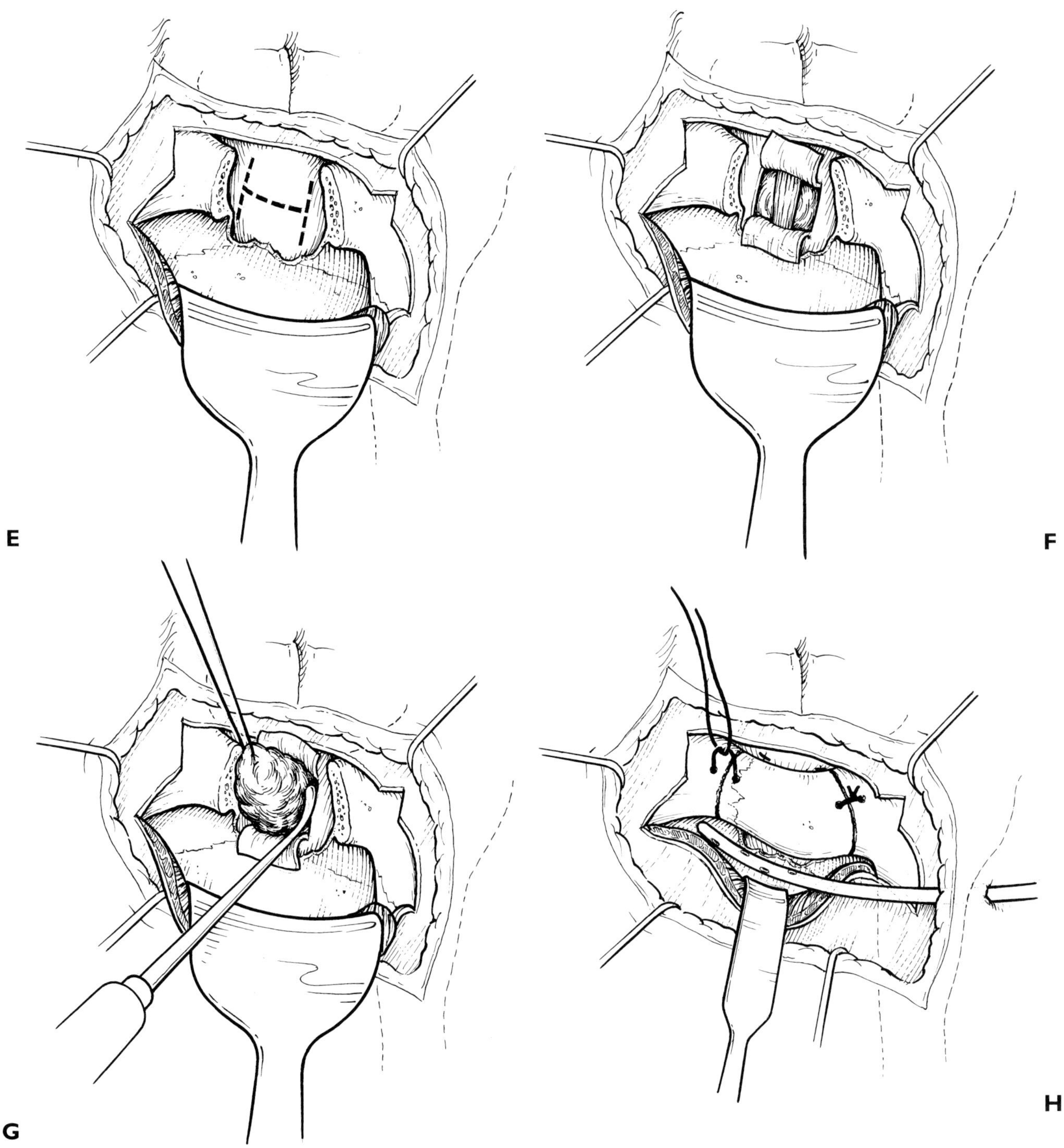

Figure 9-4 (Continued). (E) The periorbitum is opened with an "H"-shaped incision. *(F)* The lateral rectus muscle will be exposed and it is retracted as necessary to display the lesion. *(G)* Dissection and removal of tumor. *(H)* After closure of the periorbitum, the bone fragment is replaced and connected with nonabsorbable sutures. The wound is closed over a drain.

results and one has the opposite side to compare for reconstructive purposes. Indeed, a bicoronal incision is necessary if the entire arch and lateral rim need to be adequately exposed.

A bicoronal incision is made from tragus to tragus with the ability for extension into the neck. The incision should pass through the vertex of the skull not anteriorly just behind the hairline. This separates the skin incision from the craniotomy effectively placing a vascularized flap over the osteotomy; moreover, less of the scalp is denervated, the scar is better concealed and may be easily zigzagged for even greater concealment, and there is better access to the temporalis muscle, which may need to be used for reconstruction and to create larger periosteal or galeofrontalis flaps should they be required.

The dissection is subperiosteal to the supraorbital rims and continues thus into the orbits. If a periosteal flap is needed for repair, it is raised later with the adjacent areolar tissue at the time it is required. Care is taken to avoid injury to the supraorbital nerves. Medially the dissection continues to the root of the nose. If the medial canthus needs to be taken down this should have been tagged with a suture prior to starting the coronal incision. The nasolacrimal sac and duct are also dissected and retracted if needed. In the temporalis area the dissection is subgaleal until the temporal fat pad is encountered. This fat pad has anteriorly the anterior deep temporalis fascia and posteriorly the posterior deep temporalis fascia, which overlies the muscle. One must enter the fat pad and continue the dissection in this plane, deep to the anterior deep temporalis fascia, down to the zygomatic arch (Fig. 9-5). The fat pad is vascular. This maneuver avoids the possibility of injury to the frontal branch of the facial nerve. One may maintain essentially the entire fat pad on the skin flap until the level of the arch where it is transected from its buccal extension. Subperiosteal dissection then continues sharply along the zygomatic process of the frontal bone where the temporalis ends and continues along the frontal process of the zygoma as far as the infraorbital rim and malar area and continues intraorbitally to almost the apex, which lies roughly 4 cm behind the rim. Dissection of the temporalis muscle from the skull starts at the level of the zygomatic arch and proceeds superiorly. If one attempts to elevate the temporalis from above, the muscle has a greater likelihood of being torn. One should leave a small rim of periosteum along the border of the muscle superiorly in order to have something sturdy to pass a suture through.

A frontal craniotomy may now be performed with a lateral or temporal extension. Dural elevation continues until the brain is adequately retracted and protected. The superior and lateral orbital rims are removed en bloc along with lateral and superior orbital walls as needed to access a large intraorbital tumor (Fig. 9-6). The lateral osteotomy may extend onto and include the zygoma and arch. In this case one has to dissect free the masseter muscle. Clean osteotomy through the frontal sinus does not require obliteration of the sinus. Basically, one designs the osteotomy that is needed to remove the tumor.

Placing a ribbon retractor of appropriate size between the brain and the bone and another between the orbital contents and the bone, a fine blade reciprocating saw is used starting medially along the superior orbital rim and proceeding posteriorly. The direction is parallel to the medial orbital wall. Saline irrigation is liberally used. Injury is avoided to the cribriform plate. The extent is as posterior as needed but stops prior to the sphenoid. The saw is then moved laterally to cut down the greater wing of the sphenoid. Again the orbital contents are protected. The osteotomy stops upon reaching the desired inferior location. The lateral rim is then osteotomized with the reciprocating saw, again protecting the orbital contents. The lateral rim itself may be cut at a variety of levels, for example, the root of the rim itself, extend-

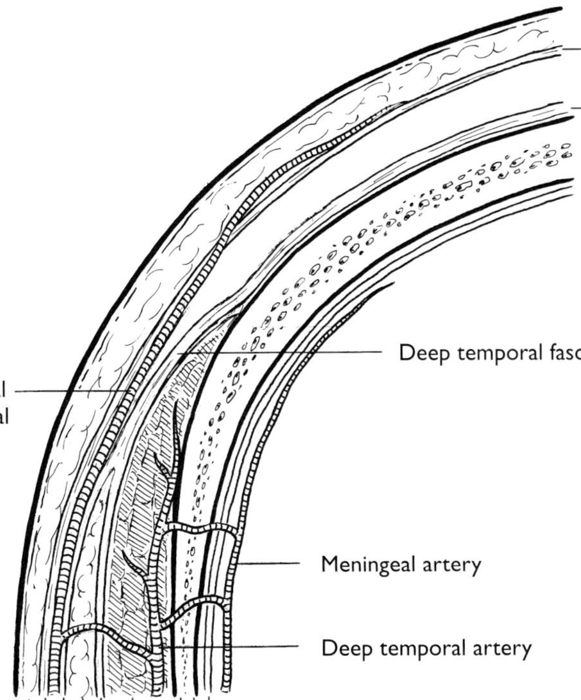

Figure 9-5. The deep temporal fascia (DTF) is very important. It is continuous with the periosteum superiorly. Over the temporalis muscle it divides into a superficial and deep layer between which is the temporal fat pad, which is continuous with the buccal fat pad. To avoid injury to the frontalis branches of the facial nerve one must enter this fat pad as the dissection continues toward the zygomatic arch. There may also be fat between the superficial temporal fascia (continuous with the galea) and the DTF, which must not be confused with the fat pad between deep and superficial layers of the DTF.

ing onto the zygoma, or through the malar eminence and including the arch. The maxillary sinus is avoided. A small osteotome is then used to connect the medial and lateral osteotomies along the roof of the orbit and the entire segment is removed en bloc. A high-speed diamond burr, rongeurs, or both are used to expose the superior orbital fissure. Removal of zygoma and arch allows access to the pterygopalatine and infratemporal fossa. Resection of the tumor begins.

In the case of fibrous dysplasia the entire diseased bone is removed. This may involve the removal of the entire anterior cranial base with opening of the optic canals and supraorbital fissures. In this case autogenous bone grafts will be required to reconstruct the orbits as necessary as well as the central portion of the cranial base where the crista galli was resected. A pericranial flap is essential to separate the brain form the nasal cavities. (See Chs. 4 and 23.)

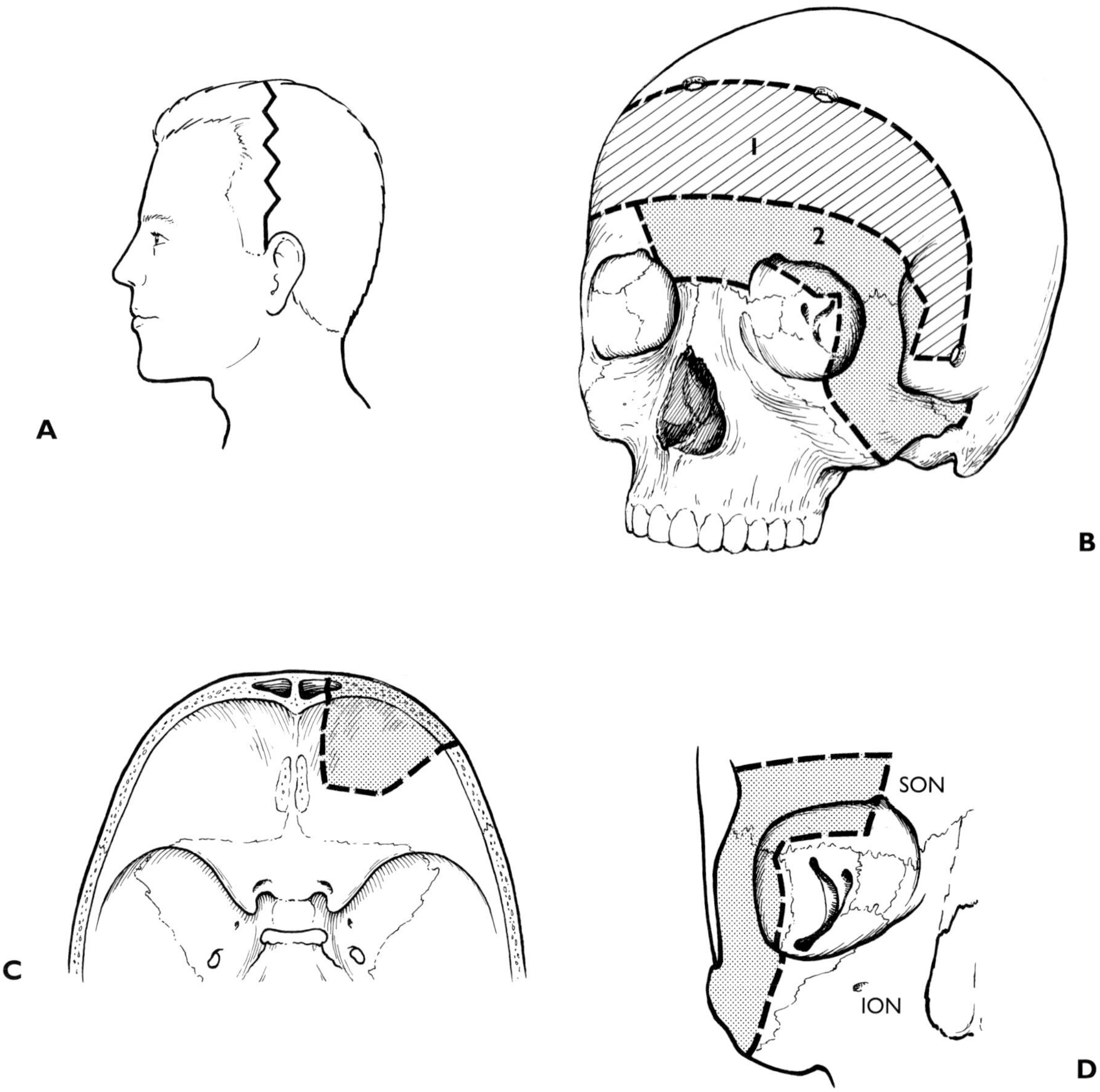

Figure 9-6. Transcranial approach to the orbit. *(A)* Zigzag coronal incision, preauricular to preauricular. The periosteum is elevated with the scalp in case a pericranial flap is needed later for repair. *(B)* The craniotomy (1) may be extended as far laterally as required and, similarly, the extent of the orbital rim osteotomy (2) is determined by the particular pathology of each case. Normally less bone removal will be required than the maximal osteotomy illustrated here. *(C)* Osteotomy of the orbital roof. *(D)* The typical extent of intraorbital osteotomy. (For explanation of abbreviations see Appendix 1, p. 373.)

One part of the orbit that is difficult to reach by conventional approaches is the area of the posterior intraconal space, inferior and medial to the optic nerve (Fig. 9-1A & C). It could be approached transethmoidally (see Ch. 6). Recently Hassler et al. (1994) have described an approach transcranially from the contralateral pterional region.

Intraorbital Dissection

In dissecting an intraorbital tumor one must avoid bleeding in order to have a clear visual field. Depending on the tumor, as the subperiosteal dissection occurs in the orbit there are a number of perforating vessels that are best cauterized at this time. These include the anterior and posterior ethmoidal arteries medially and the temporozygomatic and zygomaticofacial arteries laterally. Additionally one must make every effort to avoid injury to cranial nerves III, IV, and VI. The trochlear nerve is particularly prone to injury where it crosses from lateral to medial as it exits the superior orbital fissure and turns medially over the superior orbital muscles. The nerve needs to be retracted laterally and medially with the muscles as needed.

Face-Splitting Approach

A medial orbital malignancy such as a chondrosarcoma or ethmoidal adenocarcinoma requires a combined bicoronal and face-splitting approach. The face-splitting incision (Fig. 9-7) begins at the bicoronal incision centrally and continues down the middle of the forehead to the nose at which point it may go down the dorsum of the nose or toward the right or left medial canthus; from the canthus it continues paranasally around the ala and down the philtrum of the lip, depending on the exact location of the lesion. The medial canthi are tagged prior to raising the skin flaps. Subperiosteal dissection continues along the medial orbit. The anterior ethmoidal artery is met about 2 cm into the orbit along the medial wall followed by the posterior ethmoidal artery. Both are cauterized. The lacrimal sac and nasolacrimal duct are retracted laterally. The osteotomies (Fig. 9-8) may begin along the medial orbital wall, inferiorly, continue anteriorly into the lacrimal fossa, and, via the inferior rim, onto the maxilla and pyriform aperture. Occasionally the nasolacrimal duct (NLD) will have to be transected for wider osteotomy and exposure. Intracranially the osteotomies of the medial orbits are connected with the roof osteotomies on either side of the cribriform plate and continue anteriorly through the frontal sinus on either side. The lateral extent of the superior orbital rim osteotomy is the supraorbital notch. The roof incisions are connected on either side behind the cribriform

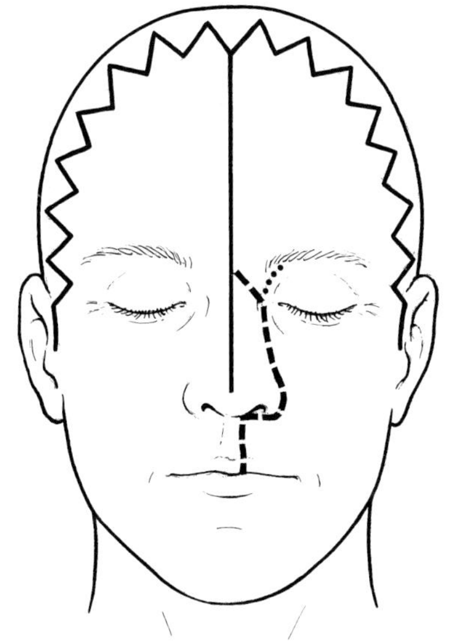

Figure 9-7. Incisions for the face-splitting approach. From the bicoronal incision, a facial incision may extend down the middle of the nose (solid line) or be diverted paranasally down to include the lip (broken line). For some smaller or benign lesions a shorter incision beginning at the eyebrow (dotted line) and continuing paranasally is appropriate.

plate. The vomer is transected. The bony segment is removed en bloc. After removing the tumor the segment is replaced and stabilized with plates and screws.

In the case of a benign tumor such as juvenile angiofibroma involving the paranasal sinuses and extending to the orbit where a paranasal incision may be used, the NLD may be exposed by unroofing of the maxilla. The skin incision (Fig. 9-7) begins below the eyebrow, continues 1 cm medial to the medial canthus, then paranasally, around the ala and down the philtrum of the lip. After the maxilla is removed the orifice of the NLD in the nasal mucosa is cut with a rim of nasal mucosa around it and the whole duct retracted. After removal of the tumor the duct is resutured to the nasal mucosa. It is helpful to inject a small amount of methylene blue (≤ .5 cc) preoperatively into the sac so as to see the sac and duct during dissection; but, as accidental opening will stain the field with the dye, larger amounts should not be used.

Orbitectomy

En bloc orbitectomies are performed for malignancies of the orbit and lacrimal gland. The goal is cure. Certain recurrent tumors of skin origin may not require removal of all the orbital contents. A normal anatomic layer beyond the tumor must be taken to reduce the risk of recurrence. This almost always means bone and sometimes dura. A bicoronal incision and anterior craniotomy are performed. The placement of the anterior incision required to access the inferior orbit and maxilla will need to be modified depending on the location and nature of the tumor. In a globe tumor the lids and even the lashes may be spared depending on the reconstruction planned. On the other hand, an ocular malignant melanoma will require skin margins that extend onto the forehead and cheek necessitating repair with a free flap. A lacrimal gland carcinoma may necessitate the removal of the eyelids, including the brow and skin innervated by the zygomaticotemporal nerve. If the maxilla is to be removed a buccal

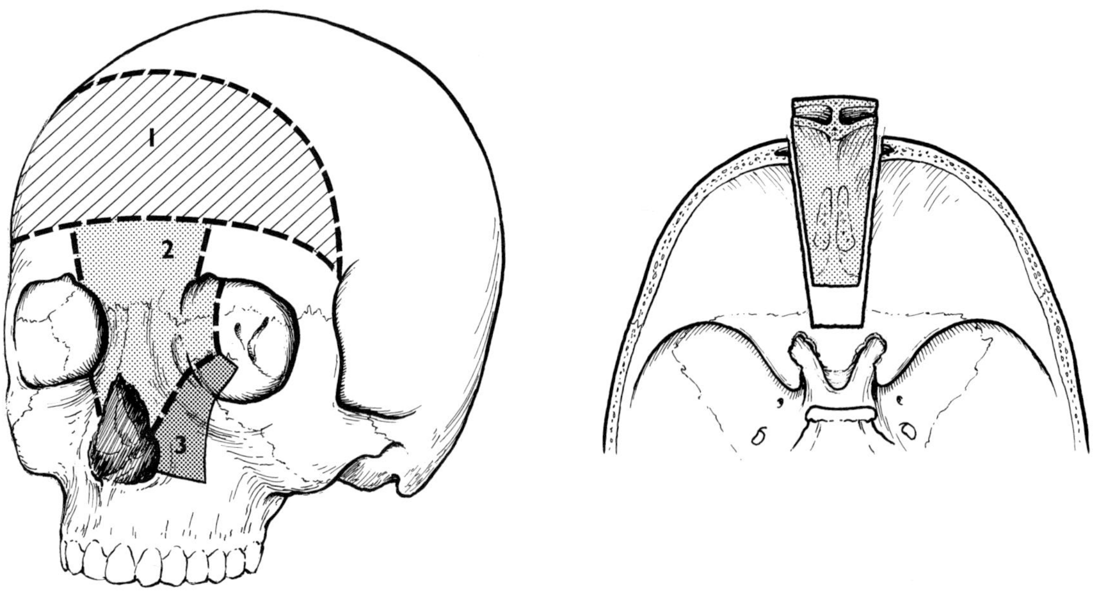

Figure 9-8. Frontonasal craniotomy. Following the elevation of the frontal flap (1), the frontonasal segment (2) is osteotomized and removed. The exposure may extend to the maxilla (3). If the osteotomy extends past the nasolacrimal duct or medial canthal tendon these must be electively reconstructed.

incision will also be necessary. The posterior extent of the orbitectomy may also vary. Sacrificed skin is left attached to bone.

An extensive orbitectomy is described (Fig. 9-9). After the bicoronal flap has been raised, the anterior (periorbital) incision is performed in the chosen area. Subperiosteal dissection is then completed and an anterolateral craniotomy is performed. The frontal dura is mobilized so as to expose the superior orbital fissure and its contents. This involves dissection along the sphenoidal wing to the anterior clinoid process and tuberculum sellae. In a lateral tumor, as in the lacrimal gland, the medial orbital wall may be spared, hence, the periorbitum is elevated along the medial wall. The osteotomy is then performed along the superomedial orbital wall junction sparing the cribriform plate. Otherwise for total orbitectomy the osteotomy is through the cribriform area so as to include the medial orbital wall. The supraorbital ridge is cut either sparing the medial wall or more medial to include it. The osteotomy continues inferiorly medial to the medial rim sparing the nasal bones then moving inferolaterally below the infraorbital nerve to include the zygoma. The zygomatic arch is cut anteriorly. A lateral osteotomy is made into the temporalis fossa and continues medially into the middle cranial fossa avoiding the lateral wall of the orbit and reaching just anterior to the foramen rotundum. This osteotomy is connected to the medial end of the superior orbital fissure and, by a cut through the anterior "body" of the anterior clinoid process (avoiding any damage to the carotid artery), to the posterior end of the medial osteotomy.

Reconstruction

Reconstruction of all defects begins during the preoperative planning stage when the approach, incisions, and osteotomies are planned. Proper planning allows the best postoperative results. The goals of orbital reconstruction include:

1. Re-establishment of stable three-dimensional framework.
2. Separation from adjacent craniofacial units (antrum, paranasal sinuses, cranium).
3. Proper positioning of the globe relative to the opposite side by adjusting orbital volume.
4. Soft tissue reconstruction to match as much as possible the opposite side.

In skull base tumors this is achieved within the broader context of separating the intracranial contents from the extracranial contents. Cerebrospinal fluid (CSF) containment and dead space obliteration are achieved with the use of local or distant vascularized flaps. This has dramatically reduced the occurrence of ascending infection and meningitis with resulting loss of nonvascularized grafts and possibly death. The most commonly used flaps are the periosteal, galeofrontalis, and temporalis muscle flaps. There are a growing variety of free flaps available (see Ch. 22).

Osseointegration techniques allow prosthetics of increased stability and are another excellent option in the reconstructive choices available. This involves the placement of titanium pins in available orbital bone followed by the attachment via magnets of the prosthesis.

Orbital Decompression

Finally, mention will be made of orbital decompression techniques, which for the most part are done for the treatment of raised intraorbital pressure due to Graves' disease. Candidates generally have proptosis and gaze limitation. CT or MRI demonstrates enlarged extraocular muscles. High-dose steroids have failed. The treatment of choice is a two-wall decompression. There are a number of options and approaches

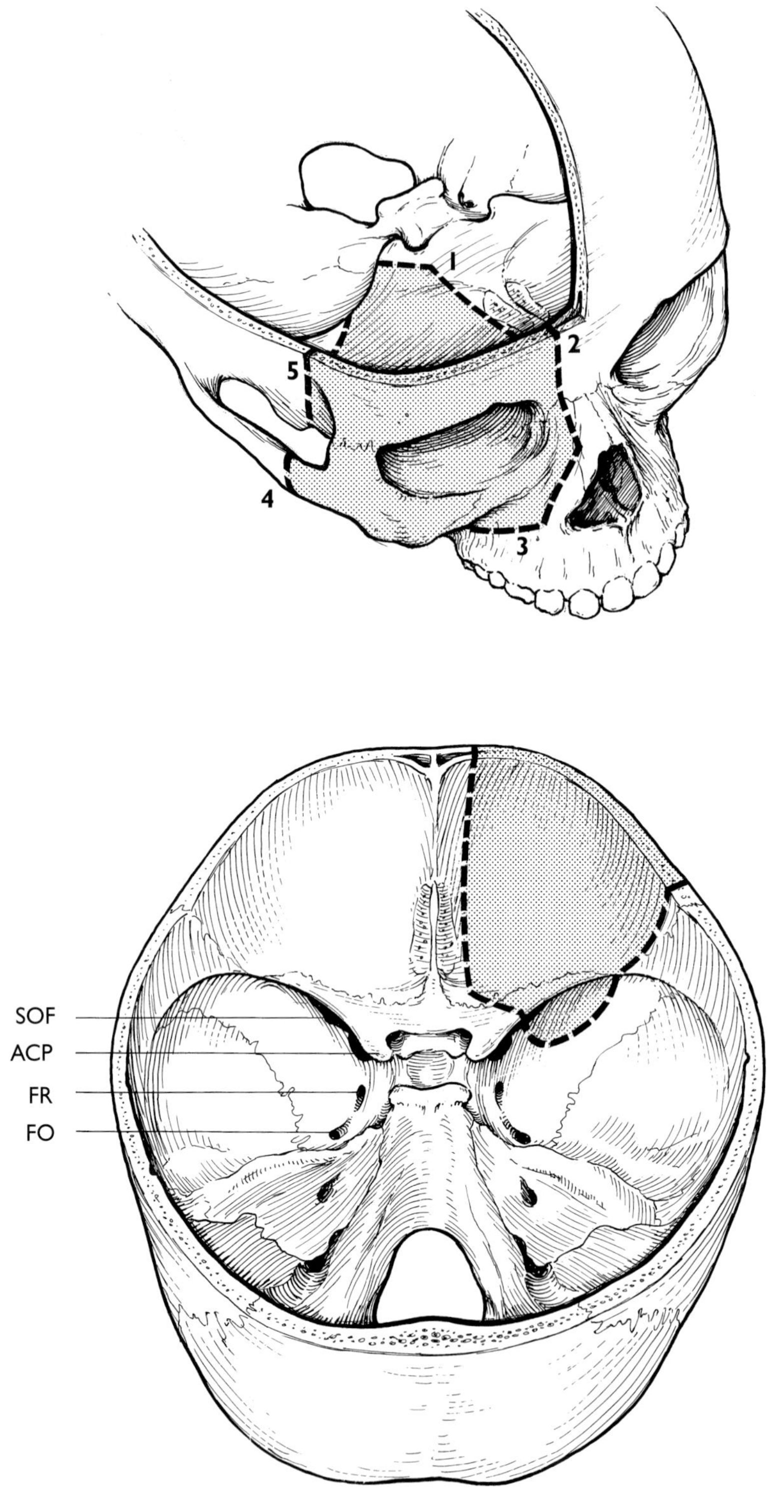

Figure 9-9. Orbitectomy. 1, Osteotomy through the anterior cranial fossa parallel to the cribriform area and ending in front of the anterior clinoid process at the region of the superior orbital fissure. 2, Osteotomy through the supraorbital ridge and nasal bones to the maxilla below the infraorbital nerve (ION). 3, The cut continues across the maxilla to include the anterior, lateral, posterior, and part of the medial wall of the maxillary sinus (but not the pterygoid). 4, The zygomatic arch is cut. 5, The greater wing of the sphenoid is cut in the temporal fossa, continuing posteromedially behind the orbit toward the foramen rotundum. This cut is joined to the first through the superior orbital fissure.

depending on one's specialty, background, and preferences. Many prefer the removal of the medial and inferior floors (Fig. 9-10), a procedure that may be performed endoscopically (see Ch. 6). The alternative macroscopic approach may be through a Caldwell Luc, ethmoidectomy, or lower lid incision. The latter may be a conjunctival incision with lateral extension or a subciliary incision. The Caldwell Luc approach results in a very high incidence of extraocular muscle imbalance presumably due to removal of more apical bone under direct vision. On the other hand, although there is minimal muscle imbalance with the lid approaches there is a slightly higher failure rate requiring supplemental surgery or irradiation. An intranasal approach to remove the medial and inferior walls is preferred by others. Those with a neurosurgical background may have a preference for removal of the superior and lateral walls through a lateral orbitotomy approach (Fig. 9-10), although without osteotomy of the orbital rim. Severe cases require a four-wall decompression. This may be done through an anterior craniotomy or a lateral orbitotomy approach in combination with the surgeon's preference for inferomedial wall removal. Three-wall decompression, that is, including the lateral with the inferomedial, has not been proven to increase success rate over a two-walled decompression.

In the lower lid approach a subciliary or conjunctival incision with lateral canthal extension is chosen. In the subciliary approach an incision is made identical to that done for blepharoplasty. Starting at the beginning of the medial lashes 1 mm below the lashes the incision extends laterally to the lateral fornix and then sharply angles downward into the crow's feet. A skin muscle flap is raised. The orbital fascia is encountered and followed down to the orbital rim. The periosteum is incised along the full length of the inferior orbital rim. Subperiosteal dissection then occurs from the nasolacrimal duct lateral to and including the lateral canthal tendon, posteriorly to the edge of the antrum and medially to the anterior and posterior ethmoidal arteries, which is the upper limit of the osteotomy. The bone to be removed is extremely thin and one may punch through it with the periosteal elevator. Care is taken to avoid injury to the inferior orbital nerve and artery, which can be seen under the floor of the orbit as a slight discoloration and posteriorly as a hump on the floor. Once the bone is removed the periorbitum is incised coronally posterior to the infe-

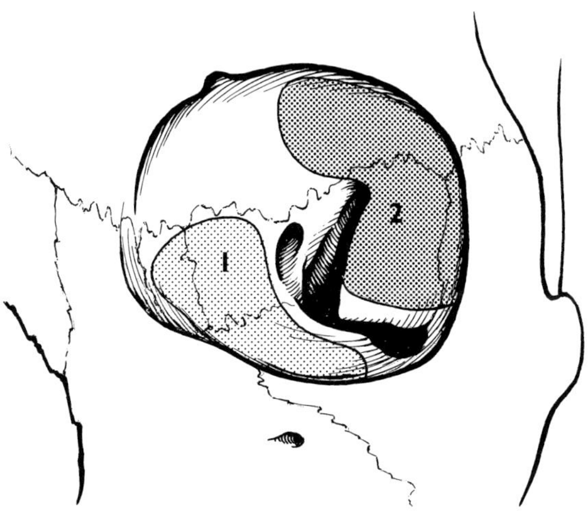

Figure 9-10. The extent of two-wall orbital decompressions. 1, Medial and inferior. 2, Lateral and superior.

rior oblique muscle and sagittally on either side of the rectus muscle. The periosteum is then peeled anterior to posterior into the maxillary sinus. Orbital fat will expand into the sinus. To prevent retrobulbar hemorrhage or neuromuscular injury avoid grasping the fat. A lateral canthoplasty is then performed by attaching the lateral canthal tendon with a Prolene or wire stitch through a drill hole in the lateral rim at the level of Whitnall's tubercle. A few sutures may be placed to close the periosteum along the inferior rim followed by 6–0 silk for the skin.

A conjunctival incision is placed just below the inferior edge of the tarsal plate. I do not take this to the lateral fornix as the scar is displeasing. One mm before the fornix one exits the lid and then continues, as for a subciliary incision, laterally and then into the crow's feet. Having incised the conjunctiva the capsulopalpebral fascia is incised and the periosteum is exposed. The procedure then continues as previously described.

For the removal of the superior and lateral walls the incision is as for lateral orbitotomy. A burr hole is made in the greater wing of the sphenoid over the confluence of the lateral wall, superior wall, and anterior cranial fossa. Periorbitum and dura are carefully elevated and, using rongeurs, the lateral and superior walls are removed.

In the Caldwell Luc approach an incision is made in the buccal mucosa on the side of the antrum to be entered. A cuff of mucosa, muscle, and periosteum on the gingival side is left so there is something to sew to at the end. Visualizing Stensen's duct prior to the incision and adjusting the lateral end of the incision accordingly will avoid injury to this duct. Generally, one need not go beyond the second bicuspid. The incision goes directly down to bone and subperiosteal dissection is accomplished. This is best done medially along the pyriform buttress and then medially along the maxillary zygomatic buttress so as to avoid injury to the infraorbital nerve, which soon comes into view with the medial and lateral dissection. An osteotome is then used to enter the sinus and the anterior wall is removed, stopping before the infraorbital foramen is reached. Enough bone is removed to visualize the infraorbital floor and medial sinus wall.

The ethmoid air cells are removed first. The thin bone makes removal easy with a rongeur or curette. They are entered behind the nasolacrimal system. The cribriform plate lies superomedial to the posterior air cells and excessive pressure in this area may result in inadvertent entrance into the cranial cavity. Once mucosa is adequately stripped the inferior two-thirds of the thin orbital plate of the ethmoid is removed. Resection then continues laterally along the floor to or beyond the infraorbital nerve, which is visualized from the sinus below. A 2-mm ledge of posterior antrum is left. The periosteum is incised as previously described.

Postoperative Care

Tumors not requiring osteotomies do not necessarily require perioperative antibiotics. Osteotomies where a sinus was not entered may be covered with a broad-spectrum cephalosporin for 24 hours. Osteotomies involving entrance into nasal or oral cavities, combined with grafts and intracranial surgery require a longer period of antibiotic use. Head elevation and ice are helpful in controlling swelling. Vision and movement are checked. Where oculomotor nerves are retracted there may be paresis. One is vigilant for hematomas and CSF leaks in intracranial procedures. If a CSF leak is probable postoperatively then a spinal drain may be placed preoperatively; otherwise, one may be required postoperatively. All drains are removed as soon as they are no longer necessary.

Complications

Blindness can occur from accidental trauma to the optic nerve particularly when operating in the posterior ethmoid sinus. Often long periods of tension and compression will result in compromise of the blood supply to the optic nerve with resultant loss of vision. Additionally, central retinal artery or vein occlusion or both, vitreous hemorrhage, or retinal detachment may occur. Finally, if orbital fat dissection is not done with extreme caution to avoid bleeding a retrobulbar hemorrhage may occur that can also result in blindness. Pupil size and reaction must be checked every 15 minutes for the first 4 hours in the intensive care unit, then every hour for 24 hours.

Meticulous technique to avoid injury to Tenon's fascia around the rotary muscles of the globe must be maintained. This will prevent adhesions with resultant limitations of movement. One must avoid aggressive manipulation of the muscle bellies in the posterior third where the nerves enter to avoid nerve injury as well as muscle fibrosis. Paralysis can also occur from injury to the oculomotor nerves. The 4th cranial nerve is particularly prone to injury because it crosses from lateral to medial and must be retracted without undue tension.

Levator palpebrae superioris dysfunction may occur if one is not careful to avoid this structure when addressing a superior orbital tumor. Damage to the aponeurosis temporally, where it fans out to divide the lacrimal gland into its orbital and palpebral portions, can result in some degree of ptosis.

One must be careful during superior wall dissection in the case of a large orbital tumor, which may have resulted in resorption of part or all of the bone, so as to avoid entering the dura with resultant CSF leak. Persistent CSF leak or inadequate separation of the aerodigestive tract from the brain may result in infection, loss of bone grafts and death. Appropriately placed flaps and appropriately chosen antibiotic regimens minimize these risks. CSF leaks may initially be treated conservatively with head elevation and bedrest. A spinal drain should be inserted if the leak does not stop within 24 hours and, if the leak persists, surgical repair may be necessary.

Intraorbital hematomas must be addressed promptly as the tight space does not allow much pressure buildup. Hemorrhage into the orbit is usually from the anterior or posterior ethmoid arteries. If they were not clipped initially they will need to be during re-exploration.

Enophthalmos is a long-term complication from inadequate filling of orbital volume. The removal of a tumor, fat atrophy, or the expansion of the orbital volume due to a large tumor are all causes. Adequate reconstruction with cranial bone grafts to the orbital walls as well as filling of the orbit with bone may need to be performed to properly position the globe. If onlay bone grafts are used for infilling one needs to overcorrect slightly as some resorption will occur. Given the inability to predict the amount of resorption that will occur reoperation may sometimes be necessary.

Telecanthus will occur if the medial canthal tendon is detached and not properly reconstructed at the end of the operation.

Injury to or transection of the lacrimal drainage system may also occur. A dacrocystorhinostomy may be performed. This involves opening the lacrimal fossa and part of the medial wall into the nasal cavity. A burr may be used as the bone is very thin. Nasal mucosa is removed. The lacrimal sac is filled with 0.5 cc methylene blue so as to outline it. A sideways "U"-shaped flap is then cut into the medial wall of the sac with the base of the flap posteriorly. This falls into the nasal cavity and if too big may be trimmed. A single suture may be placed to anchor it.

Complications of Orbital Decompression

Complications from all approaches include eyelid malposition, disturbance of eye movement, diplopia, hypoesthesia in the face, CSF rhinorrhea, sinusitis, orbital cellulitis, meningitis, late enophthalmos, blindness, failure to relieve the optic neuropathy, asymmetric correction of proptosis, and stenosis of the lacrimal system.

Upper eyelid laxity due to the inferoposterior displacement of the globe after decompression is to be expected and is not strictly a complication. Nevertheless a procedure to recess the levator aponeurosis may be necessary at a later time.

Reference

Hassler WE, Meyer B, Rohde V, Unsold R (1994) Pterional approach to the contralateral orbit. Neurosurgery 34:552–554

10

Transoral Approach to the Clivus

H. Louis Harkey

Lesions of the clivus and anterior craniovertebral junction present significant problems in terms of surgical exposure. Traditionally these lesions were treated indirectly through posterior decompression with less than optimal results overall. More recently, surgical approaches have been developed that provide direct access to the anteroinferior skull base. As experience has grown, these basic approaches to the clivus have been modified to accommodate the wide variety of pathologies that occur in this region. The transoral approach is a direct midline approach to the craniovertebral junction that can be readily modified intraoperatively to provide the degree of exposure needed for the particular individual.

The basic transoral approach to the craniovertebral junction began gaining popularity with the widespread use of the microscope and development of instruments designed specifically for this sort of procedure. It is now recognized as a relatively simple operative technique with low morbidity and excellent outcome for appropriately selected patients. There are limits, however, to the exposure gained by simply retracting the tongue and soft palate. Rostral exposure can be extended by first splitting the soft palate and then splitting or resecting the posterior margin of the hard palate if even more exposure is required. When complex lesions cross the craniovertebral junction and involve the upper clivus, the maxilla becomes an obstruction. The transoral exposure can be further extended with a maxillotomy, providing the additional exposure needed for extensive lesions of the clivus and craniovertebral junction.

Patient Selection

The transoral approach is most suitable for extradural lesions of the anterior craniovertebral junction. Most of these problems are bony in origin, either congenital or acquired. Some tumors of the clivus and upper cervical spine are amenable to transoral resection as long as they are confined to the extradural space. Only in special circumstances are intradural lesions at the craniovertebral junction suitable for transoral management.

The most common indication for transoral surgery is decompression of the cervicomedullary junction due to the ravages of rheumatoid arthritis and its effects on the atlantoaxial complex (Fig. 10-1). Transoral decompression is indicated when there is irreducible atlantoaxial subluxation with persistent neural compression due to bone or pannus. In most cases, a simple transoral approach without palatal extension is all that is required to decompress the cervical cord. However, when the inflammatory process erodes the lateral masses of the atlas, the odontoid translocates through the foramen magnum, threatening the lower brain stem, and, when skeletal traction fails to reduce this translocation, transoral decompression typically requires some surgical manipulation of the palate.

Transoral management of missile wounds and foreign bodies lodged in the clivus or upper cervical spine has been reported. Traumatic injuries of the odontoid (including os odontoidium) are sometimes associated with irreducible compression of the cervicomedullary junction and are good cases for transoral exposure. Basilar impression due to bone softening diseases such as osteogenesis imperfecta, osteomalacia, and Paget's disease is another form of acquired bony abnormality that may necessitate transoral exposure for decompression. In fact, the extreme degree of impression seen in osteogenesis imperfecta often requires mobilization of the maxilla in order to expose adequately the clivus and upper cervical spine (Harkey et al., 1990).

Vestigial bony structures, basilar invagination, and other congenital bony anomalies sometimes produce stenosis in the region of the foramen magnum. If the stenosis is primarily anterior, then transoral decompression may be the most appropriate method of treatment. The transoral approach may be appropriate even when these lesions are associated with tonsilar ectopia since Chiari malformations sometimes resolve following anterior decompression.

Tumors of the anterior craniovertebral junction that are confined to the extradural space are also readily managed via transoral exposure (Crockard and Sen, 1991).

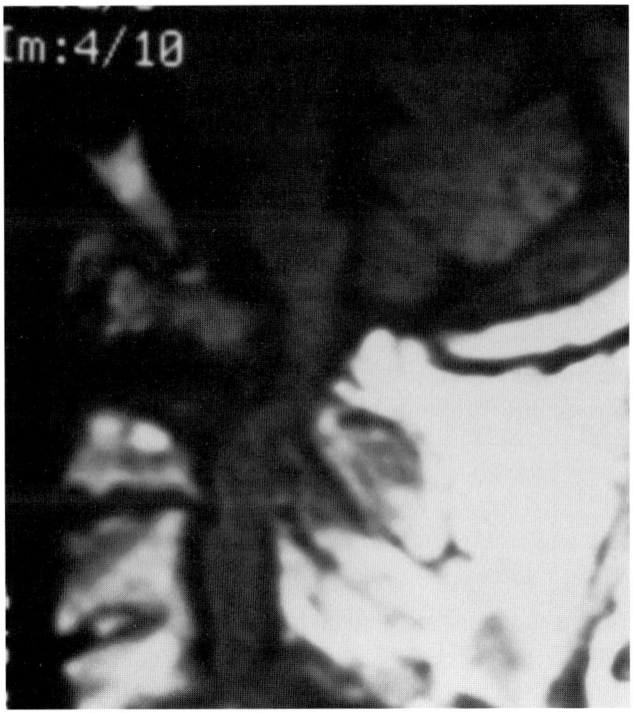

Figure 10-1. A patient with rheumatoid arthritis and severe compression of the cervicomedullary junction by a combination of atlantoaxial subluxation and pannus.

Chordomas, chondrosarcomas, fibrous dysplasia, metastases, and other bony tumors are all known to occur in this region. When such tumors are limited to the clivus and anterior components of the atlas and axis, resection may be possible. Gross total removal with tissue margins may even be achieved if the tumor does not invade the dura and does not extend too far laterally.

Successful transoral approaches for intradural problems have been reported (Crockard and Sen, 1991), but these tend to be limited to lesions that do not require a lot of microsurgical dissection of the ventral brain stem. Aneurysms of the midbasilar artery where the neck of the aneurysm is near the midline are the most suitable lesions for intradural transoral surgery (Crockard et al., 1991). Removing the clivus allows for proximal and distal control of the basilar artery and a direct view of the aneurysm's neck. Midline tumors that are anterior to the midbrain and are not adherent to delicate structures in this area can also be removed via the transoral route. The advantage of this approach for intradural lesions lies in the complete avoidance of retraction of neural structures.

Typical transoral exposure extends from the second cervical disc to the tip of the clivus. In rheumatoid arthritis, the exposure may be somewhat less if arthritis limits mandibular opening. The jaw must open so that there is a minimum of 2.5 to 3 cm between the upper and lower teeth in order to operate transorally. Otherwise, the mandible must be dislocated or the maxilla mobilized. Splitting the soft palate extends the exposure of the distal clivus. A midline osteotomy and upward fracturing of the hard palate or resection of the posterior portion of the hard palate with a Kerrison rongeur can further extend the exposure to the midclivus. If even more rostral exposure is necessary, then the maxilla must be mobilized. The rostrocaudal exposure obtained by the various transoral modifications can be dramatically altered in the presence of severe basilar impression.

Bony dissection is limited to the axis body, odontoid, anterior elements of the atlas, and clivus. The lateral limits of exposure are more confining. The atlantoaxial facets and joint are readily exposed through the mouth. As the exposure extends more cephalad, lateral dissection is limited by the hypoglossal nerve and canal, jugular veins, and carotid arteries. The carotid arteries are also a limiting factor as they exit the petrous bone prior to entering the cavernous sinus.

Preoperative Evaluation and Preparation

Magnetic resonance imaging (MRI) provides the best overall image of the anatomy and pathology of the craniovertebral junction. However, an appreciation of the bony landmarks of the skull base is crucial for transoral surgery, particularly when the anatomy is distorted by the pathologic process. For this, a supplementary computed tomography (CT) scan with three-dimensional and multiplanar two-dimensional reconstructed images is extremely helpful. Conventional and MR arteriography are optional but may be useful in demonstrating carotid or vertebrobasilar abnormalities.

Oropharyngeal cultures should be obtained preoperatively. Only pathogens are treated with antibiotics until cultures are negative, otherwise routine oral hygiene is all that is required in the days prior to surgery.

Operative Procedure

Anesthesia and Positioning

The operation begins with the patient either nasally or orally intubated depending on the type of transoral retractor to be used. I have found that awake nasal intubation over an endoscope the safest and easiest technique, when there is immobility of the mandible and hypermobility of the craniovertebral junction. Following intubation, the patient can be examined to ensure that no neurologic injury has occurred during the process. A tracheostomy is unnecessary in most cases except those requiring mobilization of the maxilla. A small feeding tube should be inserted following intubation because this will be difficult to pass at the completion of the procedure. Balanced intravenous and volatile anesthesia should be used (Marks et al., 1986). Intraoperative monitoring, if available, should be used; otherwise, the patient should be allowed to breathe spontaneously. The anesthesiologist can monitor brain stem function based on abrupt changes of vital signs.

The patient is positioned supine with the head slightly extended and secured with three-point skull fixation. Some surgeons may find fluoroscopy to be helpful but typically it is unnecessary unless there is marked distortion of normal anatomic relationships. The ventilator circuit should be passed over one shoulder allowing access to the top as well as one side of the head. The eyes should be carefully protected with adhesive dressing to allow for antiseptic preparation of the face and neck. The mouth and oropharynx is cleared and swabbed with iodinated solution and then a topical preparation of 1 percent hydrocortisone is generously applied to the lips, buccal mucosa, and tongue.

Instrumentation

Several transoral retractor systems are commercially available, each designed to perform basic functions of depressing the tongue, elevating the soft palate, and constraining the endotracheal tube. These systems also provide pharyngeal soft tissue retractor blades. The advantage of these systems lies in the fact that they are designed specifically for transoral skull base surgery and obviate the need for a tracheostomy. They anchor firmly to the upper teeth but can be modified for edentulous patients or for maxillotomy. However, it is not necessary to have these specially designed retractor systems to perform successful transoral surgery. One can rely on standard oral retractors and elevate the soft palate with stay sutures that are passed through the nostrils (Hadley et al., 1989; Menezes, 1991)

The operative field lies 10 to 12 cm below the orifice of the mouth; therefore, extra-long bayoneted instruments are necessary. The bony dissection should be performed with a high-speed drill, preferably one having an angled handpiece. Extra-long, thin foot-plated, 1- and 2-mm Kerrison rongeurs are invaluable. The surgical procedure is performed with a microscope for superior lighting and magnification. A 350- to 400-mm lens is needed to visualize the depth of the wound and allow sufficient working room for the surgical instruments.

Basic Procedure

After inserting the self-retaining oral retractor and positioning the soft palate retractor blades, the surgeon should carefully inspect the tongue and lips to ensure that they have not become entrapped between the retractor blades and the teeth (Fig. 10-2). Identifying the anterior tubercle of the atlas orients the surgeon to the midline in most cases and allows one to determine the rostrocaudal limits of exposure. If the exposure is deemed adequate, the mucosa can be infiltrated with epinephrine (1/100,000 units) and incised in the midline. This incision can then be extended with electrocautery to expose the bone. Once again, the anterior tubercle of the atlas should be identified for orientation. The longus colli and longus capitis muscles can be elevated laterally along the anterior arch of the atlas in the subperiosteal plane. As the muscle and mucosa are elevated, the base of the odontoid

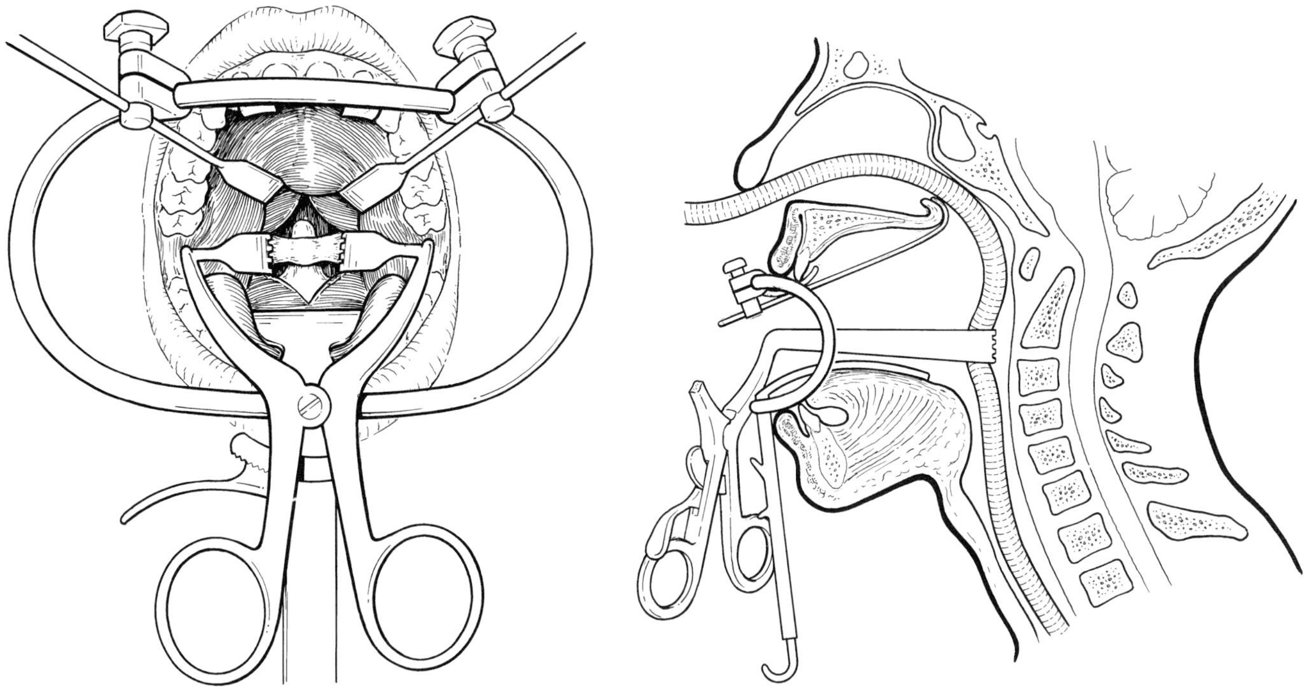

Figure 10-2. Transoral retractor in place demonstrating the basic exposure.

comes into view. The surgeon should remember that in the case of irreducible atlantoaxial subluxation the odontoid may be a centimeter or so deeper than the arch of the atlas. The soft tissue is reflected as far laterally as is necessary to expose the bone to be dissected. The exposure can extend laterally to expose the atlantoaxial facet joint. One can then release the joint capsule and simplify the atlantoaxial reduction. With the standard transoral approach the exposure can typically extend from the tip of the clivus to the second cervical disc.

Drilling begins with the atlas and removes the lower half of the anterior arch (Fig. 10-3). Only the necessary amount of bone should be removed in order to achieve the desired decompression. It is preferable to leave an anterior bridge of bone between the lateral masses, which prevents lateral displacement of the articular masses and cranial settling. If the entire anterior arch of the atlas is removed then the posterior stabilization must incorporate the skull to prevent cranial settling. If the anterior arch of the atlas is left partially intact, posterior stabilization can be limited to the atlas and axis. For most cases of rheumatoid arthritis, it is possible to remove the odontoid and pannus by working above and below the remnant arch of the atlas.

The odontoid and body of the axis are removed by first drilling the anterior cortical surface and the underlying cancellous bone. The trough is extended to the medial border of the facet and as far down into the body of the axis as necessary. A thin shell of cortical bone is left at the base of the trough and acts to protect the underlying structures and prevents the dura from prematurely herniating into the wound. The final cortical wafer can be removed with small curettes. If further lateral decompression is required, the edges can be undercut with a Kerrison rongeur. Frequently, the odontoid is amputated below the arch of the atlas. The tip of the dens can then be removed by cutting the apical ligaments free.

In rheumatoid arthritis, a substantial amount of pannus frequently compresses the dura at this point of the operation. This fibrous tissue can be removed piecemeal until

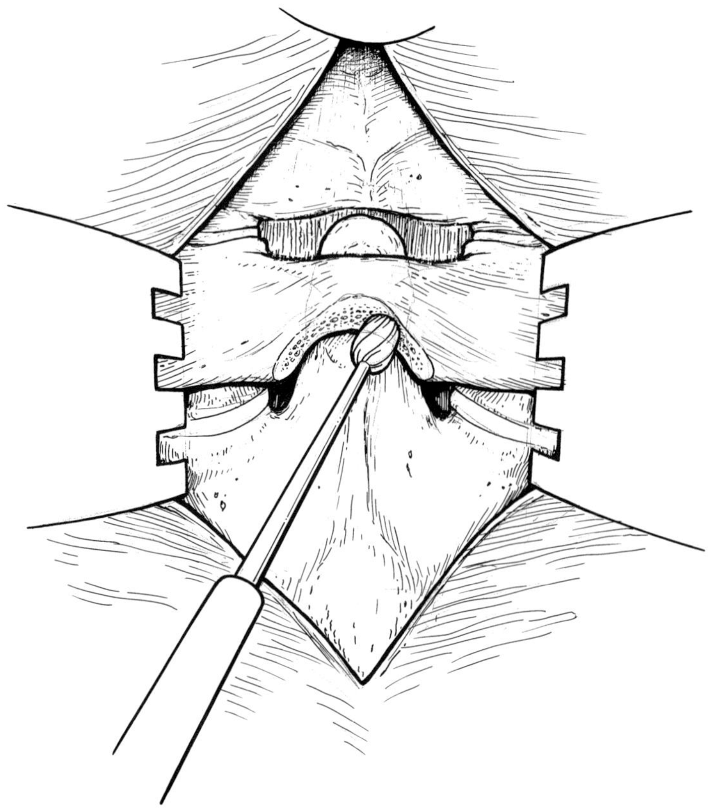

Figure 10-3. Drilling the atlas.

the dura bulges forward and begins to pulsate. It is not necessary to remove every last bit of the pannus; indeed, overly aggressive removal may result in an unnecessary dural laceration. As this tissue is removed, the surgeon will frequently encounter the thick white transverse ligament. If it is intact, it should be left as such if at all possible since it will also prevent displacement of the lateral masses of the atlas.

Extended Exposure

Splitting Palate. Additional exposure of the clivus can be achieved by incising the soft palate along the median raphe (Fig. 10-4). The incision begins at the posterior edge of the hard palate, deviating to one side at the base of the uvula. The two leaves of the soft palate are then retracted laterally and held in place with the soft palate retractors. This typically provides exposure to the midclivus and sometimes upper clivus regions, but even further exposure can be gained by relocating the hard palate. To do this, the mucosa and periosteum are incised along the midline of the hard palate and reflected several millimeters to either side. A paramedian palatal osteotomy is created to one side of the vomer with either a Gigli saw or oscillating saw. The vomer is then detached and partially resected from the other side of the hard palate. Firm pressure applied with the thumb over the osteotomy will fracture the two halves of the hard palate into the nasal cavity. Alternatively, the mucoperiosteum can be stripped from the hard palate, and the posterior rim (8 to 10 mm) can be removed with a drill or rongeur, taking care to protect both the oral and nasal mucosa covering the hard palate (Menezes, 1991).

Splitting the soft and hard palate gains an additional 3- to 5-mm exposure of the clivus with each maneuver. The midline incision can be extended into the posterior nasopharyngeal mucosa as high as the vomer. The mucosa and longus capitis muscles

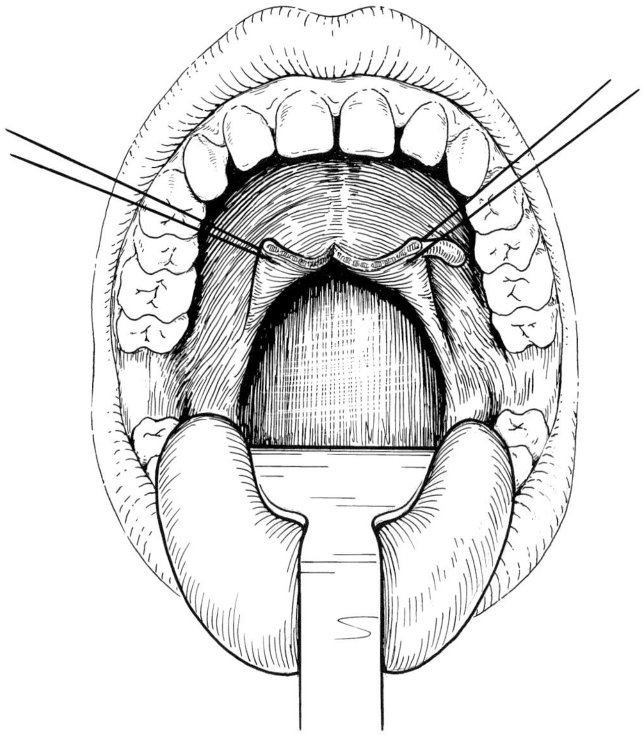

Figure 10-4. Extended exposure by splitting the palate.

are reflected as single flap in a subperiosteal plane. Bone resection begins with the anterior arch of the atlas; however, the entire arch of the atlas will generally be removed in cases also requiring clivus dissection. The distal clivus, dens, and body of the axis are drilled as needed, leaving a posterior shell of cortical bone to protect the dura. The occipital condyles should be avoided because they represent the lateral limits of exposure.

Splitting Maxilla (Anand et al., 1991; Harkey et al., 1993; James and Crockard, 1991). For the extended maxillotomy, a tracheostomy is created from the outset. The exposure begins with an incision above the mucogingival reflection similar to the incision for a sublabial trans-sphenoidal approach. This incision should extend from one maxillary tuberosity to the other (Fig. 10-5). The mucoperiosteum is elevated to expose the nasal floor and septum. Care is taken not to strip too much of the mucoperiosteum, as this helps to maintain vascularity of the maxilla. The cartilaginous septum is detached from the maxilla and vomer at this point and reflected to one side.

The transverse and midline osteotomies are marked on the exposed maxilla, and titanium compression plates are contoured to fit both maxillary buttresses and the prespinal area (Fig. 10-6). The drill holes are made, and the plates are secured before the osteotomies are made. The plates are then removed and carefully marked for replacement. This trial application of the plates ensures precise relocation of the maxilla at the completion of the procedure. An incision is made in the oral mucosa overlying the hard palate osteotomy site and reflected several millimeters. If the hard palate is substantial, plates may be applied as well; however, transosseous wires or sutures may suffice. The sagittal osteotomy in the maxilla is either midline or paramidline depending on the orientation of the teeth and the nasal septum. Osteogenesis imperfecta patients frequently have dentogenesis imperfecta because of their

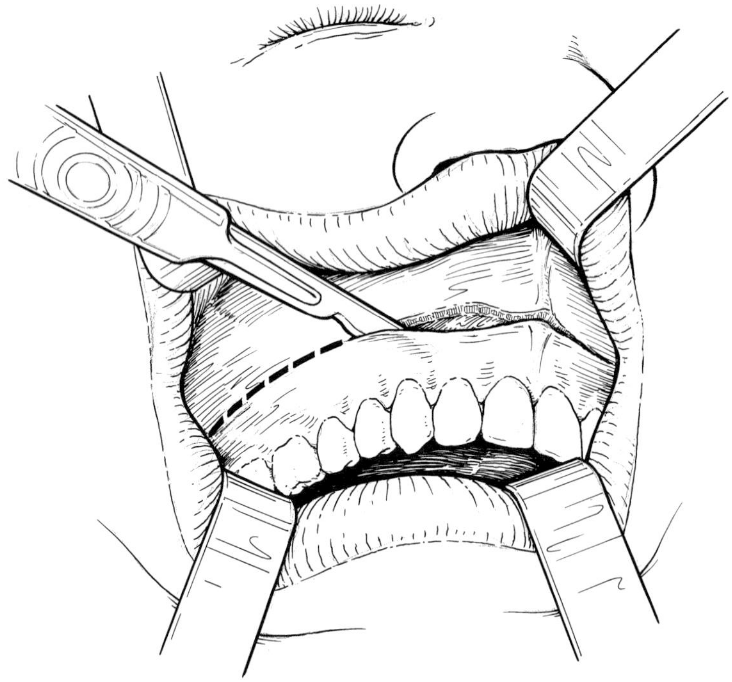

Figure 10-5. The sublabial mucosal incision for the extended maxillotomy.

malaligned teeth. It is sometimes more convenient to split between the medial and lateral incisor as opposed to the midline. The incision is then extended through the full thickness of the soft palate to the base of the uvula.

Taking care to avoid injury to the dental roots, the surgeon cuts bilateral Le Fort 1 osteotomies with an oscillating saw (Fig. 10-7). Using a Gigli saw to make the

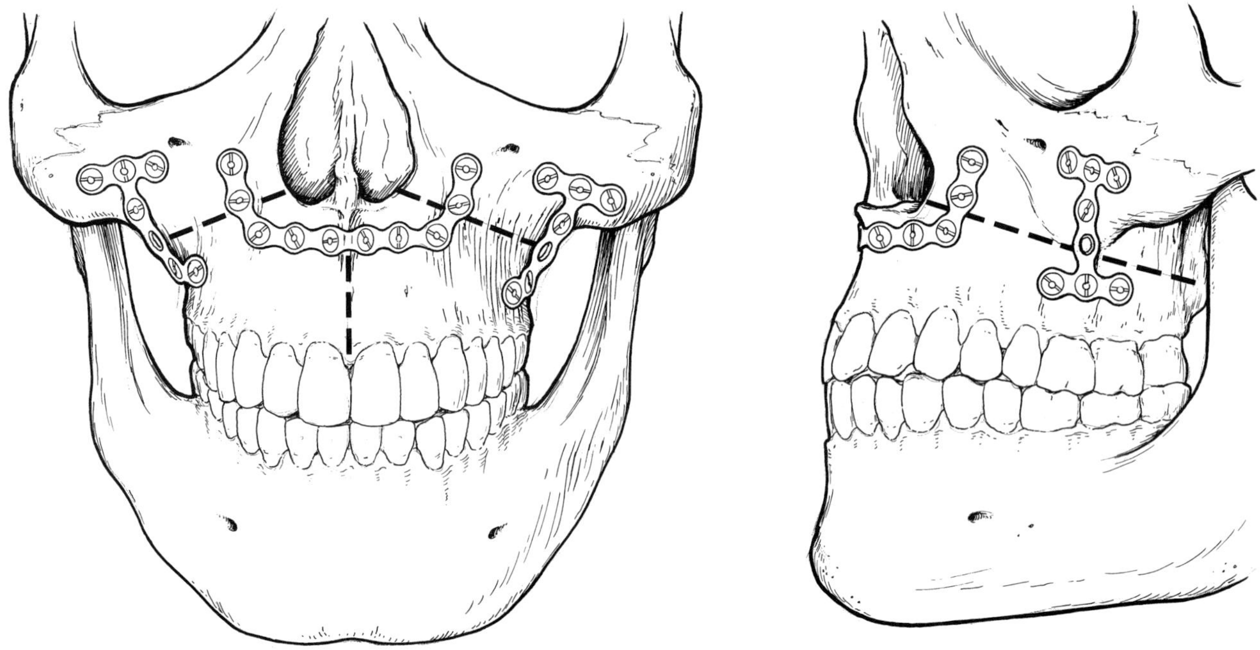

Figure 10-6. Reconstruction plates and their position relative to proposed osteotomy sites.

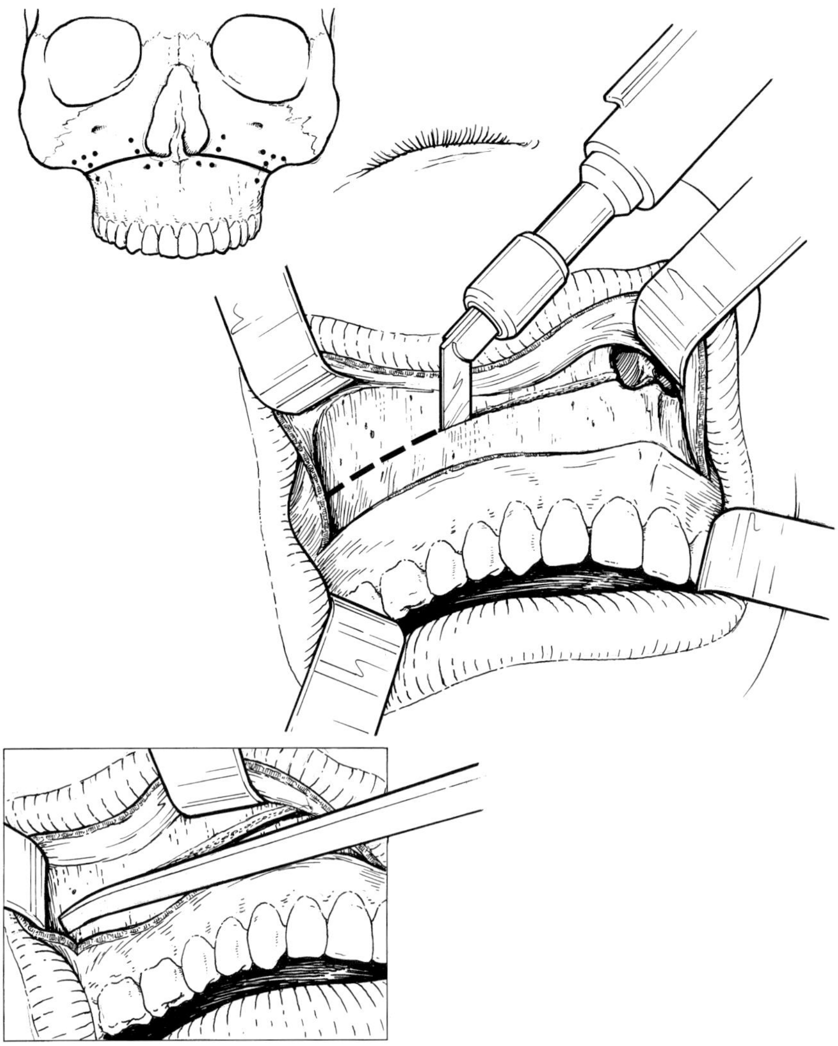

Figure 10-7. The Le Fort osteotomies extend from the floor of each nasal cavity to the maxillary tuberosity on each side.

parasagittal osteotomy, the surgeon passes along one side of the vomer and between two incisors nearest to the midline (Fig. 10-8). Finally, the maxillary tuberosities are separated from the pterygoid with a curved osteotome. At this point the two halves of the maxilla will be free to swing inferiorly and laterally (Fig. 10-9). Blood supply to each maxillary segment is maintained via the soft palate with its remaining connections to the pharynx. The vomer can be removed to expose the anterior sphenoid sinus.

The floating maxillary segments are carefully mobilized and the Crockard transoral retractor, modified with the midfacial osteotomy retractor plate, is inserted. The hard palate retractor is positioned to hold the maxillary segments out of the operative field, completing the exposure of the posterior nasopharynx from the sphenoid sinus to the upper cervical spine. The soft tissues of the posterior nasopharynx are incised and reflected in the same manner as for the less extensive transoral approaches.

Bony resection of the atlantoaxial complex and lower clivus is the same as for the less extensive exposure. Yet with this approach, rostral exposure extends to the sphenoid sinus, which can be entered as well. In order to avoid injury to vital structures, the entire width of the clivus dissection should not exceed 2 cm.

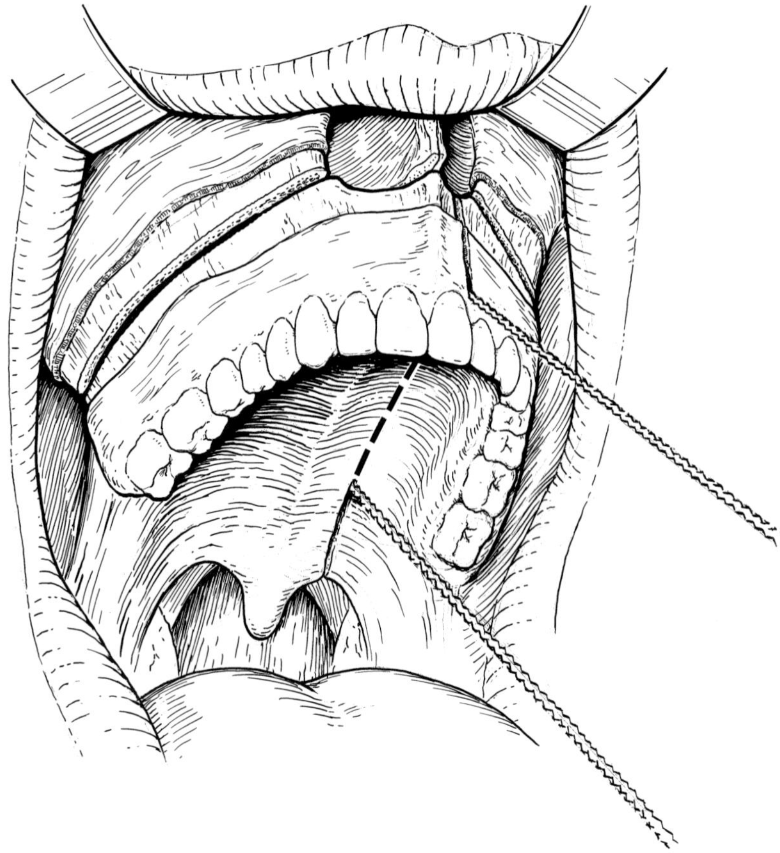

Figure 10-8. The palatal osteotomy.

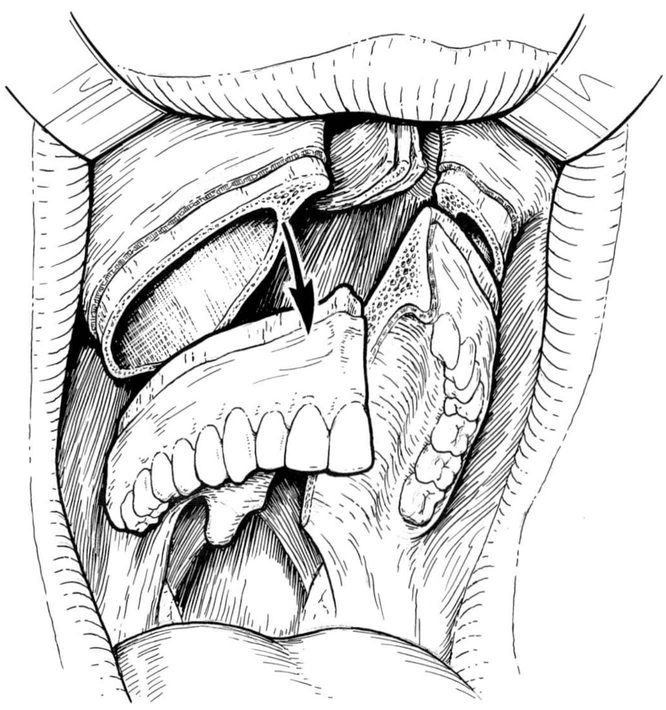

Figure 10-9. The mobilized halves of the maxilla.

Intradural Surgery

The transoral approach is best suited for bony abnormalities of the craniovertebral junction but it is also useful for selected intradural lesions, particularly if one of the extended approaches is used. When transoral surgery is strictly extradural, the problem of contamination by the oral flora is largely avoided. Once the dura has been violated, either intentionally or otherwise, the risk of meningitis increases dramatically. A watertight closure of the dura and the prevention of a cerebrospinal fluid (CSF) fistula can be quite difficult through the transoral exposure. However, if the risk of bacterial contamination of the subarachnoid space is recognized and treated appropriately, then transoral exposure may be the most appropriate route for intradural surgery at the cervicomedullary junction.

If intradural exposure is expected, a lumbar drain should be placed at the outset of surgery. The dura is opened with a cruciate or "I"-shaped incision. The circular sinus can be a source of significant hemorrhage, and aggressive attempts at hemostasis with electrocautery can shrink the dura, making it impossible to close. Therefore, the surgeon should be very careful to avoid excessive coagulation and rely on hemoclips or other methods of hemostasis when possible.

Closure

It is quite difficult to suture the dura at the depths of a transoral exposure. Therefore, it is best to close a dural incision by apposition and onlay grafting. Fibrin glue over a fascia lata, a fat graft, or both will seal most wounds if a CSF drain is maintained for 5 days postoperatively. Various vascularized grafts can be devised as well.

The soft tissue closure should be performed in two layers. The longus capitis and longus colli muscles can be reapproximated with inverted polygalactin sutures. Closing the mucosa separately results in a more complete apposition of the mucosal edges under less stress. The soft palate should also be closed in three layers: the nasal mucosa, the muscular layer, and the oral mucosa.

Closing the maxillotomy begins by repositioning and securing the two maxillary fragments with the prepared compression plates. If the hard palate is substantial, plates may be applied across the osteotomy as well; however, transosseous wires or sutures may suffice. The nasal septum is reconstructed by replacing the vomer and cartilaginous septum and repositioning the nasal mucosa with a speculum. Large-bore nasal cannulas inserted in each nostril will maintain the position of the septum and overlying mucosa until some healing occurs. Finally, the sublabial incision is closed with interrupted polyglactin sutures.

Stabilization

Many of the patients undergoing transoral surgery are unstable at the craniovertebral junction prior to surgery. Others become unstable as a result of surgery. The surgeon must recognize instability and treat it according to recognized biomechanical principles. Internal stabilization devices and rigid external braces merely act to prevent motion while bone heals across unstable motion segments. Direct apposition of decorticated bone or bone graft spanning a gap is necessary for long-term stability. Whenever possible, stabilization should be limited to unstable motion segments only.

The atlas is the focal point of stability following transoral surgery. If it remains intact by virtue of residual anterior bony arch, transverse ligament, or both then it is only necessary to restore stability to the atlantoaxial joint. When the anterior ring of the atlas is completely disrupted, the weight of the head will gradually displace the lateral masses causing the head to settle. To prevent this from occurring, the occiput should be included in the stabilization. Likewise, if the lateral masses of the atlas are compressed or significantly eroded, the occiput should be included in the stabilization. Severe basilar impression due to soft bone disease is an exception in that the craniovertebral junction is not grossly unstable even after decompression. Stabilization is necessary to spread the weight-bearing surface of the skull base in order to prevent further enfolding.

Successful anterior grafting and stabilization is possible but currently available techniques and instrumentation are not particularly successful. Therefore, posterior stabilization techniques are most suitable (Crockard, 1991).

Postoperative Management

Fortunately, the mucosa of the nose and mouth heal readily; nevertheless, unnecessary complications can be prevented with meticulous care of the mouth and nose during the postoperative period. The patient should not take any solids or fluids orally for 3 days following the surgery. During this period, nutrition and medications can be administered intravenously or through a feeding tube once bowel activity returns to normal. Hydrocortisone cream administered every 8 hours to the lips, gums, and buccal mucosa will help minimize labial edema. The tracheostomy may be removed once pharyngeal edema has subsided, usually 2 to 3 days after surgery. Nasal stents can be removed after 2 to 3 days, as well. If a lumbar drain is utilized, it should be removed after 5 days.

Broad-spectrum antibiotics directed toward normal oral flora are administered prophylactically during the immediate postoperative period. The surgeon must watch closely for signs of meningitis and change the antibiotic regimen to emphasize CSF penetration and to include anaerobic coverage at the earliest indication. An H_2 antagonist to lower gastric acidity is recommended, and antiemetics should be administered as needed to prevent regurgitation. Pain, rarely a problem following this procedure, is easily controlled with parenteral narcotics.

Complications

A spinal fluid fistula is probably the worst potential complication. If a dural puncture is recognized at the time of surgery an attempt should be made to close it primarily. If primary closure is not feasible, then the dural defect should be covered with a graft and sealed with fibrin glue. Spinal drainage is necessary postoperatively in either case.

Wound dehiscence, or improper healing of the pharyngeal soft tissue, is the most common source of complication. Retraction of the soft tissue into the anterior bony defect or palatal fenestration can result in nasal speech and regurgitation. Failure to restore and maintain preoperative dental occlusion will be a major source of complaint for the patient following maxillotomy. Some patients will experience difficulty opening their mouths following surgery because of pain and stiffness in the region of the temporomandibular joint. This typically resolves with analgesics and physical therapy.

Outcomes

Extensive experience with the transoral approach (over 350 patients) has been reported by several authors (Crockard and Johnston, 1993; Hadley et al., 1989; Menezes and Van Guilder, 1988). From these reports, the most frequent indication for transoral surgery is irreducible cervicomedullary compression secondary to rheumatoid arthritis. Nonrheumatoid, congenital, and acquired bony abnormalities make up the next largest group. Tumors, primarily extradural but a few intradural in location, comprise the third largest group of patients. The morbidity and mortality has been extremely low in each of these reports. Perioperative deaths have been primarily due to associated pulmonary complications such as pulmonary embolus or pneumonia. The majority of the reported morbidity has been limited to pharyngeal wound complications. Although CSF fistulas were reported in each series, all have been treated successfully with repair of the wound and spinal drainage. Neurologic improvement is the norm but is directly related to the preoperative neurologic function.

The transoral approach to the craniovertebral junction and clivus is a relatively safe and effective approach for extradural midline ventral lesions of the craniovertebral junction and skull base.

References

Anand VK, Harkey HL, Al-Mefty O (1991) Open-door maxillotomy approach for lesions of the clivus. Skull Base Surg 1:217–225

Crockard HA (1991) Atlantoaxial subluxation: anterior and posterior approaches. pp. 9–26 In Torrens MJ, Dickson RA (eds): Operative Spinal Surgery. Churchill Livingstone, Edinburgh

Crockard HA, Johnston F (1993) Development of transoral approaches to lesions of the skull base and craniovertebral junction. Neurosurg Q 3:61–82

Crockard HA, Koksel T, Watkin N (1991) Transoral transclival clipping of anterior inferior cerebellar aneurysm using new rotating applier. J Neurosurg 75:483–485

Crockard HA, Sen CN (1991) The transoral approach for the management of intradural lesions at the craniovertebral junction: review of 7 cases. Neurosurgery 28:88–98

Hadley MN, Spetzler RF, Sonntag VKH (1989) The transoral approach to the superior cervical spine. A review of 53 cases of extradural cervicomedullary compression. J Neurosurg 71:16–23

Harkey HL, Anand VK, Crockard HA et al (1993) Open-door maxillotomy approach for lesions of the clivus. Neurosurg Operative Atlas 3:109–118

Harkey HL, Crockard HA, Stevens JM et al (1990) The operative management of basilar impression in osteogenesis imperfecta. Neurosurgery 27:782–786

James D, Crockard HA (1991) Surgical access to the base of skull and upper cervical spine by extended maxillotomy. Neurosurgery 29:411–416

Marks RJ, Forrester PC, Calder I, Crockard HA (1986) Anesthesia for transoral craniocervical surgery. Anaesthesia 41:1049–1052

Menezes A (1991) Transoral surgery for craniovertebral junction anomalies. Neurosurg Operative Atlas 1:141–146

Menezes AH, Van Guilder JC (1988) Transoral-transpharyngeal approach to the anterior craniocervical junction. Ten-year experience with 72 patients. J Neurosurg 69:895–903

11

Le Fort 1 Osteotomy Approach with Midline Mandibular Splitting

Yoshio Tanaka
Sadao Tajima

A new modification of the Le Fort 1 maxillotomy has been developed that offers a much improved exposure of the median and paramedian skull base. The procedure involves a standard Le Fort 1 osteotomy combined with mandibular splitting (Fig. 11-1) and affords excellent exposure of the posterior half of the anterior skull base and the whole clivus (Fig. 11-2). To our knowledge, this modification of the surgical procedure has not been described previously in the literature.

Postoperative cosmetic results and occlusions are excellent using the rigid fixation method with miniplates. The Le Fort 1 maxillotomy mandibular splitting approach offers excellent exposure to the skull base and has distinct advantages in managing tumors in and around this area. The detailed procedures for this approach, and preoperative criteria regarding the necessity of mandibular splitting are described below.

Instrumentation

To ensure a relatively blood-free and widely exposed surgical field, the special requirements are as follows: (1) intravascular balloon catheter (Fig. 11-3), and (2) maxillary retractors (see Fig. 11-8).

Surgical Technique

Preoperative Treatment and Anesthesia

After oral intubation, the oronasal cavities are sterilized with diluted iodine solution. Inducing hypotensive anesthesia, in which the blood pressure is maintained below 100 mmHg, is desirable to control hemorrhage. The authors adopted an intravascular balloon technique to obstruct the maxillary artery during surgery (Fig. 11-3). The

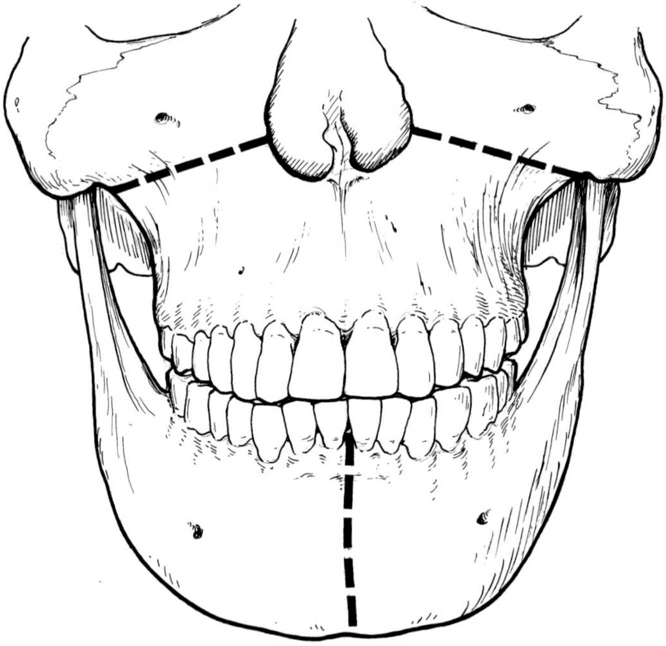

Figure 11-1. Frontal view of a skull showing the lines of maxillary and osteotomy.

balloon catheter is introduced retrogradely via the superficial temporal artery into the external carotid artery just proximal to the maxillary artery (Fig. 11-4). Ueda (1990) reported in his study that the balloon catheter should be advanced more than 3 cm from the superior margin of the external auditory canal and be maintained above a line between the anterior nasal spine and the tip of the mastoid process. Confirming pulsation of the facial artery during balloon inflation is another way of

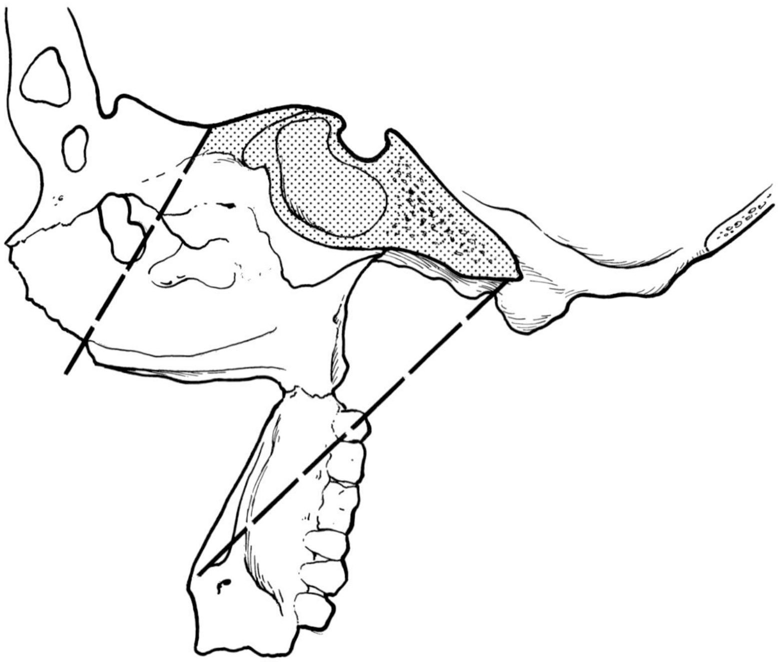

Figure 11-2. Sagittal section of a skull after Le Fort I osteotomy. The lines indicate the extent of exposure.

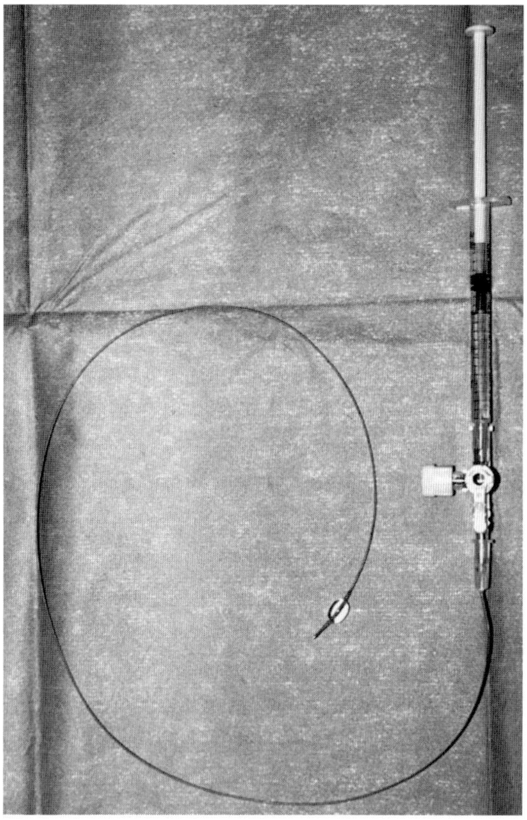

Figure 11-3. Vascular balloon catheter is made of silicone, measures 0.9 mm in diameter, and can obstruct vessels up to 5 mm in diameter.

determining that the balloon has not advanced into the common carotid artery. This intravascular balloon technique ensures a relatively blood-free surgical field and facilitates surgical procedures.

Midline Mandibular Splitting

Through a lower buccal sulcus incision extending between the second premolars, the periosteum of the mandible is completely elevated down to its inferior margin and both mental branches of the inferior alveolar neurovascular bundles, which are usually situated inferior to the root apices of the second lower premolars, are identified. Subsequently, the gingiva and interdental papilla between the central incisors are incised, and the mucoperiosteal flaps are elevated up to the tooth width to allow room for osteotomy. Prior to midline mandibular splitting, two straight miniplates with four holes, which are bent along the curve of the anterior surface of the mandible, are temporarily fixed with screws (ϕ 2 × 9 to 11 mm) across the expected osteotomy line. The miniplate should be placed at least 5 mm below the root apices of the teeth to avoid injury. To secure mechanical stability, it is preferable to place the two miniplates on different planes (e.g., one plate on the anterior surface of the mandible, and the other on the inferior margin). After all of the holes have been prepared for screws, the miniplates are removed, taking care to note their positions and orientations. When these miniplates are fixed in the same positions at the end of surgery, the mandible is accurately repositioned.

During midline mandibular splitting, a full-thickness cut is made below the root apices with a thin-blade sagittal saw. For the midline splitting between dental sockets

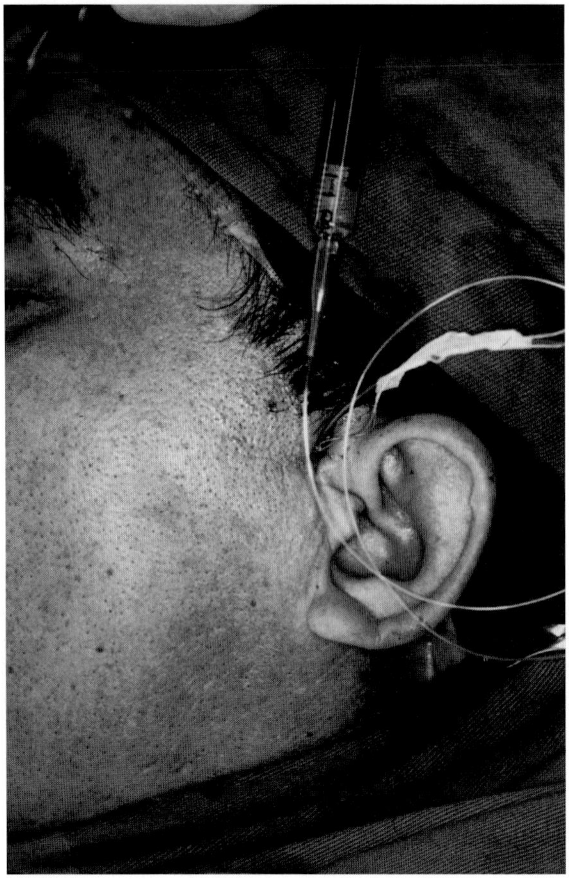

Figure 11-4. The balloon catheter is introduced retrogradely via the superficial temporal artery into the external carotid artery through a preauricular incision.

with dental roots, a sagittal saw is inserted only 3- to 4-mm deep in the midalveolar septum to prevent root injury, and the subsequent procedure for splitting is performed with a chisel. While the split stump is opened laterally with bone forceps, the lingual frenulum is incised between the sublingual caruncles. The geniohyoid muscle is then carefully separated sharply and bluntly to allow a separation and exposure of about 2 cm at this site. The endotracheal tube is transferred to the osteotomy site, and fixed by a suture.

Le Fort I Osteotomy

The upper buccal sulcus incision, extending between the distal ends of the second premolars, is made approximately 10 mm above the mucogingival junction. The rim of the pyriform aperture is elevated subperiosteally as far upward as possible, and the infraorbital neurovascular bundle is localized on the anterior surface of the maxilla. After the zygomatic buttress has been exposed laterally, the periosteum of the posterior surface of the maxilla is elevated like a tunnel taking care to avoid prolapse of the buccal fat. The dissection is taken into the pterygopalatine fossa; the pterygoid process is located posterior to the fossa. In the pyriform aperture, the mucoperiosteum of the lateral wall and the nasal floor is elevated to the anterior end of the inferior concha and the anterior nasal spine and inferior end of the nasal septum, respectively.

The septal branch of the sphenopalatine artery entering the incisor canal is cut under hemostasis. After this dissection, miniplates are temporarily fixed according to

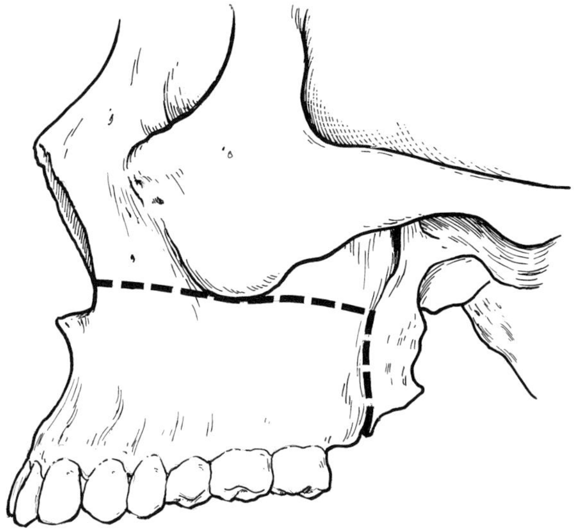

Figure 11-5. The line of Le Fort I osteotomy.

the expected Le Fort 1 osteotomy line (Fig. 11-5; it is desirable to set the line at least 5 mm above the apices of the teeth to allow room for placement of the miniplate). A total of four miniplates is used, two on each side of the maxilla. Usually, an "L"-shaped miniplate is used for the lateral margin of the pyriform aperture, and a linear or inverted "Y"-shaped miniplate is used for the zygomatic buttress (Fig. 11-6). As in the mandibular splitting, the roots at their apices must be protected against injury from a screw. The temporarily fixed miniplates are then removed.

After the lateral margin of the pyriform aperture has been cut to a depth of about 20 mm with a sagittal saw, the anterior surface of the maxilla, zygomatic buttress, and medial wall of the maxilla are cut in order. The anterior nasal spine is cut with a chisel. The nasal septum is elevated from the vomerine groove, and the vomer is cut completely from front to back with a septal chisel. Then, a curved-blunt osteotome is placed in the pterygopalatine groove and used to separate the bony connection with the pterygoid plate.

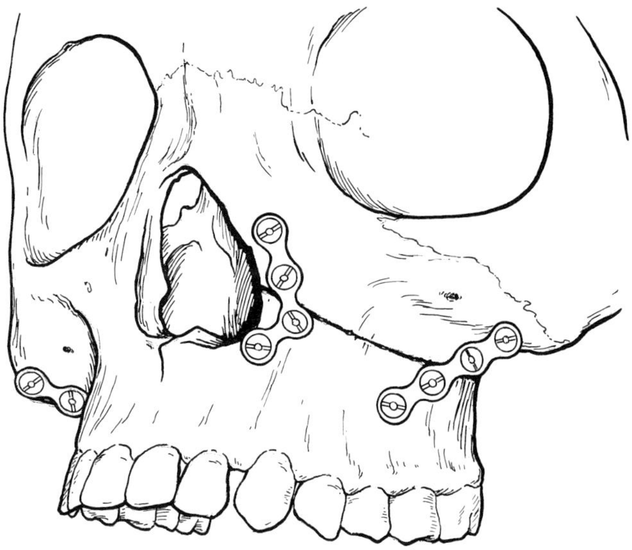

Figure 11-6. Temporary miniplate fixation at the pyriform margin and zygomatic buttress.

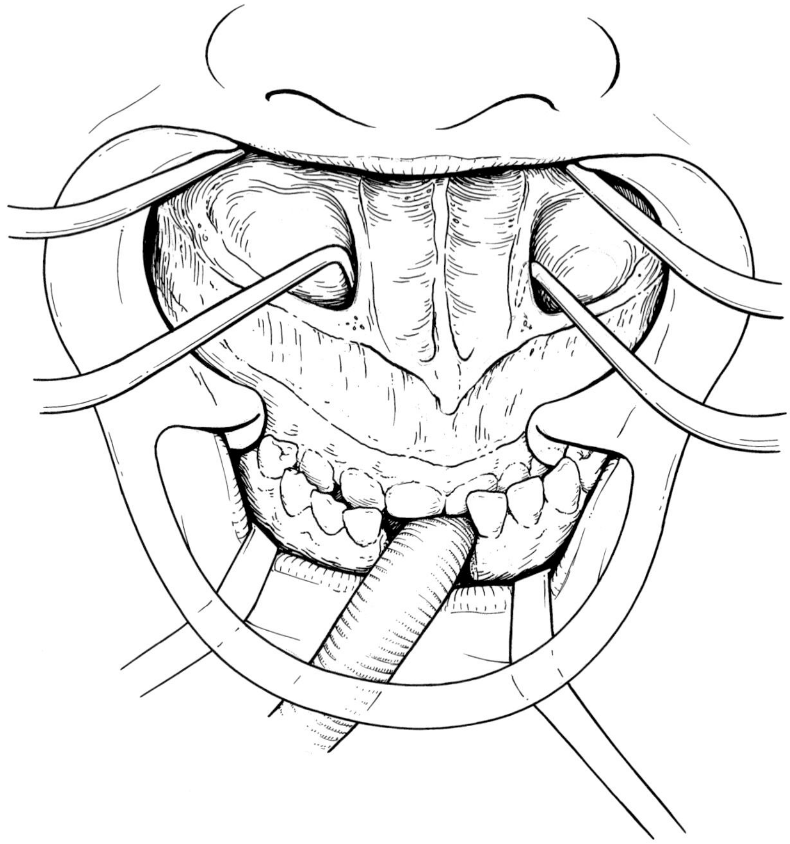

Figure 11-7. Intraoperative view. Endotracheal tube placed and fixed between the halves of the split mandible.

The maxillary segment is now connected only by the most posterior part of the medial wall of the maxilla including the descending palatine artery and vein. Mobilization of the maxilla is easily achieved by down-fracturing with maxillary forceps. While confirming that the maxilla enters the expanded mandibular arch, the surgical field is set with a maxillary retractor (Figs. 11-7 and 11-8).

Approach to the Skull Base

Anterior to the Sphenoid Sinus. The skull base is approached transseptally while separating the septonasal mucoperiosteum.

Around the Clivus. The skull base is approached by incising the posterior end of the septonasal mucosa. When an operative field including the posterior half of the clivus is considered necessary, the anterior nasal spine and nasal septum should be separated keeping the nasal floor mucosa adherent to the maxillary segment, since the elevated mucosa of the nasal floor may interrupt the surgical field.

If the inferior concha of the nose obscures the surgical field, submucosal turbinotomy may also be performed. For cases in which the surgical field requires expansion in the median to lateral direction, the field is obtained by cutting and compressing the pterygoid process under hemostasis of the descending palatine artery and vein, which are exposed as tight cords.

Wound Closure

When a dura mater defect occurs it is repaired directly if possible. The mucosa must be securely sutured. In such a case, it is useful to transfer a septonasal mucoperiosteal

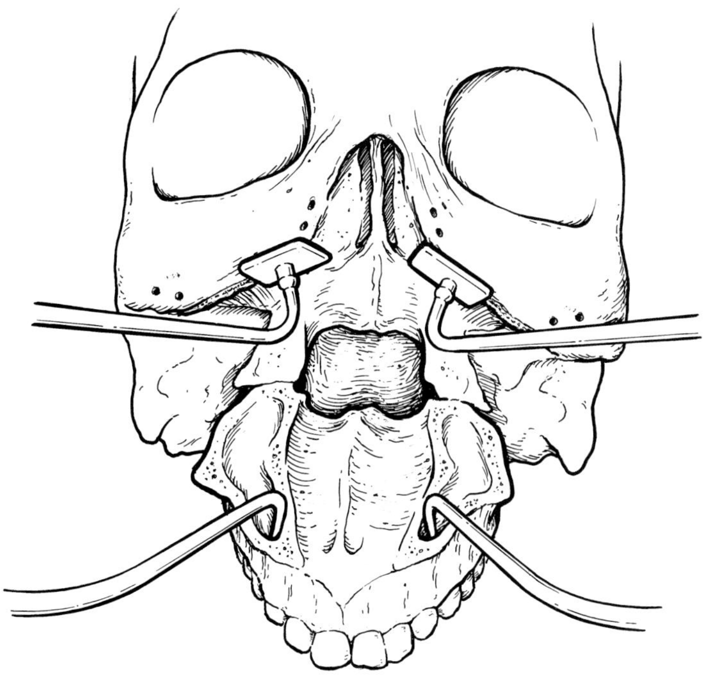

Figure 11-8. Maxillary retractors keep the down-fractured maxilla within the expanded mandibular arch and provide a wide field of exposure of the skull base.

flap. When the dura defect is large, flaps with vascular pedicles such as a galeal flap or a temporal myofascial flap can be used.

Accurate reduction and fixation of the maxilla and mandible are obtained by fixing the previously fitted miniplates in the precise positions. Since even minor changes in occlusal relationships are not acceptable, it is desirable that intermaxillary fixation should be maintained as far as circumstances permit for approximately 10 days starting from the second postoperative day.

The sensation of the teeth in the maxilla is lost due to the Le Fort 1 osteotomy, so the patient is unaware of occlusal failure until sensation is recovered. Therefore, postoperatively great care in maintaining accurate occlusion is necessary. It is said that sensation of the maxillary dental pulp and periodontal tissue recovers by 9 to 12 months postoperatively.

Discussion

Drommer (1986) reported that tumor resection by Le Fort 1 osteotomy was performed in the 1860s. The procedure, however, seems not to have been accepted because of problems such as blood loss and postoperative facial deformity. Subsequently, in the 1960s, Obwegeser reported details of the surgical procedure and clinical results of Le Fort 1 osteotomy in the treatment of facial deformity. Since then, the procedure has been widely used in oral surgery and plastic surgery.

Surgery for skull base tumor has become more common with the development of reconstructive procedures. In addition, it has become possible to control blood loss during surgery by hypotensive anesthesia and intravascular balloon techniques, and problems such as postoperative occlusal failure have been solved by the use of miniplates. With these procedures, Le Fort 1 osteotomy has been reconsidered as a surgical approach. As described by other authors (Brown, 1989; Uttley et al., 1989), approaching the skull base by Le Fort 1 osteotomy is a useful method that permits surgical access to the entire medial and paramedial portion ranging from the posterior half of the anterior skull base to the inferior end of the clivus. The surgical procedure for dividing the maxilla into two parts (Kocher's method), which provides a wider surgical field, has the following shortcomings: (1) it is rather difficult to fix the maxilla postoperatively and (2) if the descending palatine artery is ligated during surgery, circulation problems in the maxillary anterior teeth may develop. The Le Fort 1 maxillotomy—mandibular splitting approach compensates for these shortcomings.

Maxillary circulation is maintained via the random pattern of circulation from the soft palate and buccal mucosa of the posterior part and, in addition to that, by the descending palatine artery. Because the neurovascular arcade is well developed in maxillary alveolar bone, circulation to the maxillary anterior teeth is preserved even when the bilateral descending palatine arteries are cut. However, it is advisable to restore the descending palatine artery in patients with preoperative irradiation or intra-arterial infusion therapy and in those who undergo additional surgery.

Midline mandibular splitting should not necessarily be performed on all patients in whom a surgical field of 60 mm or more is required. In some patients, an adequate surgical field can be obtained without midline mandibular splitting. In our previous study (Tanaka et al., 1993), the following criteria were identified with regard to obtaining a surgical field of 60 mm or more.

1. When both maxillary and mandibular dentitions are preserved, midline mandibular splitting is essential.
2. When either the maxilla or mandible is edentulous but the maximal mouth opening is about 40 mm or less (which is measured as the distance between gum and the incisal edges of the remaining upper or lower central incisors), midline mandibular splitting is necessary.
3. In other cases, midline mandibular splitting is usually unnecessary.

References

Brown DH (1989) The Le Fort I maxillary osteotomy approach to surgery of the skull base. J Otolaryngol 18:289–292

Drommer RB (1986) The history of the "Le Fort I osteotomy." J Maxillo-Facial Surg 14:119–122

Tanaka Y, Tajima S, Tsujiguchi K et al (1993) A study on the mandible splitting effect in the Le Fort I maxillotomy–mandible splitting approach. J Jpn Soc Cranio-Maxillo-Facial Surg 7:42–49

Ueda K (1990) Intravascular balloon technique for reducing hemorrhage in cranio-facial osteotomies. J Jpn Soc Plast Reconstr Surg 10:273–281

Uttley D, Moore A, Archer DJ (1989) Surgical management of midline skull-base tumors: a new approach. J Neurosurg 71:705–710

12

Cranio-Orbito-Zygomatic Approach to the Skull Base

Kazuhiko Fujitsu

The lowest portion of the supratentorial compartment is the anterior temporal base, and extensive exposure of this portion allows the lowest possible supratentorial route to the parasellar, suprasellar, and interpeduncular region. Detachment of the zygomatic bone is helpful for this purpose (Fujitsu and Kuwabara, 1985), and detachment of the superior, lateral, and posterior wall of the orbit further helps obtain better access (Fujitsu and Kuwabara, 1986). Medial and downward compression of the orbital contents reduces the need for retraction of the brain and provides ample working space when approaching by the trans-Sylvian (pterional) and subfrontal routes.

This cranio-orbito-zygomatic approach is a very low basal approach that is produced by a combined cranio-orbito-zygomatic osteotomy. This approach is multidirectional and uses primarily the oblique anterior, but sometimes also the lateral route.

Indications

Tumors that may require this approach include sphenoid ridge meningiomas, especially of the clinoidal type, suprasellar craniopharyngiomas with superoposterior extension, huge pituitary adenomas, and other large suprasellar tumors. High-placed basilar tip aneurysms are other indications for this approach, especially when they are large or giant. However, low-placed basilar tip aneurysms are not appropriate for this approach because retraction of the brain is not reduced in these cases by using the orbitozygomatic osteotomy.

Operative Procedure

Instrumentation

Instruments required for the cranio-orbito-zygomatic approach include conventional craniotomy instruments, an oscillating bone saw with several small detachable blades, and an air drill system with several steel and diamond tip burrs. A fine tip perforating burr for bone fixation holes is also needed. As for bipolar coagulating forceps, I prefer those with a simultaneous irrigation device. These irrigating bipolar forceps have two types of tip approximation: the Malis type and the YF type. The tips of the Malis type forceps approximate at a point, and this type of forceps is suitable for point coagulation. The YF type forceps have straighter blades and are convenient for grasping vessels and coagulating in a linear fashion; these techniques are often required in aneurysm surgery. In skull base surgery I often use bayonet-shaped microsurgery forceps. The grip spring of these forceps is slightly stronger than that of the conventional microforceps and the forceps tips have three different shapes (cupped, hooked, and sharp-pointed). The cupped-tip forceps are used for grasping the tumor capsule, and the hooked forceps for grasping the basal dura. The sharp-pointed forceps are useful for microsuture of injured vessels. Malleable tip spatulas are used to avoid retraction injury to the neurovascular structures. These spatulas have varied sizes and shapes, and are coated black to avoid reflection of the microscope illumination. The ultrasonic aspiration device is quite helpful for tumor surgery, but I seldom use a laser system even in the resection of vascular meningiomas. An operating table that can be adjusted as low as 40 cm from the floor is used so the surgeon can operate sitting comfortably on a chair. The chair should have an adjusting pedal for height, and should be sufficiently light and movable for the surgeon to change his or her position easily at any time during surgery.

For skull base surgery the ceiling-type surgical microscope is preferable to the floor type because approaches in multiple directions are often required and the surgeon frequently changes his or her position during surgery.

The surgeon handles the operating microscope with one hand while the other hand always holds a sucker, which not only cleans up the surgical field but slightly displaces the neurovascular structure to seek a better angle to proceed.

For more speedy microsurgery for skull base lesions, the focus system is not as frequently required as is single-handed use of the electromagnetic unlocking system. Furthermore, for better focusing, I developed a small device that is attachable to the surgical microscope and is a motor-drive for the focus system. This device is electrically connected both to the focus system and to the electromagnetic unlocking system. While the surgeon is unlocking the microscope and looking for a better angle, the device motor-drives the focus system to return to the midposition of the focus range. The recently developed autofocus surgical microscope may be a more useful and sophisticated tool for cranial base surgery, which requires approaches from multiple directions.

Positioning

The patient is placed in the supine position with a pillow under the shoulder ipsilateral to the approach. The operating table is bent in its middle, and the rostral half of the patient's body is tilted up to make an angle of about 15 to 20 degrees against the floor. The patient's head is tilted 20 degrees, rotated 45 degrees to the contralateral side, and fixed in the rotatable head holder (Sugita et al., 1978). This head holder is useful in skull base surgery because the patient's head can be rotated easily at any time. The head holder has four pins for fixation, and is rotated by loosening the lock of the device, which is covered by the sterile drapes. Because the patient's head is tilted to the contralateral side in the initial placement (Fig. 12-1B), further rotation to the contralateral side increases the vertex down angle (Fig. 12-1C & D).

Rotation back to the ipsilateral side decreases the vertex down angle (Fig. 12-1A). By tilting up and down the rostral half of the operating table, the surgeon can further

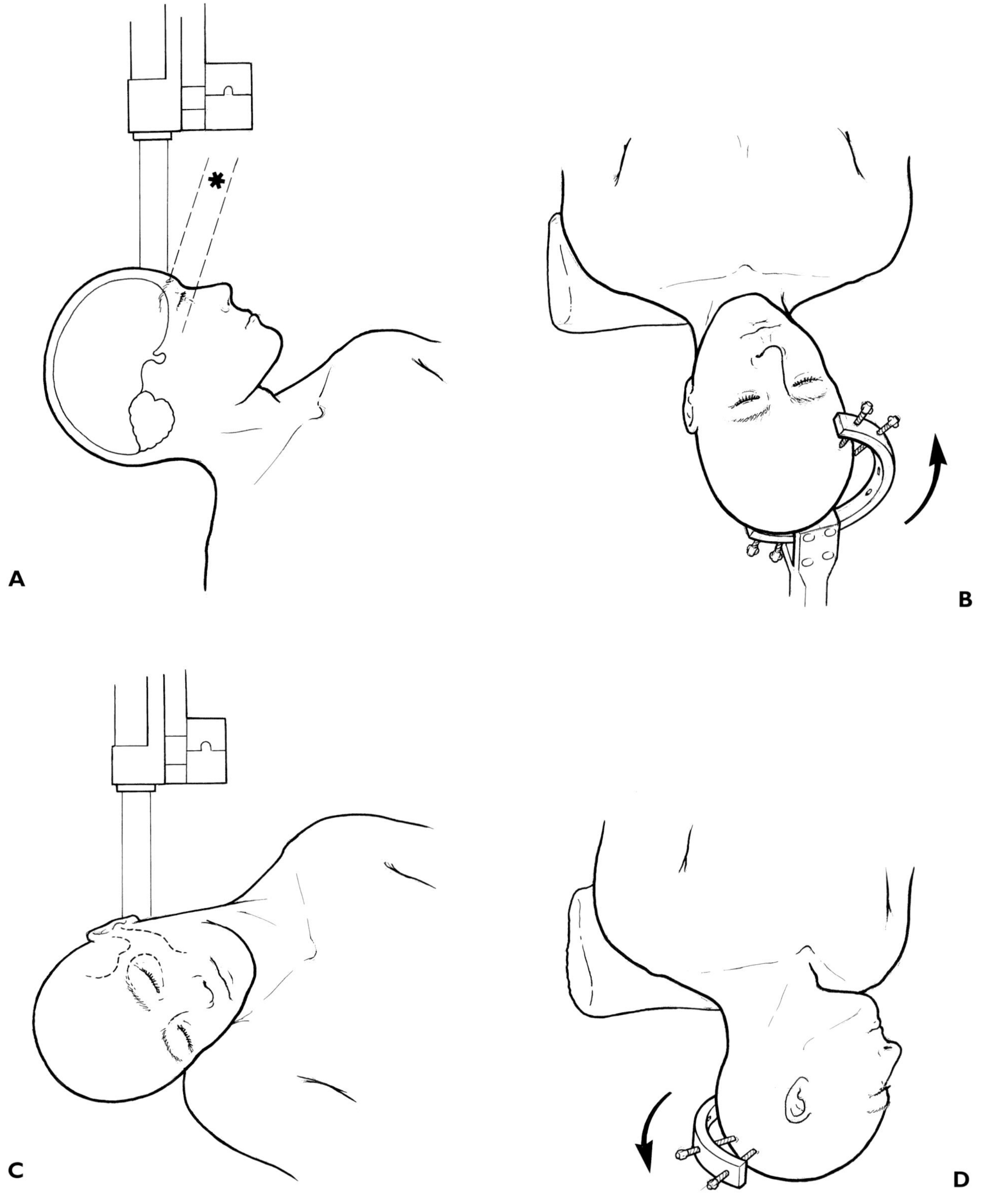

Figure 12-1. Head positioning of the patient with the rotatable head holder. *(A & B)* Position for a left anterior approach. *, Orientation of the microscope for subfrontal viewing. *(C & D)* Position for a lateral approach. For additional information see the text.

adjust the vertex down angle of the patient's head. Thus the surgeon is able to approach both from below (i.e., from the cranial base to the convexity) and from above (i.e., from the convexity to the cranial base). The rotatable head holder is quite useful not only for a multidirectional approach, but for minimizing the surgeon's fatigue and instability caused by the surgeon's uncomfortable posture.

Incision and Osteotomy

A long frontotemporal scalp incision is made, beginning on the ipsilateral side at the level of the lower end of the ear lobe, extending along the hairline to the contralateral side, and terminating at the level of the contralateral temporal line. To preserve all the branches of the facial nerve, the incision should be just in front of the ear lobe and as near as possible to the ear cartilage. Both the parietal branch and the anterior auricular branch of the superficial temporal artery are divided, and the frontal branch is preserved in the scalp flap.

The parotid gland is dissected, undermined around its posterior margin, and left attached to the scalp flap to expose the deep temporal fascia and the capsule of the temporomandibular joint (lateral ligament). The superficial temporal fascia with the areolar tissue is attached to the flap, but beyond the ipsilateral temporal line, subperiosteal dissection is carried out to expose the frontal bone. The supraorbital nerve is preserved by freeing it from the supraorbital canal, and the periorbita is detached from the superior, lateral wall of the orbit to facilitate sufficient turnover of the scalp flap (Fig. 12-2).

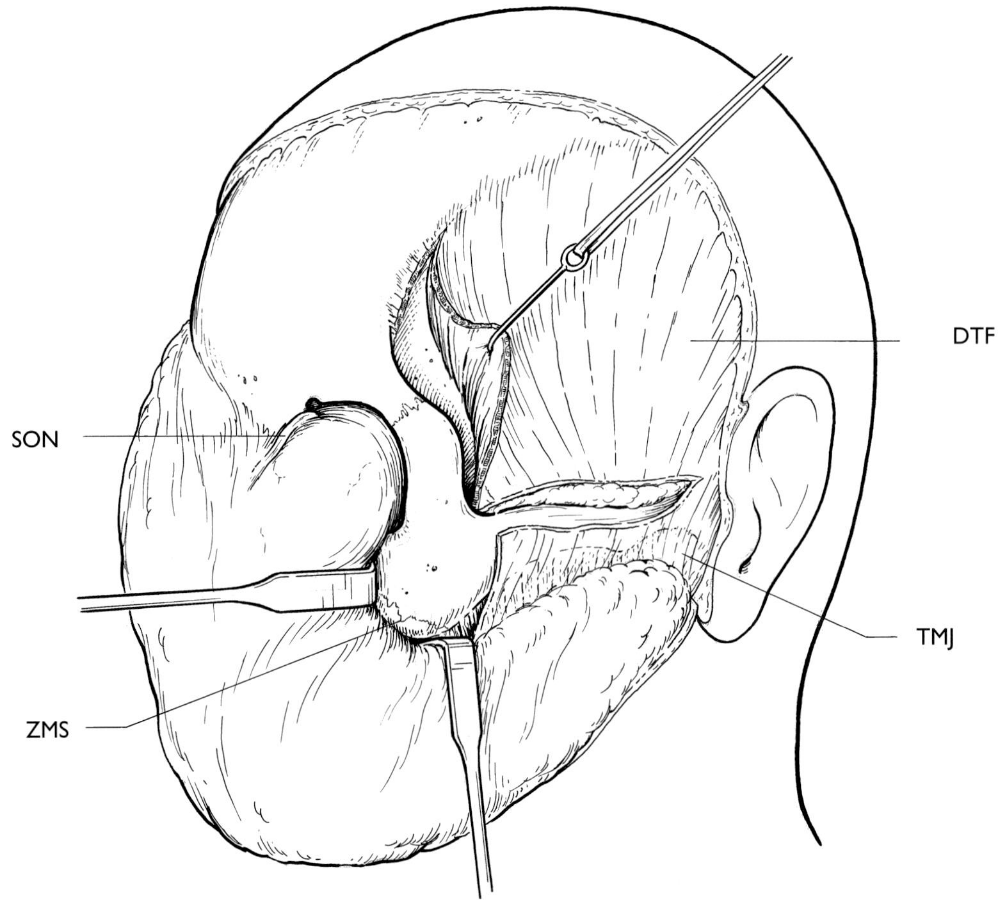

Figure 12-2. Reflection of the scalp flap. (For explanation of abbreviations, see Appendix 1, p. 373.)

After turning down the flap, the deep temporal fascia is incised along the superior border of the zygomatic arch and retracted downward to expose both the arch and the body of the zygomatic bone. The zygomaticomandibular portion of the temporal muscle is incised along the lower border of the zygomatic arch, and the zygomatic arch is undermined. The temporal muscle is detached from the lateral rim of the orbit (the frontal process of the zygomatic bone and the zygomatic process of the frontal bone), and is retracted posteriorly (Fig. 12-2). Using an oscillating bone saw in the temporal fossa, an osteotomy is made along the zygomaticosphenoidal suture (Fig. 12-3). This osteotomy begins on the base of the zygomatic process of the frontal bone, and extends downward to the inferior orbital fissure. Small holes for later bony reconstruction are drilled on both sides of the osteotomy line near the zygomatic process of the frontal bone. Likewise, with fixation holes, an osteotomy is also made near the posterior end of the zygomatic arch. On the zygomatic body, two fixation holes are made on each side of the osteotomy line for better repair in the later closure of the craniotomy.

Finally, the body of the zygomatic bone is cut about 1 cm posterior and parallel to the zygomaticomaxillary suture, and the inferior orbital fissure is reached (Fig. 12-3). Sometimes the maxillary sinus is opened and the mucous membranes are torn. In such a case the mucous membranes are sutured if possible, or pushed into the sinus, covered by a piece of muscle, and fibrin glue applied. After the zygomatic bone is detached, the temporal muscle is also detached along the temporal line and is

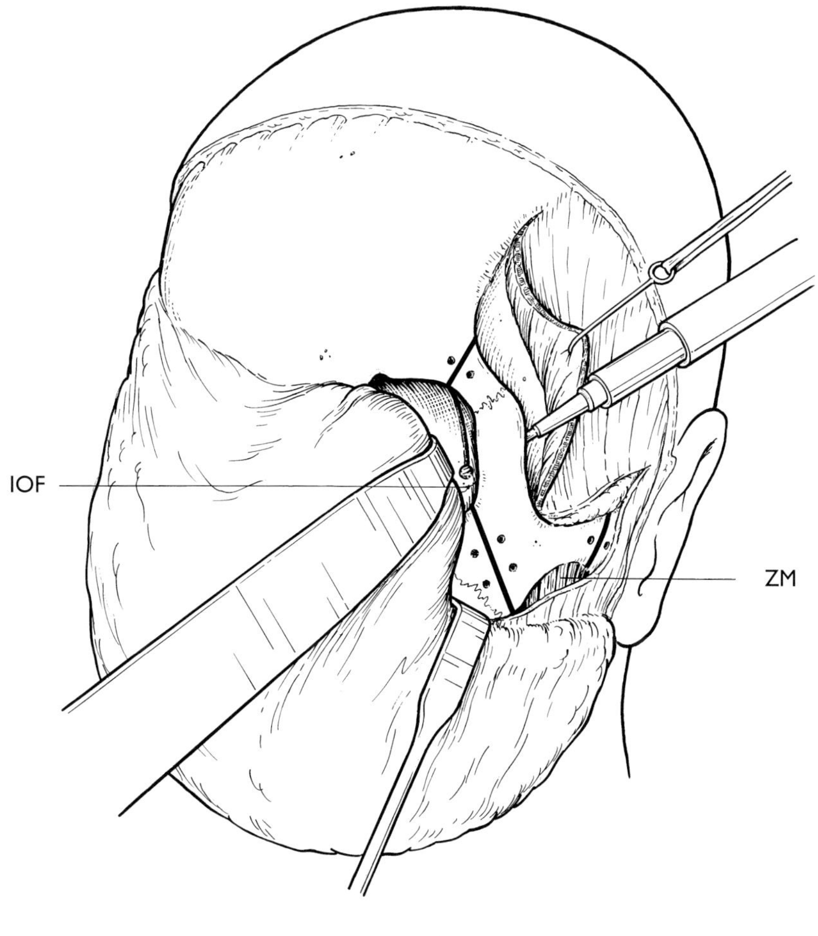

Figure 12-3. Osteotomy of the zygomatic bone.

retracted downward to expose the infratemporal fossa. Four burr holes are drilled (Fig. 12-4): the first in the frontal bone just behind the zygomatic process; the second in the sphenoidal bone, below the sphenoid wing; and the third in the temporal bone just above the pedicle of the zygomatic arch. The site of the fourth burr hole depends on the necessary size of the craniotomy, but is usually in the parietal bone about 5 cm above the third burr hole. A free bone flap is fashioned by frontotemporobasal craniotomy, with the frontal exposure being adjusted to the required extent. After the craniotomy, the third burr hole is connected with the inferior orbital fissure (Fig. 12-4).

Dural Opening and Basal Bone Removal

Before extensive removal of the basal bone, the dura is opened and some cerebrospinal fluid (CSF) is aspirated from the carotid cistern to obtain sufficient epidural working space. The dural opening is in the usual fashion; a semicircular incision is made from the anterosuperior to the anteroinferior burr hole and supplementary incisions are made toward the posteroinferior and posterosuperior burr holes (Fig. 12-5). When computed tomography (CT) scanning or magnetic resonance imaging (MRI) shows the carotid cistern packed by the tumor, lumbar drainage is placed preoperatively. After sufficient relaxation of the brain is obtained, the dura is dissected from the superior and posterolateral wall of the orbit. This dissection pro-

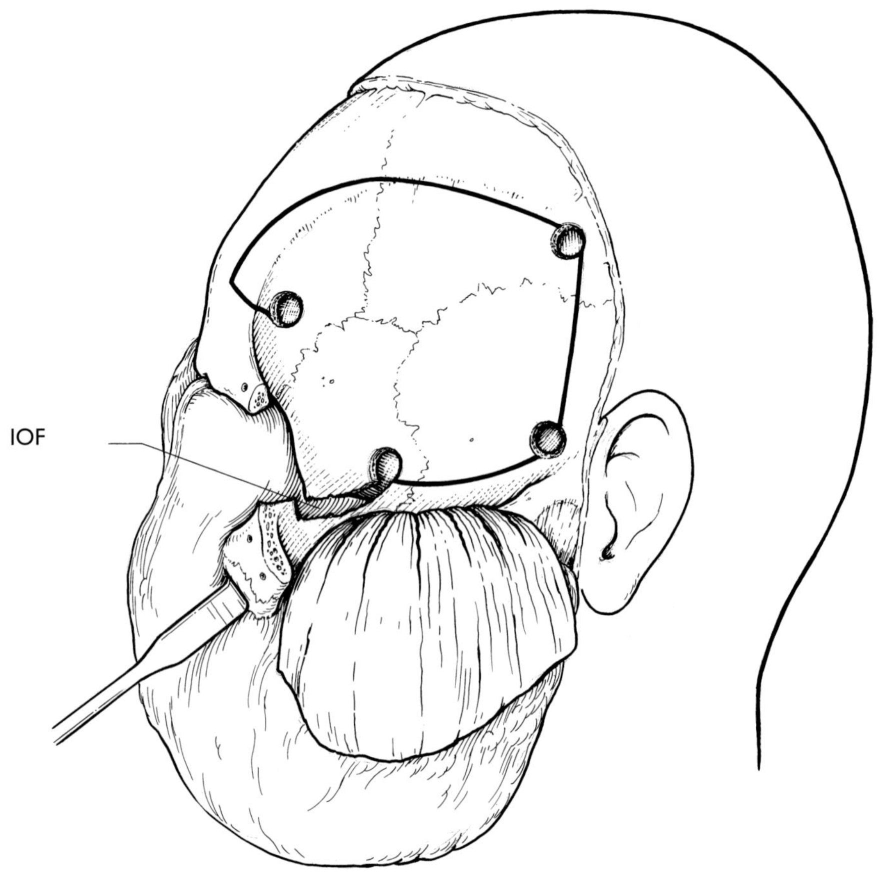

Figure 12-4. Craniotomy, the exact limits depend on the exposure required in each case.

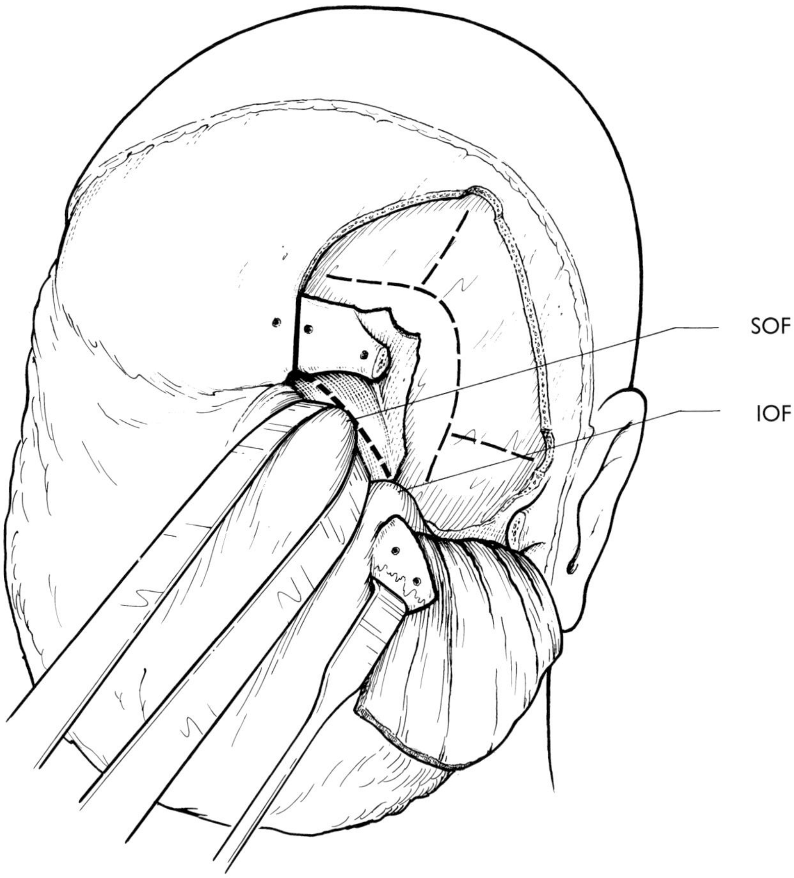

Figure 12-5. Orbitotomy and dural opening. The thick black dashed line indicates the use of a diamond drill.

ceeds along the sphenoid wing to the base of the anterior clinoid process. The orbital contents are compressed downward, and an air drill with a fine tip diamond burr is used in the space between the orbital contents and the superior, lateral wall of the orbit. The lateral end of the superior orbital fissure is connected with the inferior orbital fissure, and is also drilled toward the medial basal edge of the frontal craniotomy. For the osteotomy of the orbital rim, an oscillating bone saw is more helpful for cosmetic reasons (Fig. 12-5). During these orbital osteotomies, both the periorbita and the basal dura are protected by spatulas (Fig. 12-5). Bradycardia due to the oculocardiac reflex may be experienced when excessive compression is applied on the orbital apex. Compression upon the eyeball, however, never causes severe bradycardia that requires interruption of the procedure. Thus, the superior and lateral wall of the orbit are removed en bloc, incorporating the middle third of the sphenoid wing. This block of bone is useful for later reconstruction to prevent postoperative enophthalmos.

Drilling of other basal bones (e.g., total unroofing of the optic canal, removal of the anterior clinoid process, or decompression of the foramen rotundum and ovale) may be done in some cases. The foramen spinosum may also be reached to coagulate and cut the middle meningeal artery, and the petrous portion of the carotid artery may be exposed in the Glasscock's triangle. These extensive resections of the basal bones are required in some cases, but not necessary in others. Generally speaking, drilling of these bones is useful for epidural obliteration of the feeding vessels of cranial base meningiomas.

Surgery for Cranial Base Meningiomas

In the surgical resection of cranial base meningiomas, especially of the clinoidal meningiomas, there are two general principles of surgical strategy: early obliteration of the feeding vessels and thorough internal decompression of the tumor. To obliterate most of the feeders from the external carotid artery, thus making the tumor debulking more bloodless, the surgeon should attack the tumor attachment at the cranial base as soon as possible. As a result of the cranio-orbito-zygomatic osteotomy, the surgeon is already closer to the skull base than he or she is by conventional craniotomy. However, clinoidal meningiomas compress the basal dura tightly against the basal bone near the tumor attachment. For this reason, the anterior clinoid process and the roof of the optic canal are hardly accessible epidurally even after sufficient aspiration of the CSF. The cranio-orbito-zygomatic osteotomy enables the surgeon to approach supraorbitally and drill off these basal bones. The orbital contents are retracted medially and downward and the basal dura is peeled from the cranial base bone, creating a space between the basal dura and the orbital contents. If the space so obtained is insufficient for drilling, the basal portion of the tumor attachment is removed intradurally around the anterior clinoid process. During this epi- and subdural approach to the tumor attachment, most of the feeding vessels from the external carotid artery are coagulated and cut, making the debulking of the tumor more bloodless. The surgeon is also able to keep an easier anatomic orientation by observing supraorbitally (i.e., underneath the skull base) the bony structures around the anterior clinoid process. This supraorbital observation greatly helps to avoid the risk of injuring the internal carotid artery, which is often encased by the tumor attachment.

As the first step of the basal bone drilling, the optic canal is completely unroofed, making medial displacement of the optic nerve possible. Then, the anterior clinoid process, on which the tumor attachment is mainly based, may also be removed. The anterior clinoid process is connected to the body of the sphenoid bone by two pedicles: the roof of the optic canal and the optic strut. After the optic canal is unroofed and the optic nerve is gently displaced with its dural sheath, the optic strut can be safely drilled off with good orientation.

In some cases, however, the tip of the anterior clinoid process has another pedicle that creates a bony ring around the anterior loop of the carotid artery. This third pedicle forms the posterior semicircle of the bony ring, which makes en bloc removal of the anterior clinoid process rather difficult. In such cases, an alternative method is near total drilling off followed by piecemeal removal of the remaining thin bony shell.

As mentioned before, most of the tumor feeders from the external carotid artery are obliterated during these drilling procedures in the epidural space. However, obliteration of feeding arteries from the cerebral arteries is possible only after sufficient reduction of the bulk of the tumor. The Sylvian fissure is widely opened, the distal branches of the middle cerebral artery are identified, and internal decompression of the tumor is done by the electrocutting loop or by the ultrasonic aspirator. In parts where internal decompression is sufficiently performed, the tumor capsule is gently peeled from the surrounding brain, and tumor feeders are carefully differentiated from the cerebral arteries before they are coagulated and cut. Not only major cerebral arteries but the perforating vessels such as the striate arteries, the anterior choroidal artery, and the perforators from the posterior communicating artery, should be care-

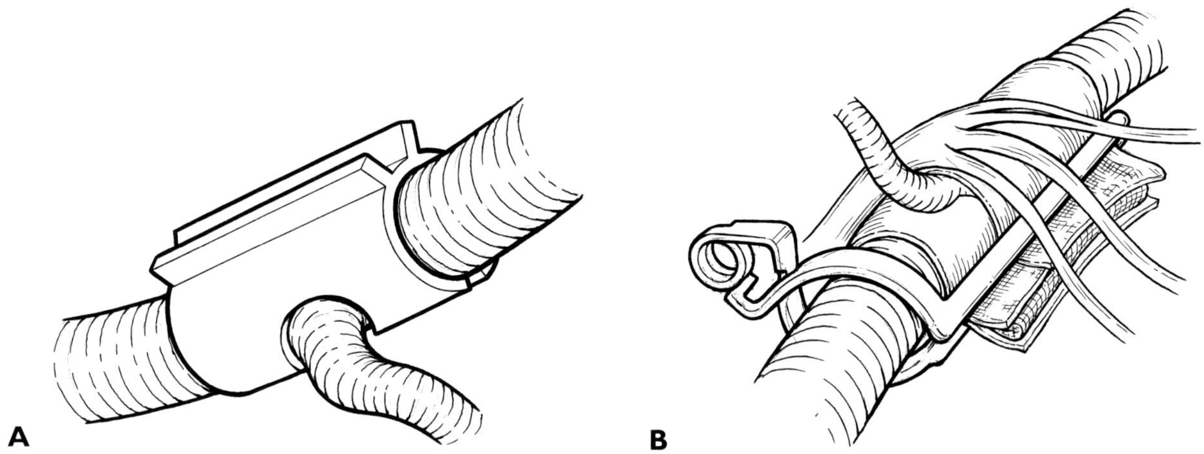

Figure 12-6. Repair methods for injured arteries. *(A)* Silastic encircling clip for hemostasis. *(B)* Wrap-clipping technique for hemostasis. For explanations see the text.

fully preserved. In cases in which the plane of cleavage between these arteries and the tumor capsule is maintained, preservation of these arteries is not difficult. However, in some cases in which the tumor invades the adventitia of the cerebral arteries, the surgeon cannot help leaving small pieces of the tumor on the vessel wall. Rupture of the vessel wall often occurs in these cases if the surgeon attempts to remove such tumor rests tightly adherent to the vessel. It is always difficult to suture the tear in the vessel wall that is invaded by the tumor. Among the alternative techniques used in the repair of injured vessels are use of a silastic encircling clip (Ishiwata et al., 1990) (Fig. 12-6A) and wrap-clipping with a Silastic sheet (Fujitsu et al., 1994) (Fig. 12-6B). The internal carotid artery is preserved and traced to the cranial base, where the surgeon can check by observing supraorbitally in the epidural space how close to the carotid artery he or she is working. If the tumor is found to infiltrate the basal dura or the lateral wall of the cavernous sinus, this dura is resected extensively until a safety margin is obtained. Margins of the resected dura are histologically checked to make sure that there is no tumor invasion.

In the surgery of cranial base tumors, the surgeon often needs to approach in multiple directions. When the surgeon attacks the bulk of a tumor that is embedded in the basal aspect of the brain, the approach is from below (i.e., from the cranial base to the convex). To approach in this direction with less retraction of the brain, a sufficiently vertex down position of the patient's head is required. With the use of the rotatable head holder, the patient's head is rotated contralaterally to increase the vertex down angle and near lateral head position is obtained (Fig. 12-1C & D). If the orbital contents are retracted inferomedially, brain retraction is further minimized and more space is obtained on the basal aspect of the brain (Fig. 12-7). On the other hand, when the surgeon attacks the tumor attachment to the skull base, the approach is from above (i.e., from the vertex to the cranial base) (Fig. 12-8). For the surgeon to approach comfortably in this direction, the patient's head should be rotated back ipsilaterally to the oblique frontal position to decrease the vertex down angle. To further decrease the vertex down angle, the rostral half of the operating table is tilted up. Otherwise, the surgeon is obliged to hyperextend his or her neck, looking obliquely upward to approach the cranial base. Such an uncomfortable posture not only increases the surgeon's fatigue but considerably disturbs the stability of the microsurgical technique. Figure 12-9

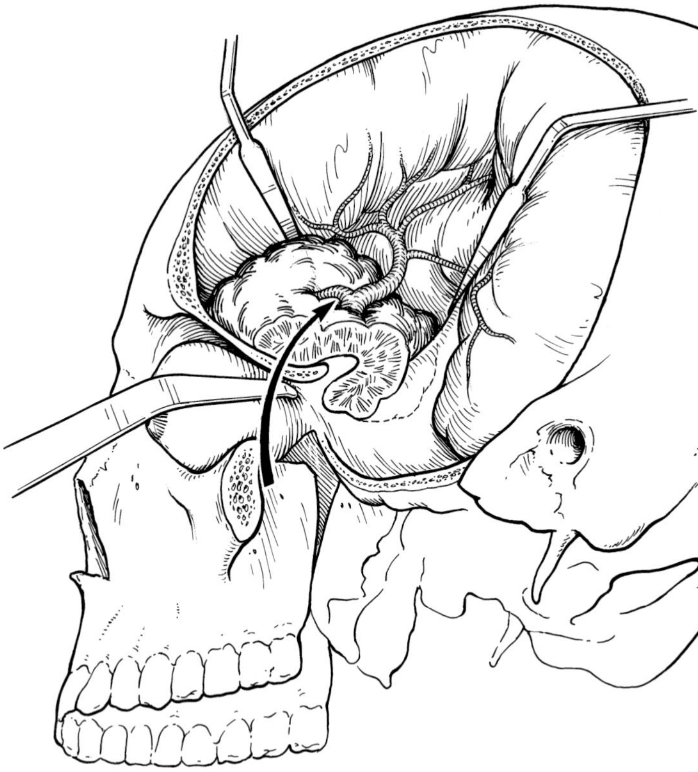

Figure 12-7. The tumor bulk in the basal aspect of the brain is attacked in the basal-to-vertex trajectory (arrow). For explanation see the text.

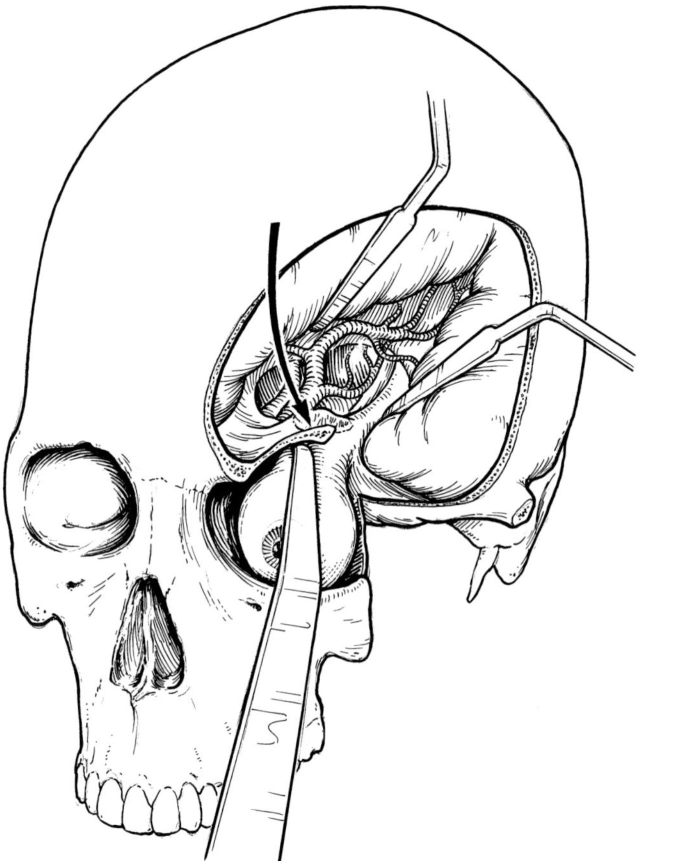

Figure 12-8. The tumor attachment on the cranial base is attacked in the vertex-to-base trajectory (arrow). For explanation see the text.

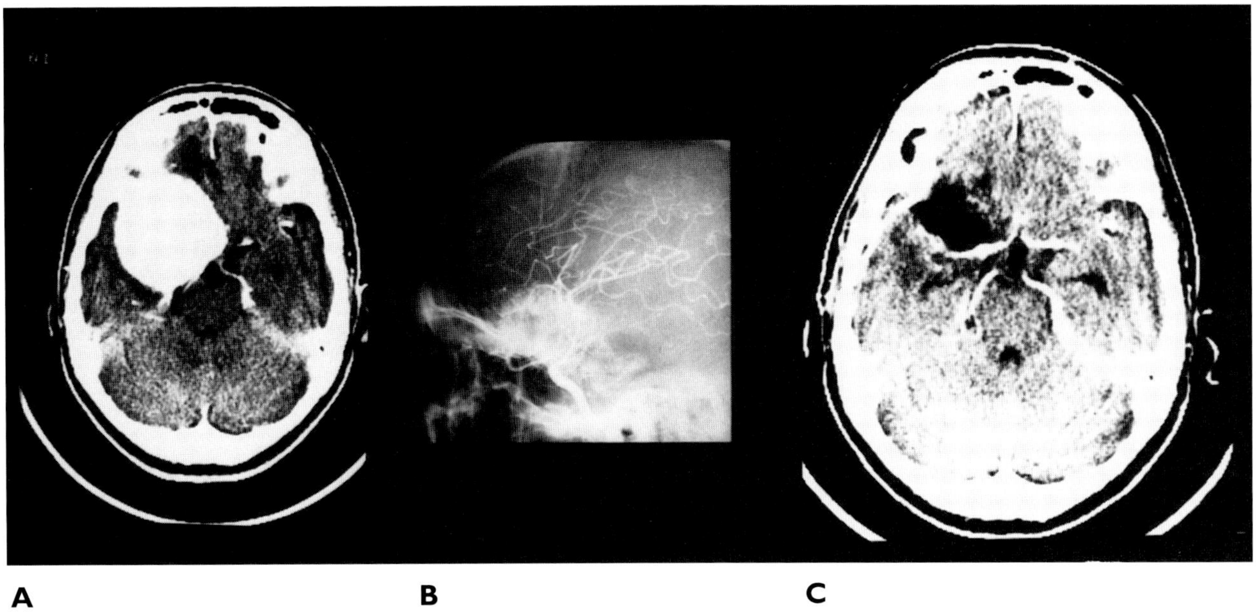

Figure 12-9. Clinoidal meningioma operated on through the cranio-orbito-zygomatic approach. (A) Preoperative CT, (B) preoperative angiogram, and (C) postoperative CT.

shows a case of clinoidal meningioma removed by the cranio-orbito-zygomatic approach.

Closure of the Craniotomy

A watertight closure of the dura mater is made in the usual fashion. When the basal dura has been extensively resected, fascia lata is obtained and is sutured to the resected margins of the basal dura. Before closure of the craniotomy, reconstruction of the orbital bone is important in order to prevent postoperative enophthalmos. Generally speaking, orbital roof decompression not associated with posterolateral wall resection does not cause enophthalmos. However, extensive resection of the posterolateral wall of the orbit always results in significant enophthalmos. To prevent such enophthalmos, the bone of the superior-lateral-posterior wall of the orbit, which was removed en bloc, is replaced and fixed to the other frontal and middle fossa bones.

Alkyl α-cyanoacrylate is then applied to the osteotomy line to reinforce the reconstruction. The craniotomy bone flap is replaced and fixed with three to four ligatures. The temporal muscle is also replaced and fixed with several ligatures on to the temporal line. The zygomatic bone is replaced and fixed using the small holes that have been made during the craniotomy.

Zygomatic Approach for High-Placed Basilar Tip Aneurysms

For high-placed basilar tip aneurysms, osteotomies other than zygomectomy are not needed unless the aneurysm is substantially large or giant. For normal-sized aneurysms on and around the high-placed basilar tip, only a portion of the orbital rim is incorporated in the zygomectomy and the frontal exposure is limited to below the level of the temporal line (Fig. 12-10). The vertex down tilt of the patient's head depends on how high placed the basilar tip is, and varies 25 to 45 degrees below the horizontal line. The sphenoid ridge is rongeured to reach the lateral end of the superior orbital fissure, and the anterior temporal base is widely exposed. However,

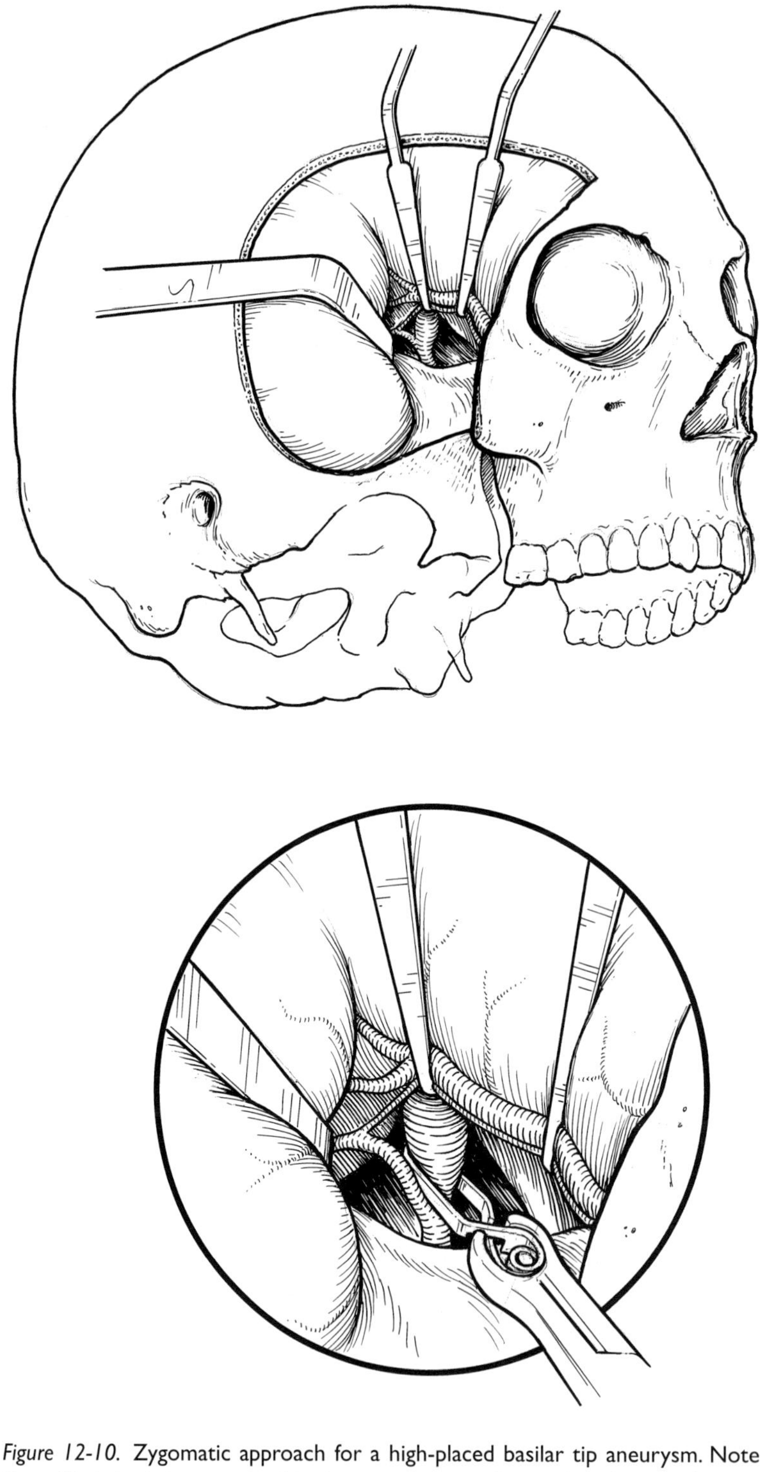

Figure 12-10. Zygomatic approach for a high-placed basilar tip aneurysm. Note only a portion of the orbital rim is incorporated in the zygomectomy. For explanation see the text.

osteotomy of the superior, lateral wall of the orbit, removal of the anterior clinoid process, or drilling of other basal bones are not necessary.

The sylvian fissure is widely opened, the bridging vein coming off the temporal lobe tip is divided, and the temporal lobe is retracted posteriorly. Usually below the posterior communicating (PCom) artery, but sometimes above this artery and between the perforators, the interpeduncular fossa is approached obliquely from anteroinferior. To obtain a more anterior view of the aneurysm and of the perforators coming off the contralateral first segment of the posterior cerebral artery (P_1), medial displacement of the carotid artery is required. A malleable tip spatula is applied on the carotid-PCom artery junction and intermittent retraction of the carotid artery is performed (Fig. 12-10). Retraction of the carotid artery should not exceed 5 minutes at one time; 5 minutes of retraction followed by 3 minutes release is recommended.

When the aneurysm points dorsally (i.e., parallel to the P_1), the aneurysmal neck is quite difficult to clip by the anteroinferior approach. In such a case the subtemporal route is more suited; the anterior half of the temporal lobe is elevated, and the ambient cistern is approached from lateral and is traced anteriorly to reach the aneurysm. Retraction of the temporal lobe is much less in the zygomatic approach than in the conventional subtemporal approach.

When the aneurysm is substantially large or giant, multidirectional approaches, including a more anterior approach, are often required. Detachment of the superior-lateral-posterior wall of the orbit and medial downward retraction of the orbital contents are helpful for this purpose. In giant aneurysms either the P_1 or PCom artery is often extremely hypoplastic near the junction of the P_1 and PCom arteries. Based on careful evaluation of preoperative angiography, either the P_1 or PCom artery can safely be divided after ligating with 8–0 monofilament nylon. To preserve all the perforators from the P_1 and PCom arteries, the use of hemostatic clips, bipolar coagulation, or braided silk should be avoided. Division of the P_1 or PCom artery serves to mobilize the carotid artery further, and provides substantial working space for safer manipulation.

I have not experienced any case of contusional hemorrhage attributable to the compromise of the bridging vein of the temporal lobe tip. Theoretically, however, this complication is possible in rare cases in which the vein of Labbé is not well developed and the venous drainage of the temporal lobe depends predominantly on the vein coming off the temporal lobe tip. In such a case, in which the aneurysm is not so large and a multidirectional approach is not needed, the extradural temporopolar approach (Day et al., 1994) may provide sufficient exposure without sacrificing this vein. In a case of a substantially large or giant aneurysm, the author recommends resection of the tip of the temporal lobe in order to preserve the bridging vein. The temporal lobe, from the pole to 3 cm posterior, is resected and the bridging vein is dissected and preserved. A giant aneurysm is approached both from above and from below this vein.

When proximal control and temporary clipping of the basilar artery is needed, the surgeon approaches in the rostrocaudal direction above the bridging vein (Fig. 12-11). On the contrary, thrombectomy of a giant aneurysm and application of the clip are usually performed in the caudorostral direction below the bridging vein (Fig. 12-12). Figures 12-13 and 12-14 show a case of a thrombosed giant aneurysm on the basilar top, operated on through the cranio-orbito-zygomatic approach, using all of the above-mentioned techniques.

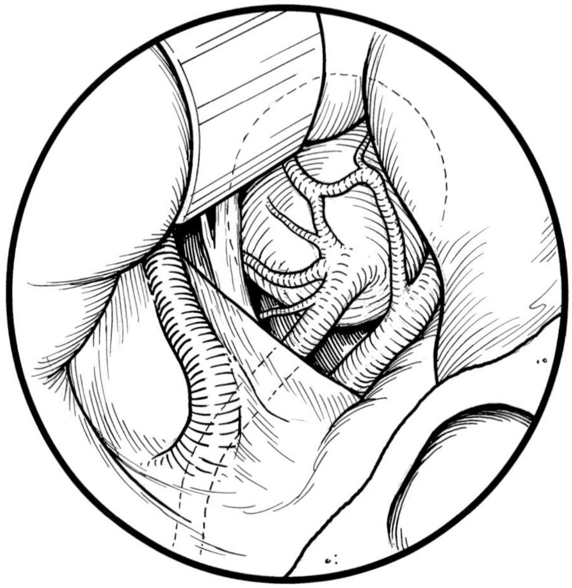

Figure 12-11. A giant, mostly thrombosed, basilar tip aneurysm. Proximal control of the basilar artery is done above the bridging vein (structures seen with the surgical microscope are magnified). For explanation see the text.

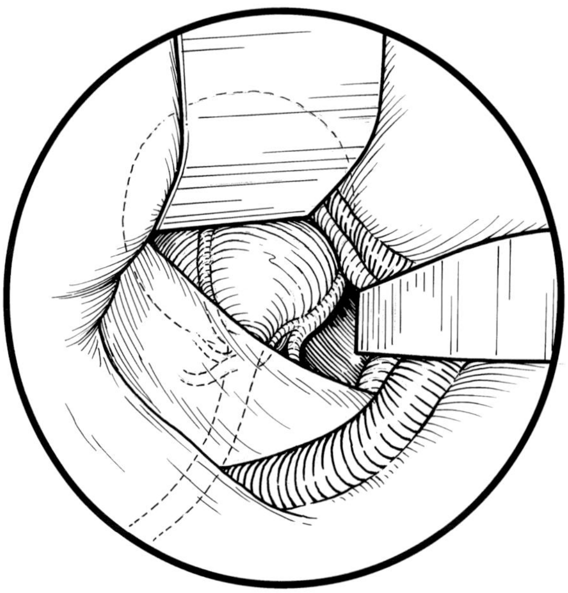

Figure 12-12. The same case as in Fig. 12-11. The head is rotated and in the basal-to-vertex trajectory, the aneurysmal neck is attacked below the bridging vein. For explanation see the text.

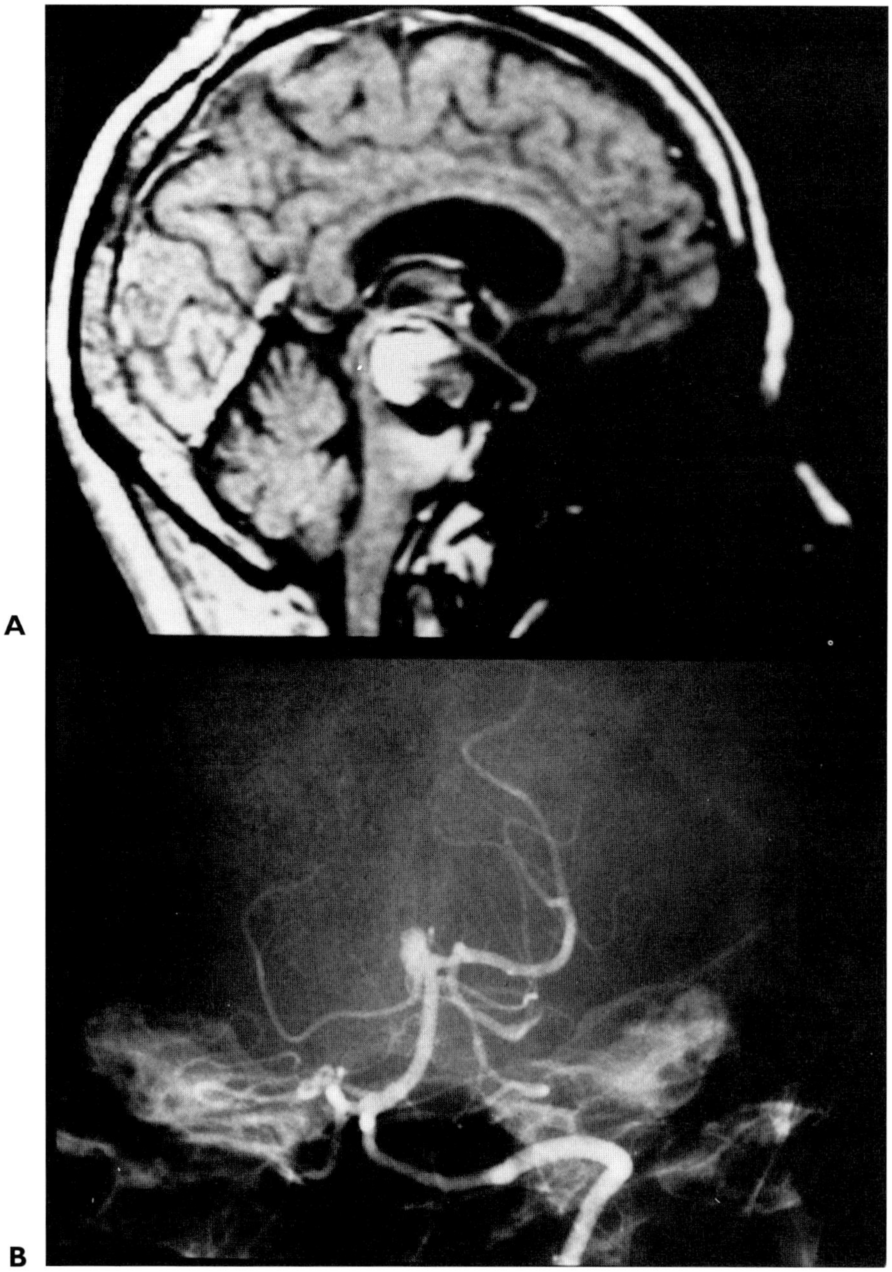

Figure 12-13. The same case as in Fig. 12-11. *(A)* Preoperative MRI and *(B)* angiogram. The left posterior cerebral artery is filled from the left carotid artery.

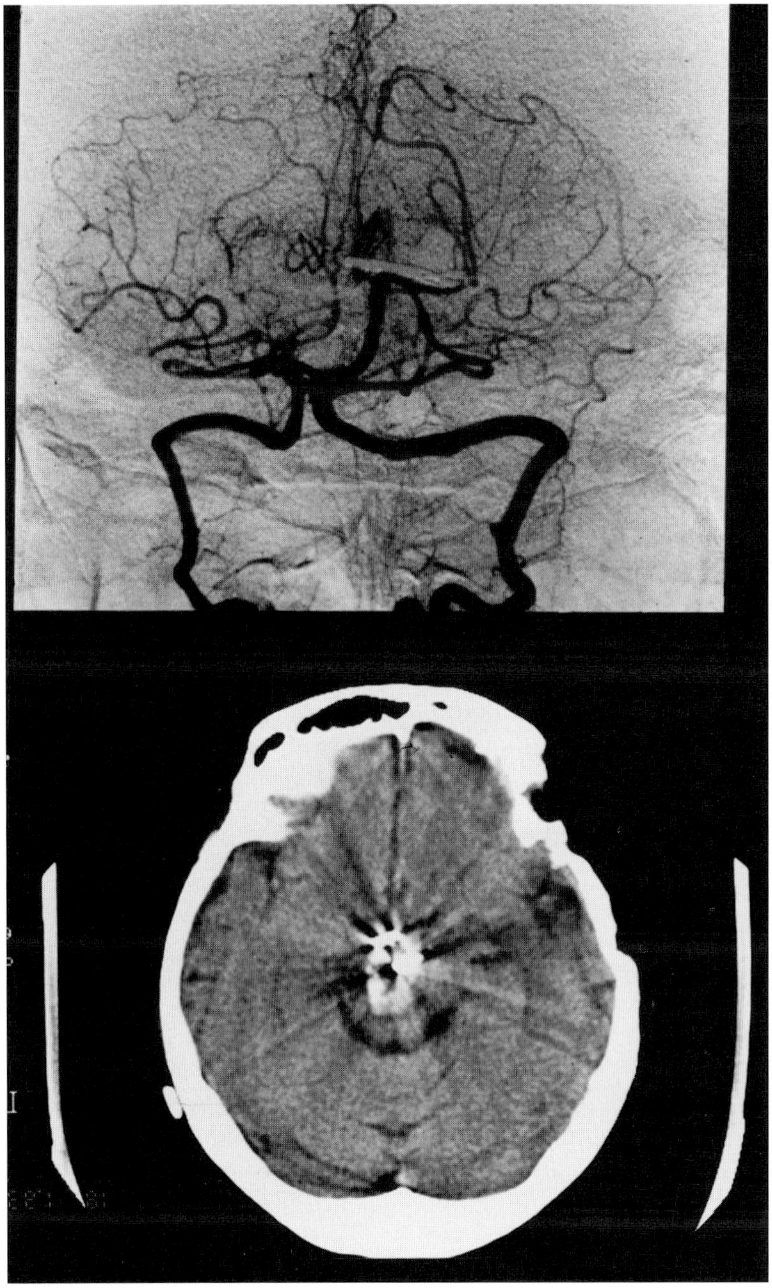

A

B

Figure 12-14. The same case as in Fig. 12-11. *(A)* Postoperative angiogram and *(B)* CT. The right-sided cranio-orbito-zygomatic approach was used in this case, and the right posterior communicating artery was divided. Consequently, both posterior cerebral arteries are filled postoperatively from the anterior circulation *(A)*.

References

Day JD, Giannotta SL, Fukushima T (1994) Extradural temporopolar approach to lesions of the upper basilar artery and infrachiasmatic region. J Neurosurg 81:230–235

Fujitsu K, Ishiwata Y, Gondo G et al (1994) Wrap-clipping with a Dacron mesh Silastic sheet. Technical note. J Neurosurg 80:336–337

Fujitsu K, Kuwabara T (1985) Zygomatic approach for lesions in the interpeduncular cistern. J Neurosurg 62:340–343

Fujitsu K, Kuwabara T (1986) Orbitocraniobasal approach for anterior communicating artery aneurysms. Neurosurgery 18:367–369

Ishiwata Y, Inomori S, Fujitsu K et al (1990) A new intracranial Silastic encircling clip for hemostasis. Technical note. J Neurosurg 73:638–639

Sugita K, Hirota T, Mizutani T et al (1978) A newly designed multipurpose microneurosurgical head frame. Technical note. J Neurosurg 48:656–657

13

Approaches to and Techniques of Surgery Within the Cavernous Sinus

Vinko V. Dolenc

The indications for surgical treatment of lesions in the cavernous sinus (CS) have been the subject of very heated debate over the last 15 years. The first direct CS surgery required extracorporeal circulation (Parkinson, 1965, 1969, 1973, 1987). Since bleeding was the main problem (Parkinson was operating on vascular lesions) it was possible to carry out such operations only in well-equipped centers. However, performance of CS surgery did not gather the expected momentum after the first successful operations. Later, with the advent of the intravascular balloon occlusion techniques in the treatment of caroticocavernous fistula (CCF) and aneurysms, CS surgery for vascular lesions was almost completely abandoned.

The first anatomic studies of the parasellar region were started half a century ago, and have since been continued (Dolenc, 1983, 1989; Parkinson, 1965, 1987; Taptas, 1949, 1960, 1982, 1987; Umansky and Nathan, 1982). The first direct surgical procedures for high-flow CCFs were performed with the help of extracorporeal circulation and hypothermia (Parkinson, 1969, 1973, 1987). Direct surgery for aneurysms and high-flow CCFs without using extracorporeal circulation and hypothermia was only possible 15 years ago. The knowledge gained was presented at the international neurosurgical meeting in Munich in 1981, but the concept was not well accepted. It then took 2 years before the obtained results could be published in the *Journal of Neurosurgery* (Dolenc, 1983). Since then, interest in CS surgery in particular, and interest in skull base surgery in general, has been steadily growing. It is interesting that there are very few topics in neurosurgery that have led to so much antagonism and difference of opinion with regard to very basic questions: Whether to operate or not and, if yes, when. For years there was a prevailing negative attitude toward direct CS surgery. However, over the last few years this attitude has almost disappeared as the young generation of neurosurgeons has become familiar with the complex normal anatomy of the CS as well as with the surgical procedures for tumorous and vascular lesions in this region.

The CS anatomy and CS vascular and tumorous lesions in particular represent the highest grade of complexity in the field of neurosurgery. This is the reason why there are neurosurgeons who are still not in favor of CS surgery. An additional reason is that endovascular procedures have been introduced that can deal successfully with many small and even medium-sized CS aneurysms as well as with CCFs, which further reduces the number of cases for direct surgical approach (Serbinenko, 1974; Vinuela and Lylyk, 1987). Embolization of meningiomas in the CS as well as γ-knife treatment of meningiomas have further postponed the final surgical solution to this problem.

There is no doubt that only direct surgery can maintain patency of the internal cartoid artery (ICA) in cases of large and giant intracavernous aneurysms, in cases of extensive laceration of the ICA causing high-flow CCFs, and also in traumatic aneurysms that, in the great majority of cases, are located on the anteromedial aspect of the wall of the anterior loop of the ICA and project inferomedially into the sphenoid sinus (Dolenc, 1990, 1991, 1994a, 1994b). This is also true for large and giant carotid ophthalmic aneurysms, and particularly those that are partially intra- and partially extradural (Dolenc, 1985, 1994b). Occlusion of large and giant vascular lesions by interventional endovascular techniques is very difficult or impossible to perform while at the same time preserving the normal lumen of the ICA (Vinuela and Lylyk, 1987). Occlusion of the ICA should not be considered as an acceptable consequence of the treatment and for this reason every effort should be made to preserve the patency of the ICA or, if this is impossible, undertake either grafting of the ICA or end-to-end anastomosis, which are nowadays only feasible with open surgery (Dolenc, 1991). γ-knife treatment of a CS meningioma, its embolization, or both represents only a temporary solution to the problem, which will later have to be resolved completely.

However, it is necessary to bear in mind that when the lesion is advanced, when the function(s) of the individual oculomotor nerves and the 5th cranial nerve are partially or completely lost, and when the ICA in the CS is not only displaced but also compressed and invaded by tumor, the problem becomes much more complex and the question must be raised as to whether the normal quality of life can still be restored (Dolenc, 1989, 1992a, 1992b, 1994c). At present, surgery can still solve many more problems than all the other modalities put together when treating these very complex and demanding CS vascular and tumorous lesions. This is the reason why normal anatomy, surgical anatomy, and surgical approaches to the CS lesions should not only be well known but also well understood and practiced, at least in the laboratory.

Surgical Technique

Craniotomy

The patient is placed in the supine position with the head in a tripoint Mayfield headrest. The head is rotated to the side opposite to the pathology, approximately 30 to 40 degrees, thus exposing the pterional area. The fronto-parieto-temporal region is shaved. The operative field is appropriately prepared, draped, and marked (Fig. 13-1) and a curvilinear skin incision is made from in front of the tragus of the ear in a superior direction toward the midline to end at a point slightly behind the hairline. The convexity of the incision line faces posteriorly. The skin flap is bluntly stripped away from the fascia of the temporalis muscle and from the periosteum in an anterior direction until the anterior edge of the orbital rim is reached. The skin flap is reflected over the eye and then fixed with a fish hook at the point where the orbital

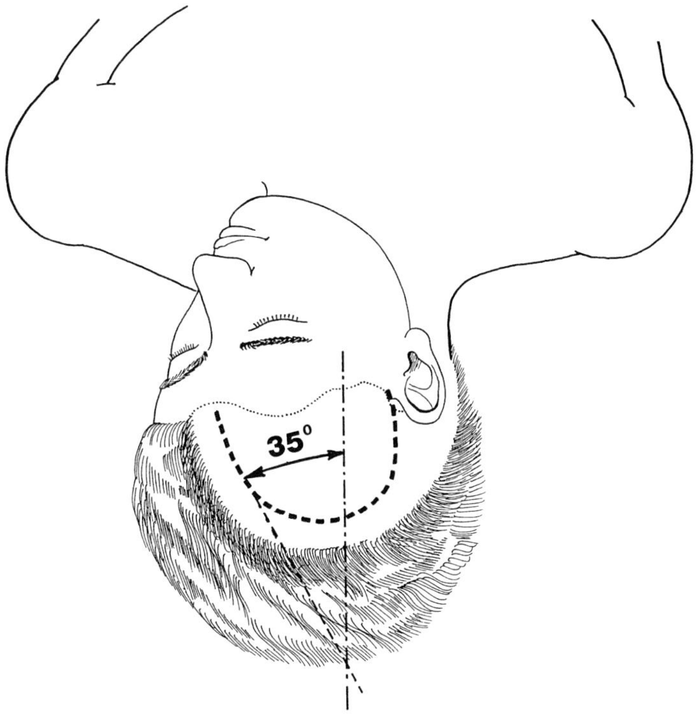

Figure 13-1. The initial position of the patient's head is shown. The ideal rotation of the head in the opposite direction to the lesion is 35 degrees, and the ideal deflection is when the orbitozygomatic junction is the highest point of the head. The veins of the neck should not be stretched on the side of the lesion or compressed on the opposite side.

rim and the zygomatic bone meet. The temporalis muscle is cut along its insertion to the bone; the muscle is then peeled off from the temporal bone and reflected laterally over the zygoma (Figs. 13-2 and 13-3). Two burr holes are made, the first at the frontoparietal junction above the temporal bone, and the second in the temporal bone (Fig. 13-4). The bone is drilled behind the junction of the zygoma and the orbital rim, where the bone is thick and continues in an inferomedial direction into the sphenoid wing (Fig. 13-4). The bone flap is then cut using a craniotome in the directions as indicated in Figure 13-4. Holes are made along the edge of the bone as well as along the bone flap which, at the end of surgery, will enable the bone flap to be fixed accordingly to the frontal bone, thus preventing the formation of a gap between the bone and the bone flap after the temporalis muscle has been resutured (Fig. 13-5). The bone flap is then lifted and the middle meningeal artery (MMA), if torn, is coagulated. The dura should be fixed with separate sutures to the edges of the temporal (posterior) and frontal (superior) bones, thus preventing postoperative epidural hematoma (Fig. 13-6).

The next step is to open the orbital roof with a diamond drill behind the orbital rim in order to expose the periorbita. Care should be taken not to damage the periorbita. The periorbita is peeled off from the orbital roof with a dissector; the dura is then separated from the orbital roof using the same technique, and so the orbital roof is isolated step by step (Fig. 13-7) and then removed on the anterior and posterior aspects of the sphenoid wing together with the sphenoid wing itself. Great caution should be exercised as it is important not to enter the frontal sinus. It is necessary to carefully inspect the edge of the resected bone of the orbital roof medialward and to check that the frontal sinus has not been opened. Once the lateral tip of the superior

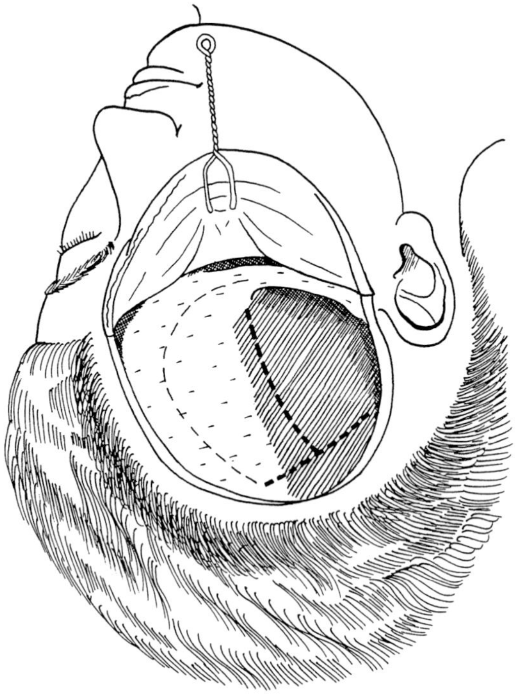

Figure 13-2. The skin flap has been reflected over the eye, and the orbital rim has been exposed. The temporalis muscle should be cut along the insertion line perpendicular to the muscle fibers over the frontal bone, and along the muscle fibers posteriorly over the temporal bone.

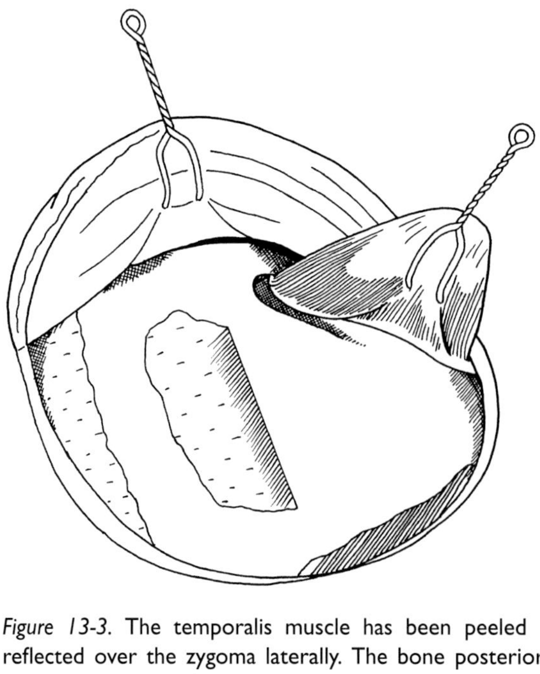

Figure 13-3. The temporalis muscle has been peeled off from the temporal bone, lifted and reflected over the zygoma laterally. The bone posterior to the junction of the zygoma and the orbital rim has been stripped off the periosteum. The periosteum over the frontal bone has been cut in a semicircular line and then separated from the bone (see Fig. 13-2).

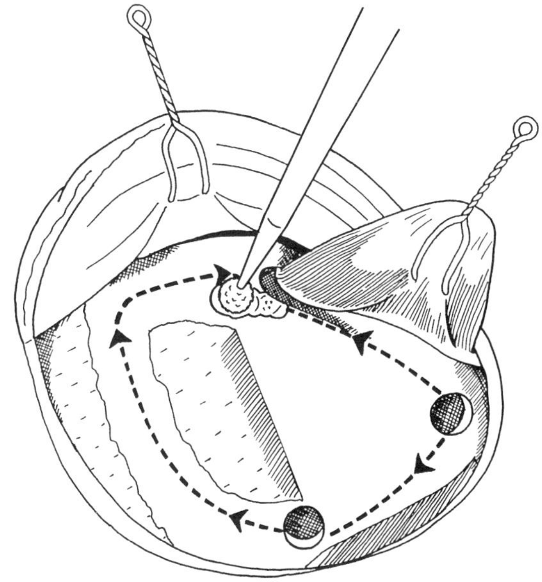

Figure 13-4. Two burr holes have been made in the posterior part of the exposed bone, and on the posterior aspect of the junction of the orbit and the zygoma the bone should be drilled away with a diamond drill in order to expose the dura as well as the periorbita. The bone flap should then be cut in the direction as indicated by the arrows.

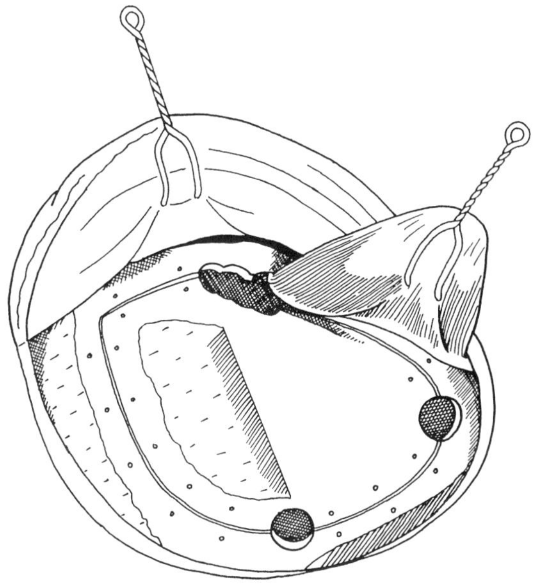

Figure 13-5. The bone flap has been cut, and before lifting it, small holes have been made at the corresponding points along both sides of the cutting line, which ensure that the bone flap is firmly fixed back in place at the end of the operation.

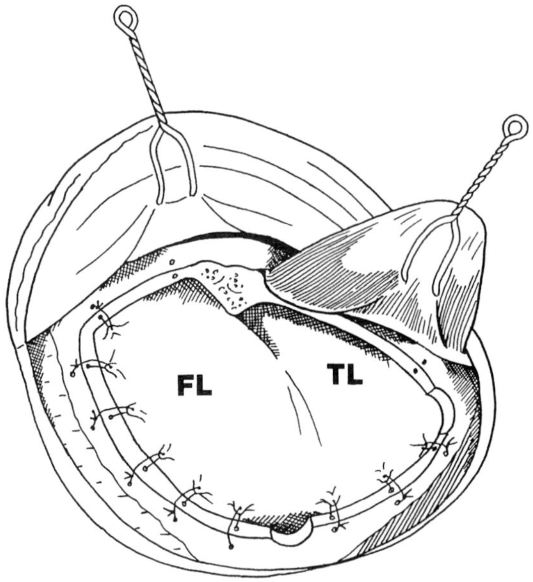

Figure 13-6. The dura has been fixed with separate sutures around the frontal and temporal bones, thus preventing epidural hematoma postoperatively. The dura over the temporal lobe (TL) and over the frontal lobe (FL) has been exposed.

orbital fissure (SOF) has been reached, the utmost care must be taken when dissecting the dura from the orbital roof anterior to the SOF, and when peeling off the periorbita from the orbital roof. This is done in order to avoid damaging the optic nerve (ON), either from the intraorbital side or from the extradural side, where it enters the optic canal underneath the falciform ligament. The orbital roof above the SOF is removed until the dorsal aspect of the SOF is completely exposed (Fig. 13-8). To achieve safe removal of the orbital roof anterior to the SOF it is wise to make an

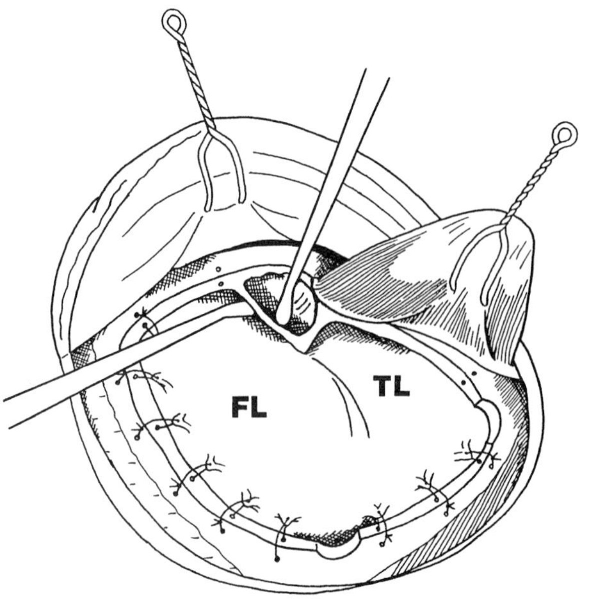

Figure 13-7. The orbit has been unroofed and the periorbita exposed. The periorbita, as well as the dura, should be separated from the orbital roof using a dissector and then the bone of the orbital roof can be carefully removed with bone rongeurs.

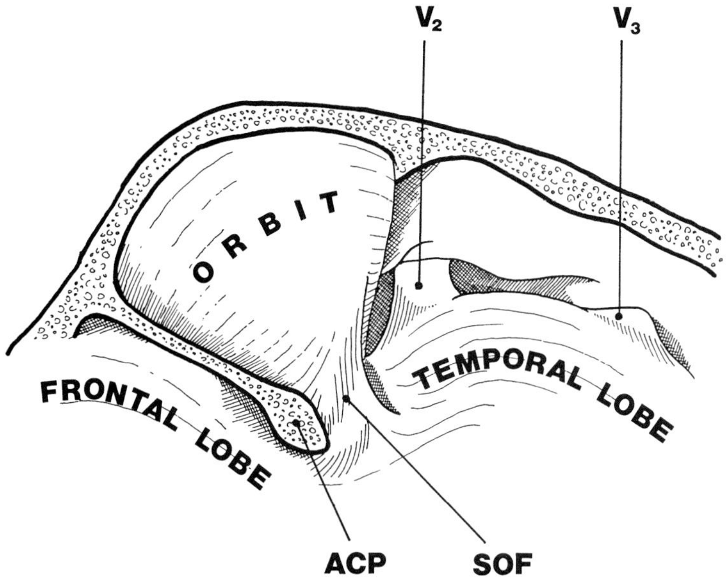

Figure 13-8. The orbit has been widely unroofed; the lateral tip of the superior orbital fissure (SOF) is free of bone on both sides (posterior and anterior). Unroofing of the orbit on the posterior aspect of the SOF is complete and extends laterally to the foramen rotundum. (For explanations of abbreviations, see Appendix 1, p. 373.)

incision of approximately 4 to 5 mm in the duplicature of the dural tent, which extends from the temporal lobe through the SOF to the orbit where it joins the periorbita (Fig. 13-9), thereby exposing cranial nerves III, IV, and V_1. In this manner the cleavage line between the two layers of the lateral wall of the CS will be reached, and the outer layer can be easily peeled away from the nerves and from the inner layer. A stay suture is placed on the outer layer to enable a better approach to the

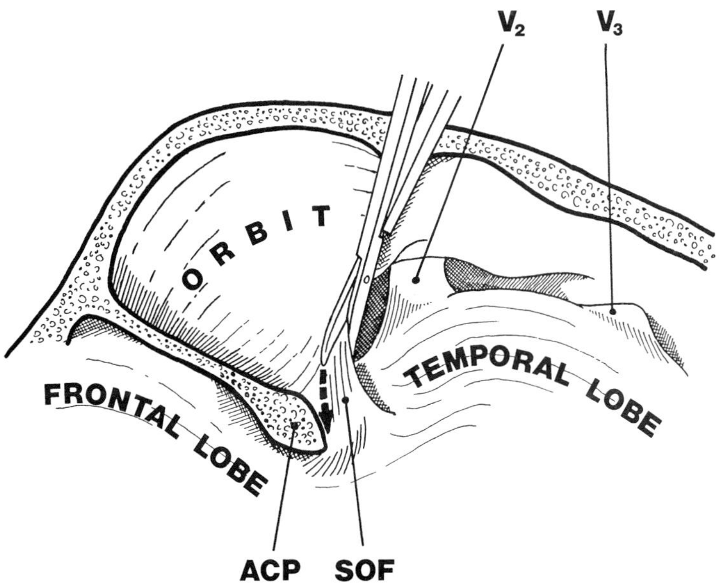

Figure 13-9. The duplication of the dural tent connecting the dura of the temporal lobe with the periorbita and overlying cranial nerves III, IV, V_1, and VI should be cut with curved scissors as indicated by the arrow. The initial incision in the indicated direction should not extend beyond 4 to 5 mm from the lateral tip of the SOF.

central portion of the sphenoid wing and the anterior clinoid process (ACP) (Fig. 13-10).

The next stage is to open the optic canal. It is important to avoid damage to the ON in the optic canal, and this is only possible if the dorsal and lateral walls of the canal are removed by careful "brushing" of the bone under the microscope, using a diamond drill. Adequate cooling of the drill must be provided by constant irrigation. A drill with an intrinsic irrigation system is preferable. If the drilling is performed by the surgeon and the irrigation by the assistant, it is of paramount importance that these two actions be synchronized. It should be clear to the assistant—as well as to the scrub nurse who prepares the syringes with saline—that irrigation during drilling is crucial in order to avoid thermal damage to the ON. It is also advisable to keep the drilling periods short. If drilling is carried out at short intervals, mechanical damage to the ON due to excessive pressure should also never occur. The ACP should never be removed by extracting it in one piece, as such a maneuver will in many cases result in injury to the ON, to cranial nerves III, IV, or both, or to the ICA along its anterior loop or in opening the sphenoid sinus. To avoid any of these four mistakes, which will lead to serious complications, it is essential to drill the ACP at its midpoint (Fig. 13-10) so that it is first hollowed, thus rendering it easy to then break its thinned walls from the outside in an inward direction and at the same time to peel off the dura from the outer surface of the ACP circumferentially. If these precautions are taken, the ON and cranial nerves III, IV, and V_1 should never be damaged. Usually a small part of the ACP remains between the ICA and ON, which continues as the optic strut, which should also be drilled off using a small diamond drill before the tip of the ACP can be removed entirely (Fig. 13-11).

Occasionally, it may be necessary to detect one of two anatomic variations. The ACP may be connected to the posterior clinoid process (PCP), or the ICA may be encircled by the ACP bone and then it sits in a canal rather than in the groove. These conditions should have been identified radiographically prior to surgery as

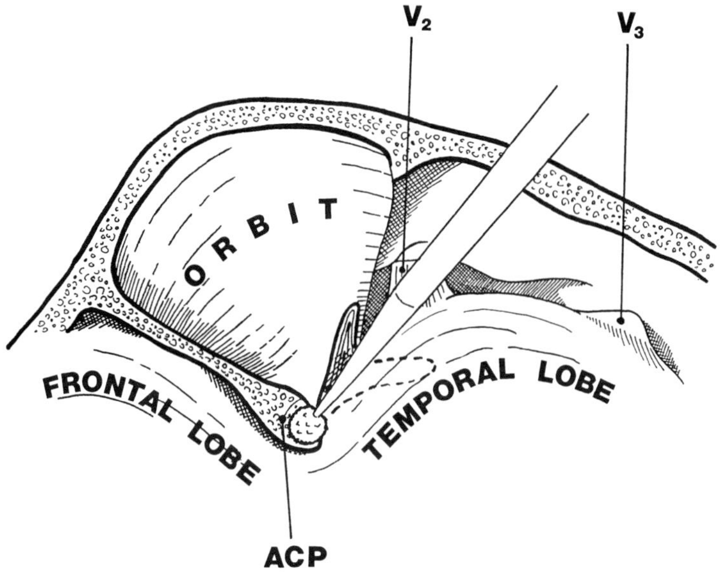

Figure 13-10. The anterior clinoid process (ACP) should be drilled with a diamond drill from the lateral side toward its center so that the surrounding structures are not damaged. Special care should be taken not to damage the 3rd cranial nerve, which is adjacent to the lateral and under aspects of the ACP and has been uncovered by sectioning the duplication of the dura.

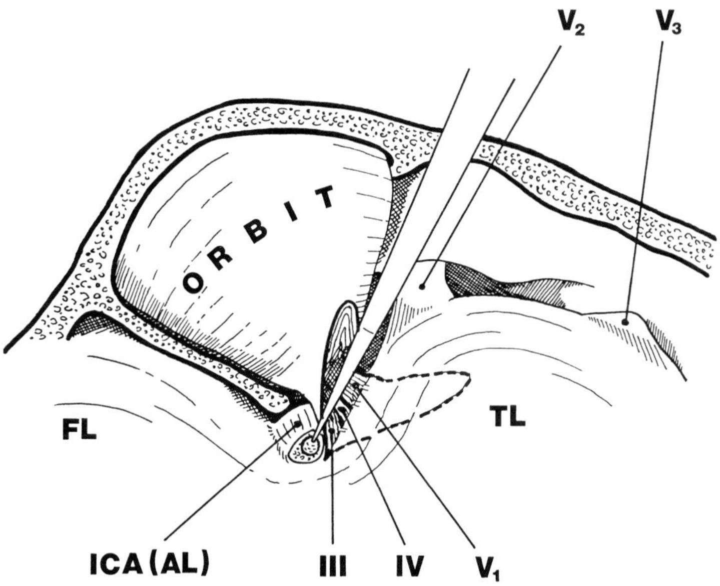

Figure 13-11. The anterior loop (AL) of the ICA has been exposed. The final piece of the ACP should be carefully drilled off. Cranial nerves III, IV, and V_1 have been exposed by separating the outer layer of the lateral wall of the cavernous sinus (CS) from them. The optic canal is still unopened.

they require additional caution. In the case of such variations it is all the more important to first hollow out the ACP rather than attempt to remove it in one piece. Finally, in order to remove the optic strut completely and to free the ICA anteromedially, it is necessary to drill off the bone along the anterior loop (AL) of the ICA in the direction of the sphenoid sinus, which should not be opened (Fig. 13-12). How-

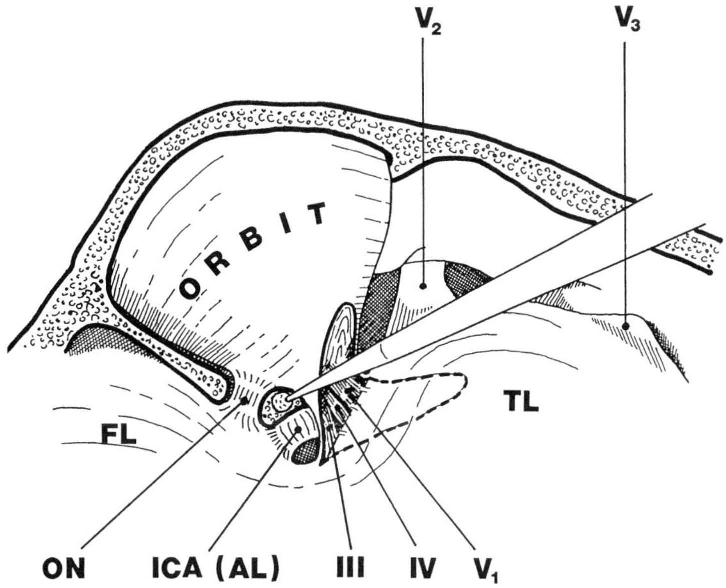

Figure 13-12. The optic canal has been opened on the superior and lateral aspects. The bone between the optic nerve (ON) and the AL of the ICA (the optic strut) should be removed meticulously using a small diamond drill and using continuous irrigation of the drill tip. The AL of the ICA has been freed from the ACP bone. The outer layer of the lateral wall of the CS has been reflected backwards and cranial nerves III, IV, and V_1 are visualized.

ever, if the sphenoid sinus is accidentally opened, care should be taken not to damage the mucous membrane. Irrespective of whether the mucous membrane is preserved or damaged, the opening in the sphenoid sinus should be closed with a piece of muscle and fibrin glue.

The temporal bone should be trimmed down to its base, and the edges of the bone should be drilled using a diamond drill, which results in optimal hemostasis of the bone. The foramen rotundum is now visible, and the canal of V_2 is then opened. However, care should be taken not to drill off too much of the bone medial to V_2 where, if complete removal of the bone is carried out, the maxillary sinus may all too easily be opened accidentally. In cases when this occurs, the maxillary sinus should be closed in a similar way to the sphenoid sinus, with a piece of muscle and fibrin glue. The outer dural layer of the lateral wall of the CS can be further peeled off from the inner layer, and V_1 and V_2 are followed centripetally (Fig. 13-13) toward the gasserian ganglion (GG). Cutting of the dura in a posterior direction is resumed until V_3 is exposed. The MMA is first coagulated, then sectioned, and its proximal stump is pushed into the foramen spinosum (FS) and plugged with Surgicel and bone wax (Fig. 13-14). Additional stay sutures are placed on the dura (i.e., on the outer layer of the lateral wall of the CS) and with these stay sutures the dura is raised and pulled gently back over the brain, and V_3 is thus exposed from the foramen ovale (FO) to the GG. Peeling the dura from the anterior surface of the temporal bone is in some cases difficult, or even impossible, because the anterior surface of the pyramid is rough and the many reef-like exostoses cause the dura to stick firmly to the bone; the dura is further fixed to the bone by several bridging veins. For this reason the veins should be coagulated and cut sharply, and the dura overlying the sharp exostotic protuberances should also be cut; the exophytes, however, should be drilled so that the

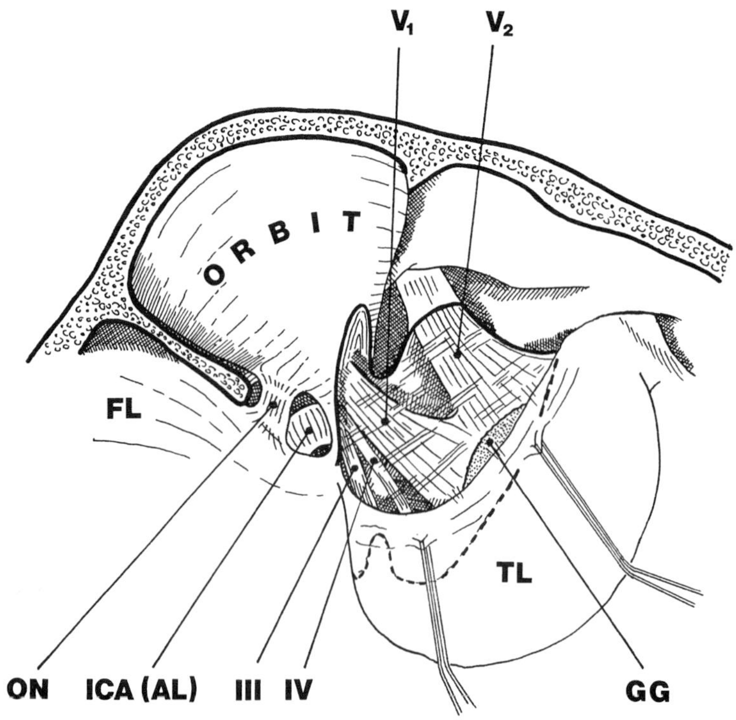

Figure 13-13. The dura has been cut along the lateral border of the CS over V_2 and further posteriorly, and then peeled off from cranial nerves III, IV, V_1, V_2, and gasserian ganglion (GG). The dura is fixed and held with stay sutures.

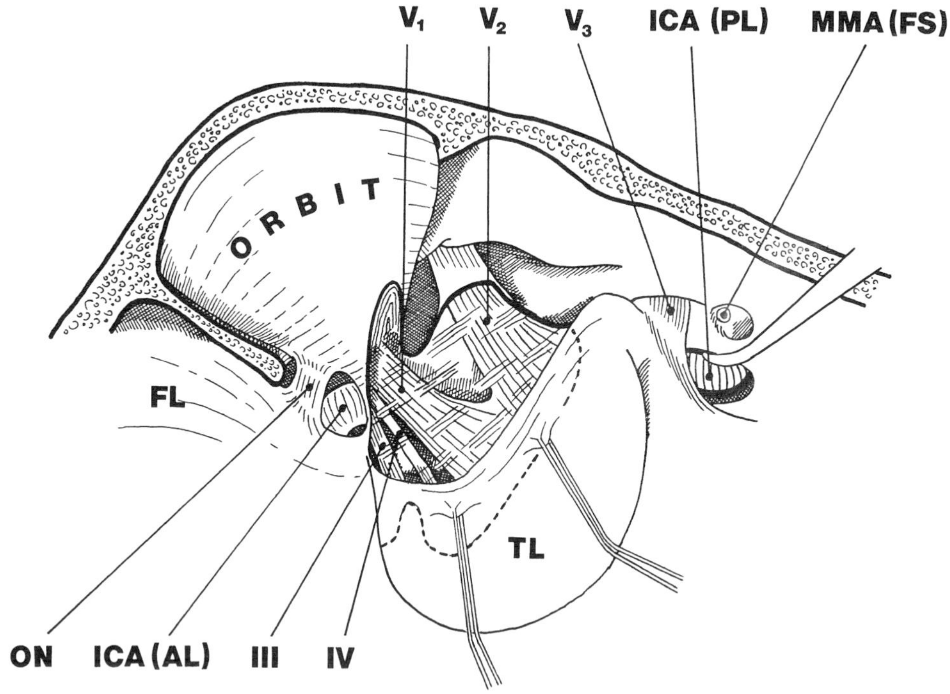

Figure 13-14. The middle meningeal artery (MMA) has been coagulated and sectioned at the foramen spinosum (FS). The carotid canal in the petrous bone has been opened and the posterior loop (PL) of the ICA exposed and separated from the walls of the bony canal.

anterior surface of the petrous bone becomes smooth, thereby completing hemostasis. Special care should be taken while dissecting the greater petrosal nerve, which should either be preserved or sectioned, but never pulled because this will damage the geniculate ganglion, thus resulting in facial palsy. Every effort should be made to preserve the greater petrosal nerve in all cases; this is absolutely vital in cases where V_1 has been damaged by the disease, in order to ensure that the ipsilateral eye has at least some degree of corneal sensory function.

The dura, which has been peeled off from the anterior surface of the petrous bone, is then further cut along the posterior aspect of V_3 and GG, as well as along the root of the 5th cranial nerve (i.e., along the posterior aspect of Meckel's cave). Thus the apex of the petrous bone and the extradural side of the superior petrous sinus on the medial aspect of the apex of the petrous bone are simultaneously exposed. At this stage, the peeling off of the dura from the bone should be stopped.

In cases where it is necessary, for example, when the whole CS is to be opened or in cases of vascular lesions, aneurysms, or CCF, the ICA in the petrous bone should also be exposed (Fig. 13-14). This may be easy when the ICA is scarcely covered with bone or is only covered with fascia. However, in cases where the ICA is fully covered with bone, drilling using a diamond drill should be started approximately 5 to 8 mm medial to the foramen spinosum and close to the posterior aspect of V_3 or GG. During the drilling of the bone at this location—Glasscock's triangle (Dolenc, 1983, 1989)—it is highly likely that the tensor tympani muscle will be first encountered (Glasscock, 1969). When this occurs, great care must be taken not to destroy this muscle (Dolenc, 1989), and drilling should be continued more medially. While drilling in a medial direction, anterior direction, or both, no important structures will be met until the apex of the pyramid has been drilled through (Fig. 13-15). However, if drilling is carried out too far posteriorly, the middle or even the inner ear

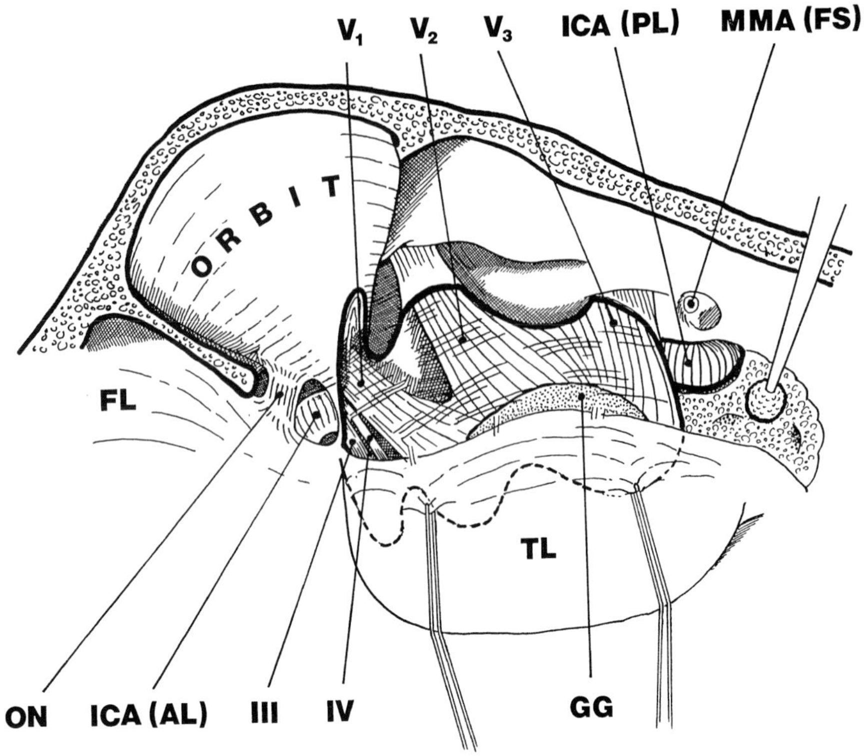

Figure 13-15. The outer layer of the lateral wall of the CS has been further peeled off from V_2, V_3, and GG, thereby exposing cranial nerves III, IV, V_1, V_2, V_3, and GG. The dura is held with stay sutures. The apex of the pyramid should be drilled off with a diamond drill.

could be opened, which will result in deafness and in some cases in cerebrospinal fluid (CSF) leak. To avoid this complication it is always wise first to drill close to the posterior aspect of V_3 until the ICA is exposed on its medial aspect. It is now much safer to drill further in a posterior direction, following the ICA toward the tip of its posterior loop (PL). The length of the ICA in the petrous bone—which needs to be exposed—depends on whether reconstruction of the ICA using a short graft is planned, or whether only a temporary occlusion of the ICA is required. In the former case, adequate exposure of the ICA is necessary, although removal of the eustachian tube is not advisable (Glasscock, 1969). In the latter case, less exposure of the ICA is necessary; it should, however, be sufficient to allow occlusion of the ICA by placing a small balloon between the bony wall of the carotid canal and the ICA itself (Spetzler et al., 1990). In cases where temporary clipping is planned, the ICA should be dissected from the bony wall circumferentially.

The removal of the apex of the pyramid is not, in most cases, a particularly difficult task; nevertheless, it is important to drill the bone from the dorsolateral aspect in an anteromedial direction and to remain close to the dorsal aspect of the GG and to the root of the 5th cranial nerve. Yet again, continuous irrigation is necessary, for it may happen that the inner auditory canal is located more anteriorly and that, with heat, cranial nerves VII and VIII might be damaged. When the apex of the pyramid has been drilled through, drilling continues in a posterior direction until the inner auditory canal is opened and the dural coat covering the inner auditory canal is exposed (Fig. 13-16). After lifting of the GG from Meckel's cave, the apex of the pyramid can be drilled off and the petroclinoid ligament (PCL) will be exposed.

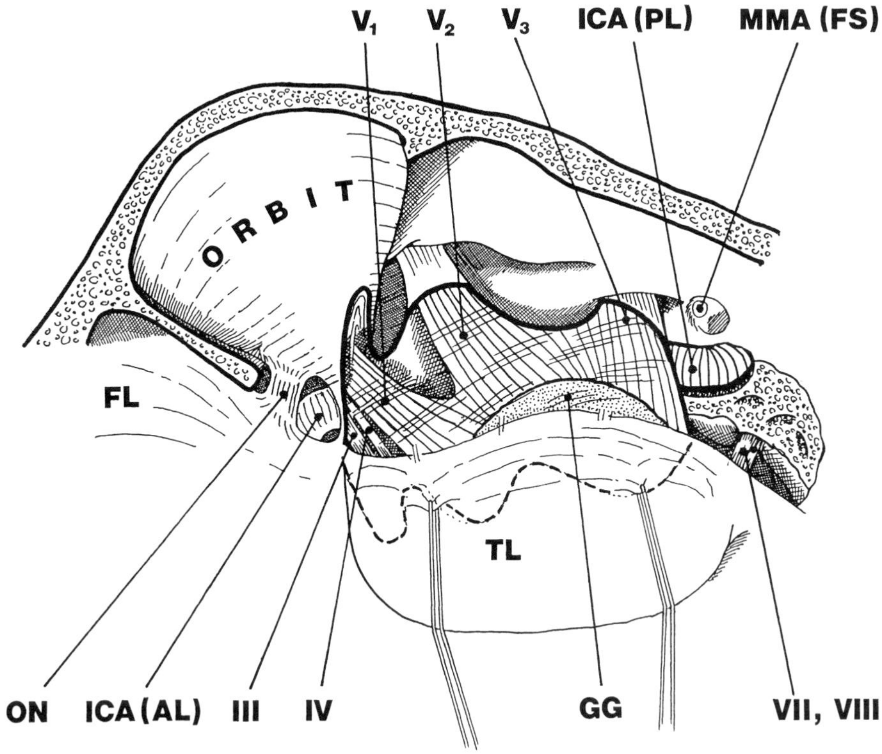

Figure 13-16. The apex of the pyramid has been drilled off and the dura on the medial aspect of the pyramid has been exposed. The internal auditory canal has been opened on the anterior side, thus exposing cranial nerves VII and VIII.

The dura is incised along the sylvian fissure, and its edges are fixed with stay sutures. The dural incision extends to the dural ring (DR) around the ICA. The next step involves the splitting of the sylvian fissure, which should be performed from the periphery toward the center (Fig. 13-17). The arachnoidea is cut on either side of the veins, which usually run along the surface of the sylvian fissure; when the veins have been dissected, a cortical artery is located and followed to the base of the sylvian fissure so that the branching point of the middle cerebral artery (MCA) is reached. The MCA is followed toward the bifurcation of the ICA. The temporal and the frontal lobes are then separated (Fig. 13-18). Because in most cases these two lobes overlap, it is much safer to begin separating them at the base of the sylvian fissure, then proceeding outward toward the surface of the brain. In cases where the lesion extends into the sella, or in cases where complete mobilization of the AL of the ICA is necessary, the DR is cut circumferentially around the ICA. Care should be taken not to damage the ophthalmic artery (Oph A), which usually branches off from the ICA very close to the DR (Fig. 13-19).

Only when the sylvian fissure has been completely split—which renders it easier to lift the temporal lobe—can the dura be cut along the medial edge of the lateral wall of the CS alongside the tentorial edge (Fig. 13-20). Cranial nerves III, IV, and VI are dissected from the lesion. Dissection of the 3rd cranial nerve is safe with a curved arachnoidal knife, cutting backward (Fig. 13-21). In this way the 3rd cranial nerve can easily be isolated from the layers of the lateral wall of the CS as well as from the tumor, aneurysm, or both. The 4th cranial nerve crosses over the 3rd cranial

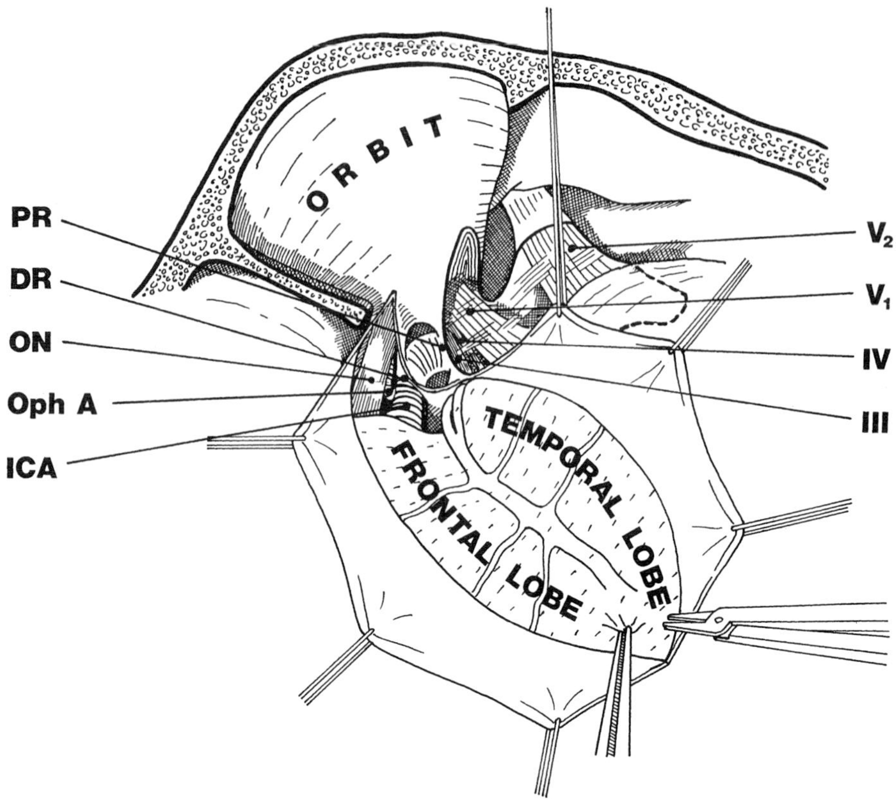

Figure 13-17. An incision of the dura has been made along the sylvian fissure from its periphery down to the dural ring and along the optic nerve. The edges of the dura have been fixed with stay sutures on both sides. The incision into the arachnoid starts from the periphery of the sylvian fissure and continues alongside the vein on the surface of the brain.

nerve and for this reason it is necessary first to dissect the 4th nerve and to expose the 3rd nerve beneath, before proceeding to dissection of the peripheral segment of the 3rd nerve to its full extent (Fig. 13-22).

Exposure of the root of the 5th cranial nerve is easily achieved by cutting the tentorium perpendicularly behind the entry point of the 4th cranial nerve (Fig. 13-23). This leads to the superior petrous sinus (SPS) being opened, the central stump of which should be closed—either by clipping or by suturing—or simply by plugging it with Surgicel. Once the tentorial edge and the walls of the SPS have been cut, the root of the 5th cranial nerve will be sufficiently exposed.

Tumorous Lesions of the Cavernous Sinus

Meningiomas. Very rarely can a meningioma of the CS be removed by using only the epidural approach without opening the dura (Dolenc, 1989, 1990, 1992a, 1992b). In most cases, the tumorous lesion is located in the CS but also extends into the orbit, sella, suprasellar area, optic canal, Meckel's cave, posterior fossa or all of these (Dolenc, 1989). Surgical approach to a meningioma in the CS requires orbitotomy; removal of the sphenoid wing and the ACP; wide opening of the optic canal on the posterior, lateral, and under aspects; and opening of the carotid canal in the petrous bone, which provides good proximal control while also allowing for reconstruction of the ICA when necessary (Fig. 13-24). In most cases the apex of the pyramid should also be resected, the SPS transected, and the root of the 5th cranial nerve exposed. After the incision of the dura along the sylvian fissure, splitting the sylvian fissure

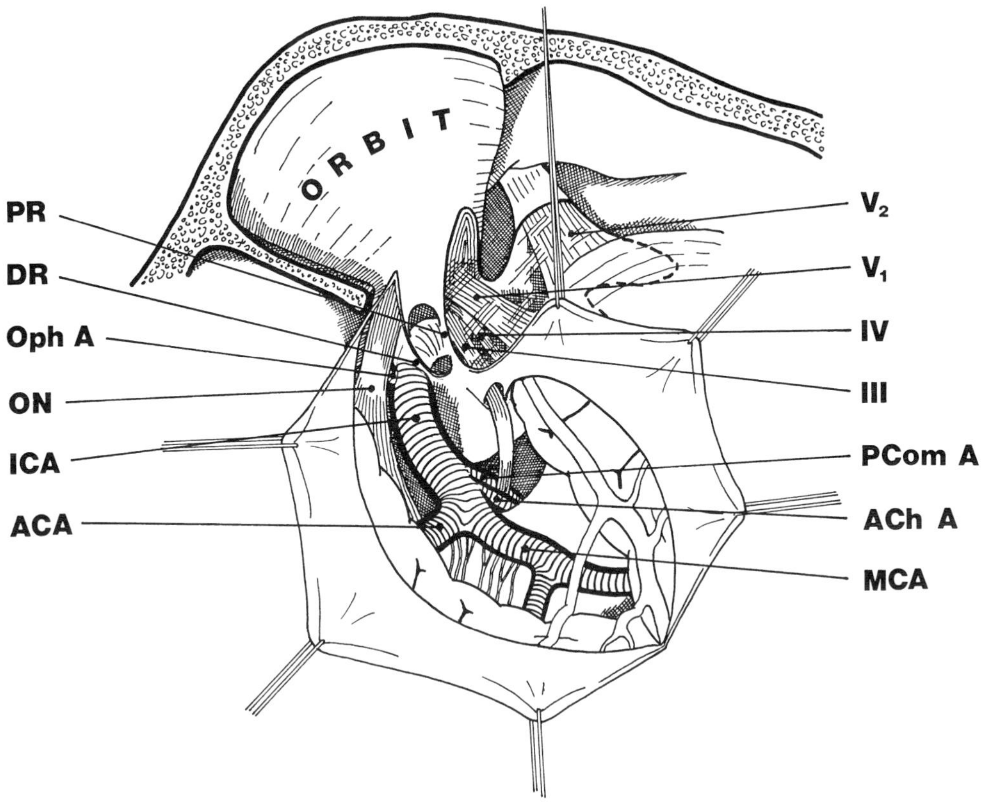

Figure 13-18. The sylvian fissure has been completely split. With slight traction of the dura medialward, the whole segment of the middle cerebral artery (MCA) with its branches, the initial portion of the anterior cerebral artery (ACA), the anterior choroidal artery (ACh A), the posterior communicating artery (PCom A), and the ophthalmic artery (Oph A) have been exposed. The intradural portion of the 3rd cranial nerve, running on the lateral aspect of the posterior clinoid process (PCP) into the dural canal in the lateral wall of the CS, is well exposed.

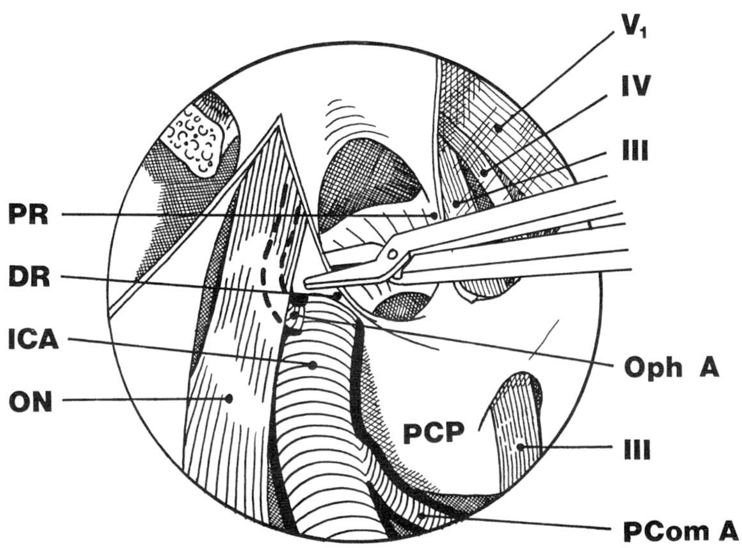

Figure 13-19. The dural ring (DR) should be cut circumferentially around the ICA allowing visualization of the initial segment of the Oph A. Complete section of the DR around the ICA enables mobilization of the distal segment of the AL of the ICA.

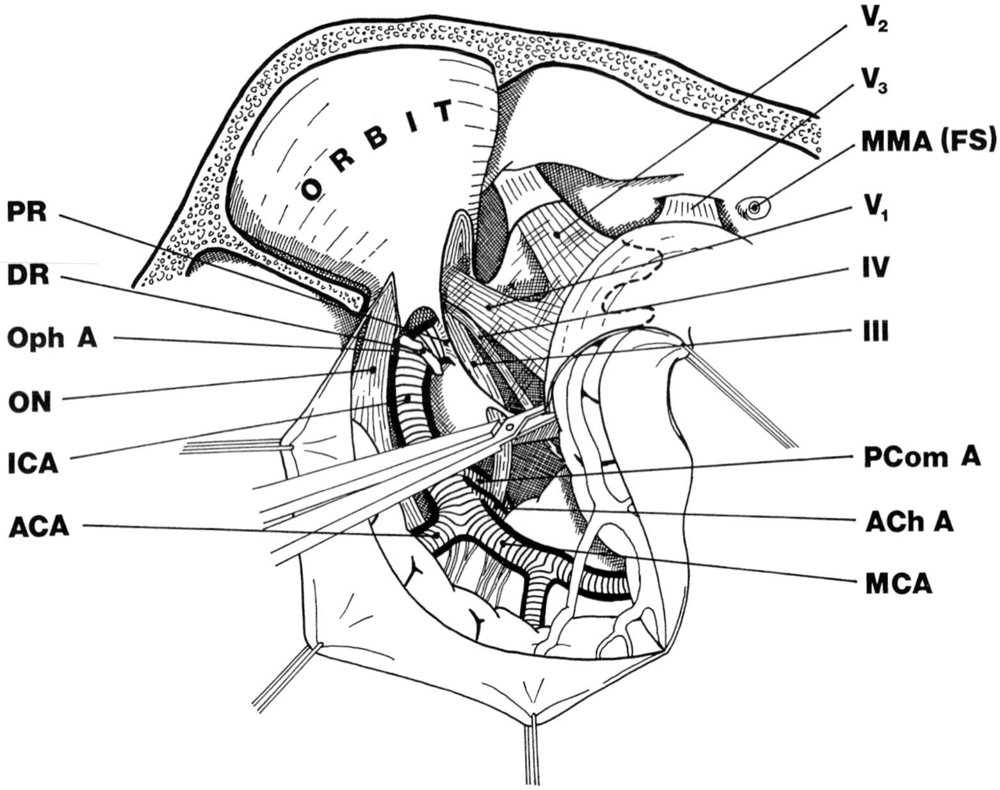

Figure 13-20. After complete splitting of the sylvian fissure, exposure of all the branches of the ICA and of the MCA, sectioning of the dural ring circumferentially around the ICA, and mobilization of the distal segment of the AL of the ICA, the dura should be cut from the orifice of the canal of the 3rd cranial nerve in a posterior direction over the entry point of the 4th cranial nerve into the lateral wall of the CS.

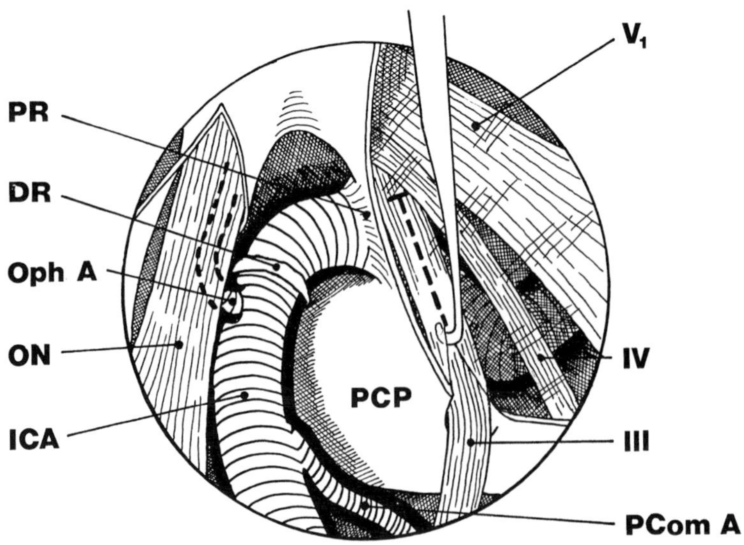

Figure 13-21. The DR has been cut circumferentially and the ICA has been mobilized. The 3rd cranial nerve has been dissected from the intradural side. The orifice of the canal of the 3rd cranial nerve should be carefully cut along the longitudinal axis of the 3rd cranial nerve using a curved arachnoidal knife. Dissection of the 3rd cranial nerve should be stopped at the level where the horizontal segment of the ICA turns medially and becomes the AL. In this way, the 4th cranial nerve where it overlies the 3rd cranial nerve will not be damaged.

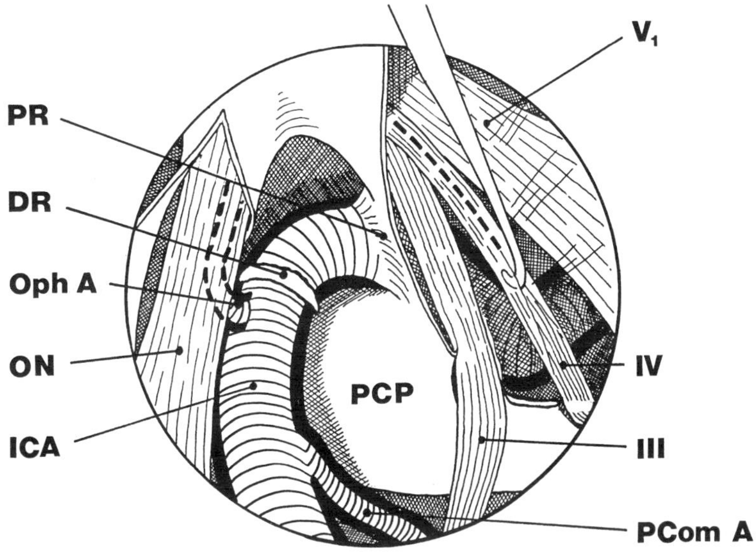

Figure 13-22. The 4th cranial nerve should be dissected in a similar way to the 3rd cranial nerve, using a curved arachnoidal knife. Dissection of the 4th cranial nerve should also be started from the intradural side and then proceed along the longitudinal axis of the nerve toward the orbit.

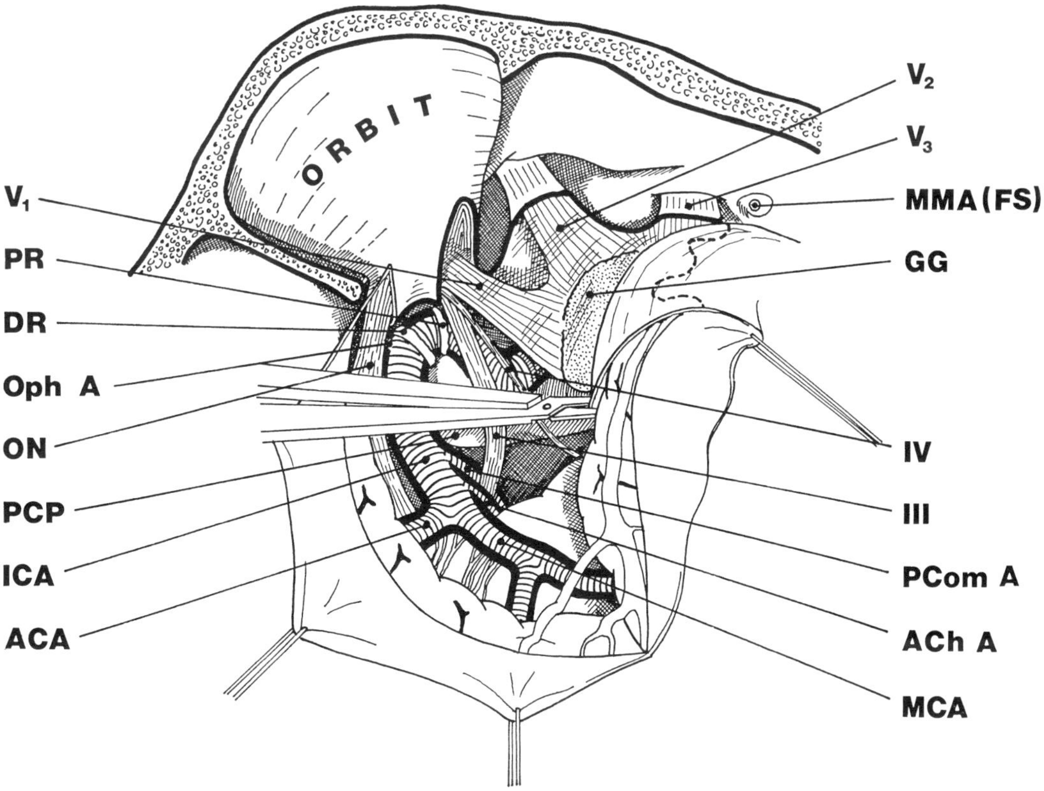

Figure 13-23. The distal ring (DR) and the proximal ring (PR) have been cut circumferentially around the ICA and the AL of the ICA has been mobilized. The 3rd and 4th cranial nerves have been dissected free both intradurally and in the lateral wall of the CS. The sylvian fissure has been completely split, and the branches of the ICA and the MCA have been exposed. The dura should be cut from the 4th cranial nerve in a perpendicular direction toward the 5th cranial nerve.

and cutting the DR circumferentially around the ICA, distal control of the ICA is also guaranteed (Fig. 13-24). Usually after the described procedure the extracavernous portion of the meningioma has already been devascularized, and its portion originating in the lateral wall of the CS and growing intradurally in the middle fossa can easily be resected along with the invaded dura (Fig. 13-25). Following this, the temporal lobe is exposed; but it is only by means of good anesthesia that undue retraction of the temporal lobe can be avoided throughout surgery.

The tumor is then removed from the intradural space on the medial aspect of the CS (i.e., from the 3rd cranial nerve, from around the posterior communicating (PCom) artery and the anterior choroidal artery (ACh A), as well as from around the ICA. In cases where the meningioma has also spread into the sella, it is removed from in front of the PCP, which is drilled off when necessary, for example when the tumor is also located on the posterior aspect of the dorsum sellae (Fig. 13-26). It is only when the tumor has been removed intradurally around the 3rd cranial nerve that dissection of this nerve is performed in a peripheral direction along the horizontal segment of the ICA (Fig. 13-21). Care should be taken not to damage the 4th nerve, which crosses over the 3rd nerve (Fig. 13-22). Therefore, the meningioma is removed from the medial wall of the CS posterior to the 3rd nerve until the 4th nerve can be visualized intradurally, encased in the tumor or overlying the tumor,

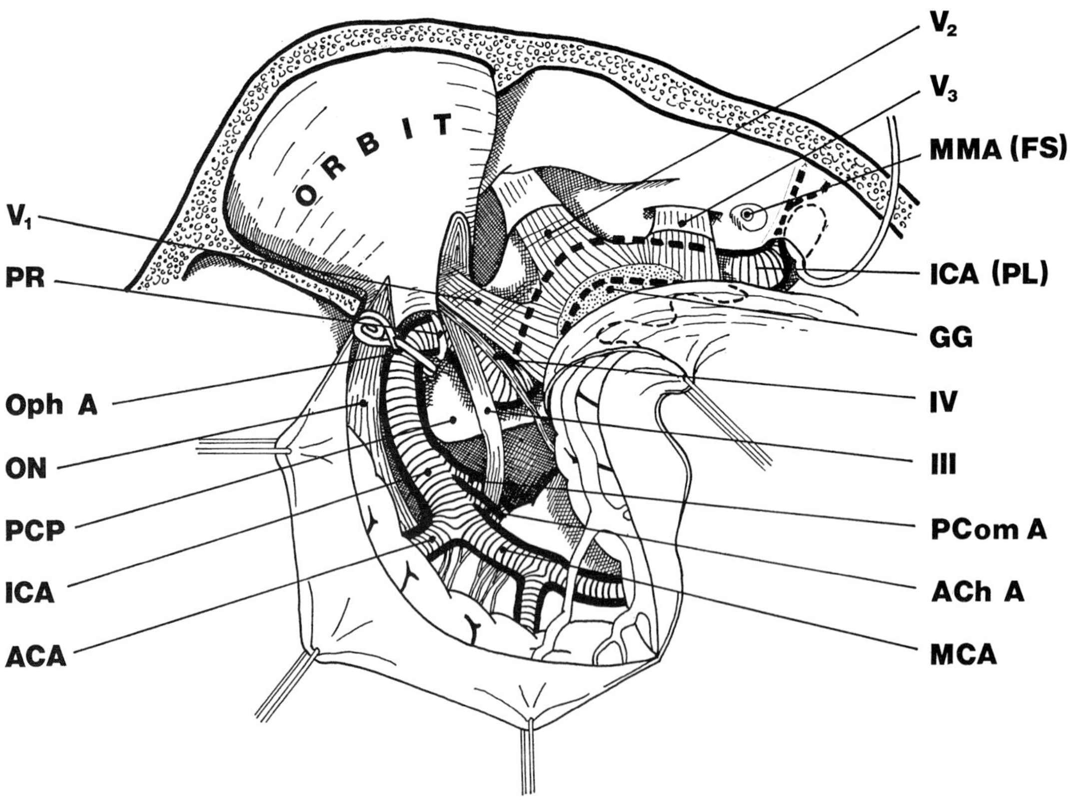

Figure 13-24. Wide exposure of the ICA at its PL and AL. A catheter with a balloon has been inserted into the petrous canal of the carotid artery and prepared for a temporary occlusion by inflating the balloon. A temporary clip has been placed proximal to the DR to provide distal control. Insertion of the balloon should be correct to enable quick inflation and to enable the flow in the ICA to be stopped, should the need arise for proximal control. For distal control, it is essential that the distal portion of the AL is completely mobilized so that the temporary clip can be easily placed, should the need arise.

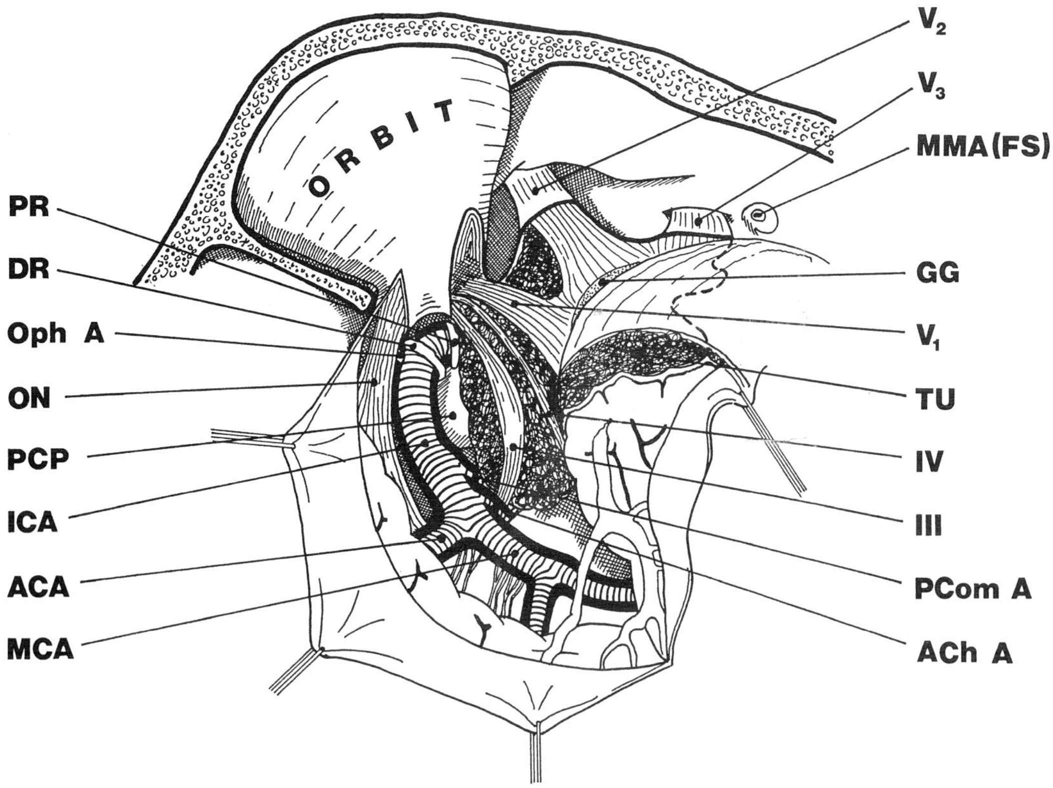

Figure 13-25. Complete splitting of the sylvian fissure has been performed. The proximal and distal dural rings have been cut circumferentially. The 3rd and 4th cranial nerves have been completely isolated from their canals in the lateral wall of the CS and dissected from the tumor intra- and extradurally. The outer layer of the lateral wall of the CS, impregnated with tumor that has grown through the dura into the intradural space, has been separated from cranial nerves V_1, V_2, V_3, and GG. The tumor, which is attached to the dura and overlies the temporal lobe, has been devascularized and can easily be completely excised together with the infiltrated dura.

and can then be followed to its entry point into the lateral wall of the CS. Then, by use of an arachnoidal knife, the canal is opened by cutting the dural ring around the 4th nerve. The nerve is further followed in a peripheral direction and dissected away from the tumor and from the 3rd nerve. Finally, the distal segment of the 3rd nerve is dissected from the tumor. During dissection of the 3rd nerve along the horizontal segment of the ICA, the proximal ring (PR) is cut and the tumor is removed on the medial aspect of the ICA facing the sella (Fig. 13-27).

The next step is removal of the tumor on the medial aspect of the 5th cranial nerve, around the apex of the pyramid and on the lateral aspect of the 5th nerve. The tumor can be resected in a posterior direction as far as the 7th and 8th cranial nerves, and in a medial direction as far as the 6th cranial nerve and the basilar artery. In most cases, the medial wall of the CS can easily be resected and the tumor can be completely removed from the horizontal segment of the ICA. The 6th nerve, which is first visualized posterior and medial to the 5th nerve over the brain stem, is then followed to its entry point into Dorello's canal. The membrane dividing Meckel's cave from the CS is cut and raised together with the GG and V_1, and then the PCP is visualized. The 6th nerve is followed throughout Dorello's canal and around the ICA. The V_1 is gently retracted in a lateral direction thus exposing the 6th nerve inferior to V_1 in its course along the horizontal segment of the ICA, lateral to the inferolateral trunk, toward the SOF (Fig. 13-28).

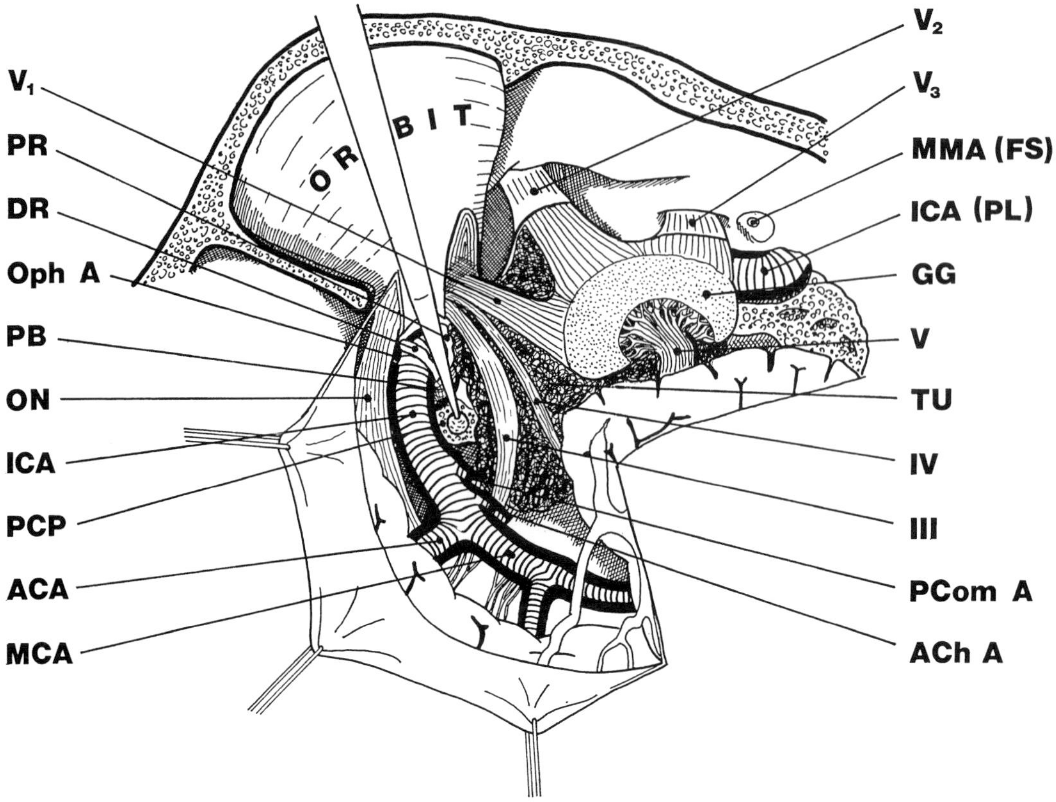

Figure 13-26. The nerves in the lateral wall of the CS have been exposed in their entirety. The dura covering the temporal lobe, impregnated with tumor, and the tumor on the inner side of the dura have been resected completely. The apex of the pyramid has been drilled off. The PL and AL of the ICA have been exposed and mobilized. When the tumor extends into the sella and over the clivus, the PCP together with the dorsum sellae should be drilled off using a diamond drill.

If the tumor is hard and adherent to the ICA, a decision should be made as to whether to leave a tumorous "coat" around the ICA or to continue with peeling away the tumor from the ICA and thus risk a rupture of the artery. In cases of evident stenosis of the ICA—and when there is good cross-flow through the anterior communicating (ACom) and PCom arteries—it is possible to resect the tumor together with the diseased segment of the ICA and to leave separate its distal and proximal stumps, which must be closed with permanent clips. However, it is much better to reconstruct the ICA with "direct" end-to-end suturing of its stumps in cases where the defect of the ICA does not exceed 5 mm. This length can be obtained by mobilizing the two adjacent loops, that is, the lateral and the anterior (Dolenc, 1991). When direct reconstruction is impossible, it is necessary to insert a graft, either a saphenous vein or a radial artery (Fig. 13-29).

In most cases of complete resection of a CS meningioma that has also invaded the dura and penetrated into the intradural space there will be a dural defect. In such cases it is sufficient to insert some pieces of the temporalis muscle or pieces of Surgicel. In addition, fibrin glue is also used to seal the dural defect. With large dural defects, strip-shaped lyodura patches should be used in order to cover the defect, which in turn should be reinforced epidurally with fibrin glue. A dural defect combined with opening of the bony sinus(es) is extremely dangerous. In such cases the repair procedure is identical, that is, a watertight closure of the bony sinus(es) and

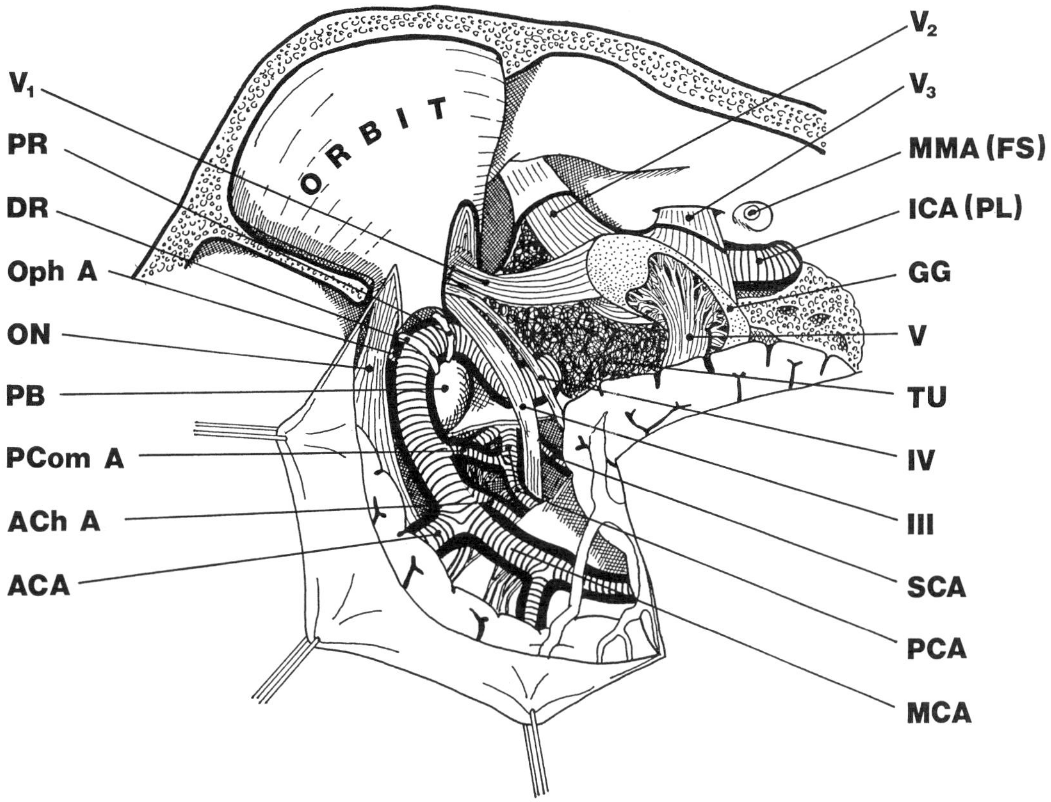

Figure 13-27. The PCP has been removed. The tumor has been completely removed from the sella, so that the horizontal segment of the intracavernous ICA can be seen on its medial aspect. The dura of the dorsum sellae and of the medial wall of the CS has been resected completely together with the tumor, thereby exposing the bifurcation of the basilar artery with both posterior cerebral arteries (PCAs), PCom A in its entire segment, and the ipsilateral superior cerebellar artery (SCA). The tumor still remains lateral to the horizontal and ascending segments of the intracavernous ICA, and around the 6th cranial nerve underneath V_1 and V_2.

the dural defect. In addition, the patient should be put on lumbar drainage for at least 1 week after surgery.

Pituitary Tumors Extending into the Cavernous Sinus. In most cases pituitary tumors with parasellar extensions are not removable by means of the trans-sphenoidal approach. It is easier to achieve complete removal of such tumors using the transcranial approach. In order to expose completely the sella and the parasellar region, it is necessary to perform orbitotomy, removal of the sphenoid wing and the ACP, and opening of the optic canal. The dural tent covering the nerves running from the CS through the SOF into the orbit must be cut, and the outer layer of the lateral wall of the CS peeled off so as to visualize cranial nerves III, IV, V_1, V_2, V_3, and GG between the two layers of the lateral wall of the CS (Figs. 13-9 and 13-13). The dura along the sylvian fissure is cut, the sylvian fissure is split, and the MCA, the bifurcation of the ICA, the ICA intradurally, as well as the initial segment of the anterior cerebral artery (ACA_1) are exposed (Figs. 13-17 and 13-18). It is also important to mobilize completely the AL of the ICA by cutting the DR circumferentially.

In some cases the pituitary tumor, which may have a very large parasellar extension, grows by extension through the canal of the 3rd cranial nerve into the intradural space. In such cases the 3rd nerve is stretched over the tumor, which is sit-

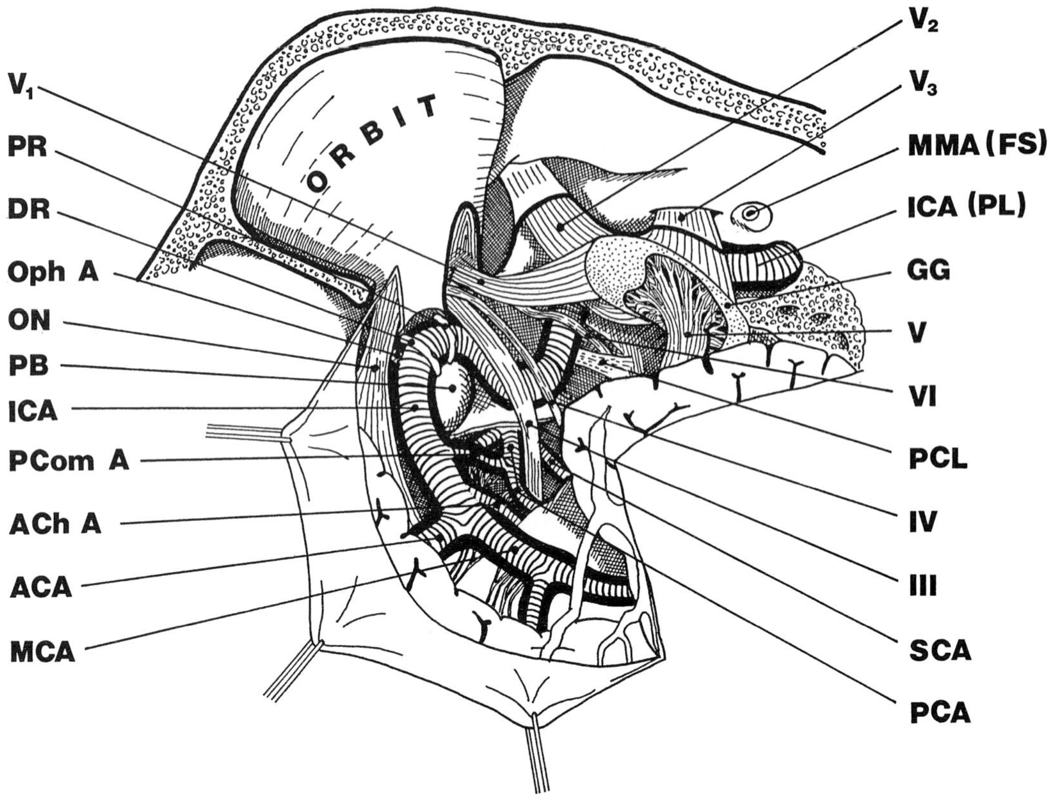

Figure 13-28. The last part of the tumor lateral to the horizontal and ascending segments of the ICA in the CS, and around the 6th cranial nerve underneath V_1 and V_2, has been completely removed. The 6th cranial nerve has been exposed at its exit from Dorello's canal—lateral to the petroclinoid ligament (PCL)—and along its course anteriorly underneath V_1, lateral to the horizontal segment of the ICA toward the orbit.

uated anteroinferior to the paper-thin 3rd nerve. It is easy to overlook the 3rd nerve and to damage it by attempting removal of the tumor, because the nerve is so overstretched that it is completely transparent.

Only after cutting the DR around the ICA (Fig. 13-19), after dissecting the 3rd nerve from the tumor and from the ICA and cutting the PR of the ICA, is it possible to enter the sella between the AL of the ICA and the PCP. At this point the tumor can be completely removed from the sella, because the floor of the sella can easily be reached. Because at the same time the pituitary stalk is also clearly visible, the diaphragma sellae can be pressed from the intradural side into the sella, and the rest of the tumor can then be removed from the dome of the diaphragm. Any remaining pituitary gland still present can easily be preserved. Because the sella is entered diagonally, care should be taken not to damage the structures of the opposite CS. The ipsilateral CS—where the tumorous extension lies on the medial and lateral aspects of the ICA—is then entered through the anteromedial, paramedian, or Parkinson's triangle(s) (Dolenc, 1989), whereby the tumor can be removed from the posterior aspect of the ascending portion of the ICA (i.e., from in front of Meckel's cave and medial to the 6th cranial nerve). After complete removal of the tumor, the dura is sutured with separate sutures. There is usually a small dural defect around the ICA at the DR, which was cut circumferentially. This defect is closed with pieces of the temporalis muscle, Surgicel, and fibrin glue.

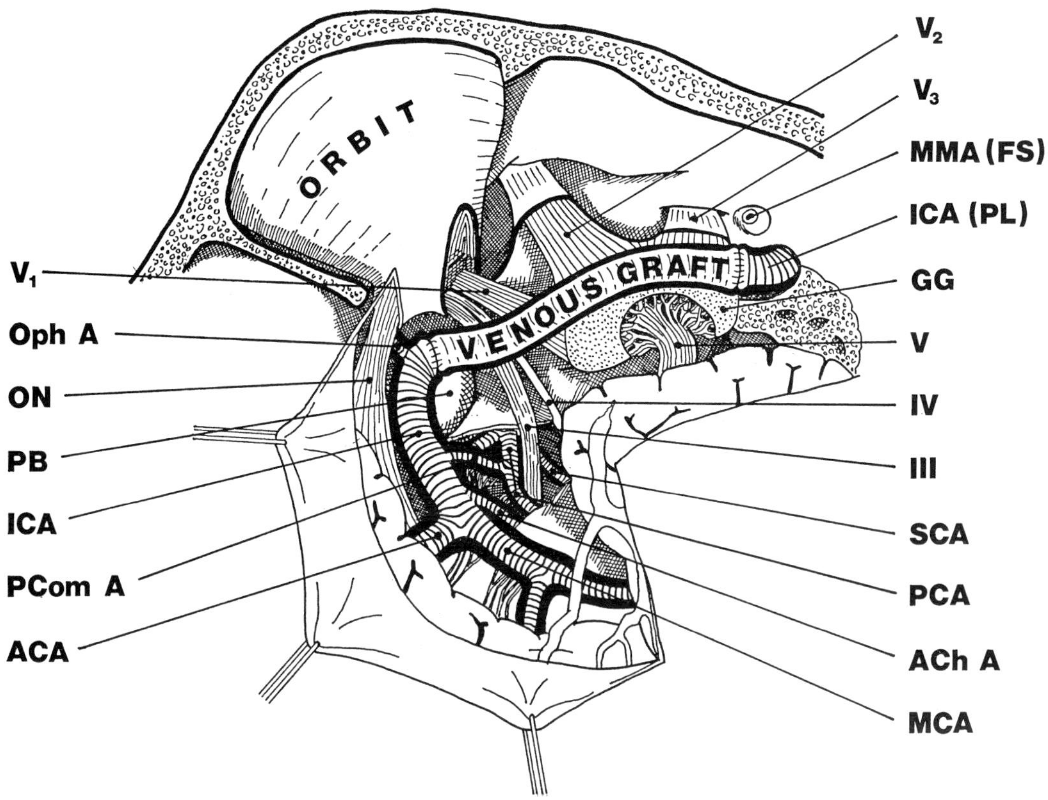

Figure 13-29. The tumor from the CS, middle fossa, clivus, and sella has been removed completely. All the cranial nerves (III, IV, V_1, V_2, V_3, GG, V, VI) have been dissected free in their entirety and have been preserved. In this case the diseased segment of the ICA in the CS—which was too long to be reconstructed "directly"—has been grafted with a venous graft from the PL to the AL. The graft has been interposed by using an end-to-end anastomosis proximally and distally.

Chordomas, Chondromas, and Chondrosarcomas. These tumors, in comparison to meningiomas and parasellar extensions of pituitary tumors, appear more rarely in the parasellar region, although in some cases they also pose a problem, especially those chondromas and chondrosarcomas that are firmly adherent to the stenotic and displaced ICA. The approach is the same as that described for meningiomas and adenomas of the pituitary gland, except that in most cases the removal of the apex of the pyramid is not necessary. In chordomas, exposure of the ICA in the petrous bone is advisable but not, strictly speaking, necessary. In chondromas and chondrosarcomas it is wise to prepare the proximal (in the petrous canal) and distal (intradural) segments of the ICA (Fig. 13-24), because the adherence of the tumor to the artery wall may be tenacious and any lesion of the ICA difficult to repair.

Chondrosarcomas usually fill the whole CS and grow into the skull base, so that after removal of the tumor a defect may be present in the wall of the bony sinus(es), thus leading to CSF leak unless measures are taken to prevent this. It is important to remember that chondrosarcomas and particularly chondromas are hard and very solid tumors; hence, in order to avoid damage to the nervous and vascular structures, they should be removed by the piecemeal technique. To take out a large "stone" from the tumor by force may easily cause damage. When removing some chondromas or chondrosarcomas from the floor of the CS, use of a diamond drill is advisable in order to break the larger pieces into smaller ones and to remove them safely without injuring the nervous or vascular structures. Because chondromas and chondrosarcomas fill the whole CS, there is no bleeding until total removal of the lesion has been completed, thereby freeing the draining channels from the affected CS to the contralateral CS and to the SPS. Following this, the bleeding points should then be packed with Surgicel and fibrin glue. The dural defect—which is in most cases very small (if present at all)—should be treated in the same manner.

Most chordomas, being soft, can be easily removed by aspiration. Because the tumor is usually only extradural, the approach is in some cases exclusively extradural, that is, the CS is entered after peeling off the outer layer of the lateral wall from the nerves and from the tumor through the anatomic windows: anteromedial, paramedial, Parkinson's, anterolateral, and lateral triangle(s). Because it is characteristic of chordomas to erode the bone, it is possible that after the removal of the tumor the defect at the skull base bone may lead to CSF leak. In cases of eroded walls of the bony sinus(es), inner ear, middle ear, or eustachian tube, it is essential to properly seal the bony defects after resection of the chordoma. It is easy to remove the bulk of the chordoma, although it is never possible to remove this tumor completely, the reason being that it lies beyond the visual field of the surgeon and that its tiny extensions into the bone always remain inaccessible. Washing out the hole after removal of the mass is useful as this will remove any free particles of the tumor, and in this way gross total removal may be achieved. Possible venous bleeding points should be packed with Surgicel, thus preventing postoperative hematoma. Because chordomas are extradural lesions, no problems should be encountered with the closure of the dura in cases where it was necessary to open the dura during the procedure.

Neurinomas of the Trigeminal Nerve. Neurinomas originating in the branches of the trigeminal nerve or in the gasserian ganglion are extradural (Dolenc, 1994c), and when they originate in the root of the 5th cranial nerve they are intradural. In almost all cases complete removal of the trigeminal neurinoma is feasible using only the extradural approach. This approach involves a pterional craniotomy; the part of the orbital roof that is situated behind the SOF must at least be removed so that the anterolateral border of the CS is visualized (Fig. 13-8). It is not necessary, in all cases, to remove the sphenoid wing, ACP, walls of the optic canal, and larger portion of the roof of the orbit anterior to the SOF. Total removal of these structures is imperative only when the trigeminal neurinoma is eroding the ACP and compressing the ON. However, it is always necessary to expose the lateral tip of the dural tent of the SOF, cut it, and then separate the outer layer of the lateral wall of the CS from the underlying tumor (Fig. 13-9). In this way the outer dural layer that covers the temporal lobe on its under aspect will be preserved, and the placing of stay sutures on this dural structure will enable the temporal lobe to be slightly lifted, thereby creating sufficient access to the CS and permitting cranial nerves III, IV, V_1, V_2, V_3, as well as the GG to be exposed. As trigeminal neurinomas are usually soft, except in rare cases, this approach will permit removal of the tumor through the anatomic windows between the individual nerves.

In cases where the neurinoma originates in the root of the 5th cranial nerve, it extends into the parasellar space and over the eroded apex of the pyramid into the posterior fossa. In such cases, after cutting the MMA, the dura should be peeled away from the anterior surface of the petrous bone and lifted with stay sutures until the SPS is exposed. In cases where the sensory function of the cornea has been lost, it is of paramount importance to preserve the greater petrosal nerve in order to protect the eye. The apex of the pyramid is then drilled off so that an access can be provided to the posterior fossa (Fig. 13-16). The dura overlying the petrous bone in Meckel's cave is cut and the root of the 5th cranial nerve, which is usually on the surface of the tumor, is thus exposed.

This procedure should be carried out with the utmost care so that all the branches of the root of the 5th cranial nerve that have not been destroyed by the tumor may be preserved. After removal of the tumor from the posterior fossa and Meckel's cave there will undoubtedly be a dural defect, and consequently CSF will have free access from the intradural into the extradural space. After complete removal of the tumor, and when hemostasis has been completed, the dural defect should be closed with a piece of muscle and fibrin glue.

Cavernomas and Cavernous Hemangiomas of the Cavernous Sinus. The initial approach to these tumors is as previously described, but it does not require the apex of the pyramid to be removed or the carotid canal in the petrous bone to be opened. Likewise, removal of the ACP and opening the optic canal is not necessary in all cases. However, the roof of the orbit must always be removed up to the lateral tip of the SOF and then posterior to it as this will enable the surgeon to cut the duplicature of the dura covering the nerves running from the CS to the orbit. Location of the cleavage line between the layers of the lateral wall of the CS will enable peeling the outer layer of the wall away from cranial nerves III, IV, V_1, V_2, V_3, and GG, and from the underlying tumor. The tumor may be removed from the CS without opening the dura, that is, using exclusively the epidural approach. Unless the highly vascular sponge-like lesion is very large, it is possible to "shrink" it by coagulation from its periphery, and then to remove it by sharp dissection from cranial nerves III, IV, V_1, and VI. In most cases it is very difficult to dissect the 6th cranial nerve from the lesion because this nerve is completely encased within it, the most affected segment being the point where the 6th cranial nerve crosses over the ICA. Whenever it is possible to "shrink" the cavernoma and remove it in one piece, loss of blood is significantly less than when the piecemeal technique is used. When the piecemeal technique is employed, extensive bleeding occurs while cutting the tumor, resulting in injury to the 6th cranial nerve during coagulation; this injury is difficult to avoid since the tumor encompasses the nerve. Therefore, the piecemeal technique is best avoided.

After detachment of the cavernoma from the floor of the CS, it is very likely that the venous channels will open, thus resulting in venous bleeding from the normally functioning CS. Bleeding from a spongy cavernoma and particularly from a cavernous hemangioma, with additional venous bleeding, leads to a situation that is very difficult to control without endangering the neural structures, especially the 6th cranial nerve. This can be avoided by working initially on the surface of the cavernous lesion (i.e., by dissecting cranial nerves III, IV, V_1, V_2, and V_3 from the lesion), then by "shrinking" the lesion by all-over coagulation, and finally dissecting it from the 6th cranial nerve and from the ICA. As the operation progresses, the venous channels should be packed so that venous bleeding does not disturb dissection of the lesion from the vital structures. The hole in the CS after the removal of the tumor is best packed with pieces of muscle/Surgicel, and then reinforced with fibrin glue.

Malignant Tumors of the Cavernous Sinus. Malignant tumors in the parasellar region should, as elsewhere, be resected beyond the frontier of the tumor, that is, until the point where healthy tissue is reached. Resection of such tumors requires en bloc resection, which will then necessitate reconstruction of the dura and, in some cases, reconstruction of the ICA and the bony defect. The main aim in this kind of surgery is to remove the tumor completely and to prevent CSF leak, and also to preserve the blood supply to the ipsilateral hemisphere, via either the preserved or the reconstructed ICA. However, surgery of the malignant tumors of the CS does not pose so much of a problem to the surgeon as does surgery of benign tumors of the CS, since in the former case the primary aim is to save the patient's life. On the other hand, surgery of benign tumors involves not only the saving of life but also preservation of the quality of life.

Vascular Lesions of the Cavernous Sinus

Vascular lesions in the CS, in most cases, cause only minimal deficits of the cranial nerves. However, one must take into account the importance of preserving the ICA. Many of these lesions cannot be dealt with by using the endovascular techniques, as they require reconstruction of the ICA in order to preserve its patency, and it is obvious that exposure of the ICA throughout the CS is necessary. For this reason, in addition to removing the orbital roof anterior and posterior to the sphenoid wing together with the sphenoid wing itself, removing the ACP and opening the optic canal on the proximal, lateral, and under aspects, it is also vitally important to expose the ICA in the petrous bone in order to prepare it for temporary occlusion while reconstructing it in the CS. Dissection of the ICA should also be made distal to the vascular lesion, particularly at the level of the DR, which should be cut circumferentially so that the ICA can be mobilized and prepared for temporary clipping in order to prevent a stroke while dealing with partially thrombosed aneurysms in the CS, and to prevent retrograde bleeding, thus enabling the surgeon to work in a blood-free field (Fig. 13-19).

In fusiform and large or giant berry aneurysms of the ICA in the CS a large segment of the wall of the ICA is involved in the neck of the aneurysm. In traumatic aneurysms located on the AL of the ICA, and in high-flow CCFs there is a large defect in the wall of the ICA. In these lesions reconstruction of the ICA may be "local," "direct" (Dolenc, 1991), or "complete" (Fig. 13-29). All the rules governing the approach to the CS for vascular lesions are different from those applied for tumorous lesions. It is imperative that no pressure should be exerted by any surgical instrument over the lateral wall of the CS before temporary clips are applied proximal and distal to the vascular lesion. Only when the ICA has been sufficiently exposed in the petrous bone, and when the DR around the ICA proximal to the Oph A has been circumferentially cut, can the outer layer of the lateral wall of the CS overlying the aneurysm or CCF be gently peeled off from the nerves that have been displaced far laterally by the aneurysmal wall.

When dissection of cranial nerves III, IV, V_1, V_2, and particularly VI has started, temporary clipping of the ICA in the petrous bone, and intradurally, should be done in order to prevent major bleeding, dislodging of emboli from the thrombus in the aneurysm, and also to prevent retrograde bleeding. The vascular lesion is then incised through one or more windows between individual nerves; blood, or a blood clot, is removed and the proximal and the distal orifice of the ICA is checked. A decision is then made as to which kind of reconstruction of the ICA is optimal (Dolenc, 1991). In cases where the neck of the aneurysm measures less than half of the circumference of the ICA and the length of the segment involved is small, a "local" reconstruction will probably be possible. However, when more than half of the circumference of the wall of the ICA is involved, and when the length of the segment from where the lesion originates is less than 5 mm, end-to-end "direct" reconstruction of the ICA is usually possible by mobilization of the two adjacent loops of the ICA. In cases of fusiform aneurysms or large lacerations of the ICA in traumatic aneurysms or in high-flow CCFs, complete reconstruction of the ICA is necessary by means of a graft (Fig. 13-29).

Postoperative Care

It is advisable that patients having undergone CS surgery be woken and extubated as soon as possible after the operation, preferably in the operating room. The patients are then transferred to the recovery room where neuroanesthesiologic supervision is necessary for 1 to 2 hours, prior to their transfer to the neurosurgical intensive care unit (NICU) for a stay of at least 24 hours. The immediate awakening of such patients after surgery is of great importance, because a great majority manifest paresis of the 3rd cranial nerve and hence a dilated pupil. If the patient is pharmacologically paralyzed, intubated, and artificially ventilated and has a dilated pupil as a result of direct surgical injury to cranial nerve III, an epidural or subdural hematoma might easily be overlooked. But if the patient is woken after surgery, carefully monitored in the recovery room, and later in the NICU, any deterioration in consciousness, changes in reflexes, or possible paresis will be more noticeable to the hospital staff, which would not be the case if the patient were artificially ventilated and pharmacologically paralyzed. It is also important that in cases when an accidental opening of the bony sinuses occurs during the operation, lumbar drainage be inserted as a preventive measure some hours after surgery and that the drainage be continued for 7 to 10 days. Accurate regulation of intracranial pressure and of the amount of drained CSF are possible only when the patient is under continuous observation in the NICU or at least in a semi-intensive unit for the required period. When lumbar drainage is necessary, the patients are also treated with antibiotics.

A drain is inserted in the epidural space in order to evacuate any epidural collection. The drain is left in place for at least 24 hours after surgery but not for more than 48 hours after surgery, depending on the amount of drained blood. In cases where resection of the diseased segment of the ICA has been carried out without reconstruction of the ICA, or where grafting of the ICA has been performed with venous or arterial grafts, it is wise to keep the patient lying flat for at least 14 days. Only then is gradual elevation of the patient's head advisable, followed a few days later by the patient sitting up in bed, and then being completely mobilized in the third postoperative week.

As a routine procedure following CS surgery, a computed tomography (CT) scan is performed on the second or third postoperative day, if it is not required earlier. A routine CT without contrast medium is performed to rule out a hematoma. If CT is not possible in the early postoperative days, it should be carried out before the patient leaves the hospital, because the possibility of a hematoma must be eliminated.

Outcome of Direct Cavernous Sinus Surgery

In the series of 1,050 patients operated on for tumorous and vascular lesions in the CS, 7 died after surgery. One patient died as a result of postoperative rupture of the ICA and fatal arterial bleeding from the artery; another died of venous bleeding from the intercavernous sinuses, which opened due to increased retrograde pressure on the eighth postoperative day when the patient suffered physical strain just as she was due to be discharged from the hospital; one patient died due to postoperative thrombosis of the ICA and complete infarction of the ipsilateral hemisphere on the 14th postoperative day; three patients died from massive pulmonary embolism during the first postoperative week (all of these patients had previously been operated on twice elsewhere and had been bedridden for many months before they underwent surgery in our hospital); and two patients died in the third postoperative month due to endocrinologic disturbances and chronic pulmonary infection.

Nine patients lost their vision in the ipsilateral eye after surgery. In two of these, mechanical injury to the ON occurred accidentally during the opening of the optic canal, whereas in the remaining seven the loss of vision could not be explained. In three patients out of these nine, vision in the ipsilateral eye was found to be preserved during the first 24 postoperative hours, but then the patients noted loss of visual perception in the eye on the side of the operation. One of these three patients was operated on for a meningioma associated with significant stenosis of the optic canal due to a bulky ACP, whereas the other two were operated on for a CS cavernoma where there was no abnormality of the optic canal or of the ACP. Because there is no obvious indication, in seven patients, that the lesion of the ON was mechanically caused, the only possible explanation might be that the lesion of the ON occurred due to excessive heat during drilling the ACP or the walls of the optic canal, or that it occurred due to depletion of the blood supply to the ON.

Out of 190 patients who had diminished vision on the side of the lesion preoperatively, only 25 experienced further deterioration after surgery, whereas the vision of the remaining 165 patients remained either the same or even improved after surgery. Contralateral hemiparesis was observed in 15 patients immediately after surgery; in 12 cases it disappeared during the first postoperative days, and in 3 cases hemiparesis has continued to persist.

Epileptic seizures were not observed in the first 3 postoperative months since all the patients were on antiepileptic preventive treatment. Antiepileptic treatment was further continued in cases where the electroencephalogram (EEG) carried out 3 months after the operation showed abnormality, but it was gradually discontinued in cases where the EEG after 3 months was normal. Twenty patients needed antiepileptic treatment for the first postoperative year, after which time it could be withdrawn; five patients, however, have remained on permanent antiepileptic treatment as their EEGs have remained abnormal.

CSF leak—which appeared in 52 patients out of the series—completely ceased after lumbar drainage in all but 6 patients, who needed surgical closure: in 4 patients this was carried out transcranially, and in 2 patients an endoscope was used. Five patients underwent an operation for epidural hematoma, and made a complete recovery.

A serious complication (although very rare) occurs after operations for meningiomas in the CS as an unpleasant, sometimes agonizing trigeminal pain. In most cases these painful sensations in the distribution of the trigeminal nerve cease during the second postoperative year. It is advisable to treat such patients with large doses of carbamazepine (sometimes as large as 800 mg/day) before any destructive procedure on the root of the trigeminal nerve is planned. In our series, two patients required a section of the root of the 5th cranial nerve in the posterior fossa. It is very dangerous to sacrifice the root of the 5th cranial nerve or the V_1—even in cases where pain is present—if the greater petrosal nerve has been damaged during the initial operation. Patients undergoing such a procedure are likely to experience ulceration of the cornea, which may lead to blindness. Fifteen of our patients had atrophic changes of the cornea; in all but one the vision was preserved by adequate ophthalmologic care.

Preoperative paresis of one or more of the oculomotor nerves was present in a group of 205 patients; in 7 patients an improvement of the oculomotor function was observed during the first 2 postoperative weeks; in 80 patients during the first 6 postoperative months; and in 40 patients during the 6 to 12 postoperative months. In the remaining 78 patients, no change of oculomotor function was observed postoperatively.

In 230 patients operated on for vascular or tumorous lesions in the CS, normal oculomotor function was preserved after surgery. In 820 patients with normal or deficient oculomotor function before surgery, paresis of nerves III, IV, VI, or all three was present after surgery, but in 420 patients the nerves regained their preoperative condition during the first 3 postoperative months, and in 350 patients during the first postoperative year. In 50 patients these nerves remained partially paretic after 1 postoperative year.

References

Dolenc VV (1983) Direct microsurgical repair of intracavernous vascular lesions. J Neurosurg 58:824–831

Dolenc VV (1985) A combined epi- and subdural approach to carotid-ophthalmic artery aneurysms. J Neurosurg 62:667–672

Dolenc VV (1989) Anatomy and Surgery of the Cavernous Sinus. Springer Verlag, Wien

Dolenc VV (1990) Surgery of vascular lesions of the cavernous sinus. Clin Neurosurg 36:240–255

Dolenc VV (1991) The necessity for intracavernous ICA reconstruction. pp. 299–307. In Sato K (ed): Neurosurgeons 10. Proceedings of the Japanese Congress of Neurological Surgeons. SciMed Publications, Tokyo

Dolenc VV (1992a) Cavernous sinus masses. pp. 601–614. In Apuzzo MLJ (ed): Brain Surgery. Vol. 1. Churchill Livingstone, New York

Dolenc VV (1992b) Surgery of tumors originating in or invading the cavernous sinus. pp. 211–221. In Long DM (ed): Surgery for Skull Base Tumors. Vol. 12. Blackwell Scientific, Boston

Dolenc VV (1994a) Intracavernous carotid artery aneurysms. pp. 659–673. In Spetzler RF, Carter LP (eds): Neurovascular Surgery. McGraw-Hill, New York

Dolenc VV (1994b) Carotid ophthalmic aneurysms. pp. 673–686. In Spetzler RF, Carter LP (eds): Neurovascular Surgery. McGraw-Hill, New York

Dolenc VV (1994c) Frontotemporal epidural approach to trigeminal neurinomas. Acta Neurochir 130/1–4:55–56

Glasscock ME (1969) Exposure of the intra-petrous portion of the carotid artery. pp. 135–143. In Hamberger CA, Wersaal J (eds): Disorders of the Skull Base Region. Proceedings of the 10th Nobel Symposium. Almqvist and Wiksell, Stockholm

Parkinson D (1965) A surgical approach to the cavernous portion of the carotid artery. Anatomical studies and case report. J Neurosurg 23:474–483

Parkinson D (1969) Transcavernous repair of carotid cavernous fistula. J Neurosurg 26:420–424

Parkinson D (1973) Carotid cavernous fistula: direct repair with preservation of the carotid artery. J Neurosurg 38:99–106

Parkinson D (1987) Carotid cavernous fistula. History and anatomy. pp. 3–29. In Dolenc VV (ed): The Cavernous Sinus—A Multidisciplinary Approach to Vascular and Tumorous Lesions. Springer Verlag, New York

Serbinenko F (1974) Wound catheterization and occlusion of major cerebral vessels. J Neurosurg 41:125–145

Spetzler RF, Fukushima T, Martin N, Zabramski JM (1990) Petrous carotid-to-intradural carotid saphenous vein graft for intracavernous giant aneurysm, tumor, and occlusive cerebrovascular disease. J Neurosurg 73:496–501

Taptas JN (1949) La loge du sinus caverneux, sa constitution et les rapports des elements qui la traversent. Sem Hop Paris 25:1719–1722

Taptas JN (1960) Loge du sinus caverneux et sinus caverneux. Rapports meninges des nerfs craniens et de l'artere carotide interne dans leur traversee de la fosse cerebrale moyenne. Sem Hop Paris 36:1853–1860

Taptas JN (1982) The so-called cavernous sinus: a review of the controversy and its implications for neurosurgeons. Neurosurgery 11:712–717

Taptas JN (1987) Must we still call cavernous sinus the parasellar vascular and nervous crossroads? The necessity of a definite topographical description of the region. pp. 30–40. In

Dolenc VV (ed): The Cavernous Sinus—A Multidisciplinary Approach to Vascular and Tumorous Lesions. Springer Verlag, New York
Umansky F, Nathan H (1982) The lateral wall of the cavernous sinus, with special reference to the nerves related to it. J Neurosurg 56:228–234
Vinuela F, Lylyk P (1987) Endovascular therapy of vascular lesions of the cavernous sinus. Experience with 129 cases. pp. 182–197. In Dolenc VV (ed): The Cavernous Sinus—A Multidisciplinary Approach to Vascular and Tumorous Lesions. Springer Verlag, New York

14

Surgery of the Intrabasal Carotid Artery

Hideyuki Ohnishi

The intrabasal carotid artery is frequently involved with tumors or aneurysms. In some patients the direct neck clipping of an internal carotid artery (ICA) aneurysm, or trapping combined with intrabasal saphenous vein graft, will be necessary in order to decompress adjacent cranial nerves and preserve ICA flow. The indications, preoperative examinations, surgical techniques, and results of a direct approach for aneurysms in and around the cavernous sinus (inferior C2 to C5 portion; Fisher, 1938) are described below.

Indications for Direct Approach to Intrabasal Carotid Artery Aneurysms

Large or giant intrabasal carotid artery aneurysms are difficult to treat only by intraaneurysmal coils because of compaction of coils and regrowth of aneurysms. The decision as to whether to perform a balloon occlusion of the ICA proximal to the aneurysm or a combination of proximal occlusion and superficial temporal artery–middle cerebral artery (STA-MCA) bypass or intrabasal saphenous vein graft bypass is based mainly on the results of an angiographic cross-flow study and balloon occlusion test of the ICA at normal blood pressure for 15 minutes (Fig. 14-1). If a neurologic deficit develops during the occlusion test, a high-flow bypass or direct neck clipping preserving the ICA flow should be done. When the patient has passed the clinical balloon occlusion test but shows local cerebral blood flow (l-CBF) in the range of 20 to 40 ml/100 g/min during a stable xenon computed tomography (CT)-CBF study or intraoperative laser-Doppler CBF study, long-term ICA occlusion seems impossible. In these patients, revascularization such as STA-MCA bypass is necessary. If the patient shows no decrease in flow at the occlusion test, reconstruction is optional. In young patients a skull base bypass is recommended because its long-term patency is higher than that of an external carotid/internal carotid vein graft bypass and it reduces the potential of hemodynamic new aneurysm formation associated with ICA occlusion.

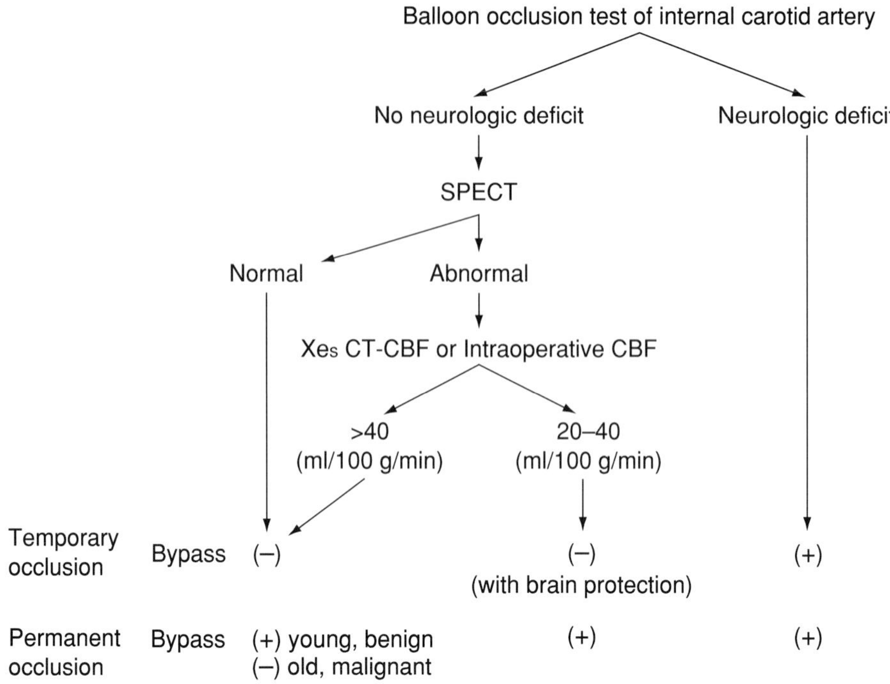

Figure 14-1. Algorithm illustrating the management of the internal carotid artery. Bypass (–) or (+) means no need or need to bypass.

In conclusion, a direct approach is selected for patients with aneurysms that may cause subarachnoid hemorrhage, patients with symptomatic intracavernous aneurysms who cannot tolerate the balloon occlusion test of the ICA, and for failed endovascular obliteration.

Special Diagnostic Considerations

The exact location and width of the aneurysm neck are very important when assessing the feasibility of direct neck clipping. For this purpose, cine- or videotape-angiography are useful. A thin slice, bone window CT is extremely important for checking the anterior and posterior clinoid processes, ethmoid and sphenoid sinuses, and calcification of the dural ring or the interclinoid ligament.

Operative Procedure

Positioning

In order to minimize blood loss from the cavernous sinus, the patient is placed in a semi-sitting position at about 20 to 30 degrees. Excess elevation of the head over 45 degrees will increase the risk of air embolism (Sugita, 1985). The head is extended slightly and rotated contralaterally about 30 degrees.

Brain Protection

During the period of temporary occlusion of the ICA, burst suppression on the electroencephalogram is maintained with thiopental infusion and the systolic blood pressure is slightly elevated to the level of 150 mmHg. Low-molecular-weight dextran

(10% dextran 40) is transfused at about 10 ml/kg and 20 percent mannitol is infused at about 10 ml/kg body weight. I have also used intravenous heparin at 80 U/kg body weight.

Monitoring

Laser-Doppler cortical blood flow and sensory evoked potentials are also monitored to check for cerebral ischemia during temporary ICA occlusion. Jugular venous oxygen saturation is monitored to check the coupling state between cerebral blood flow and global cerebral metabolism and is maintained between 55 and 75 percent. Needle electrodes are inserted into the inferior rectus, superior oblique, and lateral rectus muscles percutaneously, or after orbitozygomatic osteotomy for oculomotor, trochlear, and abducens nerve monitoring. During the surgical exploration, the oculomotor, trochlear, and abducens nerves are stimulated directly by bipolar electrodes (Fig. 14-2).

Pterional Approach

A combined epidural and subdural approach (modified from Dolenc, 1985) is used for small carotid-ophthalmic, ventral paraclinoid, or cavernous sinus aneurysms. A curvilinear skin incision is made in the frontotemporal area (Fig. 14-3A). After a conventional frontotemporal craniotomy, skull base bone is resected only on the central side of the lesser wing of the sphenoid bone (Fig. 14-4A). The resection of the bone is started at the superior orbital fissure using a rongeur. When the distal end of the optic nerve comes into sight, bone resection is then stopped and the dura is opened along the lesser wing of the sphenoid bone to the terminal point of the anterior clinoid process in order to secure the operative field. The dura, which stretches over the superior orbital fissure, is cut open partially to the level of the anterior clinoid process to get a wide operative field (Ohnishi et al., 1991b). Then bone removal is started again, this time using a diamond drill.

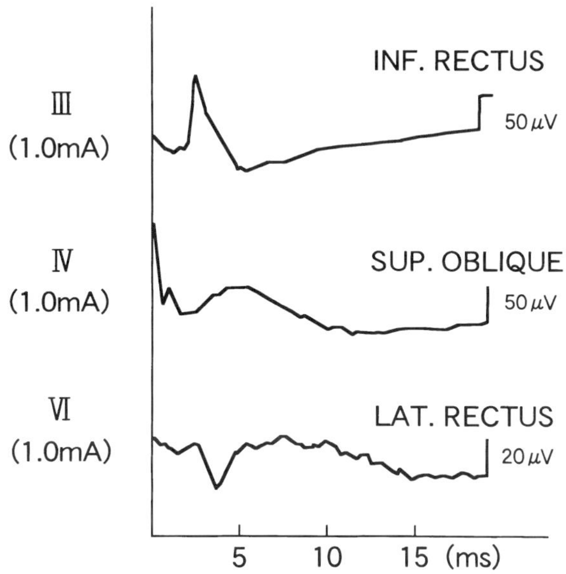

Figure 14-2. Intraoperative evoked electromyography of extraocular muscles by direct stimulation of 3rd, 4th, and 6th cranial nerves.

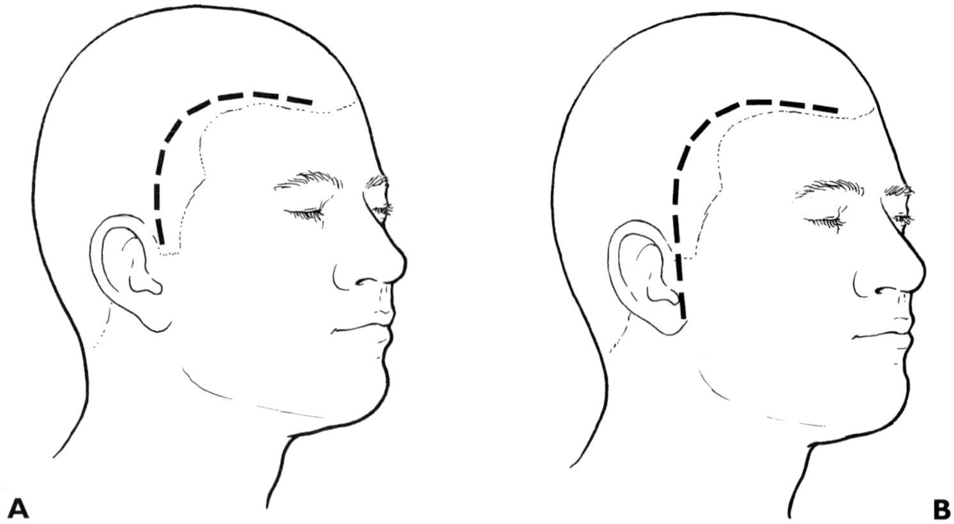

Figure 14-3. Skin incisions for *(A)* pterional approach and *(B)* fronto-temporal-orbitozygomatic approach.

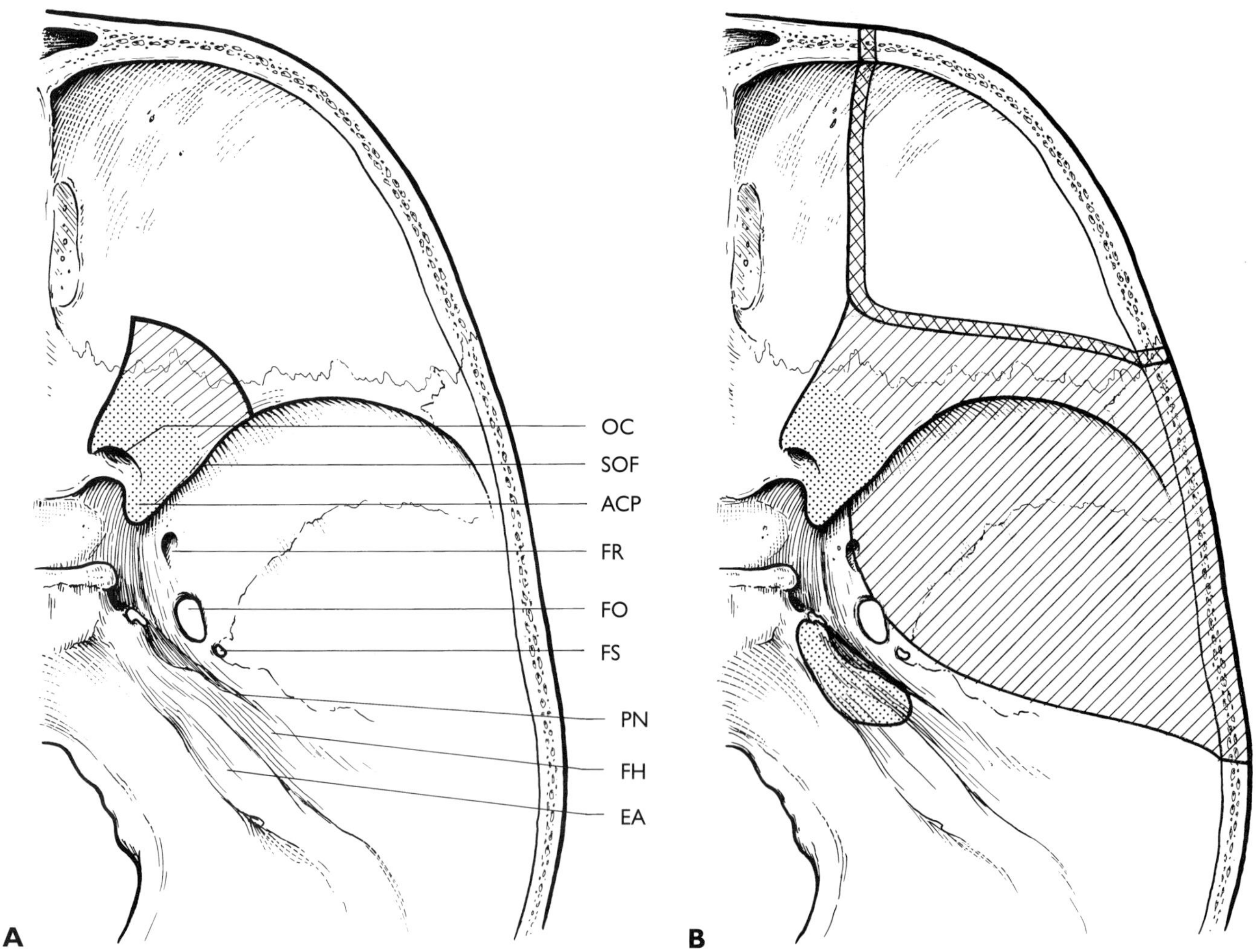

Figure 14-4. The areas of skull base bone resection for *(A)* small aneurysms and for *(B)* giant aneurysms, large tumors, and skull base bypass. The shaded part is removed with a rongeur, the crossed part with a bone saw, and the dotted part with a diamond drill. (For explanations of abbreviations, see Appendix 1, p. 373.)

Frontotemporal-Orbitozygomatic Approach

A more extensive hemicoronal skin incision is made starting from two-fingerbreadths below the zygomatic arch and extending upward along the hair line into the haired scalp (Fig. 14-3B). To avoid injuries to the frontal branch of the facial nerve and the trunk of the superficial temporal artery, the skin incision is made along the tragus. The scalp is then dissected under the temporalis fascia, which is turned down to protect this nerve. The superior orbital foramen is opened with a bone chisel and the supraorbital nerve is turned over with the scalp for protection. A frontotemporal craniotomy is performed in the standard way. The periorbita and the dura of the anterior and middle skull base are epidurally dissected. The superior and lateral walls of the orbit are drilled along a line down to the inferior orbital fissure (Fig. 14-5). This drilling is carried out as far back as possible for better reconstruction of the orbital wall. Using a bone saw, the superior orbital margin, zygomatic arch, and base of the zygomatic bone are cut. The optic canal and anterior clinoid process are drilled open with an air drill. The extent of osteotomy is illustrated in Figure 14-4B.

Exposure of the Petrous Segment of the Internal Carotid Artery

The petrous segment of the ICA is approached epidurally and exposed in the Glasscock (1969) triangle just behind the foramen ovale and the spinosum. As long as the opening of the carotid canal is limited to the gasserian ganglion on the anteromedial side, to the eustachian tube on the anterolateral side, and to the posterior wall of the carotid canal behind, the risk of injuring the cochlea can be avoided. In the cases of giant aneurysms, the lesion may hang over Glasscock's triangle and make it difficult

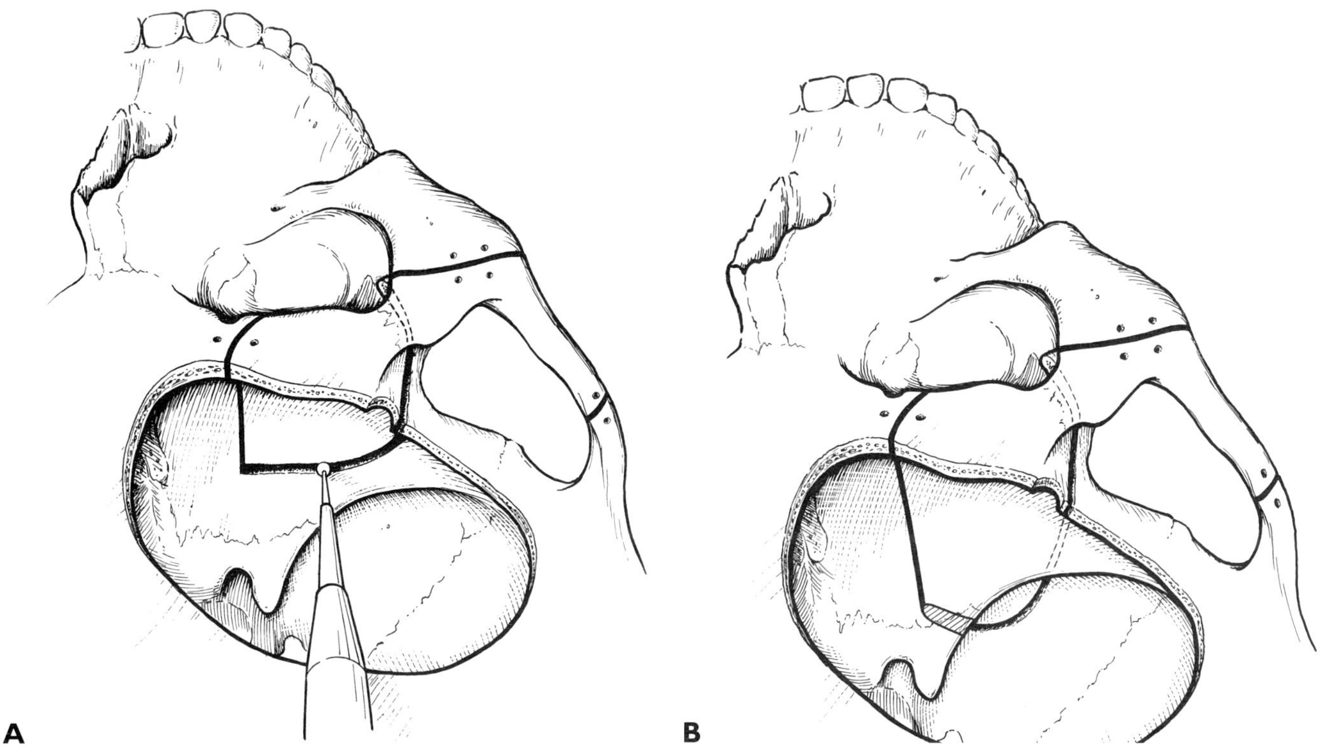

Figure 14-5. Orbitozygomatic osteotomy. Before completion of the orbitozygomatic osteotomy, small drill holes are made for microplate fixation. It is important to preserve the supraorbital nerve and the zygomaticofacial nerve. *(A)* A standard osteotomy and *(B)* an osteoplastic osteotomy for prevention of a postoperative enophthalmos.

to drill open the carotid canal. In such cases the dura is opened in a conventional way and then a longitudinal incision is made from the margin of the dural incision to the posterior end of the mandibular nerve (Ohnishi 1991A). The lesion is protected and retracted forward with a brain spatula and the canal is drilled open. The superficial petrosal nerve is amputated early so that no inadvertent retraction pressure is transferred to the geniculate ganglion. The amputation of this nerve will cause no serious problem except for a mild feeling of dryness in the eye. If the eustachian tube is opened, the endothelium is coagulated and the lumen is packed with a piece of the temporal muscle fixed with fibrin glue for prevention of cerebrospinal fluid (CSF) leakage. Tympanostomy will be performed later to treat the tubal obstruction (Sekhar et al., 1986).

Opening of the Optic Canal and Removal of the Anterior Clinoid Process

The dura is opened along the sylvian fissure in the direction of the anterior clinoid process. As shown in Figure 14-6A, the optic canal is opened under direct vision (observed from both epidural and subdural sides). It is essential that, while the bone is being drilled, the operative field must be flushed and cooled with physiologic saline solution in order to protect the optic nerve from any heat damage. Drilling should be stopped before penetrating the bone of the optic canal. When the bone becomes thin and translucent, the drilling ceases and the remaining bone layer is removed with a curette. If the ethmoid or sphenoid sinus is opened, the mucosa is pushed in and the sinus is sterilized with Isodin solution and then packed with a piece of temporal muscle or fat fixed with fibrin glue. When the anterior clinoid process and the optic strut are completely removed, the operative field will appear as in Figure 14-6B. The eyeball, the optic nerve covered with dura matter, the dura over the superior orbital fissure, and the dura on the frontal skull base form a dimple-like space known as Dolenc's (1985) anteromedial triangle. The C3 anterior loop is situated immediately below this triangle.

Opening of the Anteromedial Triangle of Dolenc and the Medial Triangle of Hakuba and Securing of the C3-C4 Portion

In the case of aneurysms of the C3 portion, the periosteum in Dolenc's triangle is opened to expose the C3-C4 portion of the ICA and Hakuba's medial triangle (Hakuba et al., 1982) is also incised backward a little to secure the peripheral C4 in case of rupture (Fig. 14-6C) before the aneurysm is approached. The passage of the oculomotor nerve within the cavernous sinus is predicted from the entering direction of the oculomotor nerve and the position of the superior orbital fissure. As long as the operation is restricted to the medial side of the oculomotor nerve in the sinus, there is no risk of damage to this nerve (Hakuba et al., 1982, 1987). With careful observation, the oculomotor nerve can be identified through the carotico-oculomotor membrane (Inoue et al., 1990). Bleeding from the sinus is controlled by packing with Biobond-soaked Oxycel or Surgicel. As tight packing will cause a palsy of the oculomotor nerve after surgery, sinus packing should be light and as little as possible. At the end of surgery, Oxycel is removed from the sinus as much as possible so that the compression of the nerve is kept minimal.

Opening of the Dural Ring and Neck Clipping

When the region proximal to the aneurysm is to be prepared, the falciform ligament attached at the posterior end of the dural sheath of the optic nerve is cut and the dural sheath is opened forward. When the operative field is extended by retraction sutures on the dura, the origin of the ophthalmic artery will be exposed. At this moment, the aneurysm is not in sight or only a small part of its dome is seen. The distal dural ring, where the ICA pierces the dura, is cut open around the ICA and then the clinoid segment of the ICA will be exposed (Fig. 14-6D). The dural ring is roughly connected with the ICA on the medial side and easily separated. Because the dural ring has been opened, the operative field can be expanded by mobilizing the ICA laterally. Direct retraction of the optic nerve should not be performed because it would cause visual disturbance after surgery. Most aneurysms are located medially below the ICA, being somewhat apart from the origin of the ophthalmic artery. They occur at the origin of the superior hypophyseal artery in most cases. Neck clipping is made with a Sugita's fenestrated curved "L"-shaped clip parallel to the course of the artery (Fig. 14-7A&B).

Exposure of the Cranial Nerves in the Cavernous Sinus

In some instances, such as the exposure of the neck of a giant aneurysm, it is necessary to expose the cranial nerves in the lateral wall of the cavernous sinus. The dura of the superior orbital fissure is opened and incised toward the middle skull base in front of the sphenoparietal sinus, preserving the draining pathway from the superficial sylvian vein (Nakase et al., 1993; Ohnishi and Karasawa, 1992). Because the dura propria on the medial side of the foramena rotundum and ovale is continuous with the superficial layer of the lateral wall of the cavernous sinus, oculomotor nerve, trochlear nerve, first, second, and third branches of the trigeminal nerve, and gasserian ganglion can rather easily be exposed by lifting off the dura from the above-mentioned area (Fig. 14-8) (Dolenc, 1983; Hakuba et al., 1989). The abducens nerve is the single cranial nerve running within the cavernous sinus and invisible from the outside so that operation should proceed carefully. For clipping of the aneurysm, it is recommended that the cranial nerves should not be all exposed but that exposure should be kept as little as possible for minimal morbidity.

Skull Base Bypass

A petrous carotid to supraclinoid carotid saphenous vein graft (Ohnishi, 1994; Ohnishi et al., 1989; Sekhar et al., 1990; Spetzler et al., 1990) for intracavernous giant aneurysms is recommended when neck clipping is impossible because of a wide neck or calcified giant dome. A saphenous vein graft is anastomosed first with 8–0 Prolene sutures to the petrous segment of the carotid artery end to side under barbiturate protection and systemic heparinization. The temporary clips are then removed to minimize the occlusion time of the ICA. The saphenous vein graft is directed to the supraclinoid region and anastomosed to the supraclinoid carotid artery end-to-end fashion with 9–0 Prolene sutures (Fig. 14-9A&B).

Closure of the Dura

To prevent postoperative CSF leakage, the dura is sutured watertight. A rotation flap is prepared by making a transverse incision in the dura and then the dura on the skull base is closed. The dead space created by the removal of the anterior clinoid process is filled with a piece of the temporal muscle. A piece of dura mater is collected and attached onto the skull base with fibrin glue. The dura defect over the frontotemporal region is closed with a freeze-dried human dura patch or fascia lata autograft. The frontotemporal and the orbitozygomatic bone flap are fixed with titanium microplates.

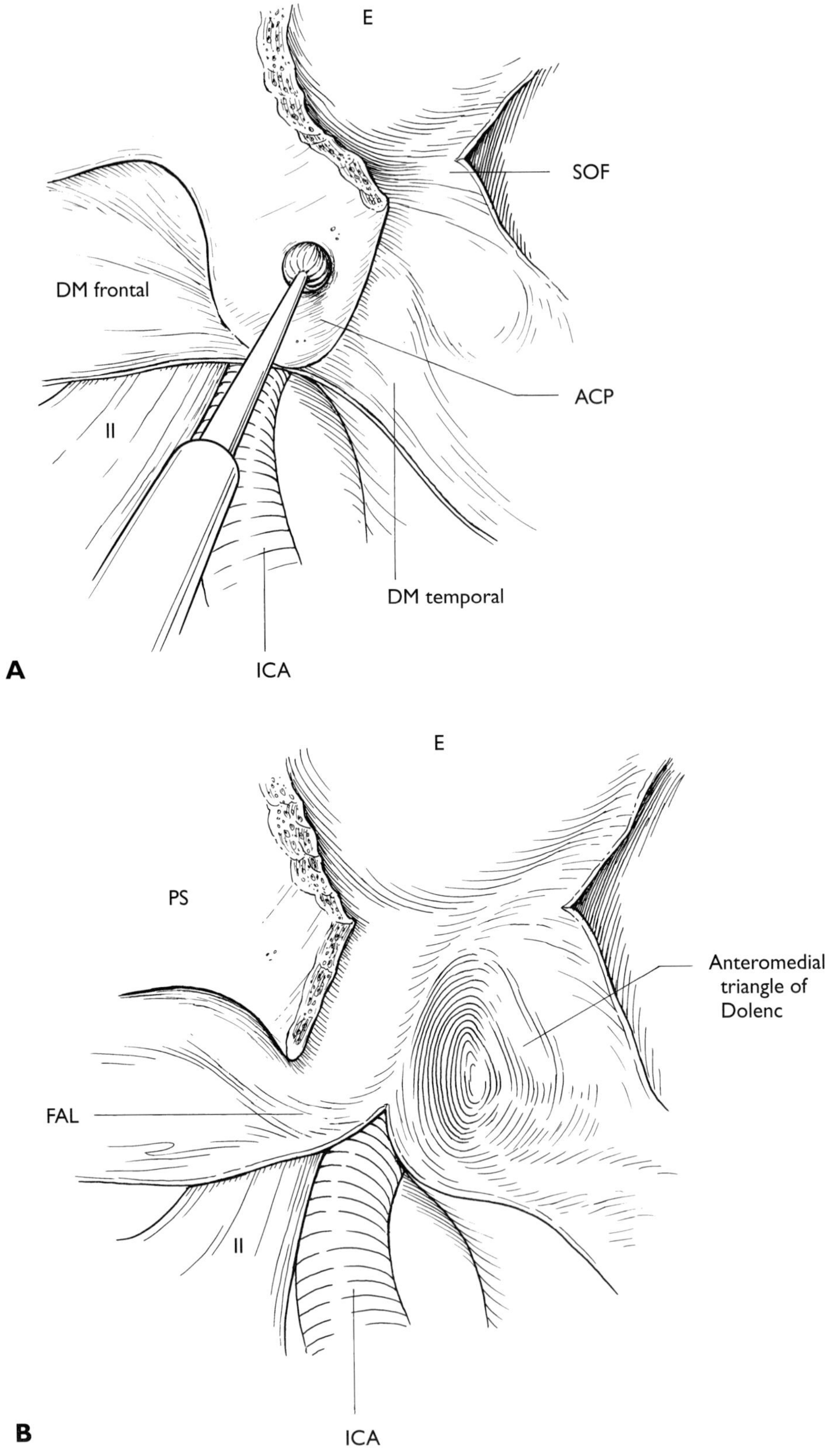

Figure 14-6. Approaches to the intrabasal carotid aneurysms. *(A)* The dural incision is extended along the sylvian fissure to the apex of the anterior clinoid process and then the anterior clinoid process is removed both intra- and epidurally. To secure the operative field, the dura of the superior orbital fissure is partly opened. C2, the C2 segment of the internal carotid artery. *(B)* The optic canal is opened and the optic strut is completely removed. *(Figure continues.)*

References

Dolenc VV (1983) Direct microsurgical repair of intracavernous vascular lesions. J Neurosurg 58:824–831

Dolenc VV (1985) A combined epi- and subdural direct approach to carotid-ophthalmic artery aneurysms. J Neurosurg 62:667–672

Fisher E (1938) Lageabweichungen der vorderen Hirnarterie in Gefassbild. Zentralbl Neurochir 3:300–312

Glasscock ME (1969) Exposure of the intrapetrous portion of the carotid artery. pp. 135–143. In Hamberger CA, Wersaall J (eds): Disorders of the Skull Base Region. Proceedings of the 10th Nobel Symposium. Almqvist and Wiksell, Stockholm

Hakuba A, Matsuoka Y, Suzuki J et al. (1987) Direct surgical approach to vascular lesions in the cavernous sinus via medical triangle. pp. 272–284. In Dolenc VV (ed): The Cavernous Sinus, Springer-Verlag, Vienna

Hakuba A, Nishimura S, Shirakata S, Tsukamoto M (1982) Surgical approach to the cavernous sinus. Report of 19 cases. Neurol Med Chir (Tokyo) 22:295–308

Hakuba A, Tanaka K, Suzuki T, Nishimura S (1989) A combined orbitozygomatic infratemporal epidural and subdural approach for legions involving the entire cavernous sinus. J Neurosurg 71:699–704

Inoue T, Rhoton AL, Theele D, Barry ME (1990) Surgical approaches to the cavernous sinus: a microsurgical study. Neurosurgery 26:903–932

Nakase H, Ohnishi H, Touho H et al. (1993) Preservation of the superficial Sylvian vein in the approach of skull base lesions. Surg Cereb Stroke 21:191–194

Ohnishi H (1994) Petrous carotid to supraclinoid carotid saphenous vein graft. pp. 678–682. In Samii M (ed): Skull Base Surgery. First International Skull Base Congress, Hannover 1992. Karger, Basel

Ohnishi H, Karasawa J (1992) Surgical approaches for tumors involving the cavernous sinus. Neurosurgeons 11:208–219

Ohnishi H, Shimomura T, Fujita T, Harada T (1989) Direct surgical approaches to intracavernous aneurysms. Neurosurgeons 8:210–221

Ohnishi H, Yuasa T, Kurokawa S et al. (1991a) Operative exposure of the petrous internal carotid artery for direct operation of intracavernous aneurysms. Surg Cereb Stroke 19:75–81

Ohnishi H, Yuasa T, Kurokawa S et al. (1991b) Transcavernous approach for infraclinoid internal carotid aneurysms. Surg Cereb Stroke 19:93–98

Sekhar LN, Schramm VL, Jones NF et al. (1986) Operative exposure and management of the petrous and upper cervical internal carotid artery. Neurosurgery 19:967–982

Sekhar LN, Sen CN, Jho HD (1990) Saphenous vein graft bypass of the cavernous internal carotid artery. J Neurosurg 72:35–41

Spetzler RF, Fukushima T, Martin N, Zabramski JM (1990) Petrous carotid-to-intradural carotid saphenous vein graft for intracavernous giant aneurysm, tumor, and occlusive cerebrovascular disease. J Neurosurg 73:496–501

Sugita K (1985) Microneurosurgical Atlas, Patient Position. p. 1. Springer-Verlag, Berlin

15

Lateral Extensive Middle Fossa Approach

Kenji Ohata
Akira Hakuba

Recent advances in cranial base surgery permit the total or near total resection of many skull base lesions with a low mortality (Hakuba et al., 1988, 1989; Mickey et al., 1988; Sekhar, 1987; Smith et al., 1990). Wide exposure of the cranial base to perform radical resection of lesions, however, may cause approach-related complications. As far as either the subtemporal or infratemporal fossa approach is concerned, these complications include (1) conductive or sensorineural hearing disturbance caused by injury to external, middle ear, or labyrinthine contents; (2) cerebrospinal fluid (CSF) leakage through the skin, paranasal sinuses, or eustachian tube that may be followed by postoperative infection; (3) trismus or malocclusion of jaw resulting from surgical insults to the temporomandibular joint (TMJ), mandible, or muscles attached to them; (4) facial nerve damage either in its intratemporal or extracranial course (Boyne, 1989; Gates, 1988; Hakuba et al., 1988; Kawase et al., 1991; Raveh et al., 1989; Sekhar, 1987). Since many neoplasms involving the middle cranial base are benign or only locally aggressive tumors, such approach-related complications must be avoided. On the contrary, excessive caution because of potential problems may cause the neurosurgeon to hesitate and lead to inadequate exposure of the middle skull base. In the middle cranial base, the TMJ, external auditory canal, and the temporal bone related to these structures may be most problematic for the neurosurgeon.

We describe an extensive middle fossa approach that has been developed for a wider exposure of the middle skull base with fewer approach-related complications.

Preoperative Evaluation

Computed tomographic (CT) scans in the axial and coronal planes, using both soft tissue and bone algorithms, and magnetic resonance imaging (MRI) are routinely performed. Magnetic resonance angiography (MRA) is also performed on all patients.

Depending on the tentative diagnosis of the lesion from imaging, conventional angiography and a sequential balloon occlusion test of the internal carotid artery (ICA) may be indicated. The occlusion test of the ipsilateral ICA and occasionally of both ICAs includes a 15-minute occlusion period with monitoring the patient's neurologic status, electroencephalogram, and stump pressure.

Preparation and Patient Positioning

On the day before the operation, a central venous line is inserted via a cephalic vein with the cut-down procedure for the management of possible air embolism during surgery. After the induction of general endotracheal anesthesia, a transesophageal echocardiography probe is inserted to detect air embolism. The superficial temporal artery and its branches are marked in the preauricular area using Doppler.

The patient is placed in a semisitting position. By using a Mayfield three-pin head-holder, the head is kept in an extended position at the craniovertebral junction, about 40 degrees, and the neck is tilted toward the side opposite the lesion, keeping the vertex of the head about 35 degrees downward. Then the head end of the operating table is elevated so as to keep the temporal region in the horizontal plane. Any obstruction of the venous return from the cranium by extension or rotation of the head should be avoided.

Surgical Technique

Skin Incision

The skin incision (Fig. 15-1) starts at the level of the earlobe and runs anterior to the auricle and is extended about 7 cm in length along the superficial temporal artery (STA). The STA is dissected with galea to form a pedicle about 1 cm in width and 7 cm in length. Care must be taken to preserve the superficial temporal vein (STV). After dissection of the vascularized STA-STV pedicle, the skin incision is extended anteriorly within the hairline to the contralateral frontotemporal region to a point

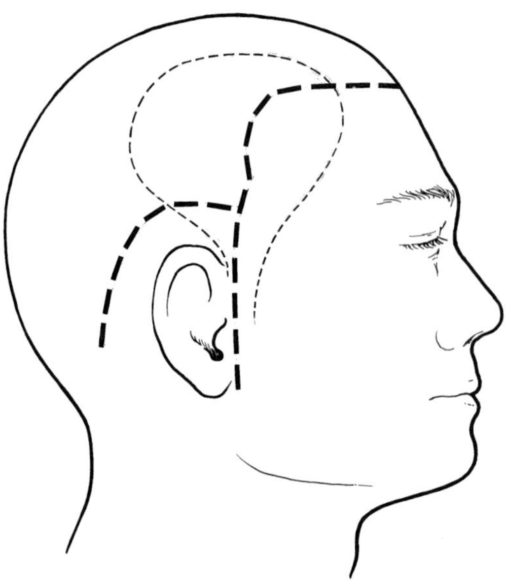

Figure 15-1. The skin incision (heavy dashed line), together with the vascularized pericranial flap (light dashed line) with a galeal pedicle incorporating the superficial temporal artery and vein, for a lateral extensive middle fossa approach.

about 5 cm above the superior margin of the opposite zygoma. An additional posterotemporal extension of the incision is made about 3 cm posterior and 1 cm inferior to the crista supramastoidea. After reflecting the skin flap, a large pericranial flap, vascularized by the STA-STV galeal pedicle, is mobilized from the frontoparietal area. Subcutaneous dissection, anterior to the vascular pedicle, is performed in a plane superficial to the deep layer of the deep temporal fascia, then extending downward to the zygomatic arch. In the posterotemporal area, posterior to the vascular pedicle, subcutaneous dissection is performed in the loose areolar tissue between the superficial temporal fascia and the superficial layer of the deep temporal fascia. The zygomatic arch is exposed subperiosteally and then the temporomandibular ligament is dissected from the overlying fascia. Care must be taken not to injure this ligament. The parotid gland is separated from the underlying masseteric fascia and from the ear cartilage posteriorly, so as to expose the condylar process of the mandible without causing injury to the facial nerve. The temporal muscle is divided along the line of the vascular pedicle down to the zygomatic arch. The posterior component of the temporal muscle is dissected subperiosteally and reflected inferiorly, exposing the superior wall of the bony part of the external auditory canal. The cartilaginous external auditory canal is transected so as to prevent an unrepairable laceration of the canal at the bone-cartilaginous junction (Fig. 15-2). This transected canal is reconstructed by suturing at the final stage of operation.

The superior and lateral orbital margins are exposed, maintaining continuity of the pericranium and the periorbita. The supraorbital nerve is preserved by freeing it

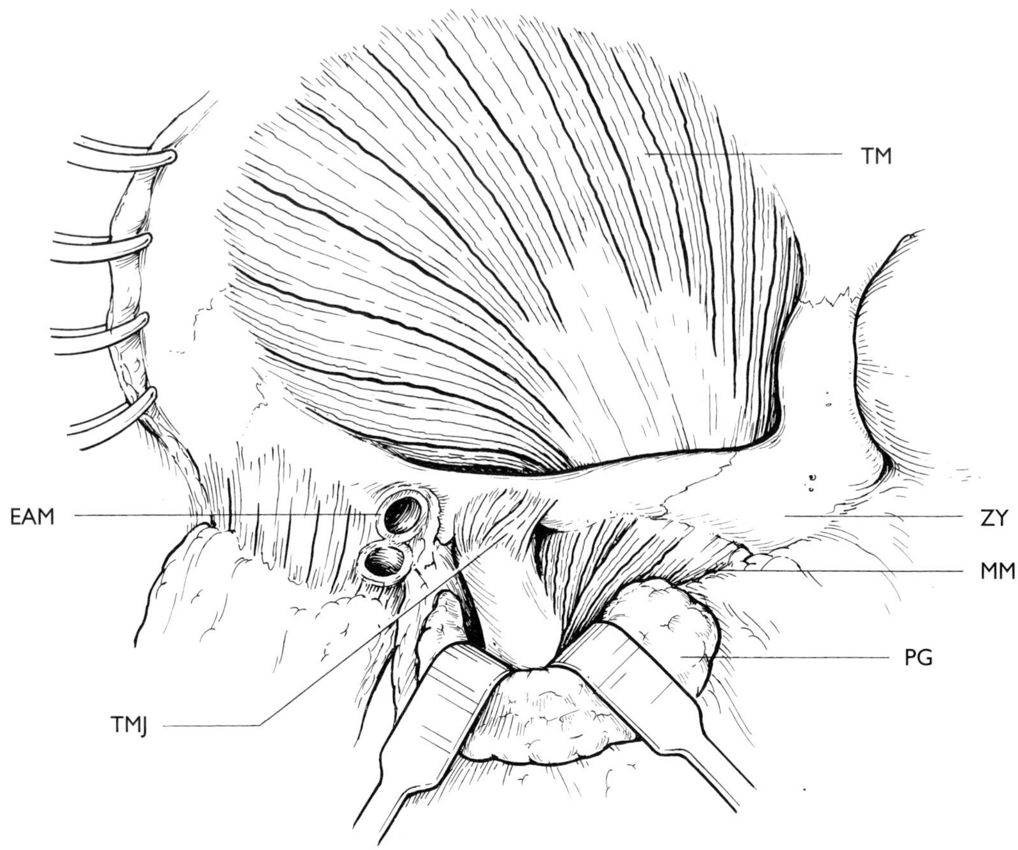

Figure 15-2. Skin flaps reflected inferiorly, separating the parotid gland from the underlying masseteric fascia and transecting the external auditory canal at its cartilaginous portion. The mandibular condyle is exposed subperiosteally by retracting the parotid gland. (For explanations of abbreviations, see Appendix 1, p. 373.)

from the supraorbital canal, which is opened with either an air drill or chisel, protecting the periorbita with a periosteal elevator.

Mandibulotomy

The masseteric fascia is used as a reference plane for the inferior extent of the dissection starting from the zygomatic arch. This dissection enables the wide exposure of the condylar process, retracting the preauricular skin flap downward with the parotid gland including the facial nerve (Fig. 15-2). The facial nerve, being left embedded in the soft tissue, is protected from traction injury. Optimal visibility of the condylar process and the mandibular incisure is crucial for the correct performance of mandibulotomy at the condylar process and the following reconstruction. After the precise application of two titanium miniplates on the condylar process, these are removed and a transverse osteotomy of the condylar process is performed using a sagittal saw (Fig. 15-3A). Care is taken to avoid injury of the temporomandibular ligament and the insertion of the lateral pterygoid muscle on the medial surface of the condylar process.

Frontotemporal Osteotomy

Seven burr holes are made: the first in the frontal bone about 5 cm above the upper margin of the orbit, the second in the "keyhole" position at the frontosphenoid suture directly behind the frontal process of the zygomatic bone, the third at the pterion, the fourth on the temporal bone just above the pedicle of the zygomatic process of the temporal bone, the fifth at the crista supramastoidea, and the sixth and seventh in the squamous bone above the fourth and third burr holes, respectively. A large frontotemporal craniotomy is first performed connecting each burr hole with a craniotome, and the bone flap is elevated (Fig. 15-3A).

Orbitozygomatic Osteotomy

The roof and lateral wall of the orbit are divided with a sagittal saw. To divide the roof, the sagittal saw is inserted from the anteromedial corner of the craniotomy, and directed posterolaterally about 45 degrees from the sagittal plane to cut the medial orbital roof for about 2 cm. Through the keyhole position the sagittal saw is then directed medially to the point at which its path meets the above cutting line. To cut the lateral wall, the sagittal saw is inserted through the keyhole and directed vertically down towards the inferior orbital fissure. The zygomatic bone is thereafter divided, from the inferior lateral corner of the orbit obliquely backward toward the inferior orbital fissure. The zygomatic arch is cut at the point of junction of its middle and posterior third. An orbitozygomatic bone flap is then hinged down on the masseter muscle.

The remaining greater sphenoid wing lateral to the superior orbital fissure, forming the posterolateral orbital wall and the anterolateral part of the middle fossa, and the posterior portion of the orbital roof are divided using either a sagittal saw or small chisel (Fig. 15-3).

Osteotomy of the Temporal Base

The remaining squamous part of the temporal bone forming the mandibular fossa is divided. Retracting the temporal dura, a sagittal saw is inserted through the epidural space in the middle fossa. Osteotomy is carried out anteromedially along the sphenosquamous suture and posteromedially along the petrosquamous fissure. Around the external auditory canal, the tympanosquamous fissure is cut from the superior wall of the external auditory canal to the posterior margin of the mandibular condyle, using a Midas Rex C1 burr and chisel. Then, the osteotomy is extended from the superior wall of the external auditory canal to the inferoposterior edge of the frontotemporal craniotomy along a line 5 mm inferior to the crista supramastoidea. Care must be taken to avoid injury of the ICA, tympanic membrane, and auditory ossicles. Then, this bone flap of temporal base, including the mandibular condyle, posterior third of the zygomatic arch and the superolateral wall of the external auditory canal, is hinged down on the temporomandibular ligament and on the masseter muscle. This hinged bone flap can be further dislocated downward with the transected condylar process by retraction. During this downward retraction, the superior outer surface of the articular disc of TMJ is denuded because the overlying mandibular fossa is rotated laterally on the temporomandibular ligament (Fig. 15-4).

The combination of mandibulotomy and temporal base osteotomy may be called an oticocondylar osteotomy.

Combined Epidural and Subdural Exposure of the Middle Fossa

The remaining medial part of the lesser sphenoid wing is then removed, and the superior orbital fissure and the optic canal are completely unroofed. The anterior clinoid process is then removed either epidurally or subdurally. The dura mater of the middle fossa is separated from the anterior wall of the petrous bone with division of the greater superficial petrosal nerve and exposure of the foramen spinosum. The middle meningeal artery is coagulated and divided near the foramen spinosum. Dissection follows the posterior and medial margins of the foramen ovale. An incision is made in the endosteal layer of dura along the lateral margin of the superior orbital fissure, superior margin of the foramen rotundum, and lateral margin of the foramen ovale. The outer layer (dura propria) of the lateral wall of the cavernous sinus is separated by blunt and sharp dissection from the inner layers consisting of the trigeminal nerve sheaths (Fig. 15-5). Venous bleeding during this procedure is controlled by quick sealing the opened venous pathway with fibrin-soaked collagen sponge.

By combined epidural and subdural approach, a wider exposure of the cavernous sinus and surrounding structures can be achieved. The dura mater is incised over the sylvian fissure, and this incision is extended along the superior dural sheath of the unroofed optic canal. Then the dural fringe of the optic nerve sheath is reflected backward, cutting the distal ring around the ICA. Thereafter, endosteal dissection along the lateral wall of the cavernous sinus is continued backward. The medial triangle formed between the ICA, the dural entrance of the oculomotor nerve, and the posterior clinoid process, comprising the superior wall of the cavernous sinus, is easily exposed. Finally, a full exposure of the lateral and superior wall of the cavernous sinus is achieved (Fig. 15-6).

The extent of this denudation is tailored according to the individual case.

Subtemporal-Infratemporal Dissection

The trigeminal impression on the petrosal tip is well exposed by retracting the temporal dura mater. By using an air drill, the petrosal bone medial to the petrosal portion of the internal carotid artery is removed until the inferior petrosal sinus is exposed between the internal auditory meatus and the petrosal tip. Care should be taken to avoid opening the cortical bone of the anterior wall of the cochlea. Dissection is continued until the ganglionic portion of the ICA is identified. Dorello's canal can be opened through this preauricular transpetrosal route.

The horizontal and the vertical segment of the petrous ICA can be exposed by drilling via an anterolateral transtemporal route after removing the bony eustachian

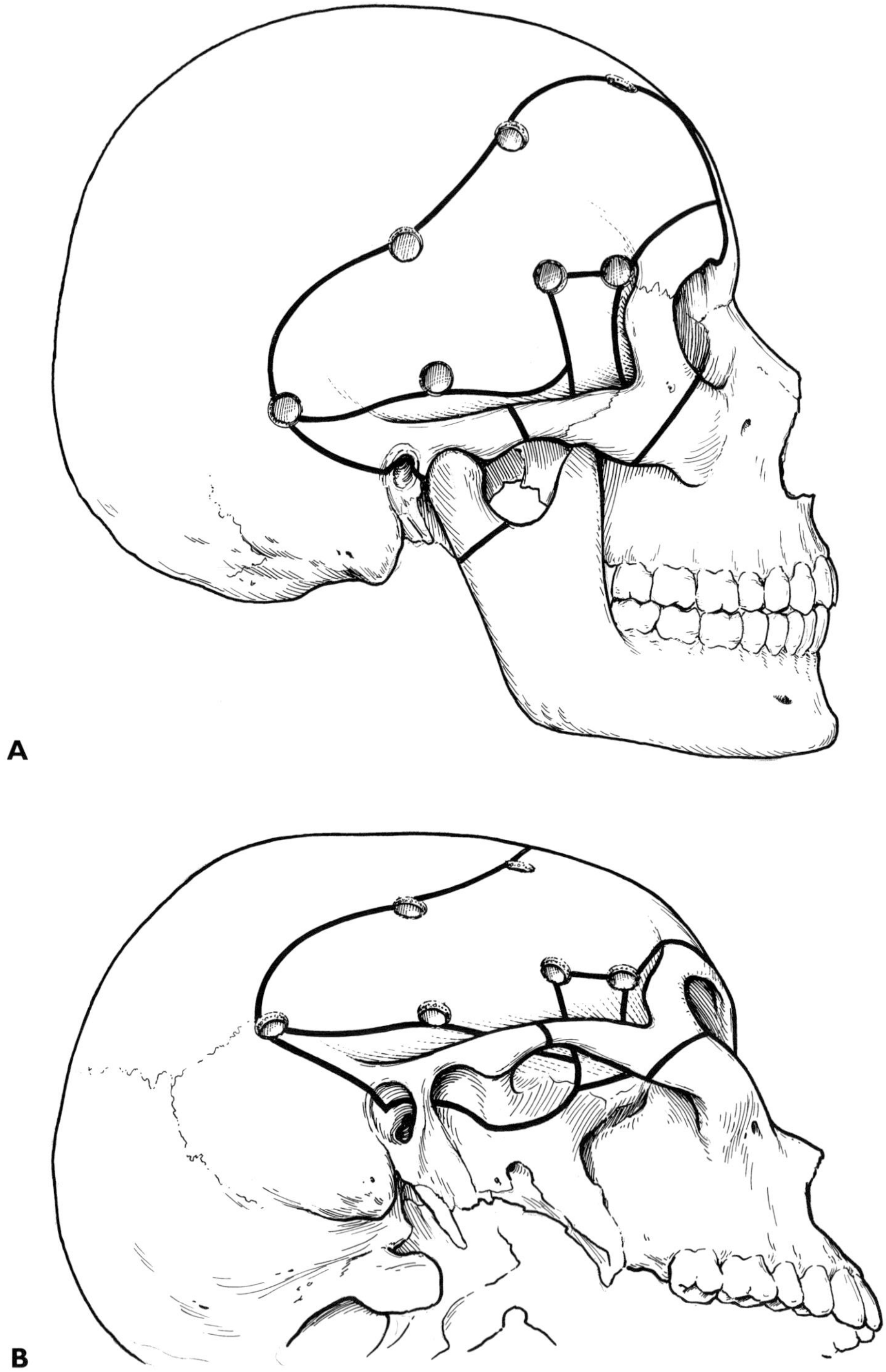

Figure 15-3. *(A)* Lateral, *(B)* inferolateral, and *(C)* superior views of cutting lines for craniotomy and osteotomy. The area of the anterior clinoid process, marked by cross-hatching, is removed later with a drill. *(Figure continues.)*

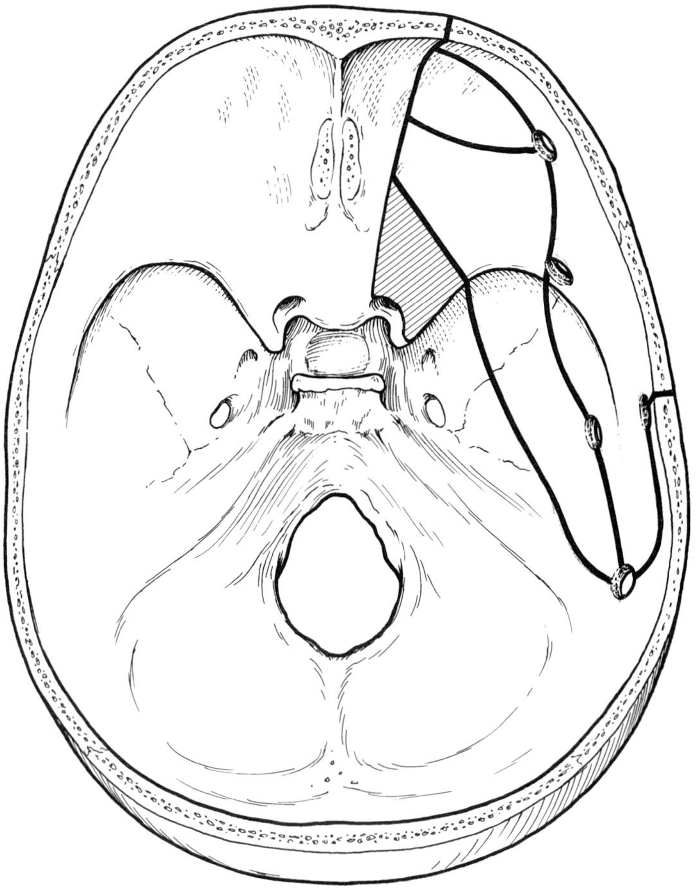

C

Figure 15-3 (Continued).

tube. The exposure of the horizontal ICA can be continued to its entrance to the petrous bone by drilling the tympanic part of the temporal bone that is anteromedial to the styloid process (Fig. 15-7).

Reconstruction

Meticulous reconstruction is crucial to avoid postoperative CSF leakage and malfunction of mandible. Any dural laceration or opening must be closed either with primary suture or with the use of a graft of vascularized pericranial flap. In deeper areas, watertight closure is not always possible. In such a situation, sutures must be placed as close as possible around the entire circumference under the microscope, followed by insertion of small pieces of fat taken from the abdominal wall. Extradural dead space resulting from tumor removal must be filled with fatty tissue. It is not necessary to use temporal muscle for reconstruction because the use of the pericranial vascularized flap combined with the abdominal fat is efficient enough. Thus, postoperative deformity of the temporal region due to the lack of temporal muscle can be avoided. When the dead space is very large, and when the removal of tumor creates a wide communication with the oropharynx, a microvascular free-flap tissue transfer is necessary.

The external auditory canal, transected at the cartilaginous site, is repaired by primary sutures from the subcutaneous side and then covered with the reflected inner layer of the posterior temporal muscle including periosteum, 2 × 3 cm in size. After

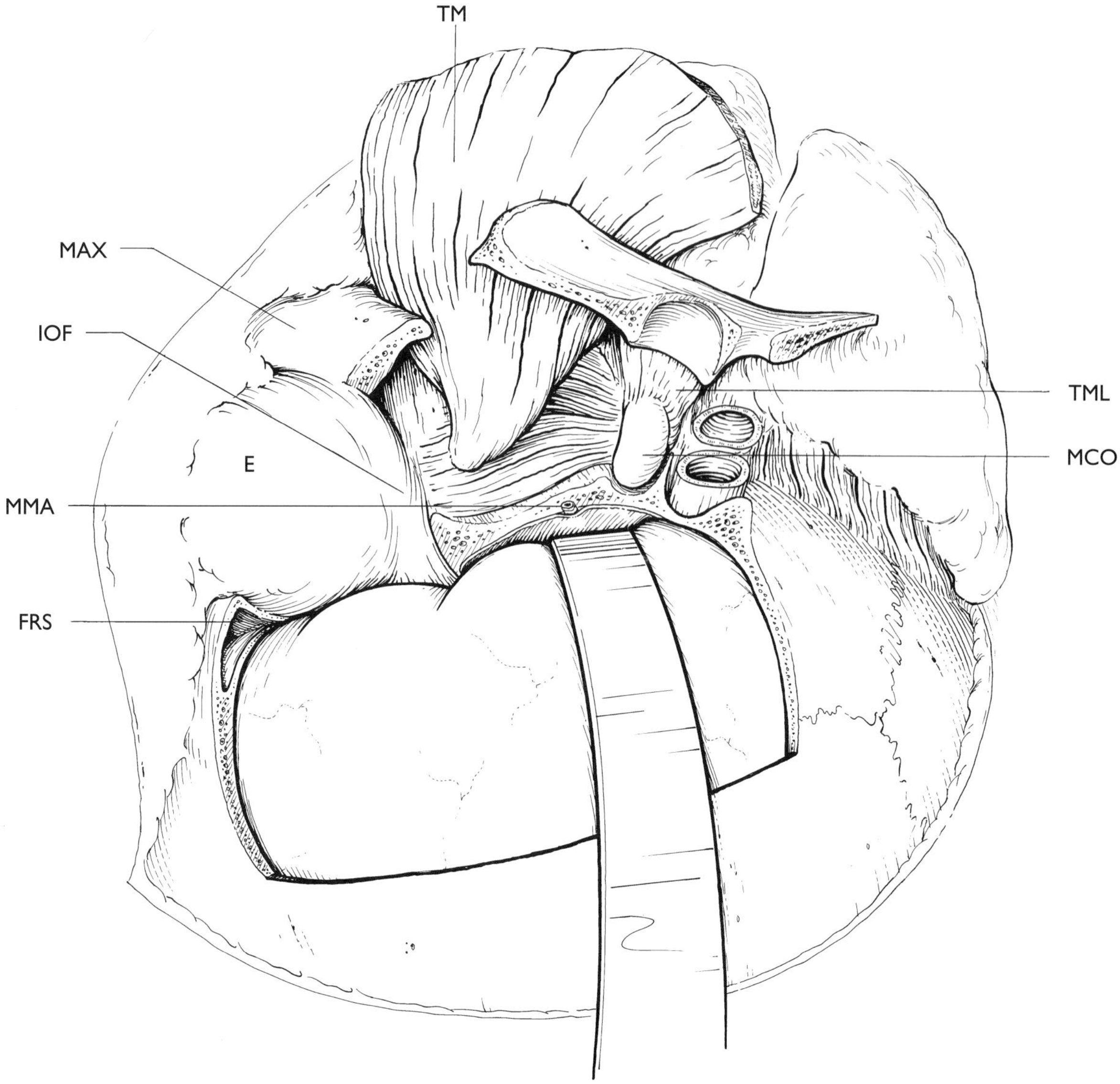

Figure 15-4. Operative view after an osteotomy of the temporal base. A bone flap of the temporal base is hinged down inferiolaterally. The temporomandibular ligament (TML) lateral to the mandibular fossa and the masseter muscle on the zygomatic arch are left attached to this bone flap. The mandibular condyle with the articular disc of the temporomandibular joint and the superior surface of the external auditory meatus are denuded.

closing the skin incision, a Silastic tube is inserted into the external auditory canal to prevent its obstruction by granulation tissue. This tube is left for 2 weeks. If the hearing is lost pre- or intraoperatively, the transected external auditory canal may be closed with sutures from the subcutaneous side and the squamous epithelium of the remaining external auditory canal medial to the point of transection must be removed.

Precise reconstruction of bony structures can be achieved by the use of miniplates. Prior to each bone cut, titanium miniplates have to be applied and fixed with screws temporarily. After removal of each miniplate and screw, the osteotomy is started. This procedure, in spite of being time consuming, permits the precise replacement of bone pieces. Intermaxillary fixation to prevent malocclusion is not necessary.

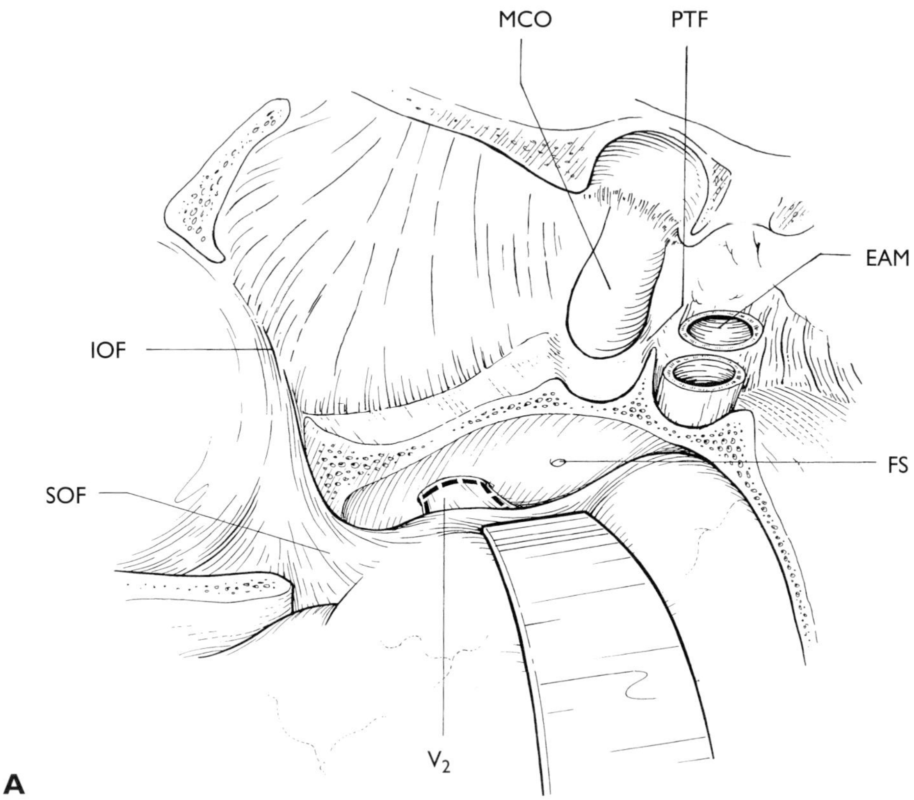

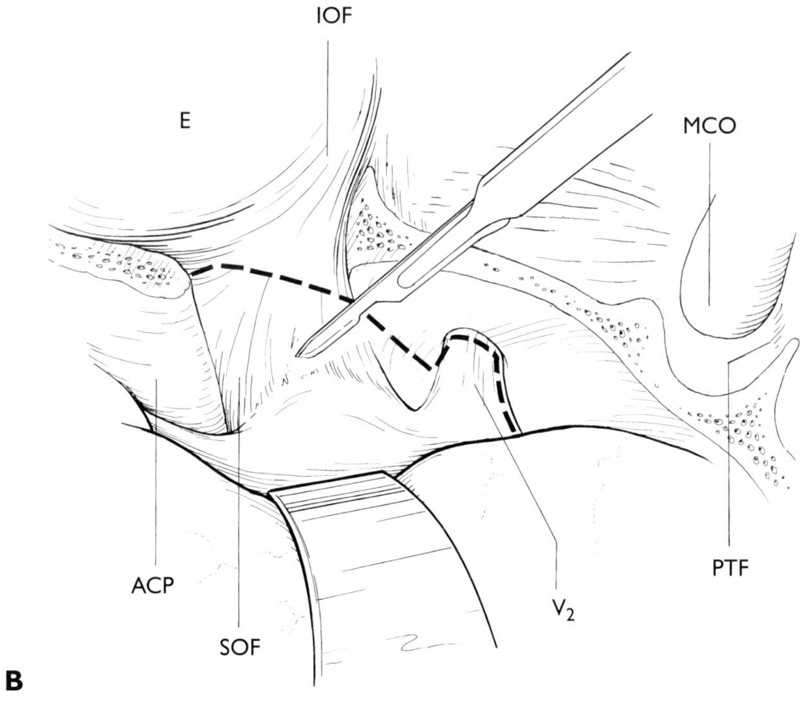

Figure 15-5. Epidural exposure of the middle fossa in the lateral extensive middle fossa approach. *(A)* Both superior and inferior orbital fissures are exposed by resecting the medial portion of the sphenoid wing. The anterior clinoid process and the roof of the optic canal have not been resected yet. An endosteal incision is started from the endosteal reflexion covering the maxillary nerve at the entrance to the foramen rotundum. Then, the dura propria is peeled off to expose the maxillary nerve toward its proximal side. The dashed line indicates the endosteal incision at the foramen rotundum. *(B)* The endosteal incision is continued in the endosteal reflexion at the lateral portion of the superior orbital fissure between the dura mater and the periorbita. The dura propria covering cranial nerves III to VI at the superior orbital fissure is peeled off toward the lateral wall of the cavernous sinus. By this means, the anterior clinoid process is fully exposed epidurally. The dashed line indicates the endosteal incision from the foramen rotundum to the superior orbital fissure.

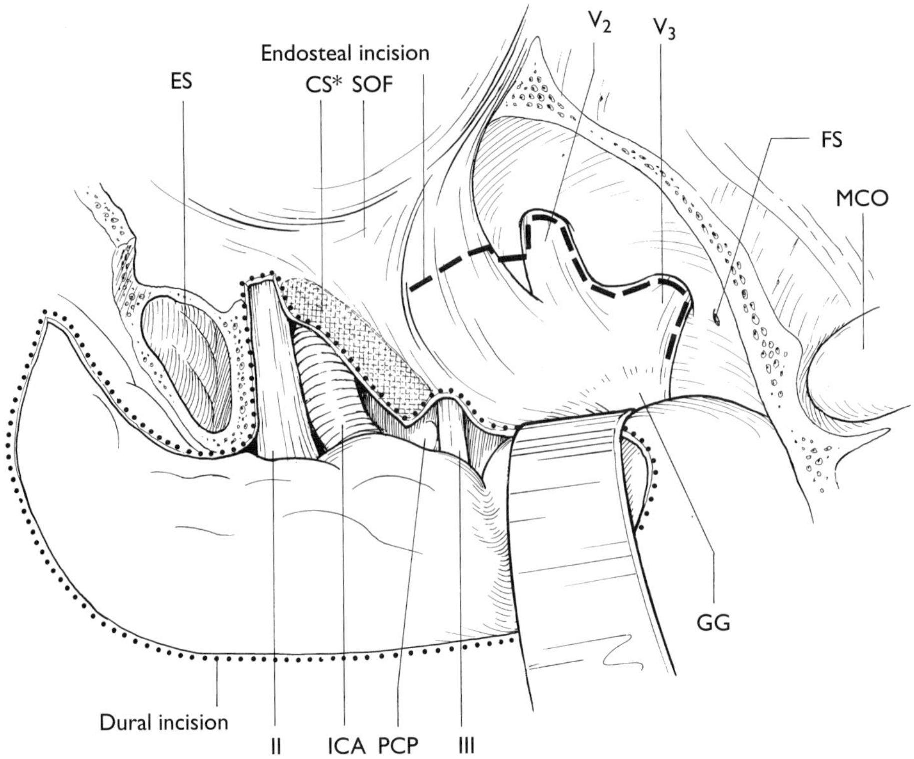

Figure 15-6. Combined epidural and subdural exposure of the cavernous sinus and the middle skull base. The anterior clinoid process has been drilled out and the dura mater incised along the sylvian fissure. The dura mater has been opened along the optic nerve and then the lateral fringe of the optic nerve sheath retracted laterally and divided along the lateral margin of the optic nerve and the carotid ring. The dura propria of the lateral wall of the cavernous sinus has been further separated backward from the deep layer and retracted back with the lateral fringe of the dura mater of the medial triangle in the superior wall of the cavernous sinus. By this means, the clinoid portion of the internal carotid artery, the canalicular portion of the optic nerve, the dural entrance of the oculomotor nerve into the cavernous sinus, and the entire lateral wall of the cavernous sinus are exposed. The middle skull base can be exposed back as far as the petrous ridge. (Dashed line, endosteal incision; dotted line, dural incision.)

Complications and Postoperative Care

Broad-spectrum antibiotics are started intravenously 12 hours before operation and continued for 48 hours after operation. The epidural drainage tube is removed within 48 hours. The patient should move as early as possible and be allowed to eat any food, regardless of its hardness, if bowel condition is good. Early mobilization of TMJ is critical to prevent complications such as trismus and malocclusion (Schobel et al., 1992). Jaw opening exercises include active hinge opening, lateral excursion, and manual stretching in front of the mirror.

The Silastic tube in the external auditory canal is left for 14 days, and then otologic care is performed every day for 1 week. Two cases who were operated on without the placement of this Silastic tube had stenosis of the external auditory canal. Clinically significant stenoses have not been experienced after its placement. CSF otorrhea via a transected external auditory canal is treated with spinal fluid drainage of 10 to 15 ml/hour for at least 4 days. During this drainage, antibiotics are continued. Three cases out of 26 of our own series had CSF otorrhea that was successfully treated by spinal fluid drainage.

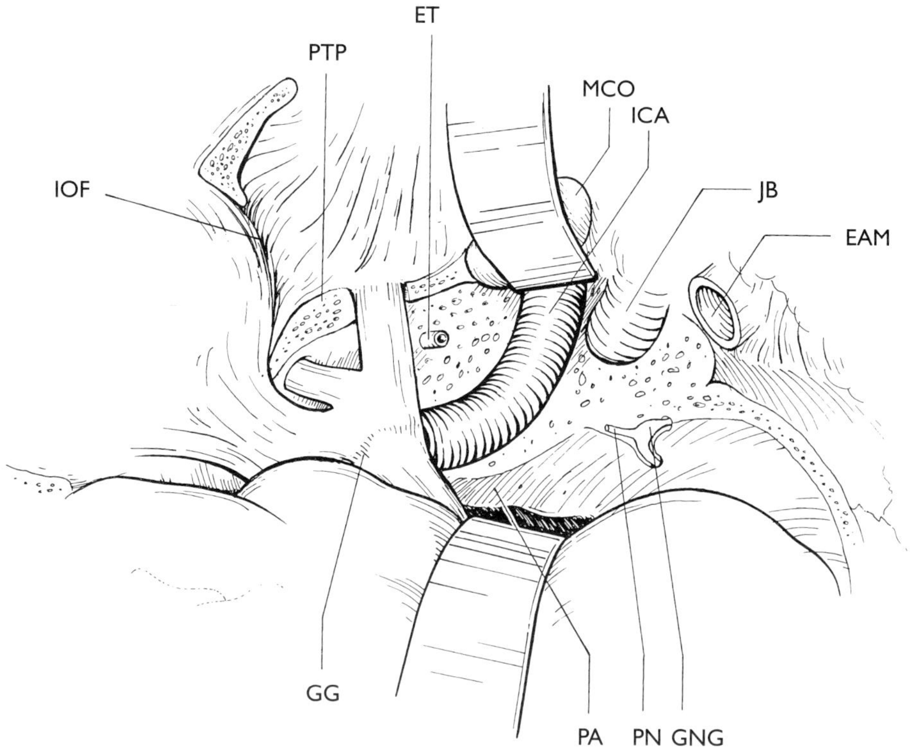

Figure 15-7. Exposure of the petrous internal carotid artery (ICA). By retracting the mandibular condyle anteroinferiorly, the anterolateral surface of the tympanic part of the temporal bone is fully exposed and then drilled out. After resecting the eustachian tube and tensor tympani muscle, drilling of the temporal bone is continued anteriorly to the geniculate ganglion. The medial part of the horizontal segment of the petrous ICA around the foramen lacerum is finally drilled out by retracting the ganglionic portion of the trigeminal nerve superiorly. By this means, the petrous ICA can be fully exposed with a minimal exposure of the facial nerve. The anterior surface of the jugular bulb can be exposed posterior to the vertical segment of the petrous ICA.

Traction or stretching of the parotid portion of the facial nerve during the mandibulotomy never causes a complete facial palsy. All patients, except for those who had direct nerve injury at another site, could cover their cornea. Facial nerve palsy caused by mandibulotomy was detected in four patients in our series, and all of them had completely recovered within 3 months after surgery. Severe facial nerve palsy resulting from direct injury requires a tarsorrhaphy.

Summary

The extensive middle fossa approach is the preferred method for removal of tumors involving the middle skull base, cavernous sinus, and infratemporal fossa. It offers direct visualization of any structure in the middle skull base from the shortest distance. Compared to other skull base approaches, every surgical step has been developed with specific consideration of the subsequent reconstruction (Raveh et al., 1989; Seifert and Diet, 1992; Sekhar, 1987). The disadvantage of this approach is its complexity both in osteotomy and in dissection of soft tissue.

We believe that the initial surgical strategy for a benign skull base tumor, even if it is invasive, is completely different from that in cases of malignancy. In the surgery of benign skull base tumors, complications related to surgical access must be avoided, and the possibility of recurrence has to be kept in mind when planning the first surgical access. Accordingly, every structure should be reconstructed, anatomically and functionally, as accurately as possible.

In order to minimize the temporal lobe damage during the surgery of the middle fossa, orbitozygomatic approaches and transpetrosal approaches have been developed by many neurosurgeons (Al-Mefty and Anand, 1990; Gates, 1988; Hakuba et al., 1988, 1989; Mickey et al., 1988; Sindou et al., 1991; Seifert and Diet, 1992; Smith et al., 1990). Although these are excellent, we have experienced several cases of temporal contusion that caused disability. An ideal route to access the middle fossa is a lateral route via the temporal bone. Some surgeons have reported the total resection of one TMJ in the surgery of benign tumors, a technique that should be indicated only for malignancy (Glasscock et al., 1983; Sekhar, 1987). Our extensive middle fossa approach is a logical and practical way to access the middle skull base.

References

Al-Mefty, Anand VK (1990) Zygomatic approach to skull-base lesions. J Neurosurg 73:668–673

Boyne PJ (1989) Free grafting of traumatically displaced or resected mandibular condyles. J Oral Maxillofac Surg 47:228–232

Gates GA (1988) The lateral facial approach to the nasopharynx and infratemporal fossa. Otolaryngol Head Neck Surg 99:321–325

Glasscock ME, Smith PG, Bond AG et al. (1983) Management of aneurysms of the petrous portion of the internal carotid artery by resection and primary anastomosis. Laryngoscope 93:1445–1453

Hakuba A, Nishimura S, Jang BJ (1988) A combined retroauricular and preauricular transpetrosal transtentorial approach to clivus meningiomas. Surg Neurol 30:108–116

Hakuba A, Tanaka K, Suzuki T, Nishimura S (1989) A combined orbitozygomatic infratemporal epidural and subdural approach for lesions involving the entire cavernous sinus. Neurosurg 71:699–706

Kawase T, Shiobara R, Toya S (1991) Anterior transpetrosal-transtentorial approach for sphenopetroclival meningiomas: surgical method and results in 10 patients. Neurosurgery 28:868–876

Mickey B, Close L, Schaefer S, Samson D (1988) A combined frontotemporal and lateral infratemporal fossa approach to the skull base. J Neurosurg 68:678–683

Raveh J, Vuillemin T, Sutter F (1989) TMJ dysfunction: surgical management and reconstruction. J Otolaryngol 18:334–343

Schobel G, Millesi W, Watzke IM, Hollmann K (1992) Ankylosis of the temporomandibular joint. Oral Surg Oral Med Oral Pathol 71:7–14

Seifert V, Diet H (1992) Combined orbito-frontal, sub- and infratemporal fossa approach to skull base neoplasms. Acta Neurochir (Wien) 114:139–144

Sekhar LN (1987) Subtemporal-preauricular infratemporal fossa approach to large lateral and posterior cranial base neoplasms. J Neurosurg 67:488–499

Sindou MP, Biol DSc, Fobe J-L (1991) Removal of the roof of the external auditory meatus in approaching the tentorial notch through a low temporal craniotomy. J Neurosurg 74:520–522

Smith PG, Grubb RL, Kletzker GR, Leonetti JP (1990) Combined pterional-anterolateral approaches to cranial base tumors. Otolaryngol Head Neck Surg 103:357–363

16

Extended Middle Cranial Fossa Approaches to the Clivus and Acoustic Meatus

Takeshi Kawase
Ryuzo Shiobara

Atkinson in 1949 pointed out the importance of the anteroinferior cerebellar artery in surgery for cerebellopontine angle tumors and since then the mortality rate associated with acoustic neuroma surgery has dramatically decreased. This was followed in 1961 by the introduction of the operating microscope by House, which was used in the middle cranial fossa approach, enabling very favorable results. Recent years have seen the further development of microsurgical and general neurosurgical techniques and the introduction and widespread application of precise physiologic and neurologic monitoring and recording systems. These tremendous advances have enabled a further decrease in the mortality rate and increase in the preservation of the facial nerve and hearing. We have also seen a lower incidence of postoperative complications, such as cerebrospinal fluid (CSF) leakage.

There are now four recognized surgical approaches to acoustic neuroma surgery: the suboccipital, middle cranial fossa, and translabyrinthine approaches, and a combination of these three constitutes a fourth approach. Neurosurgeons favor the suboccipital approach. For the most part, otorhinolaryngologists favor the middle cranial fossa and translabyrinthine approaches. The combined approach has been championed by neurosurgeons working in tandem with ear, nose, and throat (ENT) specialists (King, 1970; Morrison and King, 1973).

Since House introduced the middle cranial fossa approach in 1961, it has been used mostly by ENT surgeons. It offers the advantage of enabling an approach to the inner aspect of the temporal bone or the internal auditory canal, but because of the restricted width of the operative exposure this approach is not suitable for removal of cerebellopontine angle or acoustic tumors over 2 cm in diameter. As a result neurosurgeons tend not to use this approach except in rare circumstances. In 1975, however, Bochenek and Kukwa introduced and applied an extended approach through the middle cranial fossa, adding incisions of both the superior petrosal sinus and cerebellar tentorium following a middle cranial fossa approach. There were still many problems inherent in this approach, however, such as the restriction of the size of the cerebellopontine angle tumors that can be successfully removed; therefore, our group at Keio University further researched and developed this approach, resulting in the publication in 1977 of our extended middle cranial fossa approach (Kanzaki et al., 1977). In this chapter we describe the surgical techniques involved in these extended middle cranial fossa approaches.

Extended Middle Cranial Fossa Approaches

The extended middle cranial fossa approaches are basically expanded versions of the original middle cranial fossa approach. The approaches can be applied to a wide range of conditions, from diseases involving the internal structures of the temporal bone to the removal of large cerebellopontine angle and clival tumors. The advantage of this approach is that it eliminates the need for having to choose another approach depending on both the size of the tumor and the need for hearing preservation. For those patients with small acoustic neuromas where hearing preservation is a priority, only the upper wall of the internal auditory canal needs to be opened. In procedures for the removal of large cerebellopontine angle tumors, a wide area in the pyramidal portion of the temporal bone is drilled out followed by incisions of the tentorium and dura mater of the middle cranial fossa in that order, thus enabling an enlarged operative site. Access can be extended anteriorly into the posterior cavernous sinus. The extended middle cranial fossa approach thus allows the surgeon to open up the operative site in stages, step by step, as required. This method could also be described as a subtemporal transpetrosal transtentorial approach.

Indications

Indications include the following: (1) basilar trunk aneurysms, located between the level of the pituitary floor and the internal auditory canal on a lateral angiogram; (2) upper clival tumors, located medial to the internal auditory canal; and (3) acoustic and other cerebellopontine angle tumors.

Preoperative Assessment

This should include magnetic resonance imaging (MRI) with gadolinium, targeted petrous bone computed tomography (CT) scan, and angiography. The points to be checked from the assessments are listed in Table 16-1.

Operative Procedures

Patient Preparation

Spinal drainage may be employed preoperatively to minimize cranial hypertension as much as possible, and then immediately after the craniotomy, a further 20 to 30 ml of CSF is removed. Spinal drainage is then continued for up to 5 days postoperatively with intermittent removal of CSF to control intracranial pressure and prevent CSF leakage. If it is thought that there is a high probability of CSF leakage, then spinal drainage is carried out continuously.

Table 16-1. Diagnostic Checkpoints

Examinations	Checkpoints
Magnetic resonance imaging	
Gd	Tumor extension
T2	Arterial encasement
	Perifocal edema in the brain stem
	Tumor intensity (related to consistency)
Bone computed tomography	Size and position of air cells of petrous bone
	Internal petrous anatomy
	Bone destruction
Angiography	Feeding artery and vascularity of tumor
	Arterial narrowing

An intravenous (IV) infusion of 500 ml of mannitol (20 percent) is started at the beginning of the procedure.

Positioning

The patient's head is slightly elevated (20 degrees) and rotated to place the affected side uppermost, auricle on top (Fig. 16-1). For those patients in whom the head cannot be turned sufficiently due to obesity, old age, or other causes of lack of flexibility of the neck, then a small pillow is inserted under the patient's shoulder or the operating table adjusted to bring the head to the correct position. The importance of obtaining the correct position is that it allows the surgeon to identify accurately the angle and position of the external auditory meatus, which further forms the basis for envisaging the internal anatomy of the petrous bone. In the transpetrosal approach the dura mater is separated from the pyramidal or petrosal ridge of the temporal bone, and then, while drilling out the upper petrosal ridge of the middle skull base, the position of the tympanic cavity, vestibule, cochlea, labyrinth, or semicircular canals and the internal auditory canal can be understood relative to the position of the external auditory meatus, arcuate eminence, and so on. In particular, when hearing preservation is a priority, and a middle or extended middle cranial fossa approach (i.e., a transpetrosal approach) is indicated, it is necessary to open the internal auditory canal by drilling out only the upper canal wall, which requires correct and precise positioning of the patient's head.

Monitoring Electrode Setup

The electrodes for monitoring intraoperative facial nerve response are set up on the orbicularis oculi and orbicularis oris muscles, with other indifferent electrodes set up as necessary. In those operative procedures where hearing preservation is a priority, an earphone and electrode are set up to monitor auditory brain stem response (ABR). In patients where a cochleogram is to be recorded, following craniotomy a needle electrode is inserted from the edge of the craniotomy directly into the tympanic cavity, or through the tympanic membrane. Prior to draping, the auricle is folded forward temporarily and held with two or three sutures, thus covering the earphone and the external auditory meatus.

Instrumentation

Additional instruments to the conventional craniotomy set are listed below.

High speed air drill
Ultrasonic aspirator
Sugita's brain retractor with hooks
Dural dissector
Microdissector sets
Cellulose gauze (Surgicel)
Fibrin glue

Incision and Craniotomy

A "U"-shaped scalp incision is made above the ear (Fig. 16-1A). For the anterior transpetrosal approach to the clivus the anterior margin is straight to protect the facial nerve from injury and to create a more anteriorly based craniotomy. The upper margin is made along the sphenotemporal line, to create a fascial flap with sufficient length for use in a subsequent repair at closure. The temporal fascia is dissected off the muscle leaving a pedicle inferiorly and the muscle is retracted anteriorly (Fig. 16-1B). The craniotomy is centered low above the mandibular joint. It is created more anteriorly than that of the extended middle fossa approach to the cerebellopontine angle lesion; it is not necessary to expose the sigmoid sinus.

In the surgical procedure for acoustic neuroma or cerebellopontine angle meningioma by way of the extended middle cranial fossa approach, the skin incision is the same regardless of the size of the tumor or the priority of hearing preservation. A roughly semicircular incision is carried out centered on the auricle and external auditory meatus, starting anteriorly from the center of the midcranial skull base and extending posteriorly to the rear of the mastoid, thus ensuring adequate exposure of the midcranial skull base (Fig. 16-1C). Folding the skin flap aside, a slightly smaller incision is made in the temporal fascia, temporal muscle, and periosteum, separating them from the temporal bone all the way up to the external auditory meatus, where they are folded over with the skin flap. In the next stage, a free bone flap is constructed, extending the bone window all the way down to the bottom of the middle cranial skull base using a rongeur and a drill. At the posterior portion of the bone window, the mastoid air cells are gradually removed until a portion of the sigmoid sinus is exposed.

Anterior Transpetrosal Approach to the Clivus

The anterior transpetrosal approach to the clivus has been described by Kawise et al. (1985, 1991, 1994).

Exposure and Resection of the Pyramid

The petrous pyramid is exposed epidurally until the petrous rim is identified. The foramen spinosum, which is located in the bottom of the middle fossa, is identified and the middle meningeal artery is cut after coagulation. Minor and major petrosal nerves, which can be confirmed as having dural adhesion to the pyramid at the point posterior to the foramen ovale and course along a groove in the bone, are dissected carefully with the attached lateral dural layer. Care must be taken not to stretch the major petrosal nerve excessively, because it is connected with the facial nerve in the pyra-

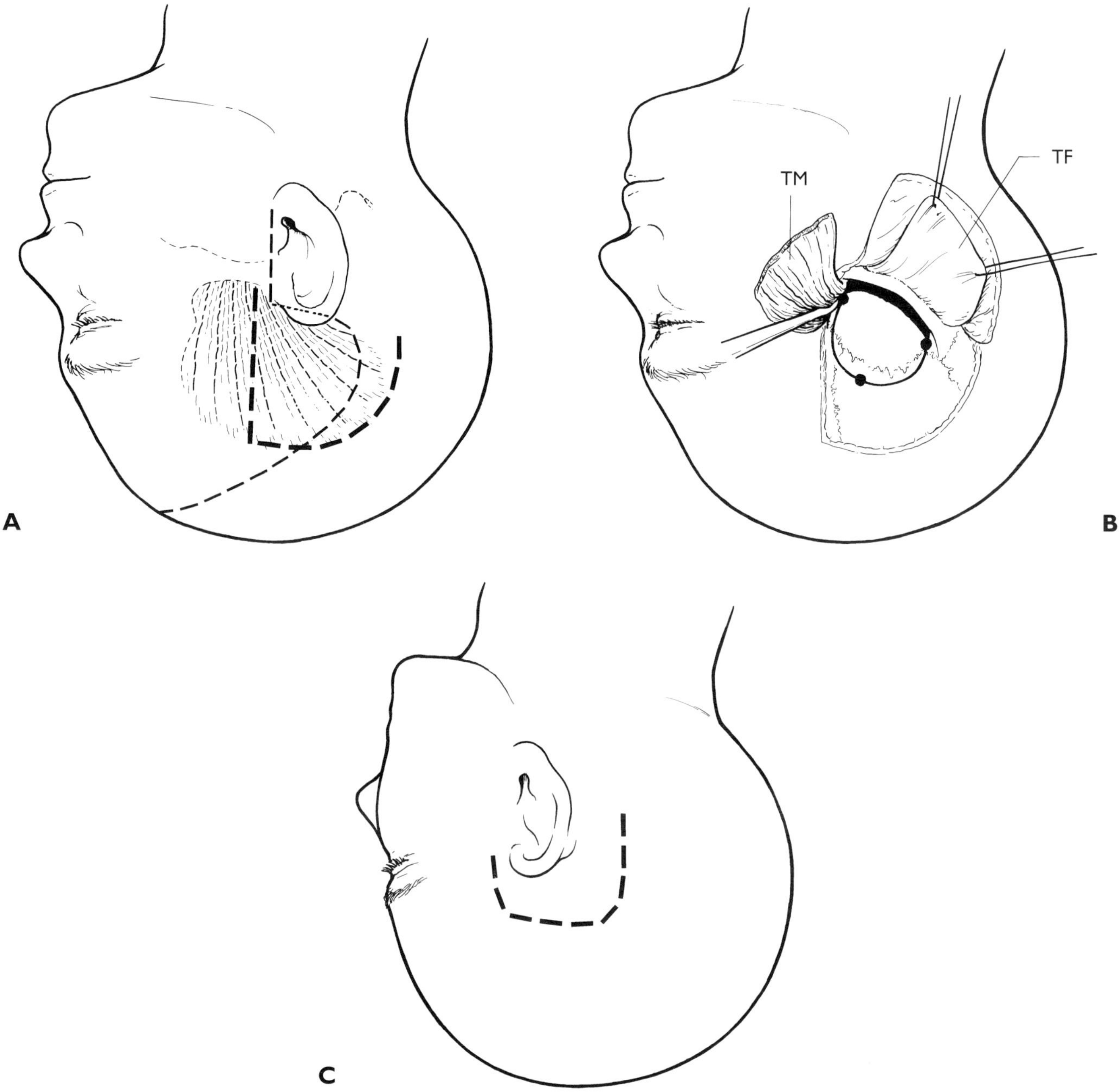

Figure 16-1. *(A)* Skin incision for anterior transpetrosal approach. The lightly dashed line represents the extent of surgical exposure when combined with pterional or zygomatic approach. *(B)* Separation of temporal fascia (TF) flap from the muscle (TM) for later dural closure. Craniotomy is centered above the mandibular joint. *(C)* The incision for approach to acoustic meatus. (For explanation of abbreviations, see Appendix 1, p. 373.)

mid. A Sugita's tapered retractor with hooks is well tolerated for strong retraction of the dura to expose the apical petrous pyramid. In the case of dura resisting retraction, CSF must be drained. The axis of the microscope is deviated to overlook the anterior part of the pyramid. On the surface of the petrous pyramid, two bone eminences are observed: eminentia arcuata posterolaterally and petrous apex anteromedially. The trigeminal impression can be seen on the apex when exposure of the pyramid has been completed (Fig. 16-2). Location of the internal auditory canal is slightly anterior to the eminentia arcuata, at a depth of 7 mm from the bone surface. The cochlea is on

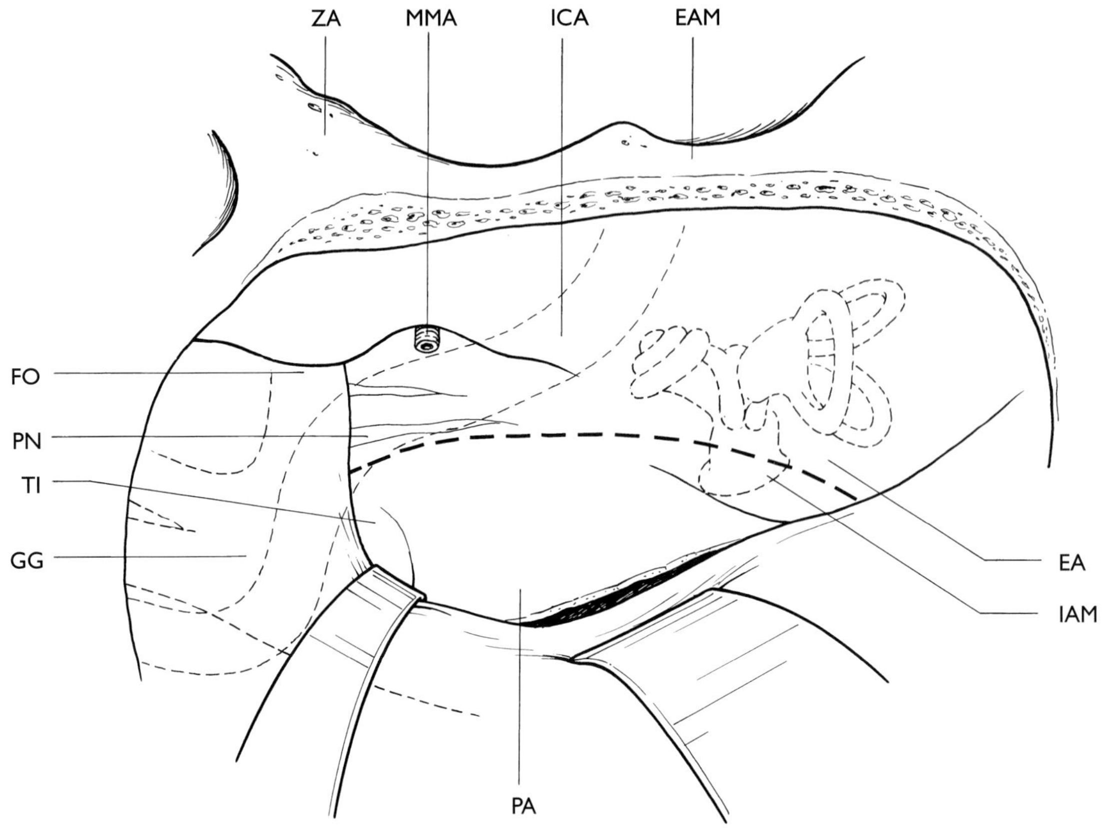

Figure 16-2. Exposure of right petrous pyramid. Location of internal auditory structures, trigeminal nerve, and internal carotid artery are overlapped. Heavy dashed line indicates maximal bone resection with preservation of auditory organs.

a line extended along the course of the major petrosal nerve. From the surgeon's viewpoint the carotid artery and eustachian tube are lateral to the major petrosal nerve.

A maximal bone resection with preservation of auditory structures is illustrated in Figure 16-2. It is medial to the major petrosal nerve, anterior to the eminentia arcuata, and superior to the internal auditory canal. The first step of bone resection is to enucleate the cancellous center of the anterior pyramid, with preservation of bone cortex of the dural side, using a small cutting burr. This is a safe way to avoid injury to the dural sinuses. Resection of the deep posterior part must be carried out carefully using a diamond burr so as not to penetrate the dura of the internal auditory canal. Resection of the bone spur of the petrous apex is important in order to mobilize the 5th cranial nerve, which courses along it. The posterior fossa dura between the 5th and 7th cranial nerves is seen after the bone resection.

Dural Incision

The basal dura of the middle fossa is incised 2 cm inward toward the superior petrosal sinus, and the incision is extended in a "T"-shape along the sinus after a brain retractor is inserted. A small dural hole is made into the posterior fossa, and the superior petrosal sinus is divided after ligation or clipping with hemoclips. This is followed by the tentorial incision (Fig. 16-3). Care must be taken not to injure the 4th cranial nerve around the free edge of the tentorium. Both sides of the tentorial leaflet are tacked back with sutures. In the case of a clival meningioma, the dural incision is made along the posterior rim of the tumor (Fig. 16-3), so that the tumor is attached to the anterior leaflet of the tentorium.

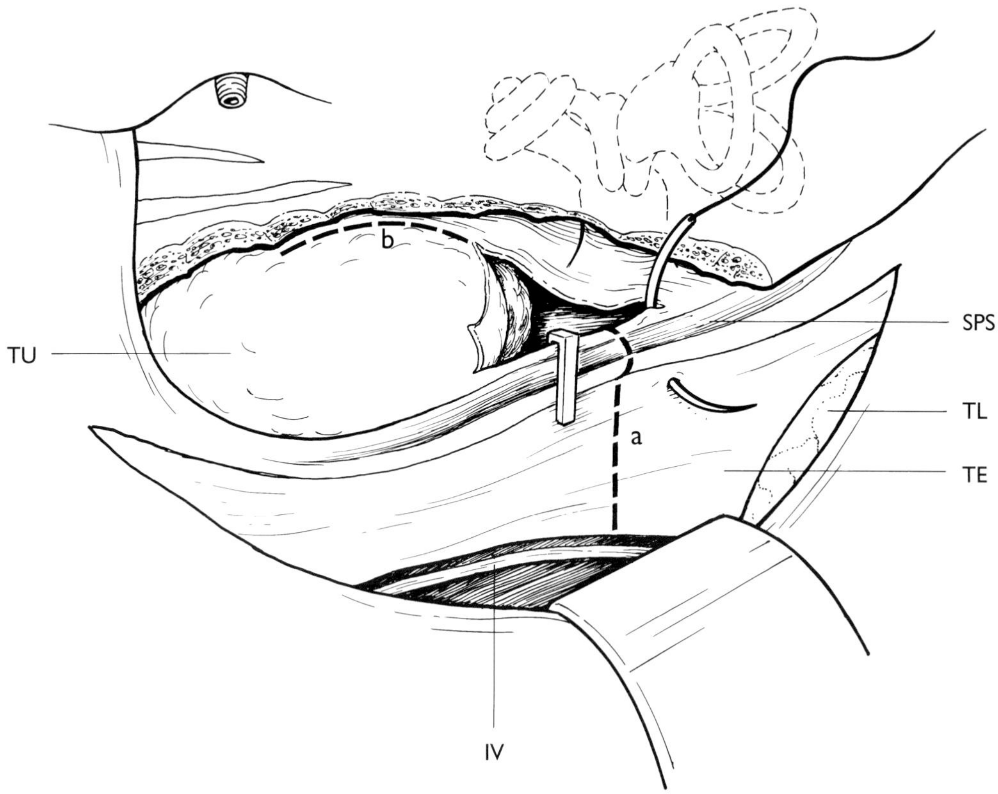

Figure 16-3. Dural incision after pyramid resection. Dashed lines indicate *(a)* tentorial incision and dural incision *(b)* of the posterior fossa along the margin of the tumor attachment.

Tumor Exposure

In the case of clival meningiomas, the 5th nerve is seen on the tumor, shifted laterally (Fig. 16-4). It is shifted inferiorly in the case of tentorial meningioma. The 3rd and 4th nerves are displaced superiorly, and the latter is commonly involved in the tumor at the point of penetration into the dural fold. Excessive stretching of the 4th nerve should be avoided. The dural incision is extended anteriorly along the 5th nerve that opens Meckel's cave, which shows a high incidence of tumor invasion. Tumor removal is started from Meckel's cave in order to increase mobilization of the 5th nerve, but note that the 5th nerve is loosely separated into individual strands in the cave, intermingled with the tumor. After mobilization of the 5th nerve, the tumor attachment is dissected from the clival dura, between the 4th and 5th nerves.

In the course of dissection, tumor feeders from the tentorial artery can be coagulated, following which bloodless surgery is possible during internal tumor decompression. Involvement of the superior cerebellar artery (SCA) and pontine perforators behind the tumor require clean dissection from the tumor. The anteroinferior cerebellar artery (AICA) is involved only in a large tumor. The abducens nerve is commonly displaced medially and found inferomedial to the 5th nerve, in the last stage of tumor removal (Fig. 16-5A). In the case of tumor extension into the cavernous sinus, the medial dural wall of Meckel's cave is incised along the superior border of the 5th nerve (V_1), and the nerve root is mobilized inferiorly to enlarge the Parkinson's triangle (Fig. 16-5B). Venous hemorrhage from the cavernous sinus is controlled by packing with Surgicel balls. The carotid siphon (C4–C5) and the 6th nerve are seen after tumor removal.

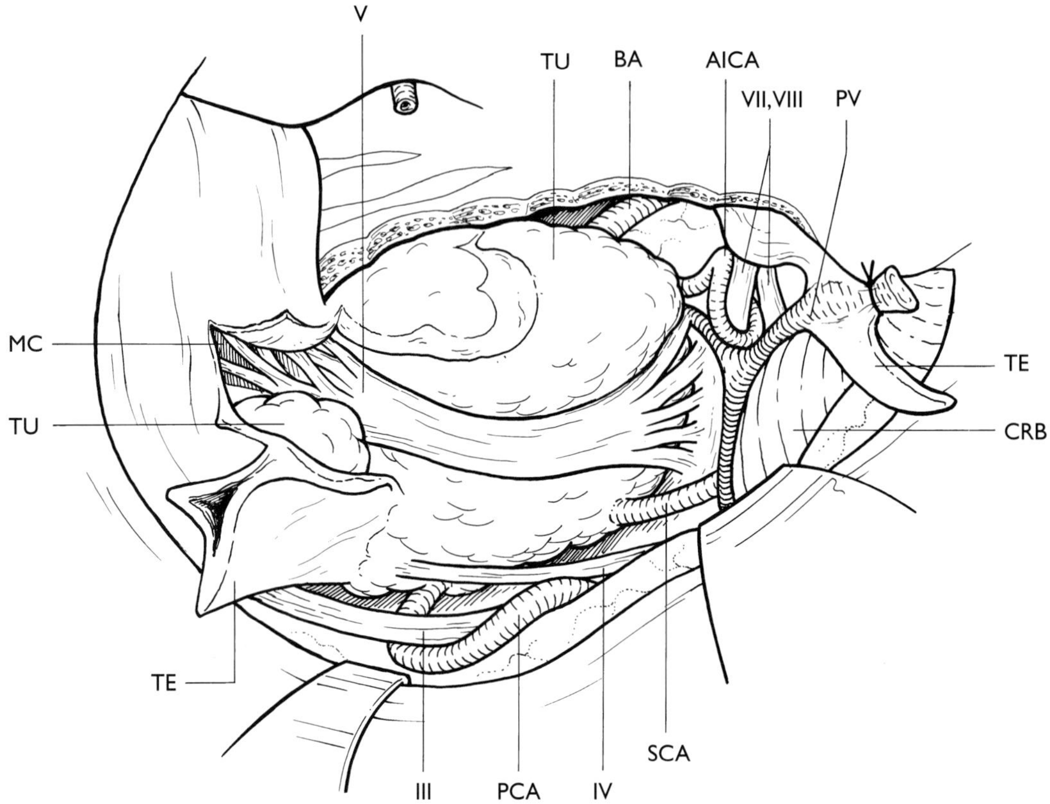

Figure 16-4. Tumor (clival meningioma) exposure after division of the tentorium.

Closure

The drilled petrous apex is covered with the temporalis fascia flap fixed by and coated with fibrin glue. In the case of large air cells, a free muscle piece is inserted into them. The dural defect is repaired by suturing the dural margin to the fascia flap (Fig. 16-6). The craniotomy is closed in the usual fashion.

Extended Middle Fossa Approach to the Cerebellopontine Angle and Acoustic Meatus

The extended middle fossa approach to the cerebellopontine angle and acoustic meatus has been described by Shiobara et al. (1988).

Epidural Approach to the Pyramidal Ridge

The middle cranial dura is separated from the midcranial skull base and elevated inwards up to the pyramidal ridge or sulcus of the superior petrosal sinus while anteriorly it is raised up to the foramen spinosum (Fig. 16-7). In the case of difficulty while employing the epidural approach to the pyramidal ridge due to tension on the dura caused by intracranial hypertension, the rate of CSF outflow from the spinal drainage can be increased. Alternatively, an incision can be made in the dura mater of the middle fossa, and then, by epidurally piercing the arachnoid membrane around the free edge of the cerebellar tentorium, CSF may be suctioned off.

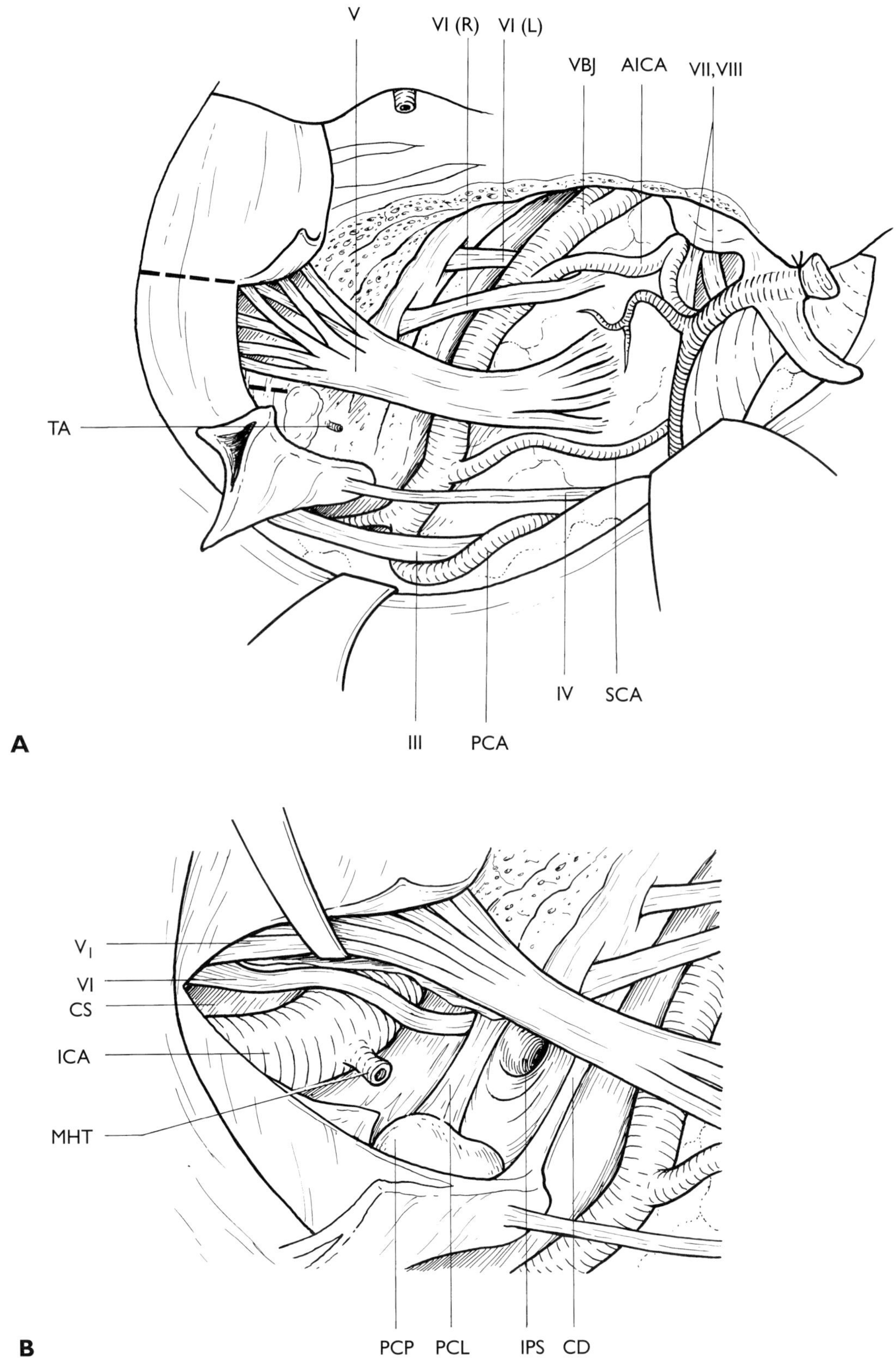

Figure 16-5. (A) After resection of the tumor. Dashed lines are additional dural openings in case of cavernous sinus invasion. *(B)* Enlarged view showing the opening of the posterior cavernous sinus. The trigeminal nerve is mobilized inferiorly, and the medial dural wall of the Meckel's cave is opened.

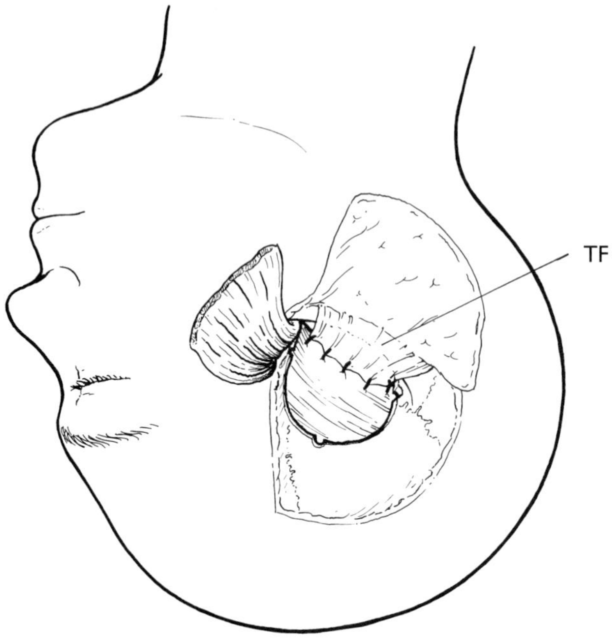

Figure 16-6. Closure. A temporal fascia flap (TF) covering the drilled pyramid is fixed with fibrin glue and sutured to the dura.

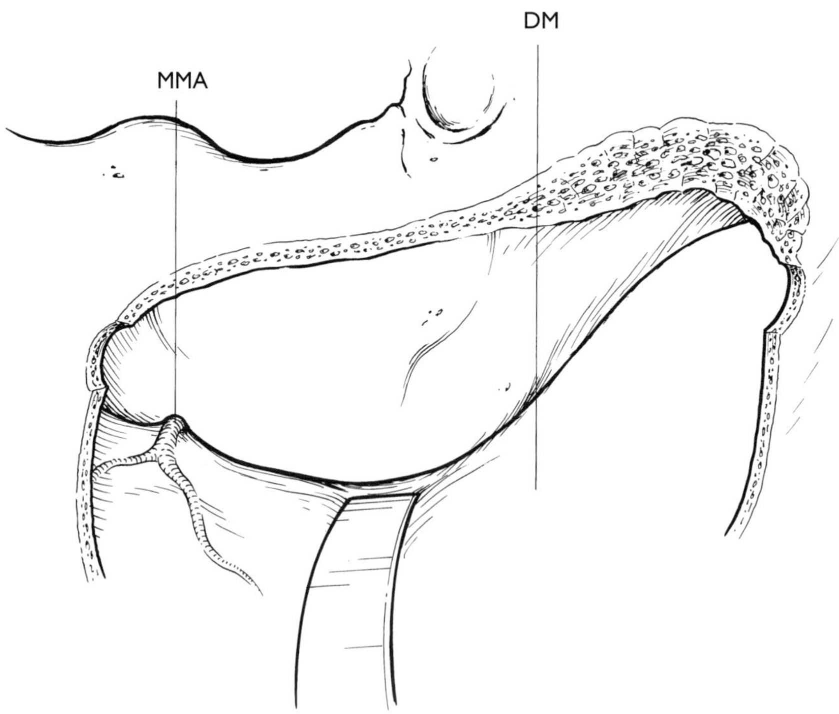

Figure 16-7. Extradural approach to the right pyramidal ridge or sulcus of superior petrosal sinus.

Operative Procedure with Attempted Hearing Preservation

Once the upper portion of the pyramidal ridge is exposed, only the upper wall of the internal auditory canal is opened (Fig. 16-8). As explained earlier, after recognizing the relative anatomy of the external auditory meatus, eminentia arcuata, and major petrosal nerve in its sulcus, the upper part of the internal auditory canal is opened by drilling along the base of the eminentia arcuata. It is important to drill with extreme

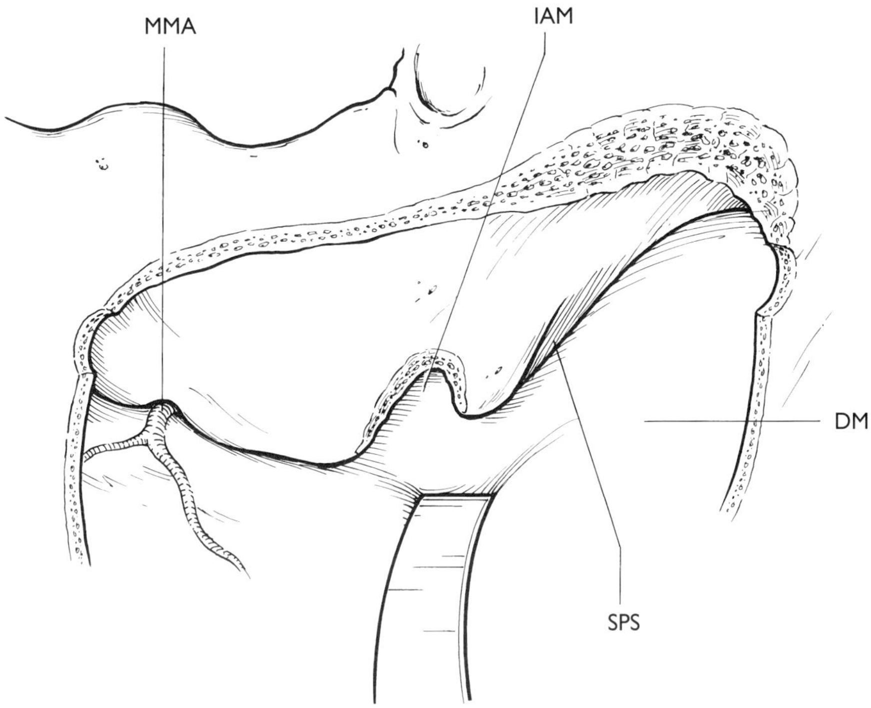

Figure 16-8. Extradural transpetrosal approach to the right internal auditory canal.

care so as not to damage the dura mater of the internal auditory canal or the facial nerve that courses along inside it. Once the internal auditory canal is successfully exposed, the dura mater is incised and the tumor resection carefully started, taking care to identify and preserve the facial and cochlear nerves (Fig. 16-9). While performing resection inside the internal auditory canal as just described, internal tumor decompression is started from the upper posterior part of the canal, identifying and

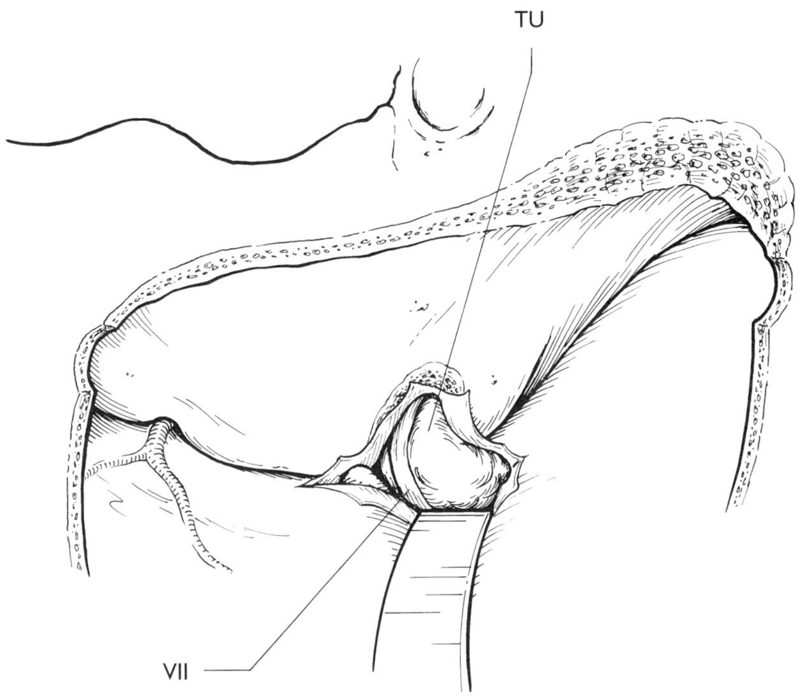

Figure 16-9. Exposed tumor and facial nerve in the right internal auditory canal and posterior fossa.

monitoring the facial nerve that is compressed against the anterior upper wall of the canal, while similarly identifying the cochlear nerve that is compressed against the anterior lower canal wall. In addition, as the resection proceeds, as much as possible of the microvasculature is spared. When the middle cranial fossa approach or extended middle cranial fossa approach are employed, the favorable view of the internal auditory canal very often allows identification of the four nerves of interest: the facial, cochlear, superior, and inferior vestibular nerves.

Operative Procedure Without Attempted Hearing Preservation

In those patients with medium- or large-sized tumors, where effective hearing has been lost preoperatively, the tumor removal is carried out following labyrinthectomy and partial mastoidectomy. Concerning the area for drilling, the internal auditory canal is opened anteriorly while the posterior pyramidal portion of the temporal bone is adequately removed from the canal. The dura mater of the posterior surface or posterior fossa surface of the pyramidal portion is exposed externally, which also exposes part of the superior petrosal and sigmoid sinuses (Fig. 16-10). Drilling in the posterior region will open the air cells close to the mastoid. Resection of the mastoid is performed as necessary, followed by a labyrinthectomy. In short, an almost complete extirpation of the semicircular canals is carried out. The middle and posterior fossa dura mater are widely excised (Fig. 16-11), while in the central region the operative area is extended to involve the free edge of the tentorium (Fig. 16-12), following which the superior petrosal sinus and tentorium are divided. The operative site is further enlarged by extending incisions anteriorly and posteriorly (Fig. 16-13). The bulk of the tumor is then able to be exposed under the cerebellar tentorium by rolling back the incised dura, cerebellar tentorium, and superior petrosal sinus (Fig. 16-14). As previously described, extirpation of the tumor will be performed while preserving and monitoring the facial nerve (Fig. 16-15).

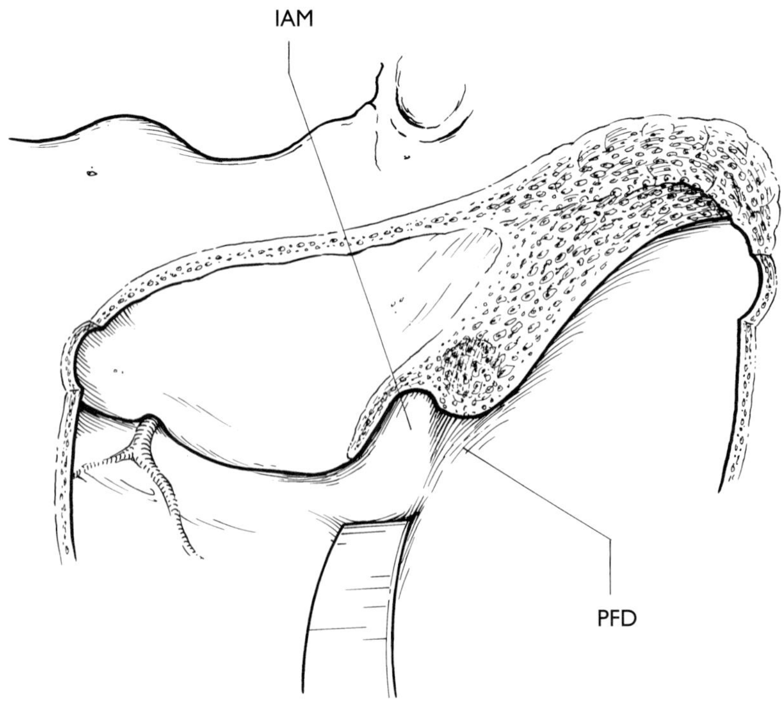

Figure 16-10. Unroofed right internal auditory canal by labyrinthectomy and partial mastoidectomy.

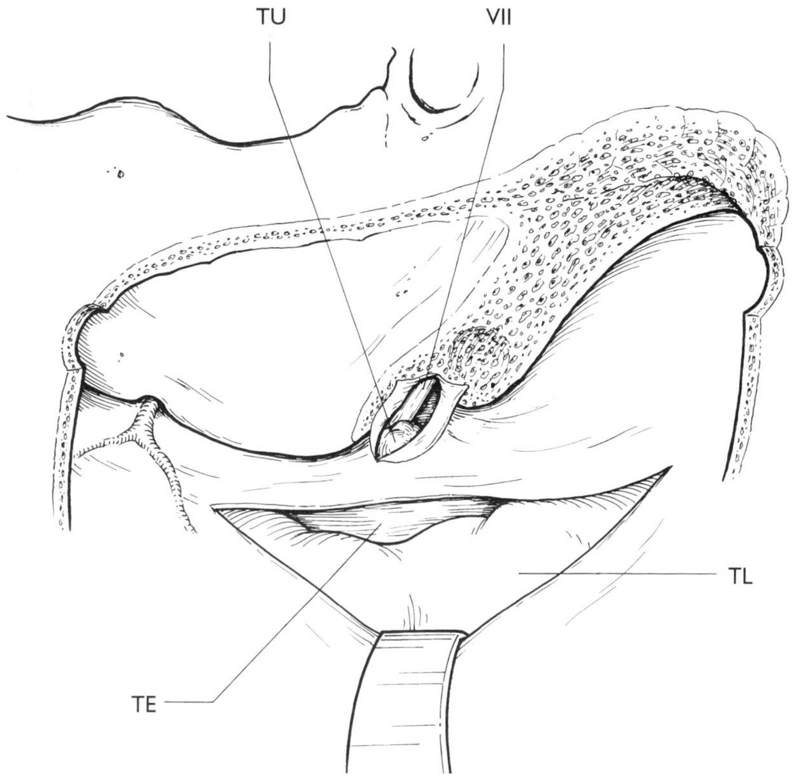

Figure 16-11. Incision of the dura mater of the internal auditory canal and middle cranial fossa.

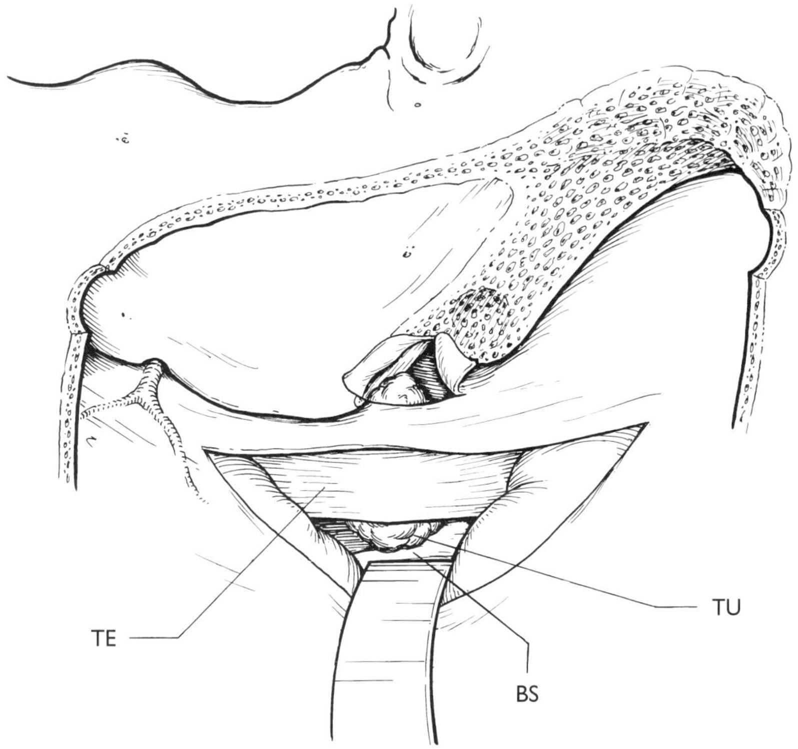

Figure 16-12. Exposure of cerebellar tentorium.

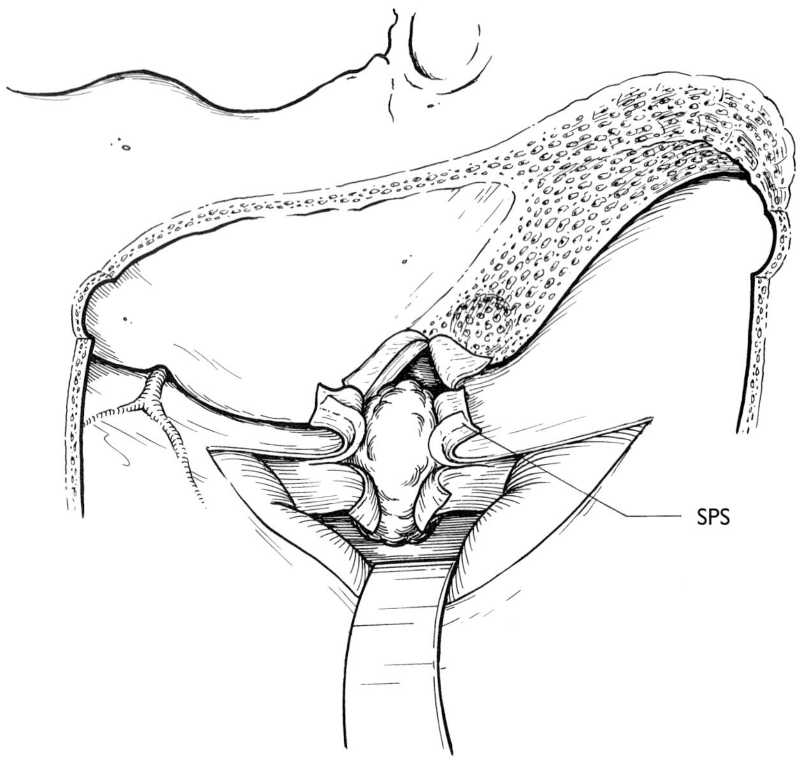

Figure 16-13. Division of the superior petrosal sinus and cerebellar tentorium.

Prevention of CSF Leakage, Skull Base Repair, and Closure

In procedures based on the extended middle cranial fossa approach in which hearing preservation has been a priority, areas of the temporal bone that have been drilled out, particularly around the internal auditory canal or the mastoid portion of the temporal bone, are sealed with fibrin glue using materials such as fat (usually harvested from the abdominal area) or temporal muscle flaps and temporal fascia flaps. In the removal of larger tumors where hearing preservation has not been attempted, it is quite possible that creating the operative site has involved drilling into the tympanic cavity itself. In such cases, after removing the incus from the middle ear, the tympanic cavity is completely packed with fat and fibrin glue. Removal of the incus makes complete packing of the cavity much easier. Following this, fibrin glue is spread over the drilled bone surface, which is sealed with a fascia flap. Any other areas of damage caused by the drilling are covered with a larger fascia flap, and all of the repair work is in turn sealed over with a pedicled temporal muscle flap thoroughly fixed with fibrin glue. These steps are necessary to prevent CSF leakage as a postoperative complication. Finally, the dura mater is sutured back together, with any damaged areas repaired with artificial dura mater and fibrin glue, the skull flap is returned to its original position, and the superficial tissues are folded down and sutured back in place.

Possible Surgical Complications

Possible surgical complications and their causes are summarized in Table 16-2. If CSF rhinorrhea occurs, 2 weeks of bedrest is recommended. Pressure-controlled lumbar drainage is commonly useful.

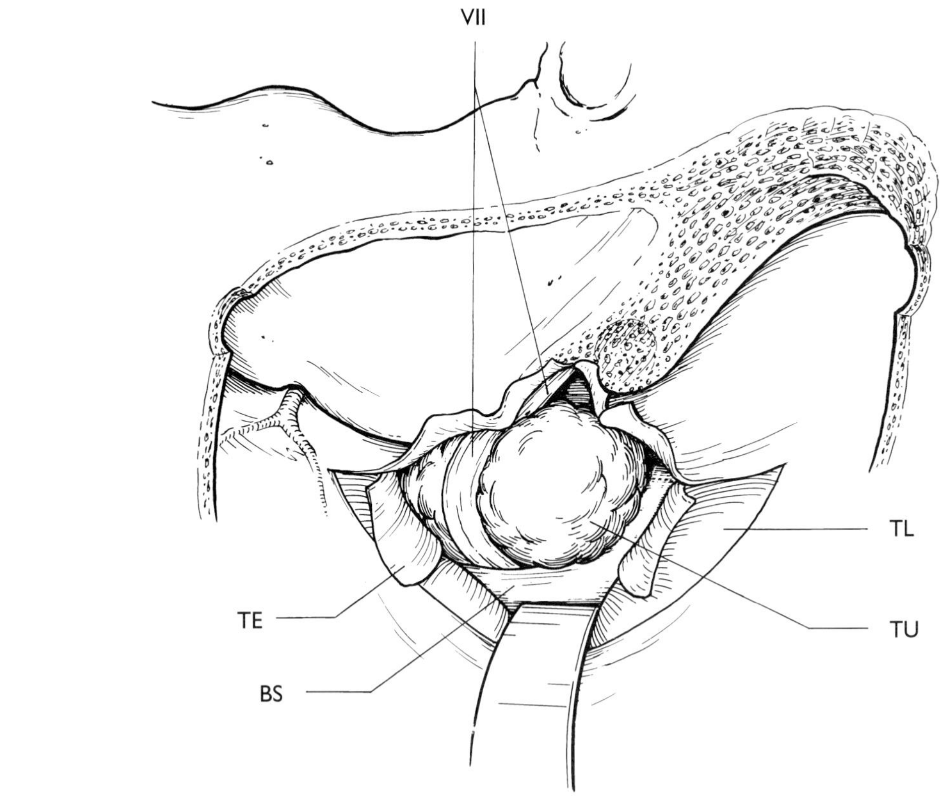

Figure 16-14. Exposed tumor and facial nerve.

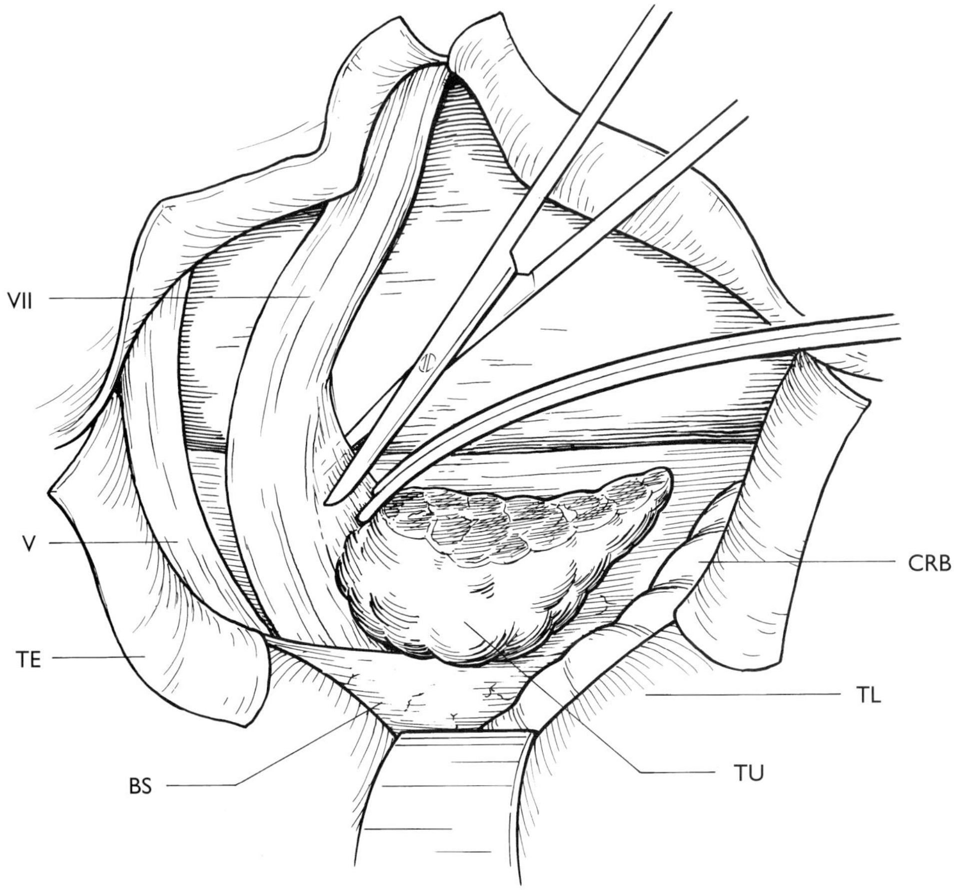

Figure 16-15. Removal of tumor with preservation of the facial nerve.

Table 16-2. Possible Surgical Complications Resulting from Surgical Approach

Complications	Cause
Cerebrospinal rhinorrhea	Incomplete petrous closure
Subgaleal fluid retention	Incomplete dural closure
Facial palsy	Retraction of petrosal nerve
	Nerve injury in internal auditory meatus or petrous
Lacrimation decrease	Sacrifice of petrosal nerve
Hearing disturbance	Opening of cochlea, and/or labyrinth
Double vision (IV)	Injury at tentorial notch
Double vision (VI)	Excessive drilling of apex

Results

In one author's (R.S.) study, involving 390 cases of acoustic neuroma, the mortality rate has been 0.5 percent, or two patients, which is comparatively low. In 471 cases of cerebellopontine angle tumors the mortality rate has been 0.4 percent. First-time patients accounted for 345 of the acoustic tumor procedures, with complete extirpation being carried out in 325 (94 percent). In these 325 patients, a success rate of 90 percent (291 cases) was achieved for anatomic preservation of the facial nerve. From 129 patients in whom hearing preservation was attempted, in 68 (53 percent) some hearing was successfully retained postoperatively, and useful hearing was retained in another 47 patients (37 percent). Spinal drainage in conjunction with fat grafts and fibrin glue sealing has been routine in this author's practice since 1991, when CSF leakage was detected in only 12 patients out of 139 operations (9 percent), in whom leakage was successfully repaired by a secondary procedure in five patients.

References

Atkinson WJ (1949) The anterior inferior cerebellar artery: its variations, pontine distribution, and significance in the surgery of cerebellopontine angle tumors. J Neurol Neurosurg Psychiatry 12:137–151

Bochenek Z, Kukwa A (1975) An extended approach through the middle cranial fossa to the internal auditory meatus and the cerebellopontine angle. Acta Otolaryngol 180:410–414

House WF (1961) Surgical exposure of internal auditory canal and its contents through middle cranial fossa. Laryngoscope 71:1363–1385

Kanzaki J, Kawase T, Sano F et al. (1977) A modified extended middle cranial fossa approach for acoustic tumors. Arch Oto-Rhino-Laryngol 217:119–121

Kawase T, Toya S, Shiobara R, Mine T (1985) Transpetrosal-transtentorial approach for aneurysms of the basilar artery. J Neurosurg 63:857–861

Kawase T, Shiobara R, Toya S (1991) Anterior transpetrosal-transtentorial approach for sphenopetroclival meningiomas: surgical method and results in 10 patients. Neurosurgery 28:869–876

Kawase T, Shiobara R, Toya S (1994) Middle fossa transpetrosal-transtentorial approaches for petroclival meningiomas: selective pyramid resection and radicality. Acta Neurochir 129:113–120

King TT (1970) Combined translabyrinthine-transtentorial approach to acoustic nerve tumours. Proc R Soc Med 63:780–782

Morrison AW, King TT (1973) Experiences with a translabyrinthine-transtentorial approach to the cerebellopontine angle: technical note. J Neurosurg 38:382–390

Shiobara R, Kanzaki J, Toya S (1988) A modified extended middle cranial fossa approach for acoustic nerve tumors. Results of 125 operations. J Neurosurg 68:358–365

17

Translabyrinthine Operation for Acoustic Nerve Tumor

T. T. King
A. Fitzgerald O'Connor

Two principal operations exist, side by side, for the removal of acoustic nerve tumors: the suboccipital or retrosigmoid approach and the translabyrinthine. Large numbers of tumors have been removed by each method with results, in general, not substantially different (Bentivoglio et al., 1988; Hardy et al., 1989; Harner et al., 1990; Sterkers et al., 1994; Tos et al., 1988).

Obvious questions that might be asked in these circumstances are why are there two methods, does a surgeon need to be acquainted with both, will one eventually displace the other, and how have the two evolved and yet survived separately?

Some of the answers can be found in the history of the techniques, and some in the shared ground the tumor occupies, ground partly belonging to ear, nose, and throat (ENT) surgery and partly to neurosurgery, each operation being identified with a different specialty.

The poor results of early surgical attempts on these benign tumors are clearly displayed in Tooth's paper of 1913. Panse (1904) was impelled to suggest an alternative approach through the petrous bone but lack of success with sporadic attempts at this route (Quix, 1912) combined with the achievements of Cushing (1917), in developing subtotal removal through the posterior fossa, and Dandy's introduction (1925, 1934) of total removal led to the tumor being wholly taken over by neurosurgeons. However, the key to improving results, early diagnosis, lay with the otologists who, however, were not in a position to exploit it until much later. In the 1950s neurosurgeons performed all the surgery and diagnosis was made by neurologists only when gross neurologic signs drew attention to the patients' plight and the tumor was very large; a significant portion of patients were actually referred from ophthalmologists because of papilledema and failing vision. Late diagnosis was therefore an important reason for the bad results that continued to be rather poor, even in the hands of the best neurosurgeons, with mortality at 20 percent (Olivecrona, 1967).

Better diagnosis by ENT surgeons at a stage when deafness and vestibular disorder were the only symptoms led naturally to their taking an interest in treatment. House was led to exume the translabyrinthine operation in a refined form made possible by the introduction of the operating microscope and high-speed drills, while neurosurgeons continued to use the posterior fossa route, taking advantage of the new technical advances that had allowed a rival to enter their field. Thus two operations existed side by side. It might have been expected that caution and medicolegal fears would have restricted otologists in developing, single-handed, the treatment of this interesting and difficult tumor and forced them to ally themselves with cooperative neurosurgeons. This has often been the case, especially in the United Kingdom, but in other countries, notably Denmark, where Tos et al. (1988) have taken a striking lead, ENT surgeons have been prepared to take over the treatment of even the largest acoustic nerve tumors as well as other cerebellopontine angle masses. The growth of interest in skull base surgery has encouraged the competitive approach and it is possible, attending meetings on this topic, to wonder if this tumor has now anything to do with neurosurgery.

The direction this matter will take in the next decade is an interesting speculation and may depend on considerations other than the relative merit of the two procedures. Diagnosis, and therefore the supply of material, is in the hands of the otologist. Neurosurgeons have a satisfactory technique that currently produces excellent results in the hands of the best surgeons (Harner et al., 1990), although an acquaintance with medicolegal practice shows that poor results still occur occasionally with surgery of this type. With even the greatest effort at open-mindedness, it is difficult to view with satisfaction ENT surgeons dealing, alone, with the problems that arise from extensive surgery in the posterior fossa. Equally there are complex skull base tumors in which a neurosurgeon, without the direction and aid of a skilled otologist, cannot provide the best treatment for the patient. Close cooperation between the specialties offers the best solution. However, if each specialty goes its own way, one or the other will presumably emerge as the dominant force, especially now that medicolegal considerations are beginning to be felt and those with only limited numbers of cases treated may be forced out of the competition. The outcome may vary from country to country but the odds, perhaps, favor the ENT surgeon.

Comparative Disadvantages and Advantages of the Translabyrinthine Operation

Disadvantages

For a neurosurgeon the first disadvantage is an inability to carry out the petrous dissection. This is not insuperable but to do both the petrous dissection and removal of a large tumor is physically taxing and it is not likely that an occasional neurosurgical exponent of this sort of work could approach the skill and anatomic knowledge of an ENT surgeon. The solution is to combine with an ENT surgeon. The advantages of this, not always easy to achieve, are more widespread than simply in the field of operative technique.

Active infection in the ear or mastoid would preclude either type of operation. Old infective ear disease may be taken as a contraindication to the translabyrinthine procedure. The technique is ruled out if the surgeon wishes to attempt to preserve hearing; in that case the neurosurgical approach would usually be preferred, because the position of the middle fossa approach is not clearly defined at the present time.

If a subtotal removal is intended because of advanced age and general disease in the patient, a translabyrinthine approach is probably too elaborate and time-consuming.

The last consideration brings us to one of the two main disadvantages of the present operation; it undoubtedly adds considerable time to the operation compared with the posterior fossa approach, probably 1 to 2 hours. The other major problem has been, in the authors' experience, postoperative cerebrospinal (CSF) leaks (Bryce et al., 1991), although these are certainly not unique to the method, being a considerable hazard in the posterior fossa approach (Bentivoglio et al., 1988; Hoffman 1994; Nadol et al., 1967). An increased risk of infection might be expected because the middle ear is opened but this has not proved a problem, with serious local or meningitic infection postoperatively being the exception.

It should be emphasized that the size of the tumor has no bearing on the appropriateness of the method, except insofar as it may be desired to preserve hearing in small lesions. The largest tumors are as easily managed through this approach as through the posterior fossa; indeed we take large sizes as an important reason for preferring the translabyrinthine approach.

Advantages

Positioning a patient on the table is straightforward compared with either the lateral (park bench) or sitting positions, in which special precautions must be taken. Simplicity of setting up is especially valuable if the patient is very large or obese.

As far as the operation itself is concerned the principal advantage is that the exposure is obtained by removal of bone, the excavation of the petrous leading directly to the tumor in the meatus and cerebellopontine angle and to the nerves in the jugular foramen. Prolonged exposure of cerebellar cortex and nerves of the jugular foramen, difficult to avoid in the posterior fossa operation, is not a problem with the translabyrinthine approach. The design of the operation has similarities with the transsphenoidal procedure for pituitary tumors or the transthoracic approach to thoracic discs, techniques that have largely displaced their rivals because they approach the lesion directly and avoid exposure of the affected portion of the central nervous system.

The translabyrinthine operation, in the late stages of the removal of the tumor, gives, in the authors' opinion, a rather shorter and more direct approach to the brain stem and to the 5th nerve as well as to the region of the tentorial hiatus.

Exposure of the lateral end of the meatus, although adequate through the posterior fossa, is better by the translabyrinthine route and, where the tumor actually arises from the facial nerve, a rare but nonetheless real possibility, especially in neurofibromatosis 2 (King and Morrison, 1990), the facial nerve can be followed along the fallopian canal and into the middle ear more easily than in the posterior fossa operation. Exposure of the intrapetrous segment of the facial nerve may be an advantage if repair or grafting must be undertaken after removal of the tumor. However, in acoustic nerve tumors this is not often needed, the distal stump of facial nerve being easily recognized in the meatus.

Local pain at the site of the incision is sometimes troublesome postoperatively after the posterior fossa operation (Schessel et al., 1992), but we have not experienced it after the present procedure.

Finally, it should be noted that the translabyrinthine dissection may be extended medially through the cochlea or upward through the tent (see below).

Preoperative Preparation

The patient should be warned that any residual hearing will be destroyed and also of the risks to the facial nerve. It is wise to discuss the risks of a CSF leak postoperatively via the nose and the need to obtain fat and fascia from the thigh in order to circumvent this risk.

No other special preparations are needed. It is unusual, even in the largest tumors, for a blood transfusion to be required, and so grouping of the patient's blood and saving of the serum is usually all that is required.

The portion of the scalp to be shaved encompasses a restricted area behind the mastoid process and above the pinna, extending a small distance forward into the temporal region.

Anesthesia

General anesthesia and controlled ventilation through an endotracheal tube are used. Intra-arterial blood pressure, electrocardiogram, end-tidal CO_2 and arterial oxygen saturation through a pulse oximeter, as well as body temperature, are all monitored. If an inhalation agent is used its concentration is measured continuously. A urinary catheter is inserted as we routinely use mannitol, infused at the end of the bone dissection. This is probably not strictly necessary in small or medium-sized tumors. It is important to minimize cooling of the patient by the use of a heating blanket. Measures against venous stasis in the legs are instituted.

Cranial Nerve Monitoring

Intraoperative monitoring of the facial nerve is essential, using one of the commercially available instruments such as the Xomed nerve integrity monitor or the Neurosign.

Position on the Table

The patient lies supine with the head turned to the opposite side. A Mayfield clamp or similar fixation device avoids prolonged pressure on the scalp that may occur if a flat headpiece is used but is not essential.

It is important that the upper half of the operating table and the patient be tilted head-up by about 15 to 20 degrees to lessen bleeding from the dural sinuses and from the veins often found on the brain stem deep to a large tumor. The patient should be secured in such a way that the table can be tilted laterally toward, and away from, the surgeon during the procedure.

If an overhead table is used, it should be placed toward the foot of the table, its cranial margin not being higher than the patient's costal margin; otherwise, it will obstruct the surgeon during those parts of the operation that require the microscope to be tilted upward toward the undersurface of the tentorium.

The surgeon is positioned behind the patient and the microscope stand is best placed on the opposite side, somewhat beyond the level of the patient's vertex.

Operative Procedure

Incision

Preliminary cannulation of the frontal horn through a burr hole is only used where there is hydrocephalus. For smaller tumors, CSF can be released from the medullary cistern in order to relax tension in the posterior fossa.

The preparation of the skin and the subsequent draping should allow access not only to the scalp around the pinna and the mastoid process but also to the upper part of the neck so that, if necessary, a nerve graft may be obtained from the great auricular nerve.

The incision (Fig. 17-1A) starts from just below the tip of the mastoid process and ascends over the middle of its outer surface to a point about 1 in. behind and above the tip of the pinna where it swings forwards into the temporal fossa like a question

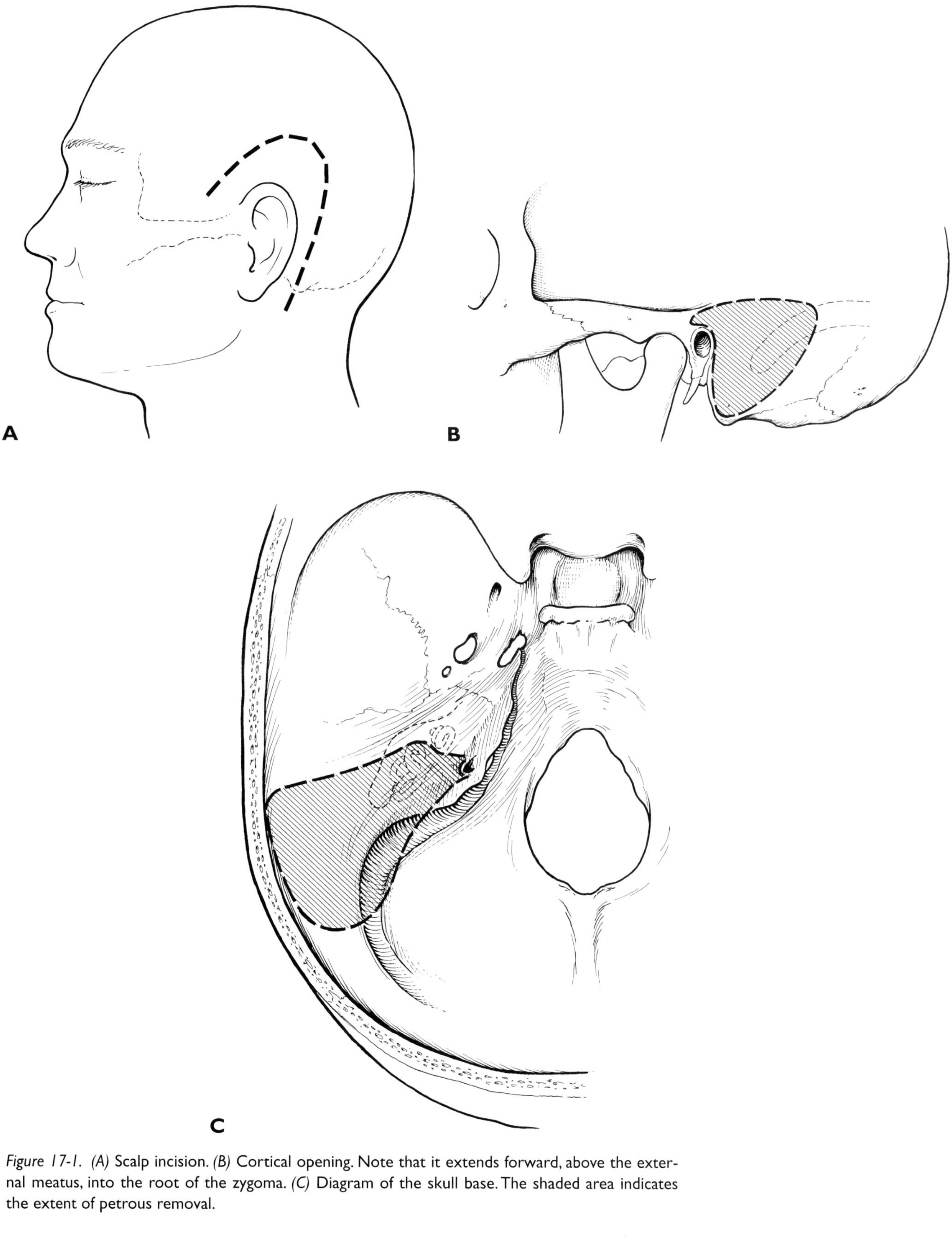

Figure 17-1. *(A)* Scalp incision. *(B)* Cortical opening. Note that it extends forward, above the external meatus, into the root of the zygoma. *(C)* Diagram of the skull base. The shaded area indicates the extent of petrous removal.

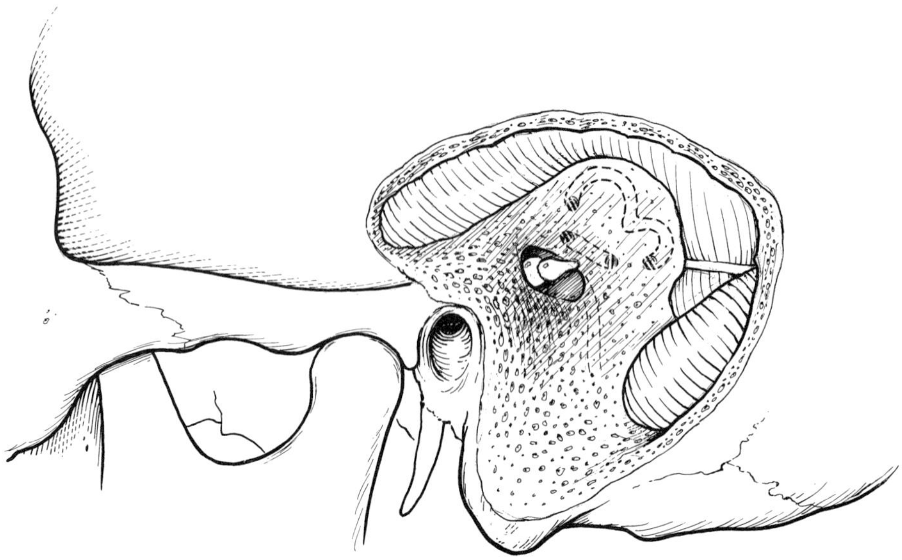

Figure 17-2. The mastoidectomy has been completed; the positions of the lateral and semicircular canals and facial nerve are indicated.

mark. Figures 17-1A–C show, schematically, the skin incision, the position of the cortical opening, and the extent of the petrous dissection. It must reach far enough anteriorly to allow the posterior and superior margins of the external meatus to be exposed when the scalp flap is turned forward. The lateral surface of the mastoid process is exposed by turning the scalp, pericranium, and temporalis muscle forward either in one or two layers. Cutting diathermy is necessary to raise the pericranium forward and backward over the mastoid area; however, further forward, the dissection under the temporalis muscle can be done with a periosteal elevator. It is essential to expose the posterior and superior rim of the bony meatus and to define the root of the zygoma, because the area on the surface of the skull just above the meatus is important in providing access to the epitympanic recess without risk to the facial nerve.

Mastoidectomy

The bone dissection is commenced by the ENT surgeon who carries out an extensive mastoidectomy (Figs. 17-1 B&C, 17-2, and 17-3). The superficial limits of this are important because a large opening is essential for ease of maneuverability during the removal of large tumors. The opening starts above the external auditory meatus, and extends upward to expose the temporal dura for a distance of about 2 cm above the floor of the middle fossa. Posteriorly the margin of the opening curves downward somewhat behind the mastoid process in order to expose the plate of bone overlying the sigmoid sinus. Removal of the sinus plate will eventually expose the whole width of the sigmoid sinus. Inferiorly the whole lateral surface of the mastoid process is unroofed as far as its tip. Figures 17-1B and 17-2 show the extent of the opening on the surface of the mastoid.

The cortex over this area is removed with a large cutting burr and the air cells exposed are then removed until the sinus plate posteriorly is exposed. When removing the bone over the inferior temporal lobe it is best to leave a thin layer of the inner cortex overlying the dura until the deeper part of the exposure is completed. The sigmoid sinus should similarly be left with a protective layer, which limits bleeding. It is important to remove all bone over the sinodural angle and the lateral portion of the superior petrosal sinus. Anteriorly, air cells between the roof of the exter-

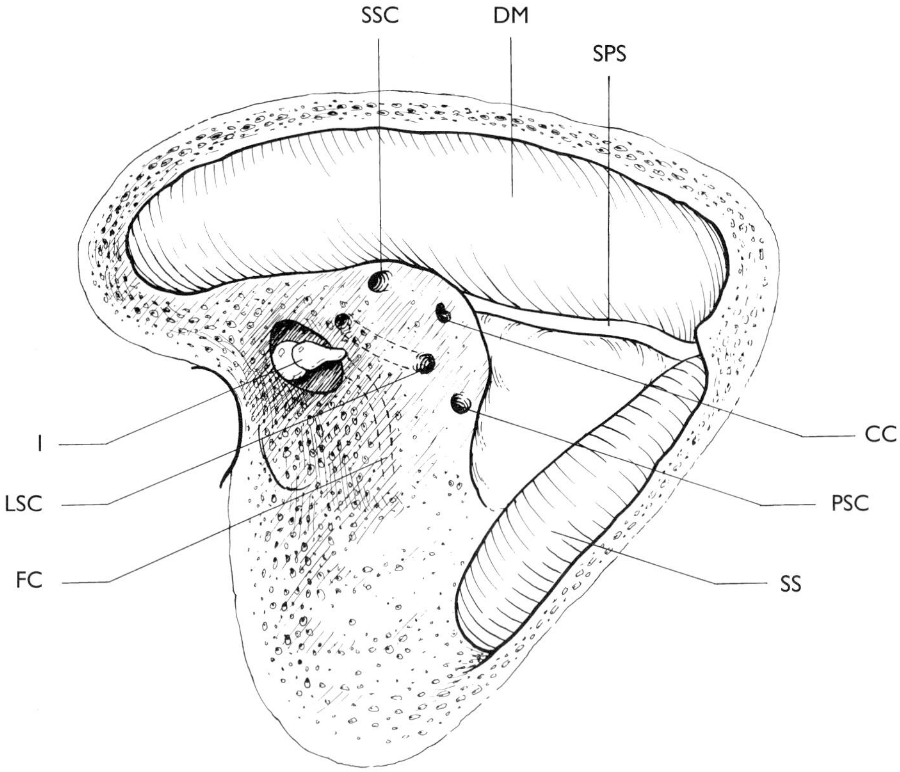

Figure 17-3. The labyrinthectomy has been partially carried out. Note the exposure of the middle and posterior fossa dura and the sigmoid and superior petrosal sinuses. (For explanation of abbreviations, see Appendix 1, p. 373.)

nal auditory meatus and the dura of the middle fossa are drilled out and the dissection is deepened until the Körner septum, an inconsistent bony septum between the lateral and medial mastoid air cells, has been removed and the epitympanic recess reached. The roof and posterior wall of the external meatus are thinned but not removed to increase the exposure of the epitympanic recess, incus, and head of malleus.

On the medial wall of the epitympanic recess the lateral semicircular canal is easily recognized as an ivory-like swelling and is an important landmark both to the labyrinth and to the facial nerve that lies in the bone almost parallel to and immediately below the canal. The incus is visible anteriorly in the ear cavity, its short process lying in proximity to the facial nerve canal. It may be removed by rotating the short process forward. The air cells in the tip of the mastoid are drilled out, exposing the deep cortex and the digastric groove. Exposure of the latter locates the stylomastoid foramen and clears bone between the sigmoid sinus and the descending facial nerve. The areas that are of particular importance to expose in doing the mastoidectomy are the middle fossa dura, sinodural angle, and sigmoid sinus because it is through these that the angle of approach during removal of the tumor may be widened. Thus by retracting the temporal lobe dura upward with the shanks of a sucker and dissecting forceps the surgeon can look downward toward the inferior pole of the tumor and the cistern around the jugular foramen nerves. Similarly via the sinodural angle the line of vision can be extended medially below the porus. By retracting the sigmoid sinus backward the view toward the apex of the petrous bone and the trigeminal nerve may be improved.

At this stage, in order to allow adequate obliteration of the middle ear cavity, the posterior tympanotomy is created. With a diamond burr, under high magnification, bone is removed between the anterolateral face of the facial nerve and the fibrous annulus of the external auditory meatus and the chorda tympani. This slot is extended downward until the round window is visible, thus allowing the footplate of the stapes to be seen. It can then be ascertained that it has not been dislocated and the ear cavity and eustachian tube can be packed under direct vision with fat and bone paté.

The superficial part of the petrous dissection now having been completed, the surgeon sets about the removal of the labyrinth (Fig. 17-3), starting by opening the lateral semicircular canal, which is followed anteriorly to the ampulla, and posteriorly, with due regard for the facial nerve lying immediately below. The canal will lead, anteriorly and posteriorly, into the vestibule. The facial nerve may, at this stage, be skeletonized in part or even exposed if the surgeon favors this maneuver, which is not essential but allows testing of the function of the facial nerve monitor on the exposed nerve. The posterior and superior canals are located by reference to the lateral and drilled out. The superior canal extends high up toward the middle fossa and its removal may require tilting of the microscope upward. The subarcuate artery, in the bone below the arc of the canal, is a useful landmark. Dissection here brings the bone removal close to the middle fossa dura, which should be left covered with a thin layer of bone as in the case of the sigmoid sinus. The posterior and lateral canals lead to the crus commune and thence to the vestibule again, posteriorly. The utricle and saccule are removed from the vestibule and the superior vestibular nerve is found protruding through the bone that separates the lateral end of the meatus from the vestibule. The endolymphatic sac is recognized below the crus commune and drilled out. The bone posteriorly is removed until the dura of the posterior fossa is identified.

The remaining dissection involves removal of the bone medial to the labyrinth and posterior to the meatus. There are few identifiable landmarks within this area except for the posterior fossa dura posteriorly and the meatus itself anteriorly. This dissection removes the posterior wall of the meatus and of the porus. The bone of the roof and floor of the meatus must also, in part, be removed using a diamond burr. The facial nerve is vulnerable during removal of the roof especially at the lateral end of the meatus. Drilling too far anteriorly here may lead to damage to the nerve as it enters the fallopian canal. Inferiorly removal of the floor of the meatus and beyond will expose the jugular bulb at its summit. An important area lies between the summit of the bulb and the dura of the posterior fossa (Figs. 17-4 and 17-5). There is a tendency to stop bone removal here for fear of damaging the bulb. Between the latter and the posterior fossa a few millimeters more of bone can be removed inferiorly because the bulb falls away leaving a ridge, removal of which gives a few extra millimeters inferiorly and this space is of considerable value in exposing the cistern around the inferior pole of the tumor. A high jugular bulb may overlap the lower part of the internal auditory meatus and interfere with removal of bone below the internal canal. If so, it should be more extensively exposed by further drilling and pushed downward with packing, as suggested by Saleh and his colleagues (1994).

The cavity thus created in the petrous bone (Figs. 17-1C and 17-4) is of pyramidal shape with a wide base on the external surface of the skull and its apex the posterior margin of the porus. The anterior limits are the posterior wall of the external meatus, the middle ear, and the descending portion of the facial nerve. Further medially the petrous segment of the facial nerve prevents further bone removal.

When exposure of the meatus and porus have been completed the facial nerve is found at the lateral end of the porus by reference to "Bill's bar." This is a vertical septum of bone separating the superior vestibular area and nerve from the facial canal. The superior vestibular nerve is divided and turned backward. In front of it a layer of bone is exposed. This is "Bill's bar." A sharp microhook with its point directed later-

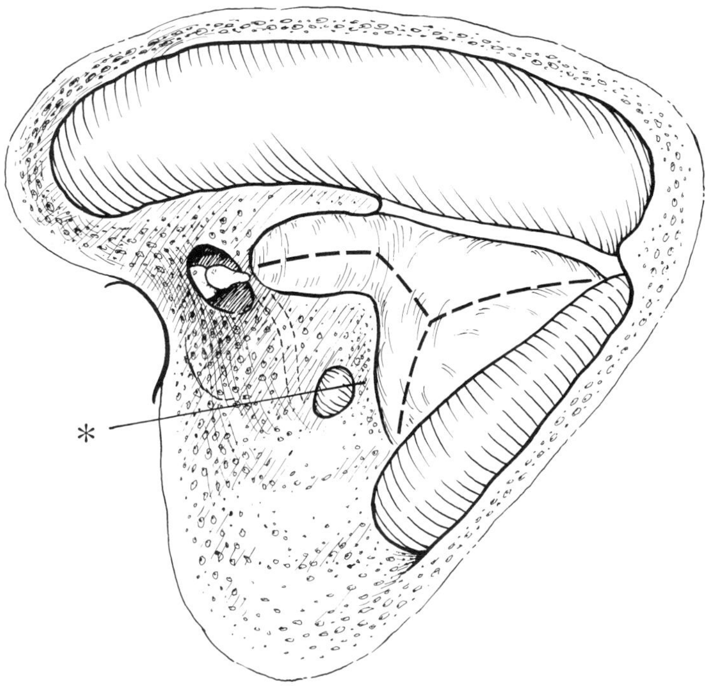

Figure 17-4. Bone removal has been completed. The dashed line indicates the dural incision. An asterisk indicates bone posterior to the summit of the jugular bulb, which must be removed to give access to the cistern around the lower pole of the tumor.

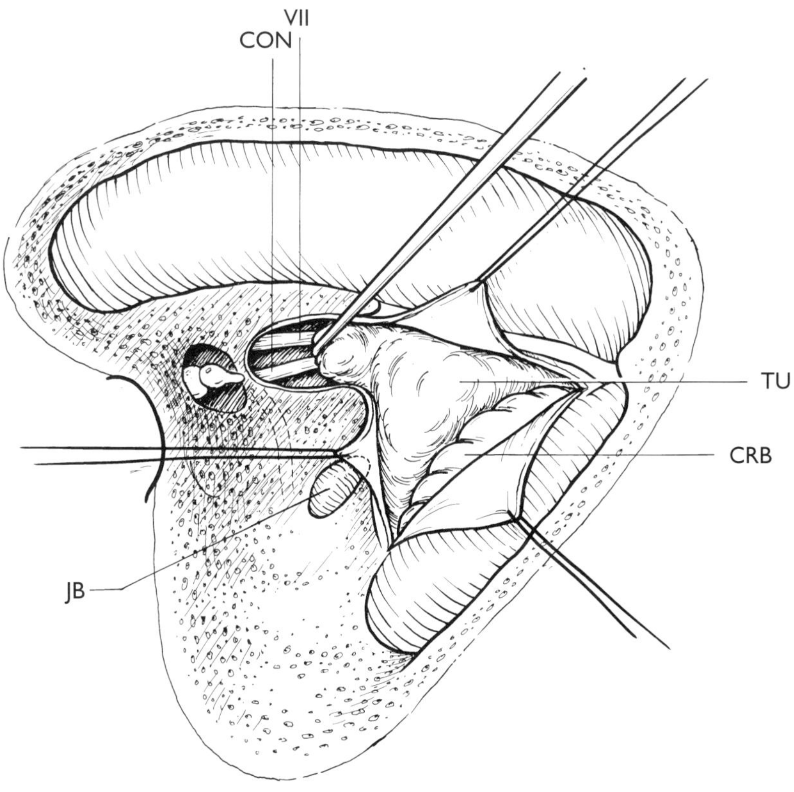

Figure 17-5. The dura is opened showing the tumor in the meatus and cerebellopontine angle. The cerebellum is just visible laterally.

ally can be slipped round the medial edge of this and, on its deep side, will enter the facial canal. Thus the position of the facial nerve is identified and it can be confirmed by using the nerve integrity monitor, the nerve being stimulated with a current of .25 mA. The bone work is finished by removal, with a curette or raspatory, of the thin layer of bone that has been left protecting the sigmoid and superior sinuses and the dura of middle and posterior fossae.

At this stage the bone dissection may be considered complete although subsequently small amounts of drilling may be necessary to improve exposure in certain areas.

Limitations of the Exposure

From the time of its introduction the translabyrinthine operation has been criticized for providing too small an opening and, therefore, leading to a high rate of subtotal removal in large tumors. Although this is disproved by surgeons experienced in the technique it is true that quite small anatomic restrictions may make the later stages of the operation uncomfortable until the cause is recognized and corrected. A millimeter or two of bone left in certain critical areas such as the sinodural angle may lead to considerable difficulty in the latter part of the operation, obstructing access to critical areas of brain.

Anatomic factors affecting exposure include the degree of aeration of the mastoid or petrous, because lack of air cells makes the bony dissection more difficult and slower and the mastoid opening may be made unusually narrow if the middle fossa dura is low or the sigmoid sinus unusually anteriorly situated, but provided these structures are divested of bone they can be retracted so as to overcome the difficulty.

The importance of unroofing the jugular bulb between its highest point and the posterior fossa dura has been discussed.

Transcochlear Dissection

In the standard labyrinthine operation the anterior and medial limits of the bone dissection are set by the external auditory meatus, middle ear, and facial nerve. These limits can be transgressed and a much more extensive removal of the petrous bone, can be achieved, up to the carotid canal and apex, if the facial nerve is drilled out in its complete length, from meatus to stylomastoid foramen (House et al., 1978). The nerve thus exposed can be physically displaced backward after mobilization by division of the greater superficial petrosal nerve or be left traversing the cavity but covered with a thin layer of bone. The posterior and superior walls of the external meatus are removed and the soft tissues divided and closed off by sutures. The middle ear is thus opened widely and its medial wall can be drilled away to expose the cochlea. Removal of this plus the medial wall of the internal meatus allows access to the petrous apex as far as the edge of the clivus and the carotid canal.

A dissection this extensive is never necessary for primary operations on acoustic nerve tumors however large but may be of considerable value in medially placed meningiomas, the attachment of which may be completely undermined, although at the cost of destroying hearing if that is present preoperatively. Mobilization of the facial nerve is likely to result in a severe or complete facial nerve palsy immediately postoperatively and the end result may be incomplete recovery to a House-Brackmann Grade III or IV.

Transtentorial Approach

Removal of the posterior part of the petrous bone includes the petrous ridge and thus exposes the superior petrosal sinus, which lies in the attachment of the tentorium. The opening in the posterior fossa dura after either a translabyrinthine or trans-

18

Surgical Treatment of Intracranial Glomus Tumors

Vinod K. Anand
Ossama Al-Mefty

Glomus tumors (paragangliomas) are usually treated surgically, but the planning and execution of surgery must follow the principles of *primum non nocere*. For glomus tumors, this implies managing tumorous involvement of the internal carotid artery, facial nerve, and the lower cranial nerves that are prone to surgical injury. Other risks of treating intracranial extensions must be weighed selectively. Factors that influence the decision to surgically remove the tumor include the following:

The size of the tumor. Smaller tumors confined to the middle ear or extending into the mastoid are relatively easy to remove through transtympanic, facial recess, or extended transmastoid approaches. The morbidity from these operations is usually minimal and may relate to conductive hearing loss or a need to move the facial nerve from the fallopian canal.

Extensions of the tumor. The presence of a cranial nerve palsy before surgery leaves little hope of preserving the nerve and, therefore, requires consideration of the appropriate reconstruction. Preservation of cochleovestibular structures and the internal carotid artery requires careful planning. The status of the cerebral venous and arterial circulation must be defined. In addition, tumor extension into the middle fossa, cavernous sinus, cerebellopontine angle, and foramen magnum requires appropriate neurosurgical considerations.

Age and medical condition of the patient. The characteristically slow growth of glomus tumors is an important consideration when planning therapy for elderly and medically infirm patients. Subtotal removal followed by radiation may be a compromise best suited to an individual patient.

Prior treatment. In patients who have undergone previous attempts at tumor removal or radiation, surgery is complicated by the presence of fibrosis. The task of neural-preservation, carotid dissection, and delineation of the tumor's boundaries becomes exceedingly difficult. Tumor embolization may not be possible, because the blood supply to the tumor may arise from posterior circulation. Reconstruction methods are also complicated, because local tissue may not provide reliable reconstruction.

Technical Factors. The availability of appropriate technical support and good skills of the operative team are paramount in dictating the outcome of the surgical treatment. Glomus surgery is facilitated by computed tomographic and magnetic resonance images that delineate the tumor's size and extent, interventional neurovascular techniques that allow assessment of the tumor's blood supply, and embolization methods. Reliable studies of cerebral blood flow, including judicious and selective use of balloon occlusion testing, intraoperative monitoring of the lower cranial nerves, and appropriate neuroanesthesia and reconstructive microvascular techniques must be available.

Preoperative Assessment

A detailed neuro-otologic examination clarifies many issues pertaining to surgery of glomus tumors. Symptoms and prior treatment, existence of additional symptomatic tumors and endocrine activity, as well as familial basis of glomus tumors must be investigated in every patient.

Physical examination almost always reveals a vascular mass in the ear, which may infiltrate the tympanic membrane. Pneumatic otoscopy may suggest some blanching. Tuning fork examinations most often suggest conductive hearing loss, although sensorineural hearing loss may suggest a more extensive tumor. Facial nerves require further functional studies when the patient has facial weakness or twitching. These include nerve stimulation tests, electroneuronography, and electromyographic studies. Cranial nerves are examined because early involvement may be asymptomatic. For example, the vocal cord may be paralyzed without significant clinical deficits.

All patients require audiometric analysis to evaluate hearing deficit and adequacy of function on the contralateral side. Tympanometric examination frequently discloses the pulsatile nature of the mass. Labyrinthine function is assessed through electronystagmography and rotary chair examination.

High-resolution computed tomography (CT) is done to assess the anatomy of the patient's temporal bone and to study the extent of bony destruction (Fig. 18-1A). The degree of temporal bone pneumatization, involvement of the middle ear ossicles, mastoid invasion, the status of the fallopian and semicircular canals and cochlea, and the degree of jugular foramen or other bony destruction from prior surgical attempts is disclosed. Extensions into the internal auditory canal, carotid canal (Fig. 18-1B), and middle or posterior cranial fossa are also delineated. Anterior extension into the eustachian orifice is visualized as well.

Magnetic resonance imaging (MRI) in coronal, axial, and sagittal planes complements the CT scans. With contrast (GDTA-gadolinium), MRI helps define intradural extension (Fig. 18-2), infiltration of the cranial nerves (Fig. 18-3), and the relationship of the tumor to the extra- and intracranial vessels (Fig. 18-4), the brain stem (Fig. 18-5), and the cavernous sinus. MRI also defines multiple tumors and postsurgical effects in previously treated patients (Fig. 18-2) and the tumor's relationship to the internal carotid artery.

A biopsy is seldom done; the required arteriographic examination generally confirms the diagnosis. Although magnetic resonance arteriography (MRA) may demonstrate the vascular nature of the tumors, it has not replaced the traditional

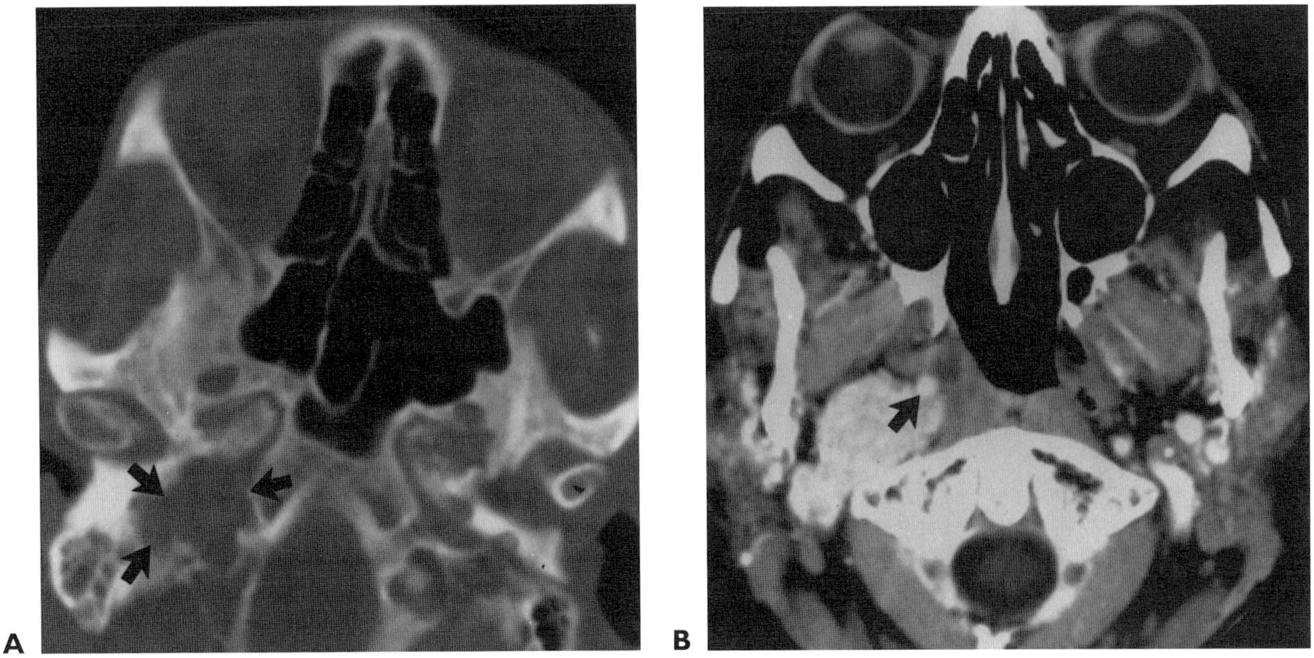

Figure 18-1. *(A)* Axial CT scan showing a large lesion with extensive bony erosion. Absence of the carotid keel and widening of the jugular foramen are apparent (arrows). The mastoid air cells are opacified. *(B)* A corresponding CT scan with contrast enhancement reveals the highly vascular nature of this lesion. This lesion is proximal to and displaces the internal carotid artery (arrow). (From Anand et al., 1996, with permission.)

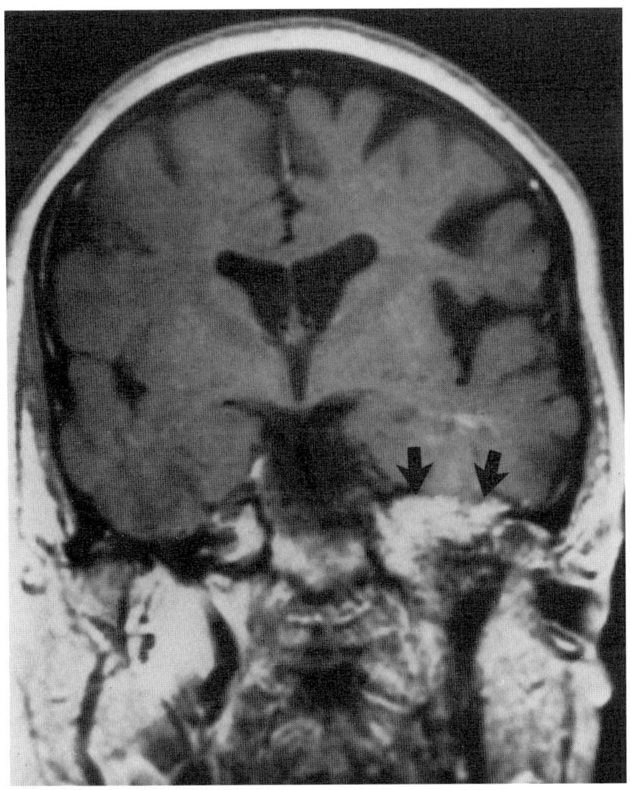

Figure 18-2. T_1-weighted coronal MRI with enhancement shows a recurrent glomus tumor (arrows) with intracranial extension. The temporal lobe is mildly atrophied and the cerebral gyri are dilated. Evidence of prior embolization is apparent along with an occluded internal carotid artery. (From Anand et al., 1996, with permission.)

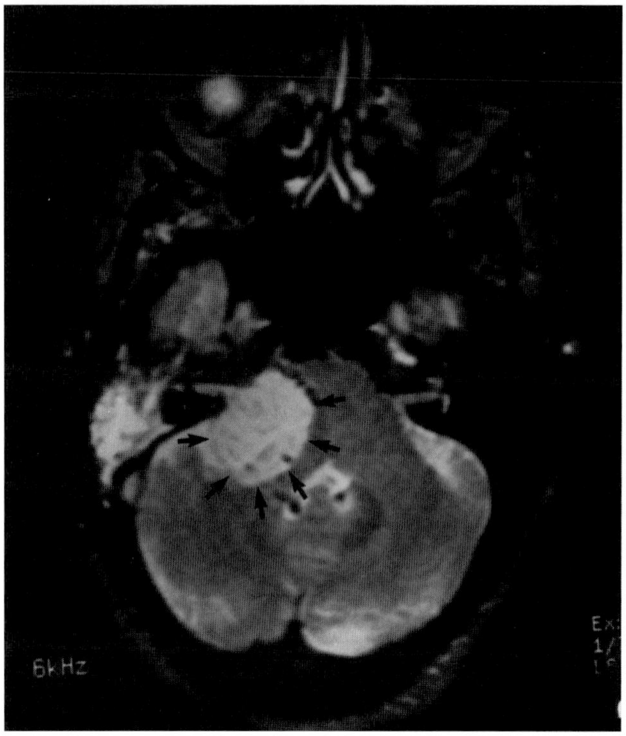

Figure 18-3. An axial T_1-weighted image (TR, 2,500; TE, 82) demonstrates the gadolinium-enhancing mass (arrows) in the temporal bone and cerebellopontine angle. Intradural infiltration is suggested with compression of the cerebellum. The 7th and 8th nerve bundles are involved as they emerge from the brain stem. (From Anand et al., 1996, with permission.)

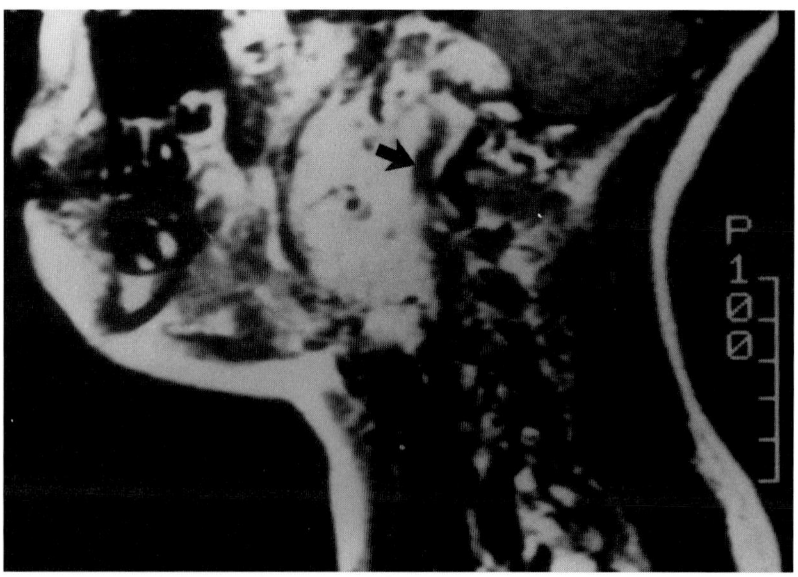

Figure 18-4. A T_1-weighted MRI shows the vertical extension of a paraganglioma from the carotid bifurcation to its extension intracranially. Extension into the region of the foramen magnum is evident on this sagittal section. The internal carotid artery is encased by the tumor (arrow). (From Anand et al., 1996, with permission.)

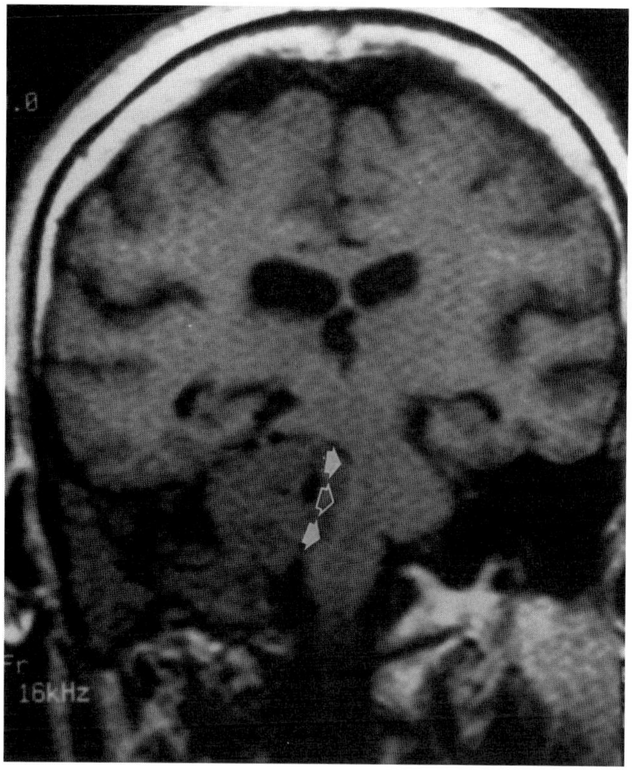

Figure 18-5. A coronal MRI shows an extensive tumor of the glomus jugulare significantly compressing the brain stem (white arrows). Note the areas of flow void within the mass, suggestive of its vascular nature. (TR, 600; TE, 11). (From Anand et al., 1996, with permission.)

invasive angiography at our institutions. Bilateral carotid angiography defines tumor vascularity, multiple tumors, and cerebrovascular anatomy in great detail (Fig. 18-6A). Most tumors derive their blood supply from the caroticotympanic branch of the internal carotid artery, and displacement, narrowing, and irregularity of the carotid artery can be assessed. The internal carotid artery is most frequently involved at the most cephalic aspect of its vertical part. In patients who have previously undergone surgical removal, the tumor's primary blood supply may emanate from the vertebrobasilar system. In these patients, embolization may not be possible. The extent of arteriovenous shunting can also be defined with angiography. During the venous phase, the sigmoid sinus should be studied for involvement and the pattern of venous collaterals assessed. Patency of the opposite sigmoid sinus and normal connection through the torcular herophili must be established.

The decision to carry out preoperative embolization is based on the findings of the angiographic examination. Embolization using polyvinyl alcohol is performed 1 to 3 days before surgery to reduce intraoperative bleeding. In previously unoperated ears, embolization generally eliminates the major blood supply to the tumor through the caroticotympanic and ascending pharyngeal branches (Fig. 18-6B&C).

When involvement of the internal carotid artery is suspected on angiographic examination because of displacement, narrowing, or irregularity of the vessel, further studies to examine cerebral blood flow are generally required. Although a number of methods are available, balloon test occlusion (BTO) in conjunction with clinical observation, transcranial Doppler, and xenon CT are most frequently done. The reliability of such testing, however, is not absolute. Moreover, a small percentage of patients undergoing balloon occlusion will have significant complications from test-

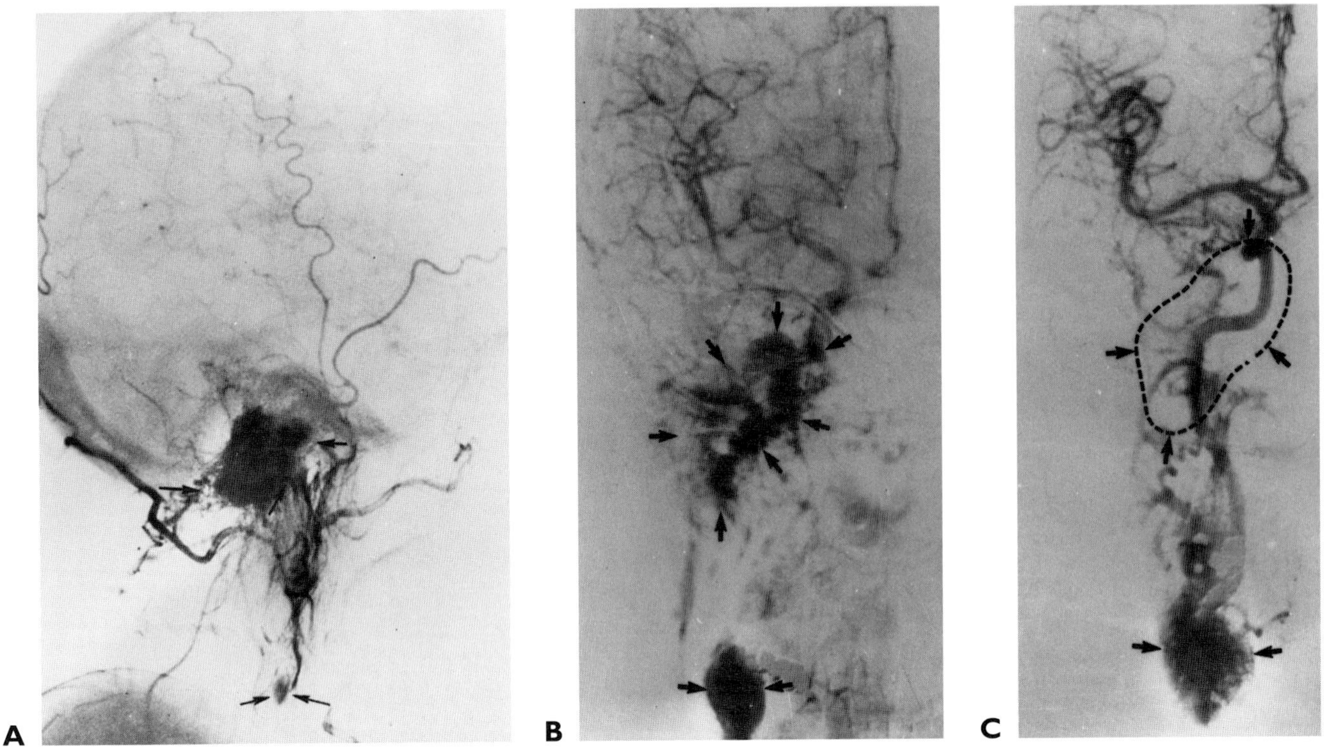

Figure 18-6. (A) Angiographic examination of a patient with a glomus jugulare tumor also reveals the presence of a carotid body tumor. The tumor encases the internal carotid artery in its petrous segment. The patient also had a glomus jugulare and carotid body tumor of the opposite side. *(B)* A late-phase angiogram showing vascular blush in the region of the carotid body tumor and glomus jugulare. *(C)* The same patient after embolization. No displacement or narrowing of the internal carotid artery is seen (tumor outline is marked by dotted lines). The carotid body tumor has not been embolized. (From Anand et al., 1996, with permission.)

ing. BTO helps identify those patients who may not tolerate internal carotid artery resection and ligation. In these patients, the need for vascular reconstruction may be determined preoperatively. Detachable intraluminal balloons are not used because the impact of interrupted blood flow in the internal carotid artery cannot be absolutely predicted even with BTO, and the tumor's dissectability from an encased internal carotid artery cannot be reliably defined preoperatively.

All glomus tumors must be suspected of catecholamine secretory activity unless proven otherwise. Routine urinary vanillylmandelic acid (VMA) and serum levels of dopamine, epinephrine, and norepinephrine are obtained. In patients with endocrinally active tumors, pharmacologic blockage with α- or β-blockers is required for 2 weeks preoperatively.

Preoperative antibiotics (vancomycin and a third-generation cephalosporin) are given to patients with infected and exposed tumors in the ear canal or intracranial extensions. Topical preparation of the wound site and ear canal are done routinely before surgery. Dexamethasone is given preoperatively to patients with intracranial tumor extension.

Anesthesia and Intraoperative Monitoring

The anesthesia team should be consulted preoperatively to discuss the appropriate control of catecholamine activity, avoidance of intracranial hypertension, and maintenance of cerebral perfusion. The induction of anesthesia should be smooth, using an agent that reduces intracranial pressure. After thiopental induction and before intubation, lidocaine can be administered intravenously to reduce the possibility of intubation-induced hypertension. Fluctuations in blood pressure must be avoided throughout surgery. Barbiturates are used for their known cerebral protective effect, if bleeding is excessive or if temporary vascular occlusion is required intraoperatively. A tracheotomy is not generally needed, but may be required in patients for whom postoperative concern for the airway is significant, that is, in patients with vocal cord paralysis and airway edema.

The internal jugular veins must be avoided during placement of the central venous line. Arterial lines are used for systemic monitoring and monitoring of pulmonary pressures. A Foley catheter measures the urinary output. Doppler oximetry is employed along with measurements of expiratory PCO_2 and arterial blood gases throughout the surgery. Blood counts, electrolytes, and coagulation profiles are routinely monitored. The facial nerve is monitored from the ipsilateral facial muscle groups, and ongoing brain stem auditory-evoked potentials are monitored throughout the procedure. The vagus and hypoglossal nerves may also be monitored if required.

Selecting the Operative Approach

Because of the vascular nature of these tumors, feeding vessels at the periphery of the tumor must be controlled before any attempt at tumor removal. Frequently, this implies gaining adequate exposure and control of the internal carotid artery. In tumors that are primarily extradural and confined to the temporal bone, more conservative transtemporal approaches including facial recess and hypotympanic approaches may permit adequate or total removal of the tumor with maximal functional preservation. Hearing loss associated with the creation of a blind pouch and removal of the ossicles or inner ear structures, facial nerve weakness from mobilization, complications of condylar dislocation, and exposure of the distal internal carotid artery can be avoided in surgery of such limited tumors. For more extensive tumors having intradural infiltration or intracranial extension with impingement against the internal carotid artery, control of the internal carotid artery becomes the crucial determinant of the surgical approach.

One-Stage Resection of Extracranial-Intracranial Glomus Jugulare Tumors

The approach described here employs the essential principles of the infratemporal approach described by Fisch (1978), allowing tumor resection from the middle fossa to the foramen magnum in a one-stage procedure. This approach has several advantages: (1) direct, proximal, and distal control of the internal carotid artery; (2) preservation of the facial nerve by its identification and transposition, whenever required; (3) control of the tumor's blood supply before the operative attack on the tumor; (4) adequate exposure to ensure control of cerebrospinal fluid leakage; and (5) the ability to remove ipsilateral carotid body tumors at the same sitting.

Positioning

The positioning of the patient, appropriate placement of the anesthesia and intraoperative monitoring team at the patient's feet, placement of the nursing team to the right of the surgeon, and preferential placement of the microscope are important in allowing the surgeon adequate space and ease of movement. The patient is placed in the supine position and the head and trunk are elevated 30 degrees (Fig. 18-7). The ipsilateral shoulder is slightly elevated and the head is somewhat extended and turned away from the side of the tumor. In this way, positional compression of the contralateral internal jugular vein is avoided. The head is stabilized in a three-point Mayfield headrest. The operative table should permit side-to-side and up-and-down head movement to facilitate exposure. Monitoring electrodes are placed in appropriately selected facial musculature. The potential donor sites for a fascia lata graft and rectus abdominis free flap are prepared and exposed (Fig. 18-7A&B). Operative sterility must be ensured throughout the procedure.

Exposing the Carotid in the Neck

The incision is marked in a reverse, upside-down, hockey-stick manner, extending from above the zygoma to a point about 2.5 cm above the external auditory meatus and then to the postauricular region down to the mastoid tip, from where it extends parallel to the anterior border of the sternomastoid muscle. If the patient has had a previous approach from this route, the incision may carefully be modified to reduce the possibility of flap necrosis. After the incision is marked, the skin is infiltrated with 1 percent xylocaine in 1:100,000 epinephrine to reduce bleeding. The incision is then made and flaps elevated. Anteriorly, one must exercise caution in the area of the frontal division of the facial nerve to avoid any injuries. Posteriorly, the accessory

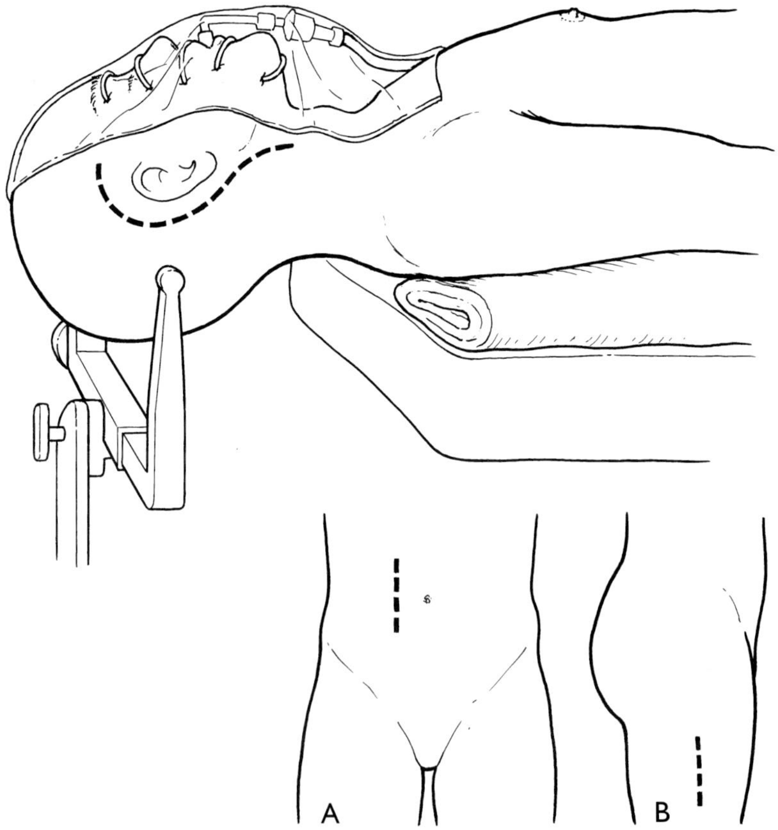

Figure 18-7. Proper positioning of the patient for surgery. The head is rotated away from the operator, hyperextended, elevated, and fixed in a Mayfield clamp. Electrodes to monitor the facial nerves are placed in appropriately selected facial musculature. *(Inset)* The donor sites for *(A)* a rectus abdominus free flap and *(B)* fascia lata graft are prepared and exposed. (Adapted from Anand et al., 1996, with permission.)

nerve can be superficial as it exits the sternomastoid muscle at Erb's point. Dissection over the mastoid periosteum is carried to the external auditory meatus. The spine of Henle is identified and the cartilaginous ear canal outlined superiorly, posteriorly, and inferiorly. The anterior border of the sternomastoid is defined. The insertions of the sternomastoid and digastric muscles into the mastoid are carefully detached and the muscle bellies reflected anteroinferiorly. The greater auricular nerve requires division; however, it must be appropriately tagged in case a graft from this nerve is required. The carotid sheath is identified and the common carotid artery, internal jugular vein, and vagus nerve are dissected superiorly (Fig. 18-8). The jugular foramen is defined. Vascular loops are placed around the internal and external carotid arteries and the internal jugular vein. If a carotid body tumor was identified preoperatively, it is now removed by microdissection.

Creation of a Blind Pouch in the External Auditory Canal

Because a closed cavity is required to control leakage of cerebrospinal fluid after tumor resection, the external auditory meatus is closed as a blind pouch. This step is done with optical loupes or microscopic magnification. The external auditory canal is infiltrated with 1 percent xylocaine with 1:100,000 epinephrine at the bony cartilaginous junction. This allows control of bleeding and adequate hydrodissection of the skin of the external auditory canal from the bony part. Posteriorly, a mastoid periosteal flap is elevated carefully (Fig. 18-8A). The cartilaginous and cutaneous layer of the external canal are elevated just lateral to the annulus. The skin is incised in a circum annular manner, after which the cartilage is carefully dissected from the skin layer, ensuring an intact epithelial layer. This permits easy eversion of the cutaneous layer. After the eversion, the skin is closed subcutaneously with Vicryl and cutaneously with 5-0 Ethilon (Fig. 18-8B). Mastoid periosteum is used to seal this closure on the medial aspect (Fig. 18-8C).

Middle Ear Exposure and Mastoidectomy

Next, the facial nerve is identified by locating its landmarks: the tympanomastoid suture line, the posterior belly of the digastric muscle, and the cartilaginous pointer. Distal dissection of the nerve requires further anterior elevation of the skin flap. Major branches of the nerve are carefully identified and protected. A simple mastoidectomy is then done, without entering the tumor. The sinodural angle and tegmen tympani are identified (Fig. 18-9A). The peripheral portion of the tumor is generally visualized at this point, and, lateral to the tumor, the facial nerve is identified in its vertical mastoid segment. The nerve is carefully drilled with a diamond drill, with copious irrigation and careful monitoring. The tumor is generally medial to the nerve and the nerve can be traced proximally by removing the bony external auditory canal and using the facial recess approach to identify the extension of the tumor in the middle ear (Fig. 18-9B). The tympanic membrane is elevated and, after incudostapedial disarticulation, the remainder of the external auditory canal, tympanic membrane, malleus, and incus are removed (Fig. 18-9C).

Facial Nerve Transposition

The middle ear and horizontal component of the fallopian canal are now directly exposed. The chorda tympani is frequently engulfed by the tumor and requires sectioning. If the chorda tympani can be preserved, traction injuries to this structure must be avoided. The bony external auditory canal is lowered, but the tumor is not yet removed from the middle ear. At the pyramidal bend of the facial nerve, bony drilling must be extremely cautious to avoid inadvertent injury to the lateral semicir-

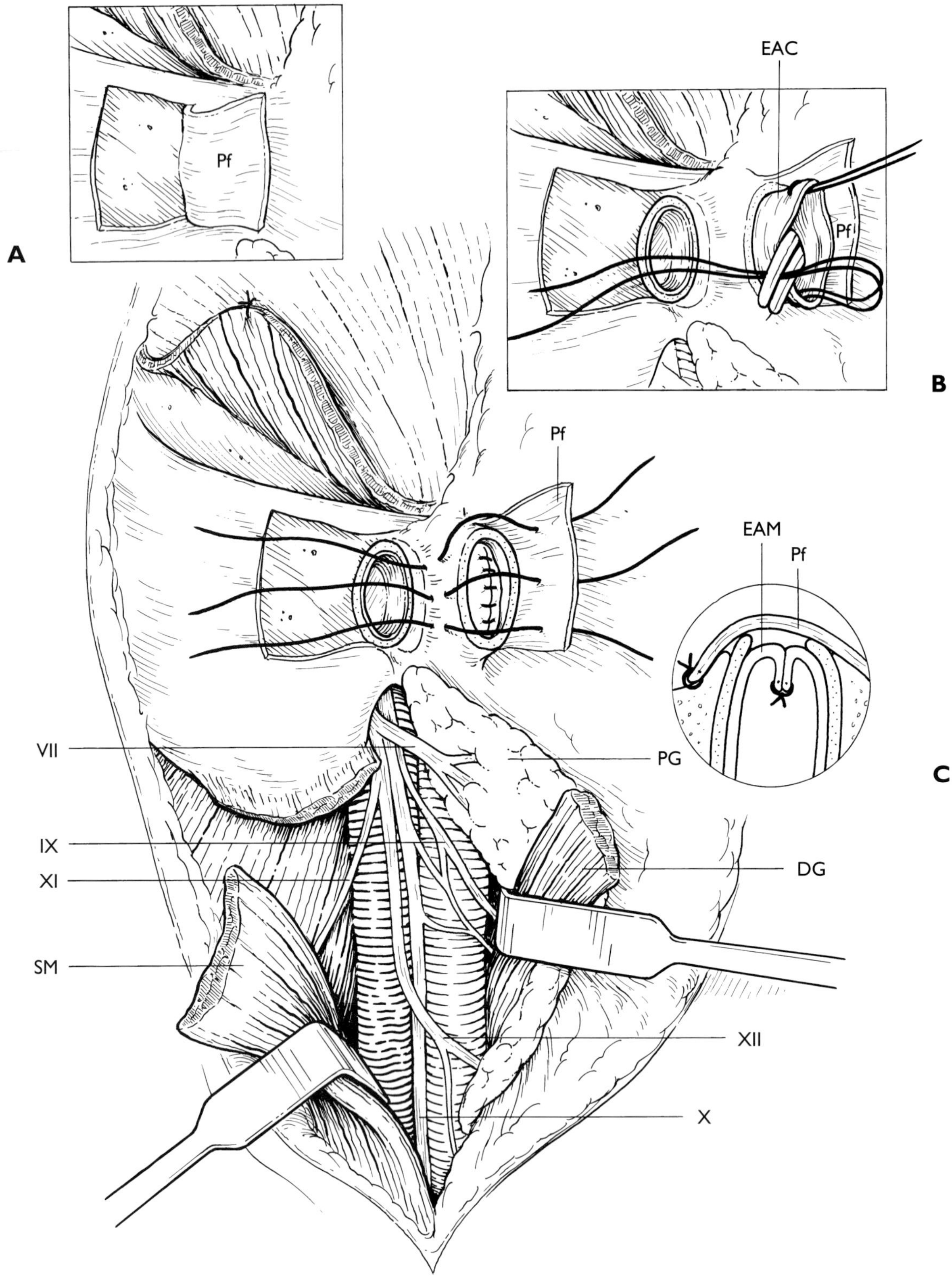

Figure 18-8. After incision, the neurovascular structures in the upper cervical region are exposed. The facial nerve is dissected in its course from the stylomastoid region to the parotid segment. The internal carotid artery, internal jugular vein, and lower cranial nerves (IX, X, XI, XII) are dissected and preserved. Double-layer, blind sac closure of the external auditory canal includes: *(A)* Elevation of the mastoid periosteal flap. *(B)* Eversion closure of the skin of the external auditory canal after the cartilage is removed. *(C)* Reinforcement of the skin closure with the periosteal flap. (For explanation of abbreviations, see Appendix 1, p. 373.) (Adapted from Anand et al., 1996, with permission.)

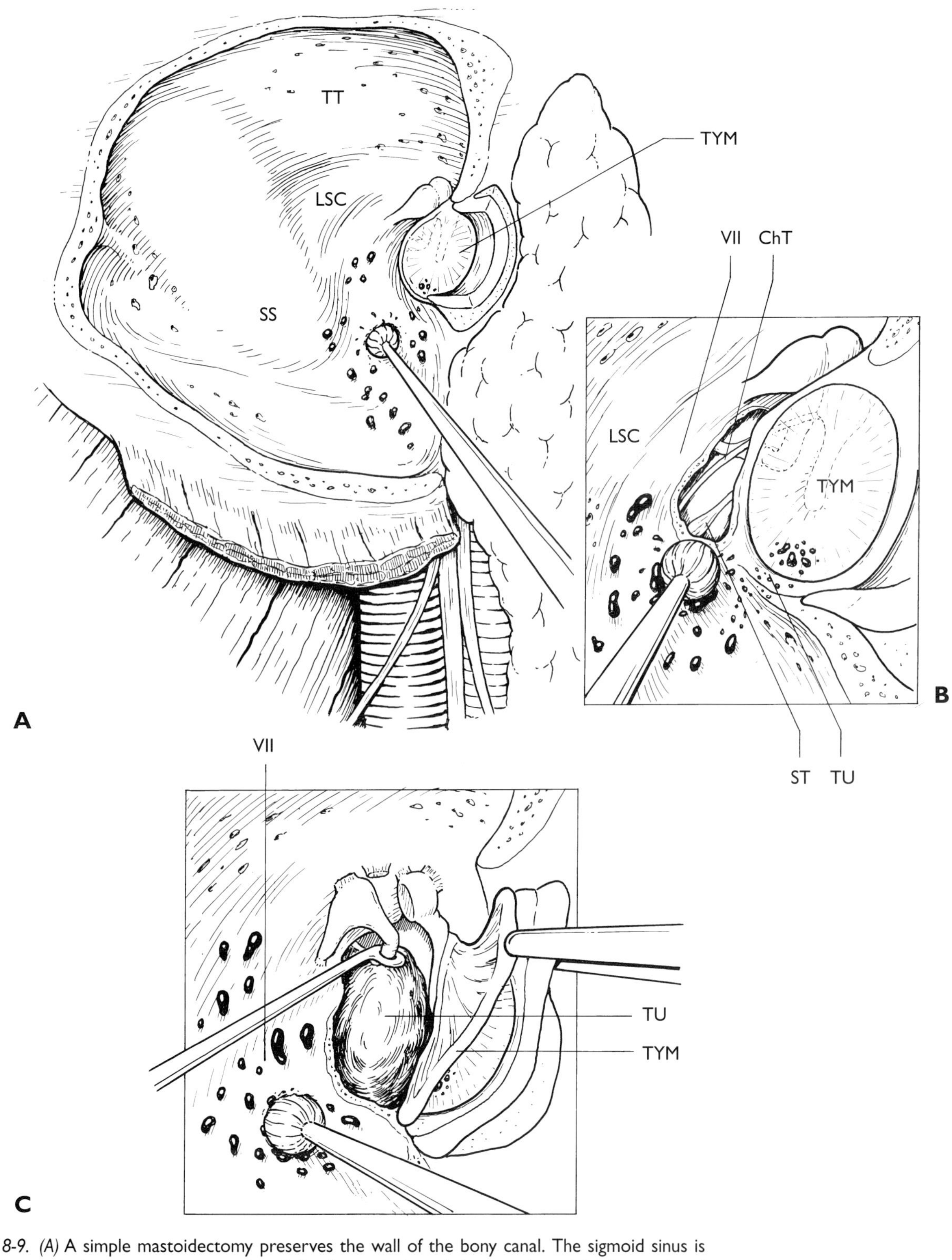

Figure 18-9. (A) A simple mastoidectomy preserves the wall of the bony canal. The sigmoid sinus is outlined posteriorly, the tegmen tympani is defined superiorly, and the lateral semicircular canal and second genu of the facial nerve are identified. *(B)* The facial recess approach to examine the middle ear cavity. *(C)* After incudostapedial disarticulation, the entire external auditory canal is removed along with the tympanic membrane and the malleus. (Adapted from Anand et al., 1996, with permission.)

cular canal. The facial nerve is mobilized after its fibrous attachments are divided with sharp dissection at the stylomastoid foramen (Fig. 18-10). After the nerve is freed in its vertical and horizontal segments, the entire nerve is transposed anteriorly if tumor extension demands it (Figs. 18-10C and 18-11). A notch is drilled in the external bony canal to lodge the transposed facial nerve. The nerve must be carefully protected by a thin, flexible, soaked telfa gauze pad throughout the remainder of the surgery. If the nerve is significantly encased and infiltrated by the tumor, selective resection of the nerve may be required and nerve grafting done after complete removal of the tumor. Neurorrhaphy requires precise microsurgical technique and absence of tension at the neurorrhaphy site to obtain the best results from nerve repair. Next, the mastoid bone is drilled along the periphery of the tumor. The sigmoid sinus is identified posteriorly in its entire length and outlined. The dura mater is exposed and delineated here. Frequently, during drill-out of the tumor, bipolar coagulation of the periphery of the tumor is required to expose the labyrinthine structures. The hypotympanic cells are frequently dense and require extensive drill-out to expose the jugular bulb completely. In selected patients, the cochlea and labyrinth may require complete removal to assure the adequacy of tumor exposure and removal (Fig. 18-10D).

Exposing the Petrous Carotid

The internal carotid artery is dissected from the neck up to its entrance into the carotid canal. This exposure requires the division of the stylopharyngeus and styloglossus muscles, as well as removal of the styloid process. The eustachian tube must be divided. The pharyngeal end of the eustachian tube is inverted and obliterated with a muscle graft or bone wax. The bony carotid canal is carefully drilled out, preserving the 9th cranial nerve as it crosses superficial to the internal carotid artery. To appropriately expose the superior portion of the vertical segment of the internal carotid artery, the mandibular condyle must be displaced anteroinferiorly. After the joint capsule is entered, the condyle of the mandible is retracted, allowing adequate exposure and seldom requiring condylar resection. The middle meningeal vessels are divided to allow dissection of the horizontal segment of the internal auditory canal. If further horizontal exposure of the carotid is needed in the cavernous sinus, clivus, or nasopharynx, the zygoma is removed and the temporalis muscle reflected downward. The mandibular and maxillary branches of the trigeminal nerve may require division to allow this anterior exposure and control of the horizontal segment of the distal petrous carotid artery (Figs. 18-10A&B and 18-12).

Exposing the Intracranial Tumor

The sigmoid sinus is skeletonized down to the jugular bulb; bipolar coagulation is used to control bleeding emanating from the periphery of the tumor. After the sigmoid sinus is exposed, the vessel loops are placed around the internal jugular vein, which is dissected from the lower cranial nerves. The sigmoid sinus is opened above and inferior to the tumor and its lumen packed with gelfoam or temporalis muscle (Fig. 18-10C). Preserving the medial wall in this manner helps preserve the function of the lower cranial nerves. If the medial wall of the sigmoid sinus is involved by the tumor, it is divided above and below the tumorous involvement, its medial wall is removed, and the intracranial extension approached as in a suboccipital approach. The superior and inferior petrosal sinuses are coagulated and transected because they bleed vigorously. The cerebellum is then gently retracted and the lower cranial nerves are exposed (Fig. 18-13A&B). The posteroinferior extent of the tumor is outlined in this manner and the dissection is carried anteriorly. The tumor is dissected from the 9th, 10th, and 11th cranial nerves and removed from the cerebellopontine angle by

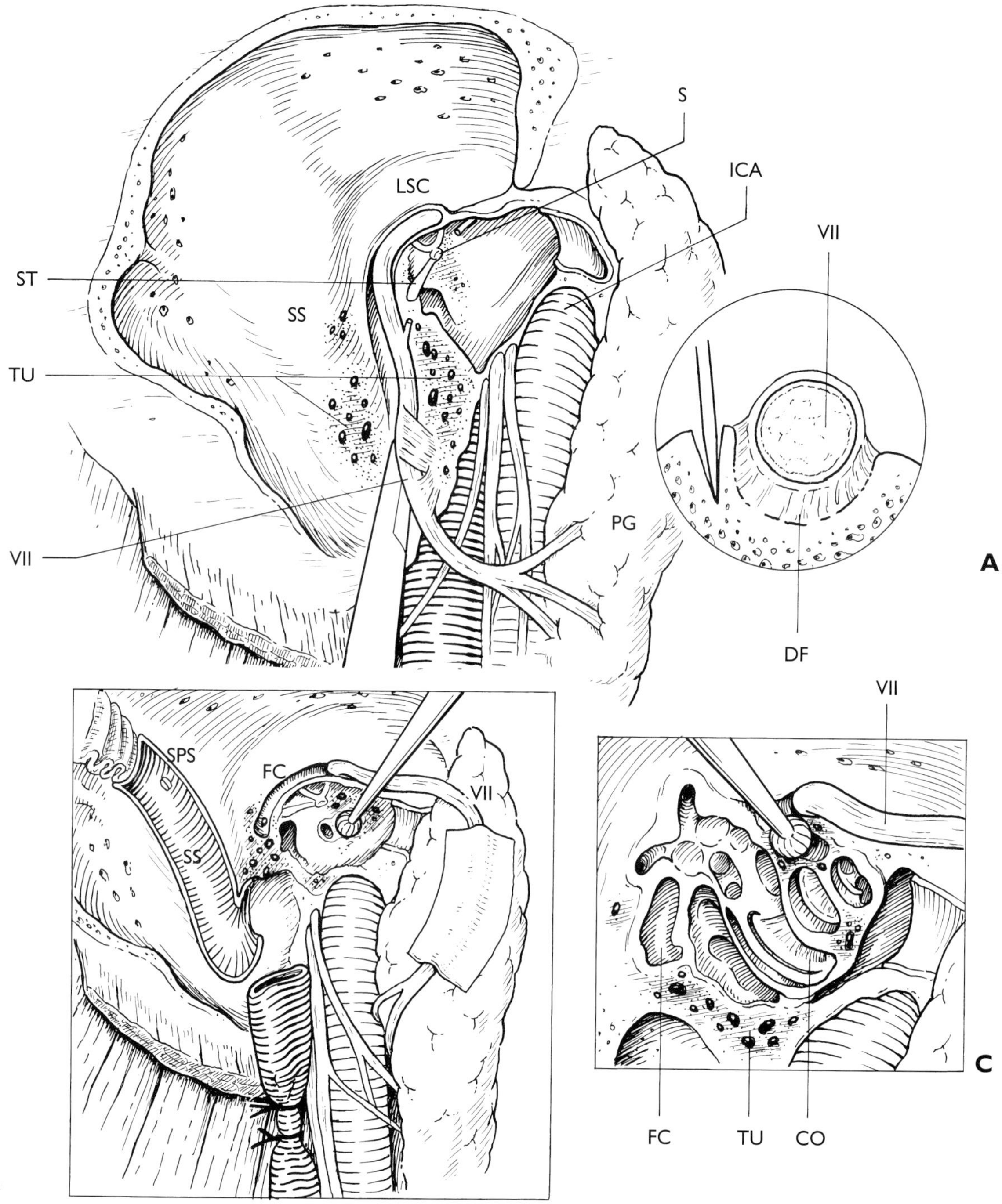

Figure 18-10. After the facial nerve is exposed in its extratympanic, vertical mastoid, and horizontal tympanic segments, a beaver blade is used to free the nerve from its dense fibrous anchorage at the stylomastoid foramen. *(A)* The spatial relationship of the nerve to the stylomastoid foramen. DF, dense fibrous tissue. *(B)* The facial nerve has been transposed and protected. The mandibular condyle is dislocated and retracted and the internal carotid artery is exposed in its vertical bony canal. Drilling achieves further cephalic exposure of the internal carotid artery. The sigmoid sinus is opened and packed superior to the most cephalad extension of the tumor. *(C)* In patients with sensorineural hearing loss, the cochlea and labyrinth are removed to expose the internal auditory canal. (Adapted from Anand et al., 1996 with permission.)

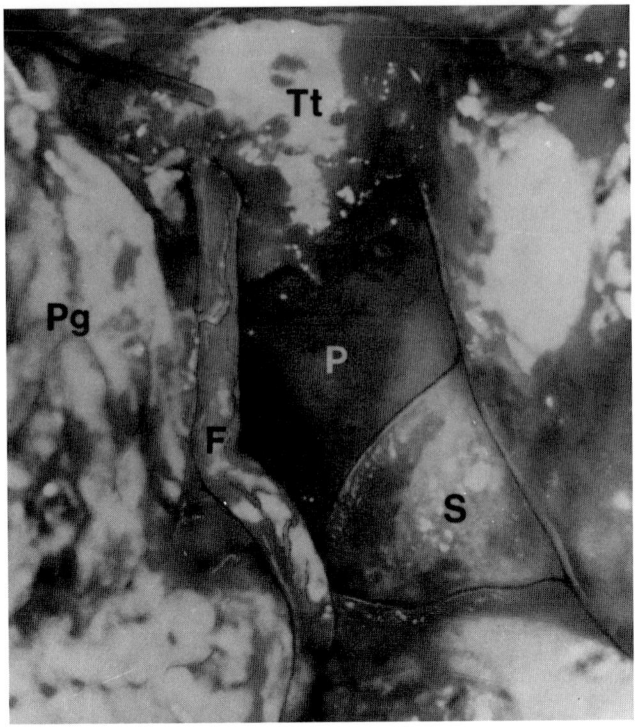

Figure 18-11. Intraoperative enhanced photograph showing anteriorly transposed facial nerve in a patient with a glomus jugulare tumor. F, facial nerve; Tt, tegmen tympani; S, jugular bulb; Pg, parotid gland. (From Anand et al., 1993a, with permission.)

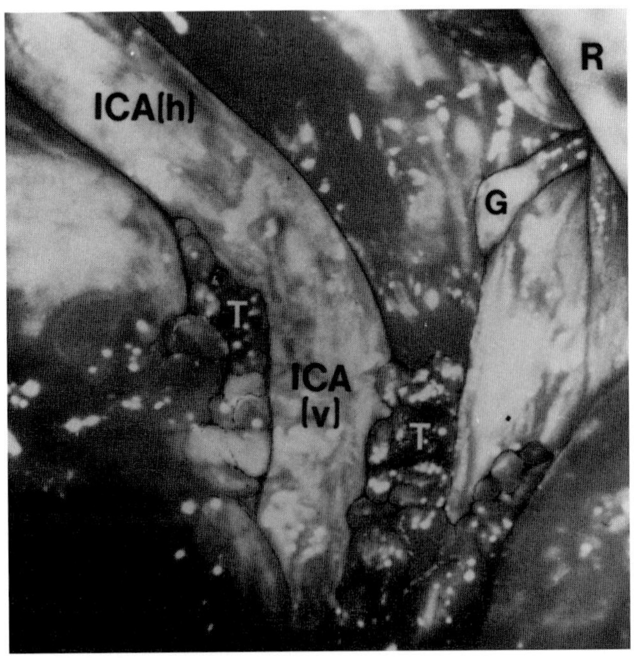

Figure 18-12. Intraoperative enhanced micrograph shows that the tumor has been dissected from the internal carotid artery, which is preserved. R, retractor; T, tumor; G, geniculate ganglion. (From Anand et al., 1993a, with permission.)

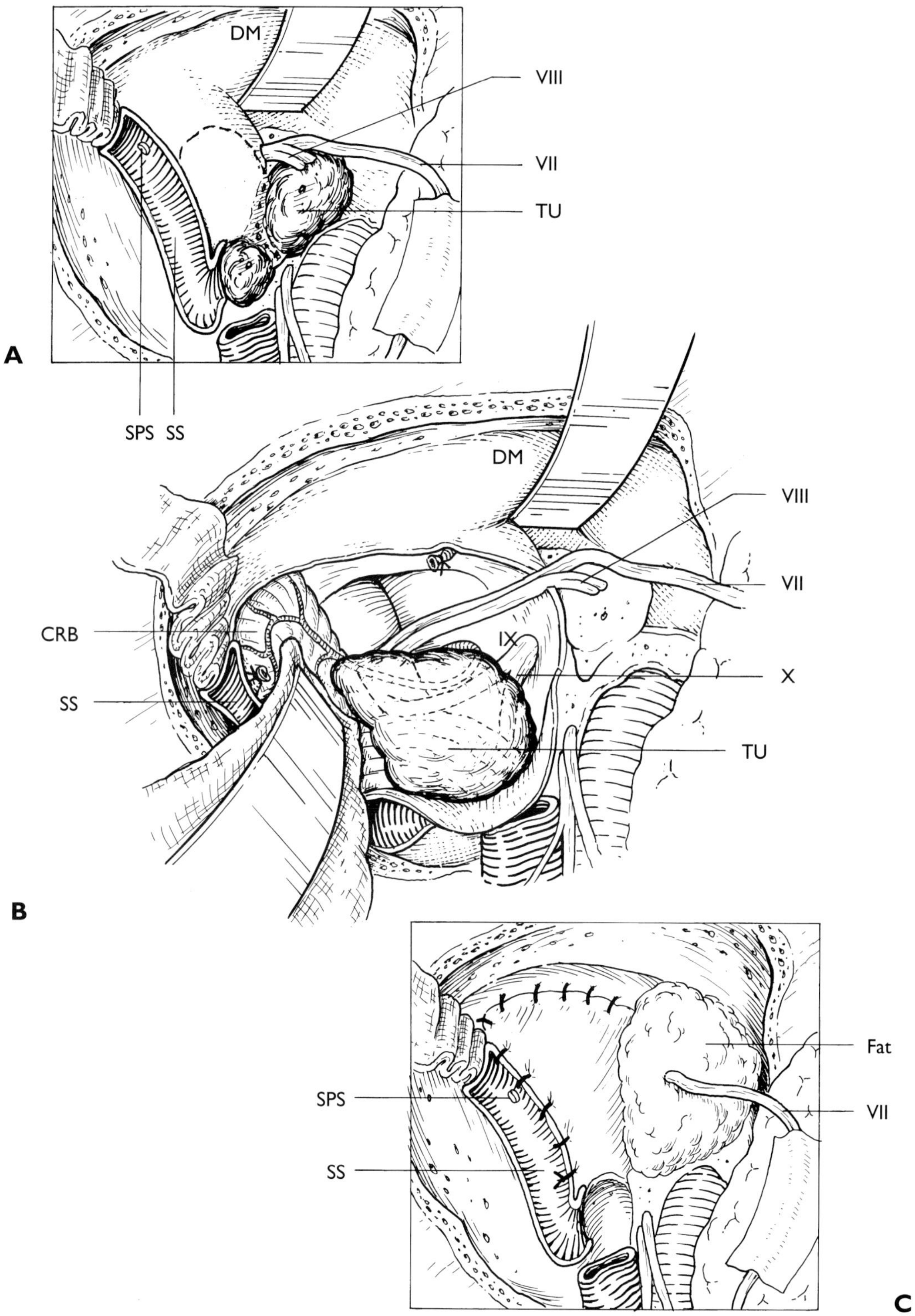

Figure 18-13. *(A)* The dura mater of the middle cranial fossa is elevated with the temporal lobe to expose middle fossa extensions of the tumor. Note the divided stump of the vestibulocochlear nerve. *(B)* The posterior fossa is exposed. After the dura is incised, the cerebellum is retracted and the extension of the tumor into the cerebellopontine angle is exposed. The relationship of the lower cranial nerves to the tumor is shown. Microsurgical techniques are used to remove the tumor from important neurovascular structures. *(C)* The dural defect is closed watertight with a fascia lata graft (Fg). Closure is augmented by the placement of fat (Ft) to prevent small leaks of cerebrospinal fluid around the internal auditory meatus. Fibrin glue is often used. (Adapted from Anand et al., 1996, with permission.)

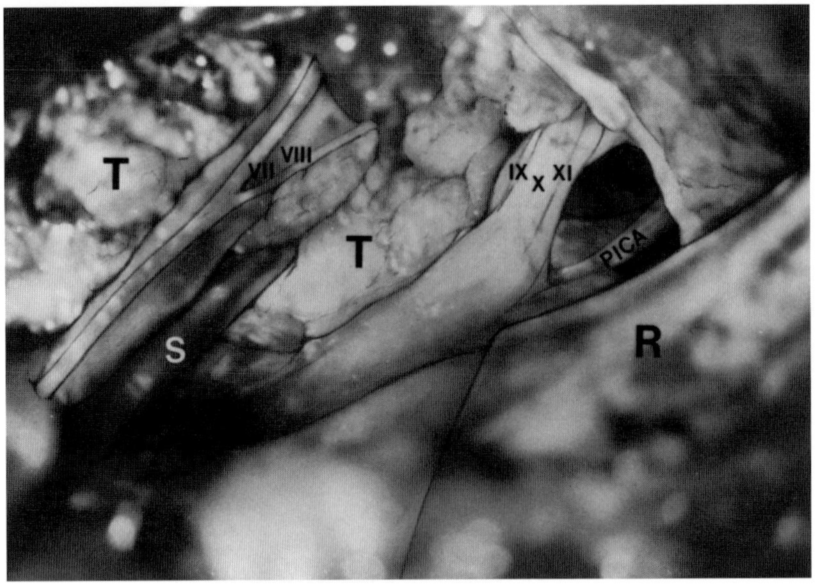

Figure 18-14. Enhanced operative micrograph of an intradural glomus lesion showing the tumor dissection from important neurovascular structures. S, suction; T, tumor; R, retractor. (From Anand et al., 1993b, with permission.)

mobilizing it anterolaterally. Gentle dissection is required to avoid hypertension bradycardia from vagal stimulation. The tumor is further devascularized by coagulating the small arterial feeders. When the tumor is small or moderate in size intradurally, the 7th and 8th cranial nerves are usually stretched posteriorly and are easily identified. When the tumor is large, however, these cranial nerves may be engulfed and dissection can be extremely difficult (Fig. 18-14). The posteroinferior and anteroinferior cerebellar arteries may also be embedded in the tumor. The tumor is debulked with microscissors, bipolar coagulation, or a CO_2 laser. Maintaining dissection within the arachnoidal planes is crucial to preserve the neurovascular structures.

Closure

The dura is closed in a watertight manner. If a large segment of the dura is missing, a fascial graft is used to close the defect (Fig. 18-13C). To avoid a postoperative cerebrospinal fluid leak, the eustachian tube is packed with muscle, adipose tissue, or bone wax after the mucosa is inverted. The temporalis or sternomastoid muscle is then reflected to close the surgical defect. In patients with a history of previous surgery or radiation therapy who have extensive dural defects, the transfer of a microanastomosed free flap from the rectus abdominis over the patched dura may be required to avoid postoperative cerebrospinal fluid leak. A lumbar drain for 5 days or longer helps prevent a postoperative leak. The soft tissues are closed in multiple layers.

Complications

Prevention and early detection of complications is crucial in achieving a successful outcome for patients requiring this surgery. Intensive neurosurgical monitoring is required for a few days after surgery. Complications can develop for a variety of reasons and early detection and prompt therapeutic response must be instituted.

Removing intracranial tumors of the glomus jugulare carries with it all the potential risks of intracranial surgery. Manipulation of the brain stem and interruption of its blood supply must be diligently avoided. This complication occurs more often when the anteroinferior cerebellar artery loops deeply into the internal auditory canal and the collateral circulation is poor.

Altered cerebral spinal fluid dynamics may lead to postoperative leakage of cerebrospinal fluid, pseudomeningocele, and hydrocephalus. Acute hydrocephalus that develops postoperatively is generally obstructive due to mass effect (edema, hemorrhage). On the contrary, delayed hydrocephalus is generally communicating and related to poor absorption of the cerebrospinal fluid or scarring of the basal cisterns. A CT scan is generally diagnostic and treatment includes a shunt. Postoperative leakage of cerebrospinal fluid is a significant risk and can be avoided through the following steps: (1) watertight closure of the dura; (2) meticulous control of the eustachian tube orifice with muscle and bone wax; (3) appropriate closure of the dead space with viable muscle flaps such as the temporalis or sternomastoid; and (4) meticulous closure of the blind sac of the external auditory canal. Postoperative cerebrospinal fluid leakage is associated with an approximately 20 percent incidence of meningitis. Head elevation and spinal drainage are required to abolish the leak. The use of prophylactic antibiotics remains controversial. If postoperative leakage persists, cisternography with contrast enhancement can determine the site. Surgery may be required to close the dura with a fascial graft or to place a shunt if hydrocephalus exists.

Complications related to the internal carotid artery can be sudden and are most serious. They include vasospasm, thrombosis, and hemorrhage. Postoperative heparinization is not routinely employed. Previously radiated patients or those in whom dissection from a deeply encased internal carotid artery is difficult must be monitored. In patients who require removal of the internal carotid artery and replacement with a saphenous venous graft, appropriate vascular management is instituted. The primary risk of glomus tumor surgery is injury to the cranial nerves; morbidity from facial nerve paralysis can be substantial. Eye protection must be promptly rendered in these patients. Meticulous microscopic technique and intraoperative monitoring of the facial nerve, however, greatly assist in preserving facial nerve function. The loss of the 9th and 10th cranial nerves can be associated with the life-threatening potential complications of postoperative aspiration and pneumonia. The loss of the 9th and 10th cranial nerve function is better tolerated by younger than by older patients. Problems with swallowing and loss of sensation in the palate are a rule in patients with extensive glomus tumors. A cricopharyngeal myotomy and silastic thyroplasty, which medialize the paralyzed vocal cord, generally ameliorate clinical symptoms and must be considered immediately. The problem of aspiration is significantly worsened by a hypoglossal nerve deficit, which may occur in these patients.

Although conductive hearing loss generally exists in patients preoperatively, it is usually not worsened after surgery. The cochlea, labyrinth, and 8th cranial nerve are generally not injured. To avoid severe hypoacusis, the blood supply to the cochlea through the anteroinferior cerebellar artery and its branches must be preserved.

References

Anand VJ, Al-Mefty O, Leonetti JP (1993a) Complications of skull base surgery and how to avoid them. pp. 323–339. In Johnson T (ed): The Academy of Otolaryngology—Head and Neck Surgery Instructional Courses. Mosby-Year Book, St. Louis

Anand VK, Leonetti JP, Al-Mefty O (1993b) Neurovascular considerations in surgery of glomus tumors with intracranial extension. Laryngoscope 103:722–728

Anand VK, Schenk MP, Leonetti JP, Al-Mefty O (1996) Surgical treatment of intracranial glomus tumors. pp. 117–124. In Rengachary SS, Wilkins RH (eds): Neurosurgical Operative Atlas, Volume IV. American Association of Neurological Surgeons; Park Ridge, IL

Fisch U (1978) Infratemporal fossa approach to tumors of the temporal bone and base of the skull. J Laryngol Otol 92:949–967

19

Petrosal "Presigmoid" Approach to the Clivus

Georges F. Haddad
Ossama Al-Mefty

Surgical access to the clivus and petrous apex remains a formidable challenge. Numerous approaches have been designed to reach lesions at this deep-seated and vital location. Intradural tumors affecting the clivus may be divided into three categories depending on the area primarily involved by tumor. The first area comprises the dorsum sellae, the posterior wall of the sphenoid sinus, and the petrous apex down to a horizontal line joining the acoustic meati. Tumors in this location are best dealt with via a cranio-orbito-zygomatic or an extended middle fossa approach. The second area extends from the spheno-occipital synchondrosis to the level of the jugular foramina. This area is best approached through a petrosal (lateral presigmoid) or a transtemporal approach. The third area comprises the remainder of the clivus down to the anterior rim of the foramen magnum. It is reached best via a transcondylar approach (Table 19-1). We discuss in detail the approach to the second area.

The petrosal approach is best suited for patients with intact hearing on the side of surgery. In deaf patients a transtemporal approach is selected. The petrosal approach is centered on the petrous bone, creating several advantages: (1) the cerebellar and temporal lobes are minimally retracted; (2) the operative distance to the clivus is shortened by 3 cm as compared with a standard subtemporal approach; (3) the surgeon has a direct line of sight to the lesion and the anterior and lateral aspects of the brain stem; (4) the neural and otologic structures, including the cochlea, labyrinth, and facial nerve, are preserved; (5) the transverse and sigmoid sinuses, as well as the vein of Labbé and the basal veins are preserved; (6) the tumor's vascular supply is interrupted early in the procedure; and (7) multiple axes for dissection are provided.

Preoperative Assessment

The necessity of a preoperative angiogram or magnetic resonance (MR) venous angiography is obvious. The position and displacement of the arteries should be studied. Particular attention should also be paid to the venous pattern because venous

Table 19-1. Approaches to Intradural Clival Tumors

Tumor Location	Additional Factors	Approach
Upper clivus	Involvement of cavernous sinus	Cranio-orbito-zygomatic
	No involvement of cavernous sinus	Extended middle fossa
Midclivus	Hearing preserved	Petrosal
	No hearing	Transtemporal
Lower clivus		Transcondylar

infarction of the temporal lobe has grave sequelae. How big is the vein of Labbé? Is it the dominant venous drainage of the temporal lobe? Are there other basal temporal veins that may be equally vital? Does the patient have two transverse sinuses, and do these sinuses connect at the torcular herophili?

Positioning

The patient is placed supine with the ipsilateral shoulder slightly elevated (Fig. 19-1). The face is turned toward the contralateral shoulder and the vertex inclined toward the floor, thus placing the petrous base at the highest point of the operative field. The head is fixed in this position with a three-point Mayfield headrest. During the operation, the surgeon's line of sight can be altered by rotating the table from side to side or up and down.

Surgical Technique

A reverse question-mark incision is made, starting at the zygoma in front of the ear, circling above the ear, and descending 1 cm behind the mastoid process (Fig. 19-1). The skin flap is elevated and reflected anteriorly and inferiorly. Care is taken not to

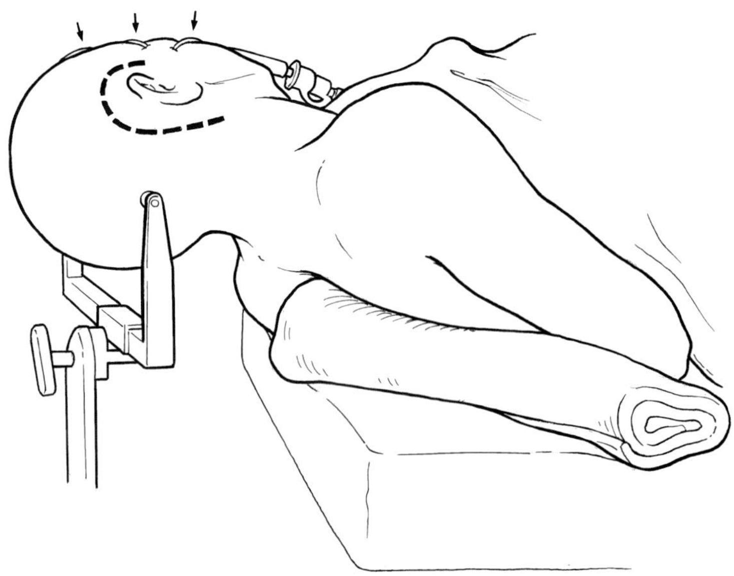

Figure 19-1. The position of the patient and the location of the incision for a right-sided petrosal "presigmoid" approach to the clivus. The arrows indicate electromyography needle electrodes for the monitoring of facial nerve function.

injure the temporalis fascia. This fascia is cut anteriorly and superiorly and dissected from the underlying muscle. The fascia is kept in continuity with the periosteum and the fascia of the sternocleidomastoid muscle. After the insertion of the sternocleidomastoid is detached, the temporalis fascia, periosteum, and sternomastoid muscle and fascia are reflected as one unit inferiorly and posteriorly (Fig. 19-2). The temporalis muscle is detached from its origin, using the cautery. The muscle is reflected anteriorly. The bony surface of the temporal fossa mastoid and lateral posterior fossa are thus exposed.

Four burr holes are made, two on each side of the transverse sinus (Fig. 19-3). The first hole is made just medial and inferior to the asterion. It opens into the posterior fossa below the transverse-sigmoid sinus junction. The second hole is located at the squamal and mastoid junction of the temporal bone, along the projection of the superior temporal line. It opens into the supratentorial compartment. The burr hole at each of these two points will flank the sigmoid sinus. The other two burr holes are placed slightly more medial than the first two and closer together, flanking the transverse sinus. The temporal bone and a portion of the parietal bone above the tentorium, as well as the occipital bone below the tentorium, are incised between burr holes using the foot attachment of the Midas Rex drill (Fig. 19-3). The foot attachment is not used to cross over the sinus. The burr holes flanking the transverse sinus are then connected using a thin rongeur or drilled with the Midas Rex drill (Fig. 19-3). Particular attention should be paid to avoid tearing the wall of the venous sinus. The bone may be severely adherent to the dura where the sigmoid and transverse sinuses meet. The craniotomy flap is then carefully elevated, freeing the aforementioned adhesions.

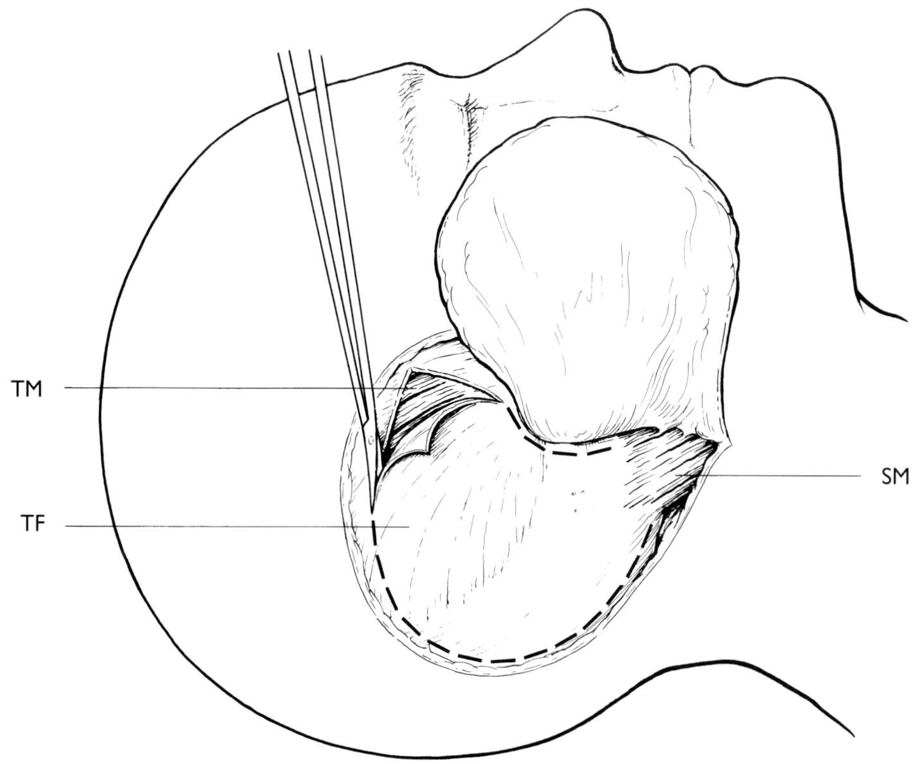

Figure 19-2. A large triangular flap consisting of temporalis fascia and pericranium is elevated maintaining an intact vascular base by its attachment to the fascia of the sternocleidomastoid muscle. (For explanation of abbreviations, see Appendix 1, p. 373.)

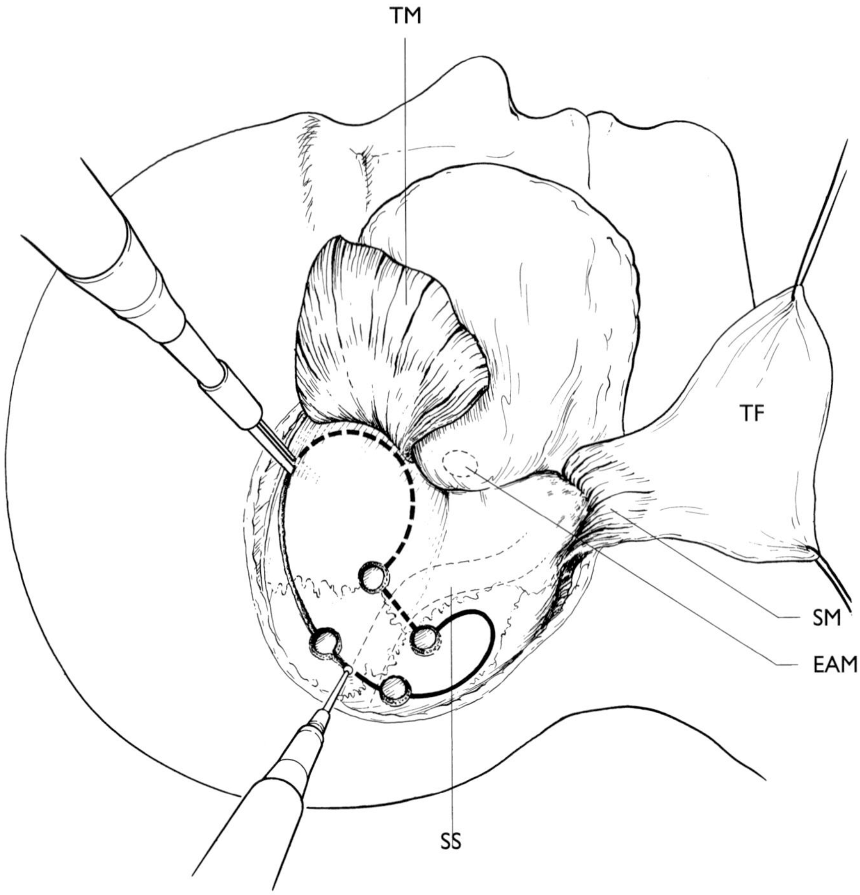

Figure 19-3. The temporalis muscle is elevated and retracted forward. The sternomastoid is detached from its insertion. On each side of the transverse sinus two pairs of burr holes are drilled as shown, each pair being connected across the sinus by drilling with a small diamond burr. The temporal and occipital sections of the flap are cut with a craniotome.

A thorough knowledge of the anatomy of the petrous bone and surrounding structures is required to drill the temporal bone (see Ch. 3). The orifice of the external acoustic meatus lies below the posterior root of the zygomatic arch. Along the superior wall of the external acoustic meatus is the suprameatal spine. Above this spine lies the temporal line, which extends posteriorly from the zygomatic root. The area between these two lines is the suprameatal triangle, which is used as a guide in locating the mastoid antrum 1.5 cm medially within the bone. The facial (fallopian) canal and the inner ear structures including the semicircular canals lie deep and anterior to the antrum. The first level of mastoidectomy can be performed quickly using a cutting drill. The mastoid cortex overlying the antrum is first drilled. Once the antrum is identified, the drilling is confined in a posterior direction. At this stage, the two structures that must be preserved are the sigmoid sinus posteriorly and the facial nerve inferiorly as it emerges from the stylomastoid foramen, medial to the digastric notch.

The rest of the mastoidectomy is performed with a diamond drill under the microscope. An area of denser bone, the "solid angle," is identified just medial to the antrum. It is characterized by a noticeable increase in bone density, and houses the three semicircular canals. The facial canal is exposed and identified just below this solid angle. The sigmoid sinus is skeletonized down to the jugular bulb. Opened air cells are obliterated with bone wax.

Two dural incisions are performed, one supratentorial along the floor of the middle fossa, the other anterior to the sigmoid sinus (Fig. 19-4). The two incisions are joined at the sinodural (Citelli's) angle, which identifies the position of the superior petrosal sinus. The superior petrosal sinus is clipped or coagulated and transected, the incision is continued through the tentorium, parallel to the pyramid, and is extended through the incisura. This last step opens up the way to the clivus widely. During this maneuver, the surgeon should preserve the trochlear nerve by keeping the incision through the tentorial notch behind the area where the 4th cranial nerve enters the tentorial dural fold. Opening the tentorium allows excellent exposure of the upper pole of the tumor and the anterior and lateral aspects of the brain stem. A retractor is placed to support the posterior part of the tentorium and the overlying temporal lobe. Care must be taken not to injure the vein of Labbé. Another retractor holds medially the sigmoid sinus and the cerebellum.

When the lesion is large and extends significantly in both supra- and infratentorial compartments, the dura of the posterior fossa is opened along both sides of the sigmoid sinus (Fig. 19-4). The sigmoid sinus need not be transected; exposure may be obtained by alternating the visualized field above and below the tentorium.

Further relaxation is obtained by opening the arachnoid of the cerebellopontine cistern and draining cerebrospinal fluid (CSF). The tumor is devascularized by coagulating its insertion on the pyramid and its meningeal feeders over the tentorium. When the tumor is small or moderate in size, the 7th and 8th cranial nerves are usually stretched posteriorly and are thus easily identified. When the tumor reaches a large size these nerves may well be engulfed in the tumor. A suitable area on the tumor is selected and the arachnoid over the tumor is opened. The tumor is then

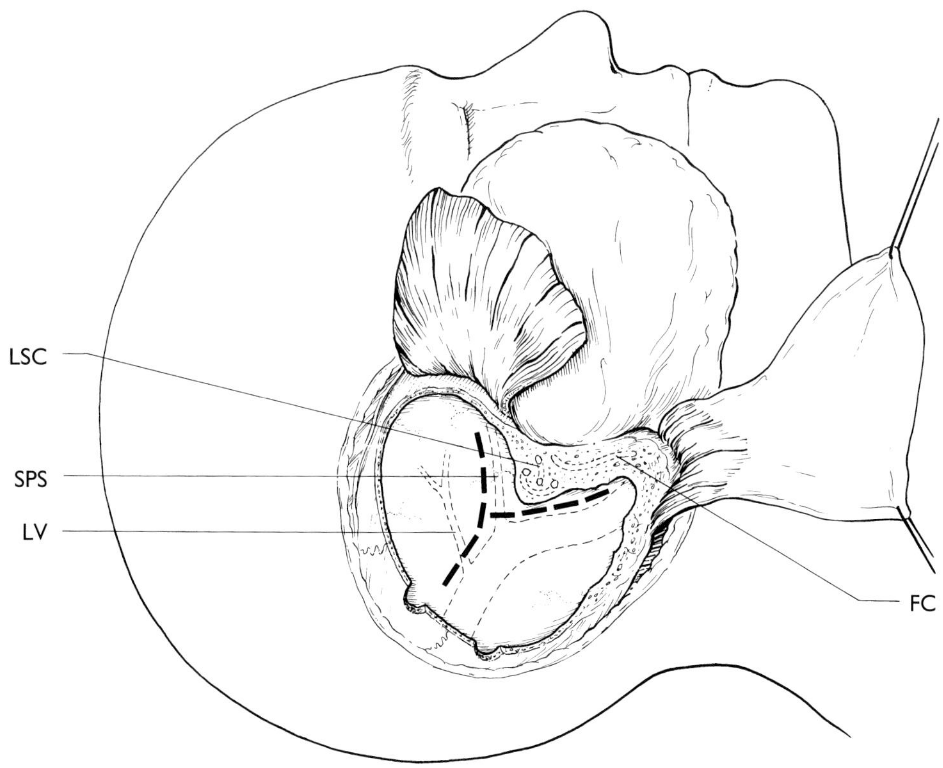

Figure 19-4. The petrous bone has been drilled away exposing the sigmoid sinus and the presigmoid dura mater with preservation of the labyrinth and the facial nerve within its canal. The positions of potential dural incision are marked. The temporal incision may expose the vein of Labbé, depending on its position and the extent of exposure required. If it is exposed it must be carefully dissected from the cortical surface to avoid traction, obstruction, and damage. The retrosigmoid dura may be incised to obtain extra exposure by working above and below the sinus.

debulked with extreme caution because the 7th and 8th cranial nerves, as well as the posterior inferior cerebellar artery (PICA) and anterior inferior cerebellar artery (AICA) may be embedded in the tumor. The trigeminal nerve rootlets are found under the tentorium, frequently stretched and splayed by the tumor (Fig. 19-5).

The tumor capsule is dissected free from the surrounding structures. Maintaining dissection within the arachnoidal planes is crucial to preserving the vital neural and vascular structures. The cut edge of the tumor should not be allowed to slip away lest the plane of cleavage be lost. The lower cranial nerves are dissected off the inferior pole of the tumor through the infratentorial avenue. Gentle dissection is required to avoid hypotension and bradycardia from vagal stimulation. If it is not embedded in the tumor, the basilar artery is usually displaced to the opposite side. The preservation of the main and small branches of the basilar artery cannot be overemphasized. If the tumor has extended into the internal auditory meatus, the meatus wall is drilled posteriorly and the tumor removed. Because the petrous apex contains no vital structures, it can easily be drilled away, exposing tumor attachments and facilitating dissection of the 5th and 6th cranial nerves. The area that can be removed extends from the internal auditory meatus to Meckel's cave and medial to the petrous carotid artery.

The dura is closed watertight. A fascia lata graft is used if necessary. The mastoidectomy cavity is filled with fat taken from the thigh. The temporal muscle is then rotated over the defect and sutured to the sternomastoid muscle, and the temporalis fascia flap is brought back to its original position and sutured into place (Fig. 19-6). The soft tissues are closed in layers.

If the tumor is large and a bigger access is needed, the amount of bone drilling can be increased to encompass the vestibule and semicircular canals (translabyrinthine) and even the cochlea (transcochlear) and adjoining air cells (transotic). All of these procedures sacrifice hearing for a better access to the tumor. In our practice, when hearing is absent, the translabyrinthine and transcochlear routes are always coupled to the petrosal craniotomy as described above.

Complications

Brain Stem Infarction

Ischemia is caused by surgical damage to vessels, which emphasizes the need for meticulous technique.

Temporal Lobe or Cerebellar Swelling

Temporal lobe or cerebellar swelling is precipitated by undue retraction and damage to the draining veins, especially the vein of Labbé and the basilar occipital veins, which must be protected.

Hematoma

Exact hemostasis is essential. Venous hemostasis may be deceptive when the veins are collapsed or with low pressure due to elevation of the head. Jugular vein compression and a Valsalva maneuver are essential to check hemostasis.

Cranial Nerve Injury

Although any cranial nerve deficit can cause unpleasant morbidity the most serious problem is injury to the jugular group of nerves. These may be more vulnerable

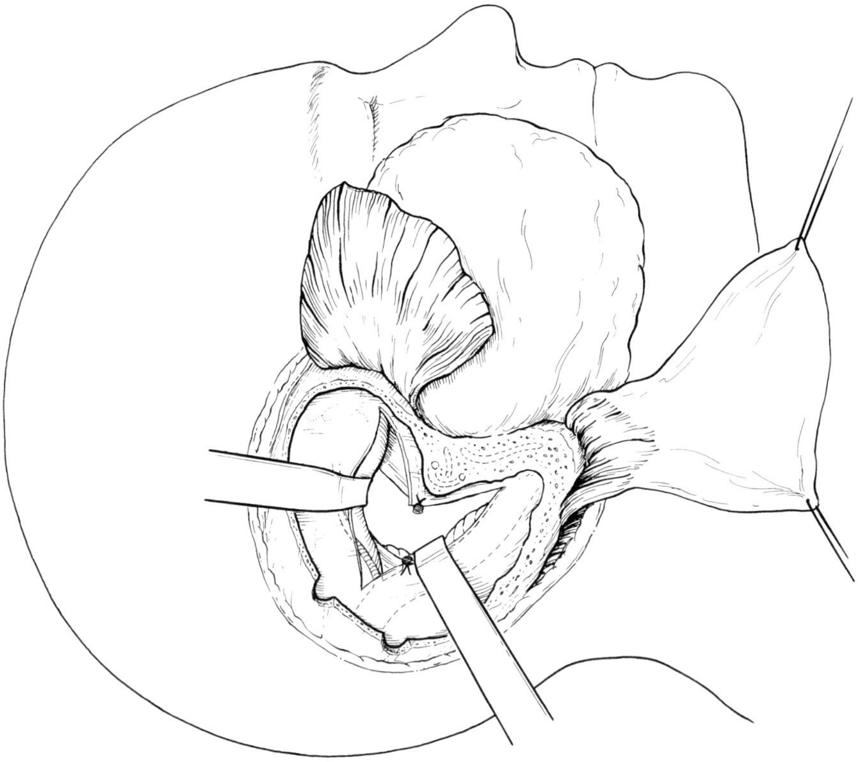

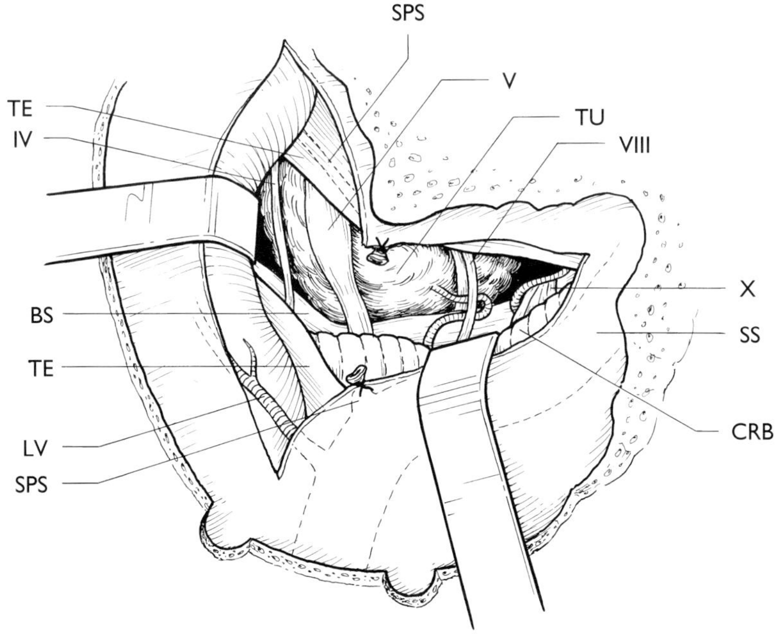

Figure 19-5. Following incision of the dura and section of the superior petrosal sinus the tentorium is incised forward and medially to the hiatus, avoiding the 4th cranial nerve. The tumor is exposed by retracting the temporal lobe superiorly and the cerebellum together with the sigmoid sinus medially.

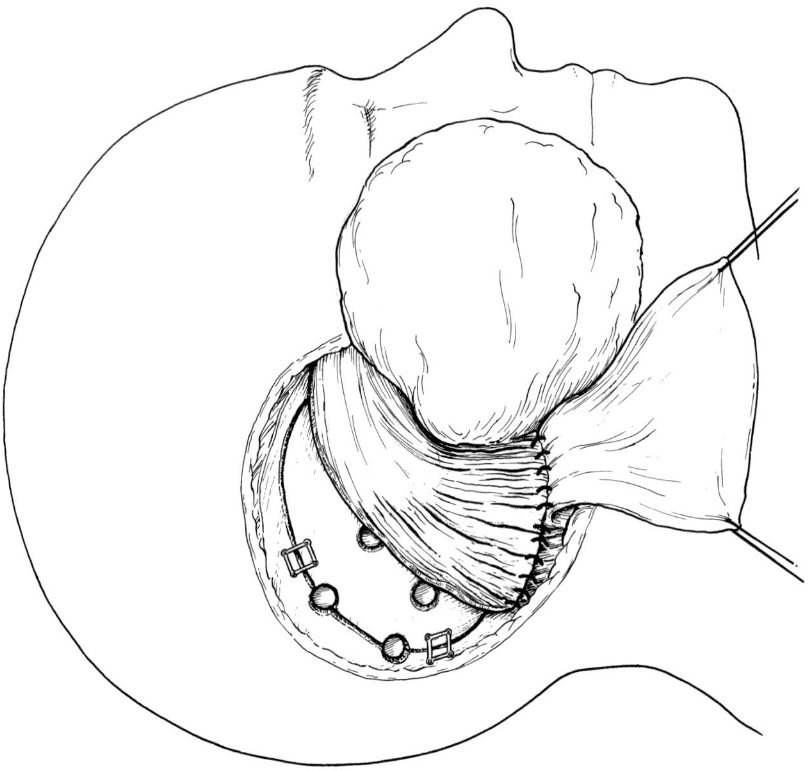

Figure 19-6. Closure. The free bone flap is replaced and fixed with microplates. The temporalis muscle is sutured to the sternomastoid and suboccipital muscles, thus covering the drilled area of the petrous bone. The temporalis fascial flap is returned to its original position.

because they run as separate rootlets. Intraoperative manipulation can cause bradycardia and hypotension. Paresis may precipitate aspiration pneumonia postoperatively. Nonadherent patties or wrapping with film helps protect the nerves intraoperatively.

CSF Leakage

CSF leakage is a serious complication associated with a 20 percent incidence of meningitis. It is best avoided by careful closure technique. The dura should be watertight, with patching and fibrin glue used as necessary. The petrous bone must also be watertight and waxing the surface may not be enough. The antrum or eustacian tube should be electively closed with fat and covered with a muscle patch and fibrin glue as necessary. The pericranial flap, fat, or both may be placed over the drilled area. The use of prophylactic spinal CSF drainage is wise in cases where the repair is unsatisfactory and is essential if a CSF leak is observed on more than one occasion. If hydrocephalus is an underlying factor then shunting is required.

20

Suboccipital Approach to Acoustic Neuromas

Yuichiro Tanaka
Shigeaki Kobayashi

The acoustic neuroma accounts for approximately 80 percent of cerebellopontine angle tumors and most of the acoustic neuromas originate from the vestibular nerve. The total length of vestibular nerve in the subarachnoid space is approximately 25 mm, consisting of a 10-mm segment in the internal auditory canal and a 15-mm segment in the cerebellopontine angle (Lang, 1991). The Obersteiner-Redlich zone, which is the border zone between the glial myelination and Schwann cell myelination, exists around the porus acusticus. Therefore, the tumor usually starts growing in the canal, because the tumor originates from the Schwann cell.

Three surgical approaches are mainly used: translabyrinthine, middle cranial fossa, and posterior fossa. The first two approaches were mainly developed by otolaryngologists and the third by neurosurgeons. The translabyrinthine approach has the advantage of allowing close observation of the intracanalicular portion of the tumor and the disadvantage of difficulty due to restricted visibility when removing a large tumor. The middle cranial fossa approach usually provides better access to the internal auditory canal than the posterior fossa approach. The middle cranial fossa approach, however, has a risk of temporal lobe contusion and postoperative cerebrospinal fluid leakage especially when applied to a large tumor.

The posterior fossa approach has the advantage of being applicable to tumors of all sizes. The surgical result is influenced by the following factors: size of the tumor, consistency of the tumor, whether cystic or not, direction of tumor growth, degree of adhesion between the tumor and nerves, and the surgeon's experience (Cohen et al., 1986; Ebersold et al., 1992; Fisher et al., 1992; Glasscock et al., 1993; Whittaker and Luetje, 1992; Yokoh et al., 1993). In this chapter, we describe our most familiar approach: the retrosigmoid suboccipital transmeatal approach (Rand and Kurze, 1968) with which 179 tumors have been treated during the last 16 years in our institute and affiliated hospitals.

Classification of the Acoustic Neuroma

The relationship between the internal auditory canal and tumor is important because, with the retrosigmoid suboccipital transmeatal approach, it is difficult to expose the tumor in the canal fully without damaging cochlear function. The tumor remnant left in the canal regrows more often than tumor left in other sites. The degree of tumor extension in the canal determines how far the canal should be exposed by drilling from the porus acusticus. On the other hand, the overall size of the tumor is a dominant factor influencing the preservation rate of postoperative facial and cochlear nerve function. We consider that two factors, extension of the tumor in the canal and tumor size, should be noted preoperatively as important factors determining the surgical strategy.

We classify acoustic neuromas into four types according to the extension of the tumor into the internal auditory canal and three tumor sizes from the surgical point of view (Fig. 20-1). Type I is the intracanalicular tumor without extension of the tumor into the cerebellopontine angle. Type II is a most common type entirely occupying the internal auditory canal with extracanalicular extension. Types III and IV, which were described as medial type tumors by Tos et al. (1992), leave a tumor-free space in the internal acoustic canal. In type III tumors, the internal auditory canal is partially filled with the tumor (Fig. 20-2). In type IV, the tumor grows exclusively in the cerebellopontine angle cistern without tumor extension into the internal auditory canal. The type III and IV tumors have the following characteristics: (1) the tumor tends to reach a large size when diagnosed, (2) preoperative hearing level is

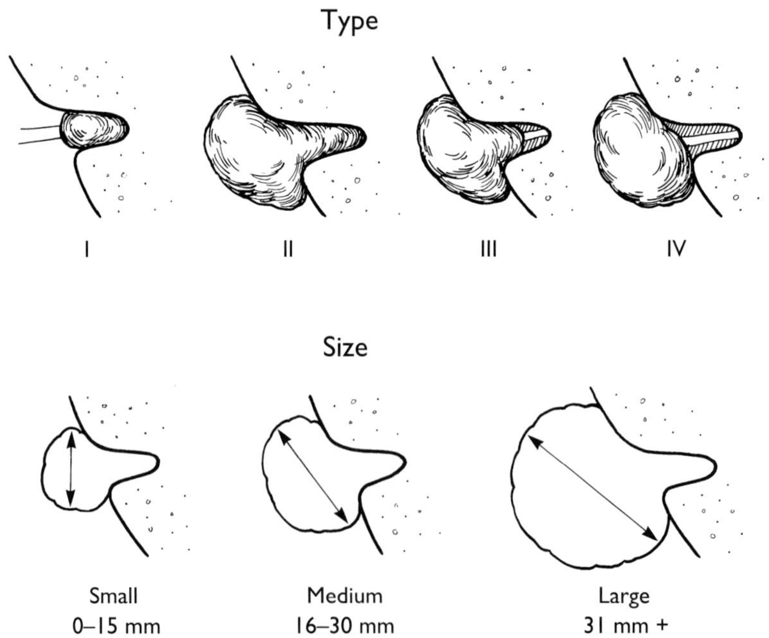

Figure 20-1. Classification of acoustic neuromas into four types according to the extension of the tumor into the internal auditory canal and three tumor sizes from the surgical point of view. Type I is an intracanalicular tumor without extension of the tumor into the cerebellopontine angle. Type II is the most common type, entirely occupying the internal auditory canal with extracanalicular extension. Types III and IV leave a tumor-free space in the internal acoustic canal. In type III tumors, the internal auditory canal is partially filled with the tumor. In type IV, the tumor grows exclusively in the cerebellopontine angle cistern without tumor extension into the internal auditory canal. The maximum diameter of the extracanalicular portion in the horizontal slice of CT scan or MRI is determined as the size of the tumor and is classified into three categories: small, medium, and large.

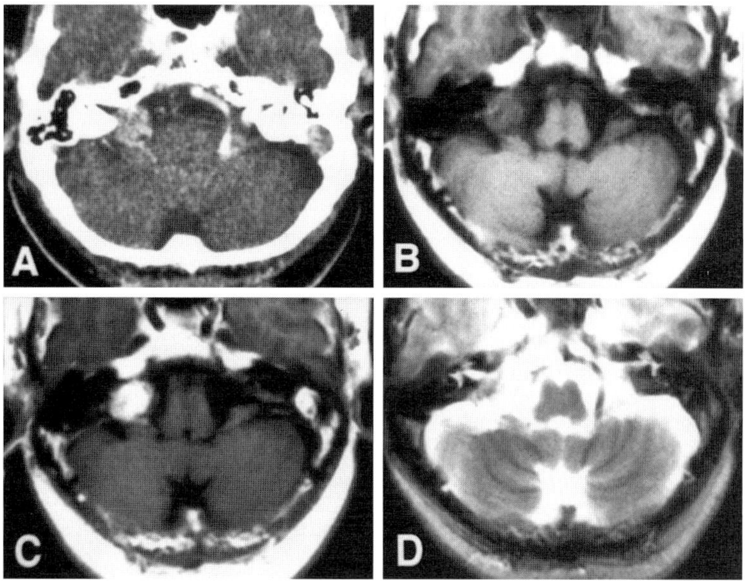

Figure 20-2. A case of type III-M tumor in a 61-year-old woman. *(A–C)* The internal auditory canal was partially filled with the tumor, leaving a high intensity area at the fundus in a T_2-weighted image *(D)*. The maximum diameter of the extracanalicular part of the tumor is 22 mm. *(A)* A CT scan with contrast enhancement. *(B)* An MRI T_1-weighted image without contrast enhancement. *(C)* An MRI T_1-weighted image with contrast enhancement.

relatively good, and (3) preservation of hearing is difficult unless the preoperative diagnosis of acoustic neuroma is exactly established.

The size of tumors is classified by the maximum diameter of the extracanalicular portion based on the preoperative computed tomography (CT) or magnetic resonance imaging (MRI) of axial slice across the internal auditory canal and is divided into three groups: small (less than 15 mm), medium (between 15 and 30 mm), and large (more than 30 mm).

The incidence of each type in our surgical series was 0 percent in type I, 81 percent in type II, 13 percent in type III, and 6 percent in type IV. Duvoisin et al. (1991) reported the incidence of type I as 21 percent, type II as 47 percent, type III as 27 percent, and type IV as 5 percent based on MRI findings. Tos et al. (1992) described the incidence of medial type tumor, corresponding to type III and IV, as 12 percent of their 400 surgical cases. Koos and Perneczky (1985) reported that 8 percent of acoustic neuromas were of the extracanalicular type (type IV). Preoperative diagnosis of the tumor as type IV is important to allow preservation of facial and cochlear nerve function. As the porus does not often enlarge, early identification of the porus acusticus during surgery is sometimes difficult in type IV tumor with the nerves having an increased likelihood of injury.

Positioning and Monitoring

Variable positioning of the patients has been reported, including lateral, three-quarter prone (park bench), prone, sitting, and supine lateral positions. We prefer the lateral position because of less incidence of air embolism and of a wide horizontal working space for the surgeons (Kobayashi and Sugita, 1987; Sugita and Kobayashi, 1982). The patient's head is fixed in the Sugita's headholder using four pins and with the following precautions. The head is elevated higher than heart level and maximally flexed anteriorly, but not to the degree that the endotracheal tube is compressed; the head is then rotated 30 to 45 degrees with the face downward to keep

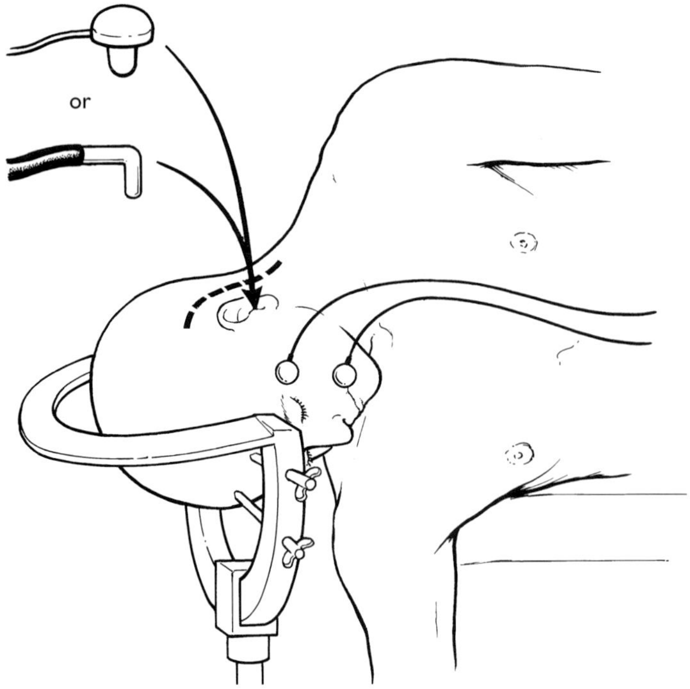

Figure 20-3. The patient's head position and skin incision (dashed line) for a left acoustic tumor. Two motion sensors are placed on the orbicularis oris and oculi, respectively. An earphone or illuminator of the mastoid air cell is put in the external auditory canal for an intraoperative auditory-evoked potential or for surgical orientation at the time of craniotomy.

the posterior margin of the petrous bone vertical and the patient's shoulder on the tumor side is stretched downward.

A facial nerve monitoring system consisting of a stimulator and tremograms to detect facial muscle movement is routinely used. Auditory brain stem responses (ABR) are recorded intraoperatively in the case of serviceable hearing according to the 50-50 rule (Fig. 20-3).

Skin Incision and Craniotomy

In the retrosigmoid transmeatal approach, the size of the craniotomy is recommended to be large enough to drill away the posterior lip without opening the vestibule and semicircular canals (Fig. 20-4). To accomplish the large craniotomy, an S-shaped skin incision 12 cm long is made 3 or 4 cm behind the hairline and 5 cm from the mastoid process. Illumination of the mastoid air cells (Tanaka et al., 1995), in which an illuminating fiber cable is placed inside the external auditory canal, is helpful for estimating the position of the sigmoid sinus (Fig. 20-5). In the majority of cases, the posterior margin of the illuminated air cell indicates the position of the sigmoid sinus. A gap between the posterior margin of the mastoid air cells and the position of the sigmoid sinus is easily identified from the CT findings.

Tumor Removal of the Extracanalicular Portion

Meticulous manipulation to peel off the arachnoid fold covering the tumor from the side of the porus acusticus to the brain stem is the first step in preserving the vessels

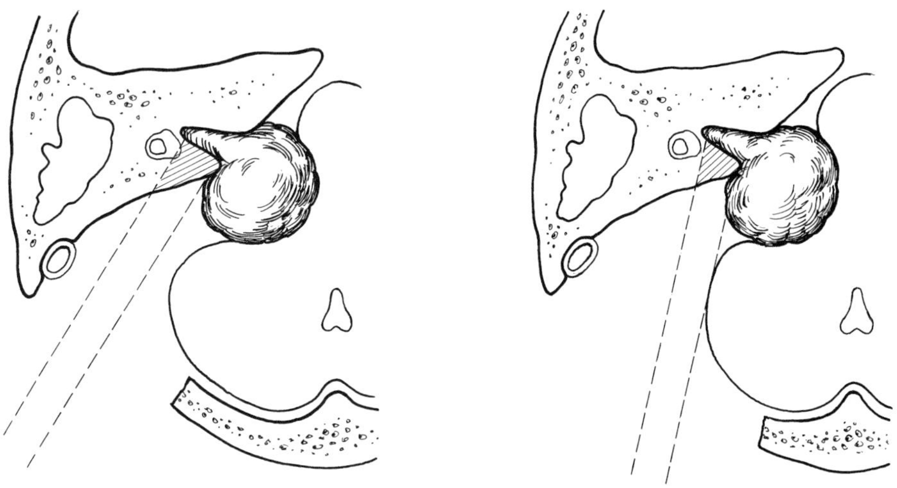

A B

Figure 20-4. Relationship between the size of the craniotomy and the direction of the approach route to the internal auditory canal. *(A)* When the size of craniotomy is small, resection of the posterior lip may injure the vestibule or semicircular canal. *(B)* A large craniotomy affords the proper angle to accomplish the bone removal without damaging the labyrinth.

over the cerebellum. Identification of the facial nerve at the root exit zone is not difficult in a small tumor. In a medium or large tumor, internal decompression of the extracanalicular portion should be done before trying to find the facial and cochlear nerves at the junction with the brain stem. In a patient with useful hearing preoperatively, intraoperative identification of the cochlear nerve should be performed in the early stage of tumor dissection to help achieve functional preservation.

Crossing of the facial and cochlear nerves is a good landmark for identifying the location of the cochlear nerve especially in medium and large tumors (Fig. 20-6). The facial nerve is usually detected at the caudal end of the tumor and is confirmed by electrical stimulation. It is essential to keep the surgical field free from blood in order to find and follow the facial and cochlear nerves on the surface of the tumor. Silicone (Silastic) sheet and tubing are useful to protect the cerebellum, cranial

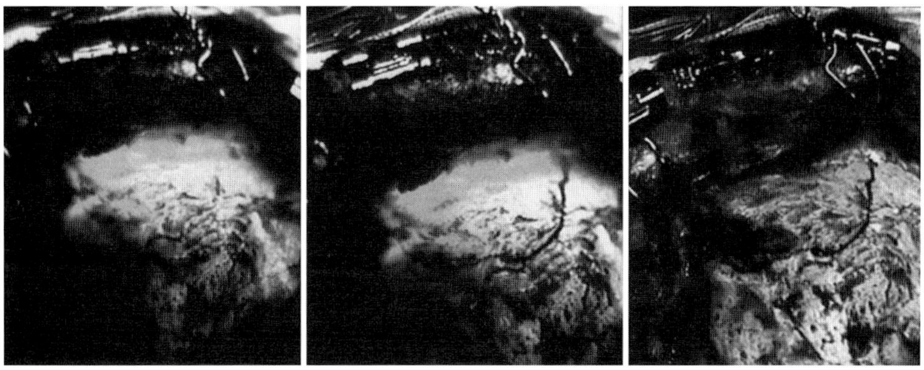

A B C

Figure 20-5. The surface of the left mastoid and occipital bone showing the illumination method to delineate the posterior margin of the mastoid air cell. *(A)* The mastoid air cell is illuminated through the outer table of the skull. *(B)* The posterior margin of the illuminated air cell is delineated by nontoxic ink and *(C)* the illumination is turned off. This method is helpful for estimating the position of the sigmoid sinus at the time of craniotomy.

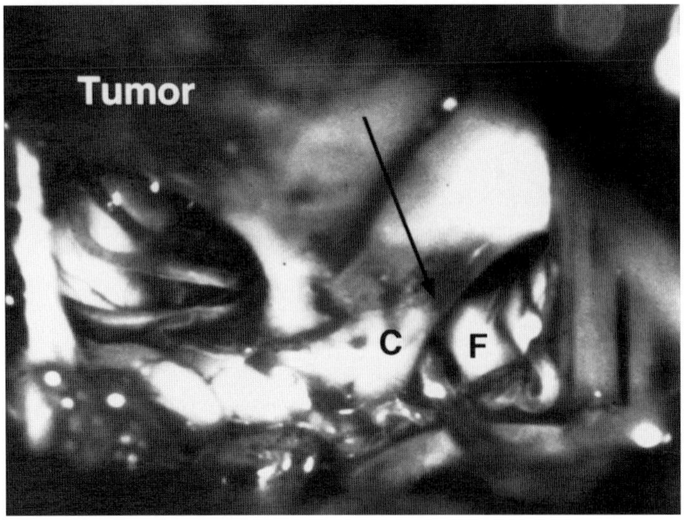

Figure 20-6. An intraoperative photograph showing the crossing (arrow) of the facial (F) and cochlear (C) nerves at the caudal side of the tumor. This relationship is maintained even in the large tumor. The cochlear nerve can be identified after confirming the facial nerve by electrical stimulation.

nerves, and vessels from damage by surgical manipulation (Shibuya et al., 1991; Tanaka et al., 1993) (Fig. 20-7). We use either a cotton sheet or a silicone rubber sheet to protect the brain, nerves, and vessels when mechanical injuries are anticipated. The silicone sheet enables us to observe the underlying tissue because of its translucency, and to avoid electrical injury, adhesion to tissue, and the catastrophe that may happen if a cotton patty is rolled up by drilling.

A rake retractor is helpful for keeping the tumor away from the nerves. We developed several different kinds of rake retractors, of which the most suitable type is chosen depending on the tumor consistency, tumor size, and direction of retraction (Fig. 20-8). Several different kinds of microdissectors should be prepared and the

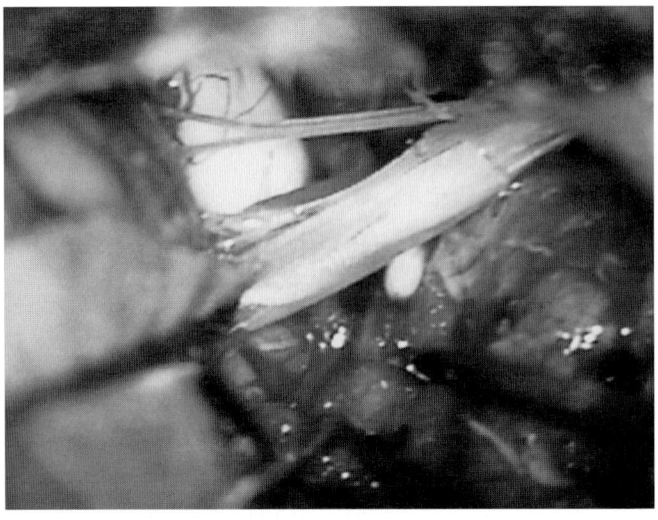

Figure 20-7. An intraoperative photograph showing a Silastic tube applied to the 9th, 10th, and 11th cranial nerve complex to avoid an inadvertent injury by surgical manipulation.

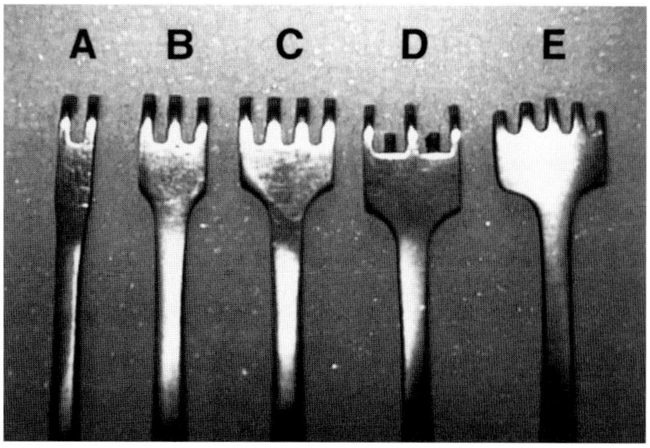

Figure 20-8. Various shapes of rake retractor. The most suitable one should be selected depending on the consistency of the tumor. A retractor with zigzag nails (D) is useful to retract a soft tumor to minimize the destruction of the tumor.

most suitable one is selected based on the situation during dissection of the nerves from the tumor. We prepare silver dissectors of variable angles, shapes, and sharpness that can be remodeled during the operation if necessary (Fig. 20-9).

An ultrasonic aspirator with a light-weight handpiece is very helpful for removing a part of the tumor tightly adherent to the nerves (Fig. 20-10). Compared with the previous model, the weight has been reduced approximately to half, allowing the surgeon to make quick and delicate movement as if using an ordinary suction tube. The more recent design enables us to change the tip of the aspirator to a smaller caliber (1.2 mm in outer diameter) for removing the intracanalicular tumor and to a larger caliber (1.8 mm in outer diameter) for performing internal decompression of the extracanalicular part. Excessive traction of nerves can be avoided by use of the aspirator when removing a tumor tightly adherent to the nerve.

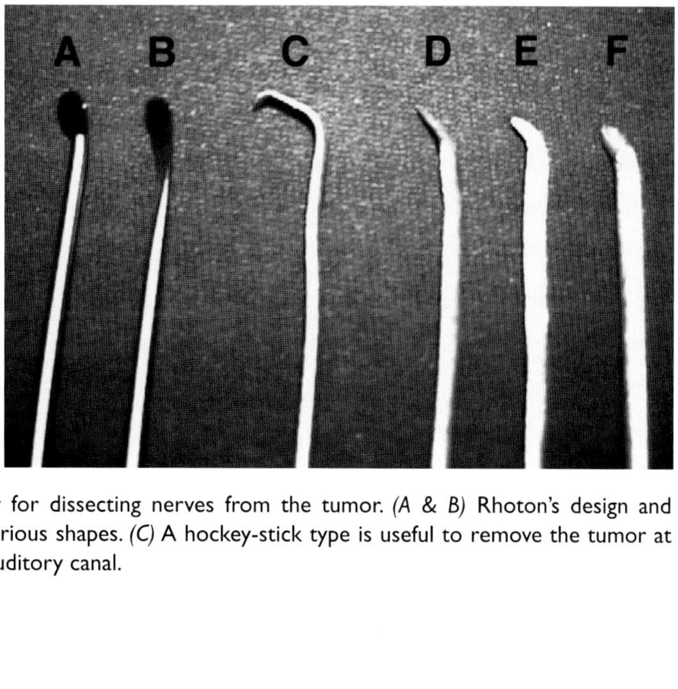

Figure 20-9. Microdissector for dissecting nerves from the tumor. *(A & B)* Rhoton's design and *(C–F)* silver dissectors of various shapes. *(C)* A hockey-stick type is useful to remove the tumor at the fundus of the internal auditory canal.

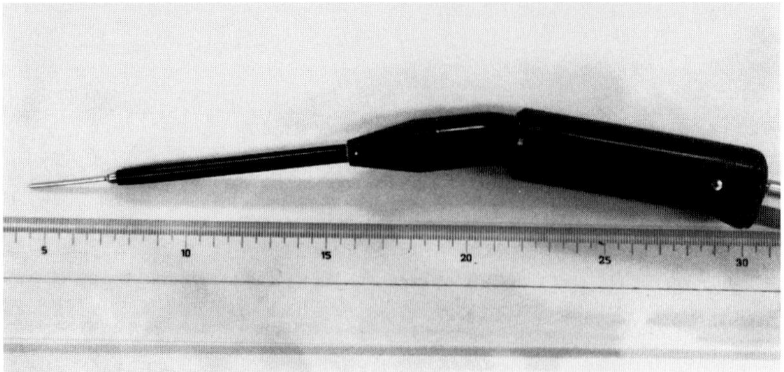

Figure 20-10. A micro-ultrasonic aspirator (Microsonop) specially designed for acoustic neuroma surgery. The instrument is characterized by an ultra-lightweight and an exchangeable tip of different calibers.

Tumor Removal of Intracanalicular Portion

As much bone resection of the posterior lip should be done as possible to accomplish total removal of the tumor in the canal. Staged drilling is recommended to remove the posterior lip effectively without injuring the facial and cochlear nerves, removing the bone grossly with a 3-mm drill head first, incising the dura and removing the tumor partially, and finally resecting the bone further with a 1-mm drill head using a tapered spatula or Silastic sheet to protect the nerves (Fig. 20-11). The common crus is most prone to damage. In some cases, the mastoid air cell extends into the posterior lip and the jugular bulb reaches up to the level of the internal auditory canal. The preoperative high-resolution CT scan is essential for performing the removal of the posterior lip with precision and safety (Tantagiba et al., 1992).

When the posterior lip is not fully resected, a microsurgical mirror is useful for observing the fundus of the canal. An illuminated mirror is helpful for close observation (Fig. 20-12). An illuminated mirror has the advantage of allowing a clearer view

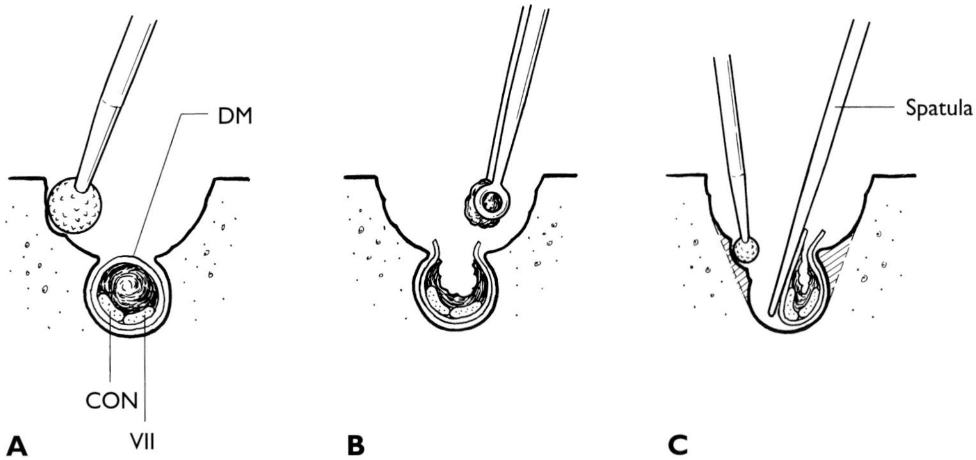

Figure 20-11. Diagrams showing a method of staged drilling of the posterior lip of the internal auditory canal. *(A)* Drilling of the posterior lip is started with a 3-mm drill head. *(B)* After incising the dura (DM) and debulking the tumor in the canal, *(C)* a 1-mm drill head is used to remove further bone with protection of facial (VII) and cochlear (CON) nerves by a tapered spatula (right).

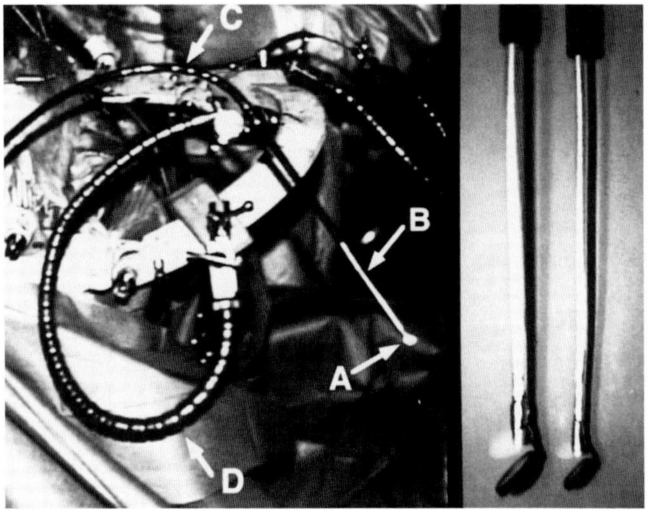

Figure 20-12. A flexible illuminating mirror system. (A) A mirror with a (B) malleable rod that contains illuminating fibers is sustained with a (D) self-retaining retractor to keep the mirror consistently in the proper position. (C) Fiber optic cable conducting the light.

without cloudiness than a regular mirror. When the mirror is attached to the self-retaining retractor, a hockey-stick type silver dissector is useful for removing the tumor without damage to the nerve in the canal (Fig. 20-10). A malleable rod that contains illuminating fibers does not disturb the visual access to the lesion.

Surgical Results and Complications

Between August 1978 and March 1995, 179 unilateral acoustic neuromas had been operated on in our institute and affiliated hospitals. Seven patients were first treated in the other hospitals and referred to ours. The other 172 patients, who were initially admitted to our institutes, were analyzed regarding the overall surgical result. The age ranged from 17 to 82 (mean 52.8 ± 12.9) years and the female to male ratio was 116:56. The side of the tumor was almost even: the right side in 85 patients and the left in 87. The size of the tumor varied from 5 to 60 (mean 32.0 ± 12.7) mm. The surgical approach was by the suboccipital route in 170 patients and by the subtemporal route in 2 patients.

Major complications were encountered in three patients: one patient was severely disturbed due to cerebellar contusion caused by technical failure handling an air drill, another patient remains in a vegetative state due to postoperative hemorrhage, and the last died of meningitis. The latter two cases were experienced in the early period of the present series. The extent of removal was classified into the following four grades; total removal (100 percent), nearly total removal (99 percent, leaving a small fragment of tumor capsule), subtotal removal (90 to 99 percent), and partial removal (less than 90 percent). In our surgical series, total removal was accomplished in 95 cases (55.2 percent), nearly total removal in 49 (28.5 percent), subtotal removal in 27 (15.7 percent), and partial removal in 1 (0.6 percent).

Recurrence or regrowth of the tumor occurred in 8 cases (4.7 percent). The extent of removal of the tumor in the initial surgery was "total removal" in 2 patients, nearly total removal in 4, and subtotal removal in 2. The interval between the initial operation and the second operation ranged from 2 to 9 (mean 5.1) years. Cyst formation (5 of 8) was the characteristic CT and MRI finding when tumor recurrence was detected. The tumor entirely occupied the internal auditory canal at the time of the second operation in all 8 cases. Therefore, the tumor is suspected to recur from a remnant left in the internal auditory canal. It is recommended that MRI follow-up be performed 10 years after operation even if the tumor is thought to be removed totally.

Facial paresis was observed preoperatively in 13.4 percent of the cases (House and Brackmann grade 2 in 22 cases and grade 3 in 1). Anatomic preservation of the facial nerve was accomplished in 97.1 percent of the cases. End-to-end anastomoses were performed intraoperatively in 4 of the 5 cases where the facial nerve was interrupted. The final functional outcome of facial movement was normal (grade 1) in 43 percent, mild paresis (grade 2, 3) in 30 percent, moderate paresis (grade 4, 5) in 16 percent, and severe paresis (grade 6) in 11 percent. Useful hearing (pure tone average less than 50 dB) was recorded preoperatively in 45 cases (26 percent). Anatomic preservation of the cochlear nerve was achieved in 32 cases (71 percent) and functional preservation of hearing in 8 (25 percent). Recent advances in technology and surgical techniques encourage us to improve the functional outcome even in the large tumor (Torrens et al., 1994).

References

Cohen NL, Hammerschlag P, Berg H et al. (1986) Acoustic neuroma surgery: an eclectic approach with emphasis on preservation of hearing. Ann Otol Rhinol Laryngol 95:21–27

Duvoisin B, Fernandes J, Doyon D et al. (1991) Magnetic resonance findings in 92 acoustic neuromas. Eur J Radiol 13:96–102

Ebersold MJ, Harner SG, Beatty CW et al. (1992) Current results of the retrosigmoid approach to acoustic neurinoma. J Neurosurg 76:901–909

Fisher G, Fisher C, Rémond J (1992) Hearing preservation in acoustic neurinoma surgery. J Neurosurg 76:910–917

Glasscock ME III, Hays JW, Minor LB et al. (1993) Preservation of hearing in surgery for acoustic neuromas. J Neurosurg 78:864–870

Kobayashi S, Sugita K (1987) Acoustic neurinoma surgery by lateral suboccipital craniectomy. Neurosurgeons (Jpn) 6:192–198

Koos WT, Perneczky A (1985) Suboccipital approach to acoustic neurinomas with emphasis on preservation of facial nerve and cochlear nerve function. pp. 335–365. In Rand RW: Microneurosurgery. Mosby, St. Louis

Lang J (1991) Clinical anatomy of the posterior cranial fossa and its foramina pp. 83–91. Thieme, Stuttgart

Rand RW, Kurze T (1968) Preservation of vestibular, cochlear, and facial nerves during microsurgical removal of acoustic tumors: Report of two cases. J Neurosurg 28:158–161

Shibuya M, Sugita K, Kobayashi S (1991) Intraoperative protection of cranial nerves and perforating arteries by silicone rubber sheets. J Neurosurg 74:677–679

Sugita K, Kobayashi S (1982) Technical and instrumental improvements in the surgical treatment of acoustic neurinomas. J Neurosurg 57:747–752

Tanaka Y, Kobayashi S, Hongo K, Oikawa S (1993) Intraoperative protection of cranial nerves and arteries by split silicone tube. Neurosurgery 33:523–525

Tanaka Y, Kobayashi S, Unoki T et al. (1995) Illumination of mastoid air cell for suboccipital craniotomy: Technical note. Neurosurgery 39:1049–1051

Tantagiba M, Samii M, Matthies C et al. (1992) The significance for postoperative hearing of preserving the labyrinth in acoustic neurinoma surgery. J Neurosurg 77:677–684

Torrens M, Maw R, Coakham H, Butler S (1994) Facial and acoustic nerve preservation during excision of extracanalicular acoustic neuromas using the suboccipital approach. Br J Neurosurg 8:655–665

Tos M, Drozdziewicz D, Thomsen J (1992) Medial acoustic neuromas. A new clinical entity. Arch Otolaryngol Head Neck Surg 118:127–133
Whittaker CK, Luetje CM (1992) Vestibular schwannomas. J Neurosurg 76:897–900
Yokoh A, Kobayashi S, Tanaka Y et al. (1993) Preservation of cochlear nerve function in acoustic neurinoma surgery. Acta Neurochir 123:8–13

21

Far Lateral Approach to the Foramen Magnum

Gerald F. Tuite
H. Alan Crockard

Diagnosis and treatment of foramen magnum lesions has long proven challenging. They produce nonspecific and sometimes misleading signs and symptoms and diagnosis is difficult based on clinical findings alone (Stein et al., 1963). Until recently, radiographic imaging of this area has been limited. Once diagnosed, these lesions have been difficult to approach surgically, with access limited by bone and important neurovascular structures. However, with advances in imaging and surgical techniques, they are now more easily diagnosed and approached more safely and successfully.

There is a broad spectrum of surgically treatable pathology in this area, both intradural and extradural. Foramen magnum tumors account for 5 percent of all spinal and 1 percent of all intracranial neoplasms. Meningiomas and neurinomas account for over 90 percent of the tumors in this area, with the former occurring twice as frequently as the latter. Other intradural tumors include epidermoids, gliomas, and neurenteric cysts. Extradural tumors include chordomas, chondromas, chondrosarcomas, and metastasis (George et al., 1993). The area may also be affected by vascular diseases such as posterior circulation aneurysms or arterovenous malformations; by inflammatory conditions such as rheumatoid arthritis; by metabolic diseases such as the mucopolysaccharidoses or osteogenesis imperfecta; or by traumatic conditions such as atlantoaxial rotatory subluxation or occipitocervical dislocation (Crockard, 1993; Crockard and Johnston, 1993; Crockard and Rogers, 1995; Crockard et al., 1991; George et al., 1993; Harkey et al., 1990; Kuttner, 1917; Meyer et al., 1984; Stein et al., 1963).

The entire circumference of the foramen magnum may be affected by disease, but the bulk of pathology that compresses the neuraxis is ventral or ventrolateral in position. Sixty-five percent of meningiomas and neurofibromas are located ventrolateral to the spinal cord (Stein et al., 1963). To be able to best treat this wide range of lesions the surgeon must be proficient with several approaches.

The far lateral approach is ideally suited to a wide variety of lesions of the craniovertebral junction. However, a thorough knowledge of the anatomy of this area is necessary to avoid potentially devastating complications. The bony and neurologic structures are familiar to most surgeons, but the course of the vertebral artery is the most important and least familiar anatomic course to master.

Anatomy Relevant to the Far Lateral Approach

After originating from the subclavian artery, the vertebral artery traverses the transverse foramina of the upper six cervical vertebrae to its dural entry at the craniovertebral junction. From a posterior perspective, the artery is well protected between C6 and C2 as it passes ventral to the facet joints and the 7th through 3rd cranial nerve roots. The artery is more accessible at the C1-C2 intertransverse space as it takes a lateral course to the transverse foramen of the atlas. At this level, the artery can be consistently found caudal to the inferior oblique muscle, which originates on the spinous process of the axis and inserts on the transverse process of the atlas (Henry, 1973). Under this muscle there is a rich venous plexus and the C2 nerve root; as with the other spinal levels, the artery consistently lies ventral to the primary ventral ramus of the nerve.

After looping laterally between the atlas and the axis, the artery passes through the transverse foramen of C1 and courses medially along the cephalic surface of the C1 lamina, within the sulcus arteriosus (George and Laurian, 1987; Lang, 1986; Lister et al., 1982). After a short medial course, it enters the dural sac ventral to the lateral border of the atlanto-occipital membrane. Between the atlas and the foramen magnum, the C1 nerve root passes caudal to the artery within the sulcus arteriosus and then dorsal further laterally.

Intradurally, the artery passes superomedially and joins the contralateral vertebral artery to form the basilar artery (DeOliveira et al., 1985). The arteries join near the pontomedullary junction, but the precise level is variable due to variations in the size and tortuosity of the vertebral artery.

The artery has many branches along its course. Intradurally, the anterior spinal artery is usually formed from the most distal portion of the vertebral arteries, although a single vertebral origin augmented by vertebral radicular branches at C2 or C3 is a common variant (Lang, 1986). The posteroinferior cerebellar artery (PICA) is usually the most proximal major branch of the intradural vertebral artery, but it may originate occasionally from the extradural segment of the artery (DeOliveira et al., 1985). The posterior spinal artery has widely variable origins, from either the PICA or the intra- or extradural segments of the vertebral artery. Branches of the extradural vertebral artery are variable and plentiful between C2 and the dural entry: they usually include the anterior and posterior meningeal arteries as well as a variable number of radiculomuscular branches (Lang, 1986). It is important to remember that in patients with lesions at the craniovertebral junction, the vascular supply of the upper cervical spinal cord can be variable, with collaterals obtained from the extradural segment of the vertebral artery.

The vertebral artery passes from the dorsal to the ventral surface of the medulla. Throughout its course, the 6th through 12th cranial nerves generally pass dorsal to the artery. However, individual variation exists and some rootlets may pass ventral to this vessel. The facial and vestibulocochlear nerves arise from the pontomedullary junction, dorsal to the vertebral artery, and pass through the internal auditory meatus. The glossopharyngeal and vagus nerves arise from the dorsal margin of the medulla and pass laterally, through the jugular foramen. The spinal accessory nerve arises from the upper spinal cord and lower medulla: the spinal rootlets pass cephalad, dorsal to the dentate ligament, through the foramen magnum and jugular foramen. The medullary rootlets of the spinal accessory nerve pass directly through the jugular foramen. The hypoglossal nerve originates from the lower part of the medulla, in line with the ventral spinal rootlets, to pass laterally through the hypoglossal canal (DeOliveira et al., 1985; Rhoton and DeOliveira, 1991). There are connections between the hypoglossal, glossopharyngeal, spinal accessory, and C2 nerves that may give rise to a variety of "neck and tongue" syndromes (Orrell and Marsden, 1994).

The dentate ligament originates from pia mater on the lateral part of the spinal cord, between the ventral and dorsal nerve rootlets. The first dentate ligament attaches to the pia mater at the level of the foramen magnum, dorsal to the vertebral artery. The second dentate ligament has its pial attachment between the first and second nerve rootlet dural exits. The dorsal rootlets of C1 arise from branches of the spinal accessory nerve, but all other dorsal and all ventral rootlets arise from the corresponding levels of the spinal cord (Rhoton and DeOliveira, 1991).

Advantages and Disadvantages of the Approaches to the Foramen Magnum

The principal factors restricting access to lesions of the craniovertebral junction are its dense bony encasement and the presence of vital neurovascular structures. Extensive bony exposure is often necessary to allow optimal visualization of lesions without retraction of the neuraxis. The posterior midline approach allows lengthy sagittal exposure from the skull base through the entirety of the spine, but lateral exposure is restricted by the danger involved in the removal of ventrolateral bone without good visualization or control of the vertebral artery (Stein et al., 1963). The transoral approach provides easy access to the lower clivus and first and second cervical vertebrae: with addition of an extended maxillotomy or labiomandibulotomy and glossotomy it can provide access from the top of the clivus to the midcervical spine (Ashraf et al., 1991; Crockard et al., 1991, Crockard and Sen, 1991; Crockard and Johnston, 1993; Harkey et al., 1990). However, the lateral bone removal is limited through the transoral route by the vertebral and carotid arteries at the spinal and clival levels, respectively. At the foramen magnum the vertebral arteries are only separated by an average of 14 mm (Crockard and Johnston, 1993). The far lateral approach, however, provides both a lengthy and wide exposure from the skull base down the length of the cervical spine (Bertalanffy and Seeger, 1991; Crockard and Rogers, 1995; George, 1989; George et al., 1988; Gilsbach, 1991; Heros, 1986; Kratimenos and Crockard, 1993, 1994; Perneczy, 1986; Sen and Sekhar, 1990, 1991; Spetzler and Grahm, 1990; Verbiest, 1968). This approach allows more extensive bone removal because of early visualization and proximal control of the vertebral artery and improved access to the ventral and dorsal spine (Table 21-1).

The need for concomitant stabilization and fusion may become necessary as a result of the primary disease or because of iatrogenic instability secondary to surgical

Table 21-1. Advantages and Disadvantages of Approaches to the Foramen Magnum

	Posterior Midline	Transoral	Far Lateral
Access to lateral lesions	Limited	Limited	Excellent
Vascular control	Limited	None	Excellent
Risk of meningitis with intradural lesions	Low	High	Low
Concomitant bony stabilization	Possible	Limited	Possible

bone removal after any craniovertebral procedure (Spetzler and Grahm, 1990). The standard posterior midline and far lateral approaches infrequently result in instability, but the transoral approach is usually followed by dorsal fusion because of the propensity for postoperative instability. In cases of instability, the posterior midline and far lateral approaches are well suited for concomitant fusion and stabilization. However, fusion or instrumentation through the transoral exposure is difficult, unreliable, and fraught with complications; if stabilization and fusion are necessary after transoral procedures, a separate posterior approach is usually performed (Table 21-1).

Lesions of the foramen magnum often encase or are supplied by the vertebral artery. The posterior midline approach allows visualization of a short segment of the vertebral artery within the sulcus arteriosus, but control distal to its dural entry or proximal to the atlas is difficult from a strictly posterior approach. Vascular control through the transoral route is nearly impossible because of limited exposure and bony impediments. The far lateral approach offers extensive control and visualization of the vertebral artery, without retraction of the spinal cord or brain stem. With knowledge of the pertinent landmarks, the vertebral artery can be readily exposed, controlled, and mobilized through this approach (Table 21-1).

Removal of intradural pathology can lead to difficulties with cerebrospinal fluid (CSF) leaks through any approach. The posterior midline and far lateral approaches provide a tight seal through layered muscle and skin closure. CSF leakage can be particularly problematic after the transoral approach: the dura is difficult to repair, there is a limited soft tissue closure, and the CSF is exposed to the bacterially colonized pharynx (Table 21-1) (Crockard and Sen, 1991).

Choosing the Most Appropriate Surgical Route

Before the best surgical approach can be chosen, a thorough radiographic investigation should be completed in each case. Magnetic resonance imaging (MRI) is the study of choice for detailing the relationship of the lesion to the neurovascular structures. Computed tomography (CT) is necessary to delineate the bony anatomy. MR angiography is useful to determine the patency and position of the vertebral artery, but the vascular supply of the lesion and neuraxis is best studied with cerebral angiography. Suspected instability can be evaluated by plain radiographs and CT scanning in flexion and extension. Each study is useful in the preoperative surgical planning; the exact type will depend on the presumed pathologic diagnosis and bony stability of the craniovertebral joints.

These radiographic studies provide detail about the relative position of neurovascular structures, the origin of the lesion, and the vascular supply. All of these factors are important in choosing the most appropriate approach. However, minimizing or eliminating spinal cord and brain stem retraction are of paramount importance in choosing the best route; other factors should be considered secondarily (Fig. 21-1).

Lesions that lie in the midline, dorsal to the spinal cord, displace neurovascular structures ventrally and can be exposed through the posterior midline approach. For most surgeons, the relative ease, familiarity, low risk of CSF leak, and the diversity of possible fusion techniques make this an attractive approach to dorsal midline lesions. Similarly, midline ventral lesions displace neurovascular structures dorsally and can be approached transorally. Extradural and bony lesions that lie in the ventral midline, without vertebral artery involvement, are particularly well suited for this approach. However, both the posterior midline and transoral routes should not be used if retraction of the neuraxis, vascular control, or vertebral artery mobilization are necessary to address ventral or lateral components of the lesion (Fig. 21-1).

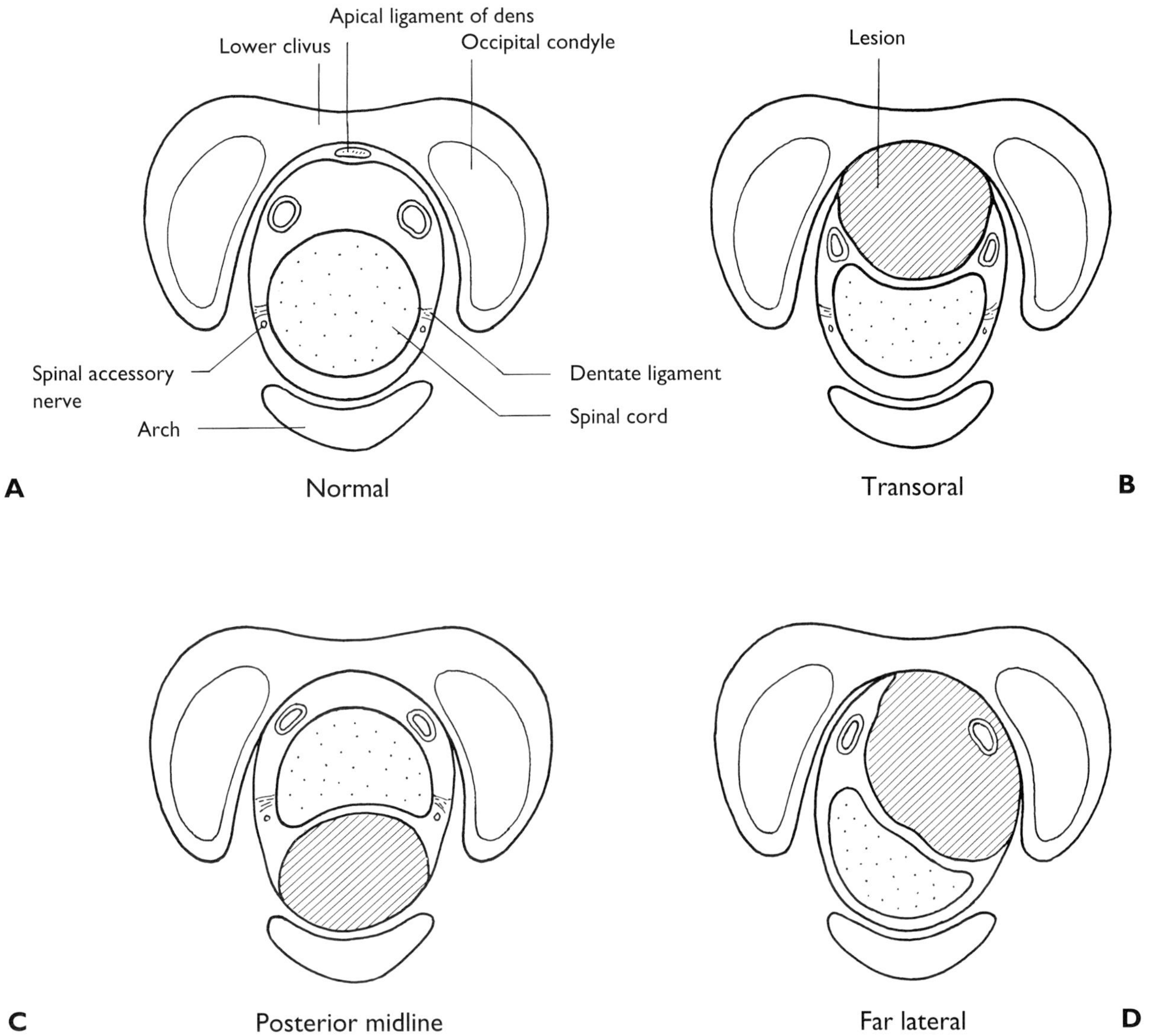

Figure 21-1. The choice of the appropriate surgical approach to lesions of the foramen magnum is primarily determined by the location of the lesion relative to the neuraxis. *(A)* Normal relationship of the neuraxis and vertebral artery relative to the bony aperture. *(B)* Typical extradural lesion best approached transorally. *(C)* Intradural lesion suitable for the posterior midline approach. *(D)* Ventrolateral lesion best approached through a far lateral approach.

Ventrolateral lesions of the foramen magnum, the most common lesions in this area, can displace neurovascular structures in various directions. Their relative position is variable, but the spinal cord is often displaced dorsomedially, the cranial and spinal nerves are pushed dorsally, and the vertebral artery and its branches are displaced ventrally (Fig. 21-1). The far lateral approach offers the widest, most direct, and versatile route to these lesions.

Operative Technique: The Far Lateral Approach

Intubation, Monitoring, and Positioning

If there is any cervical deformity or instability, awake fiberoptic nasotracheal intubation is essential (Calder et al., 1995). For intradural pathology, a lumbar CSF drain is inserted prior to final patient positioning. Somatosensory evoked potential and lower cranial nerve monitoring is then positioned and recorded throughout the operation.

The patent is placed in the true lateral position with an axillary roll and the head fixed in the Mayfield headholder. The head is placed in slight lateral tilt, contralateral to the lesion, with 10 degrees of anterior flexion (Fig. 21-2). Once in position and well-padded, the patient is secured by generous taping and bracing. Elevating the head of the operating table can reduce venous bleeding. Lowering the head of the table combined with angling the microscope from caudal to cephalad allows greater intracranial visualization and can lessen the necessary bone removal (Fig. 21-3). Exposure in the axial plane can be improved by using the lateral tilt function to improve access ventral and dorsal to the neuraxis (Fig. 21-3). These maneuvers to improve visibility and hemostasis are only possible if the patient is firmly secured to the operating table. Skin preparation is performed on the neck and dorsal skull. The iliac crest and distal lower extremity are also prepared in anticipation of possible fusion or vascular repair.

Skin Incision, Exposure, and Bone Removal

The skin incision is begun 4 cm above and 2.5 cm medial to the mastoid tip, descending in a gentle curve dorsal to the sternocleidomastoid muscle, down to the C4 level (Fig. 21-2). Dissection is then carried through the subcutaneous tissues, to the muscular fascia. Access to the lateral spine is then gained through a fatty plane that was originally described by Henry (1973). This plane is defined by dorsal musculature consisting of the splenius capitis, semispinalis, and longissimus capitis. The ventral musculature is composed of the levator scapulae and the scalene muscles. Blunt dissection through this plane provides free access to the transverse process of C1 and the lateral masses of the lower cervical vertebrae, while mobilizing the bulky dorsal musculature dorsomedially and providing a true lateral, unobstructed view to the craniovertebral junction (Fig. 21-4).

After exposure of the suboccipital skull, foramen magnum, laminae, and lateral masses of the atlas and axis, the vertical section of the vertebral artery is exposed in the C1-C2 intertransverse space. The artery is located by following the dorsal primary ramus of the C2 nerve root proximally to the primary ventral ramus. The vertebral artery can consistently be found ventral to the nerve, just caudal to the inferior border

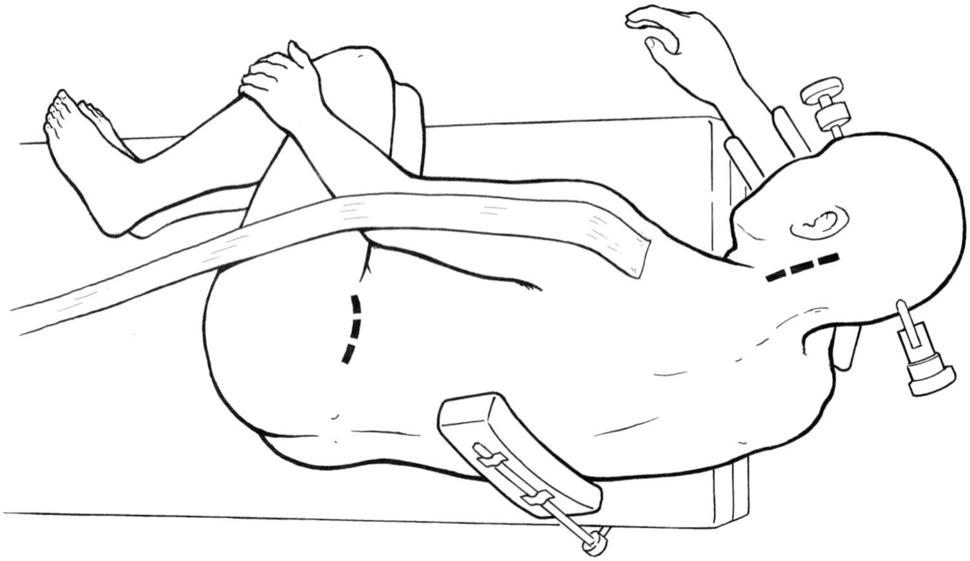

Figure 21-2. Positioning and skin incision for the far lateral approach.

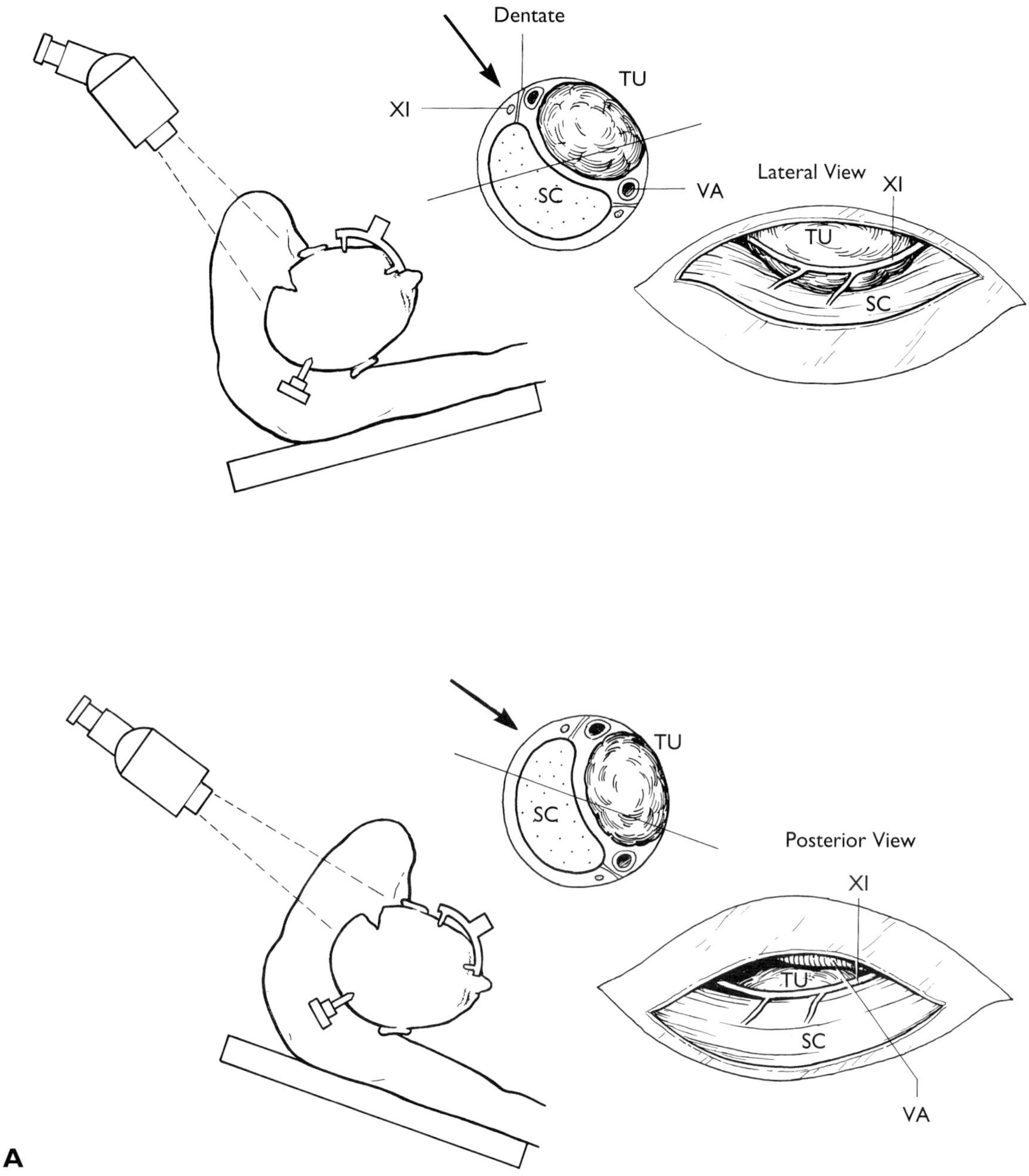

Figure 21-3. Visibility can be improved in the axial and sagittal planes by altering the operating table position and microscope position. *(A)* Using the lateral tilt function on the operating table can improve axial plane exposure by improving visibility anterior to the spinal cord. (*left*) Patient position, table tilt, and microscope angle; (*middle*) cross-section of dural tube (arrow indicates the direction of the surgeon's view); (*right*) operative view. *(B)* Angling the operating microscope from caudal to cephalad improves intracranial exposure, thus minimizing bone removal. (For explanation of abbreviations, see Appendix 1, p. 373.) *(Figure continues.)*

of the inferior oblique muscle. The rich venous plexus that surrounds the artery in this location and the transverse foramina of C1 can also be useful landmarks (Fig. 21-5). Using a subperiosteal dissection along the lamina and lateral mass, the vertebral artery is then freed from the sulcus arteriosus of C1 and isolated to its entrance into the dura.

Once the muscular mobilization and the vertebral artery dissection have been performed, the bony exposure is dictated by the location and extent of the lesion. For exposure of lesions of the spine and foramen magnum, a hemilaminectomy of the

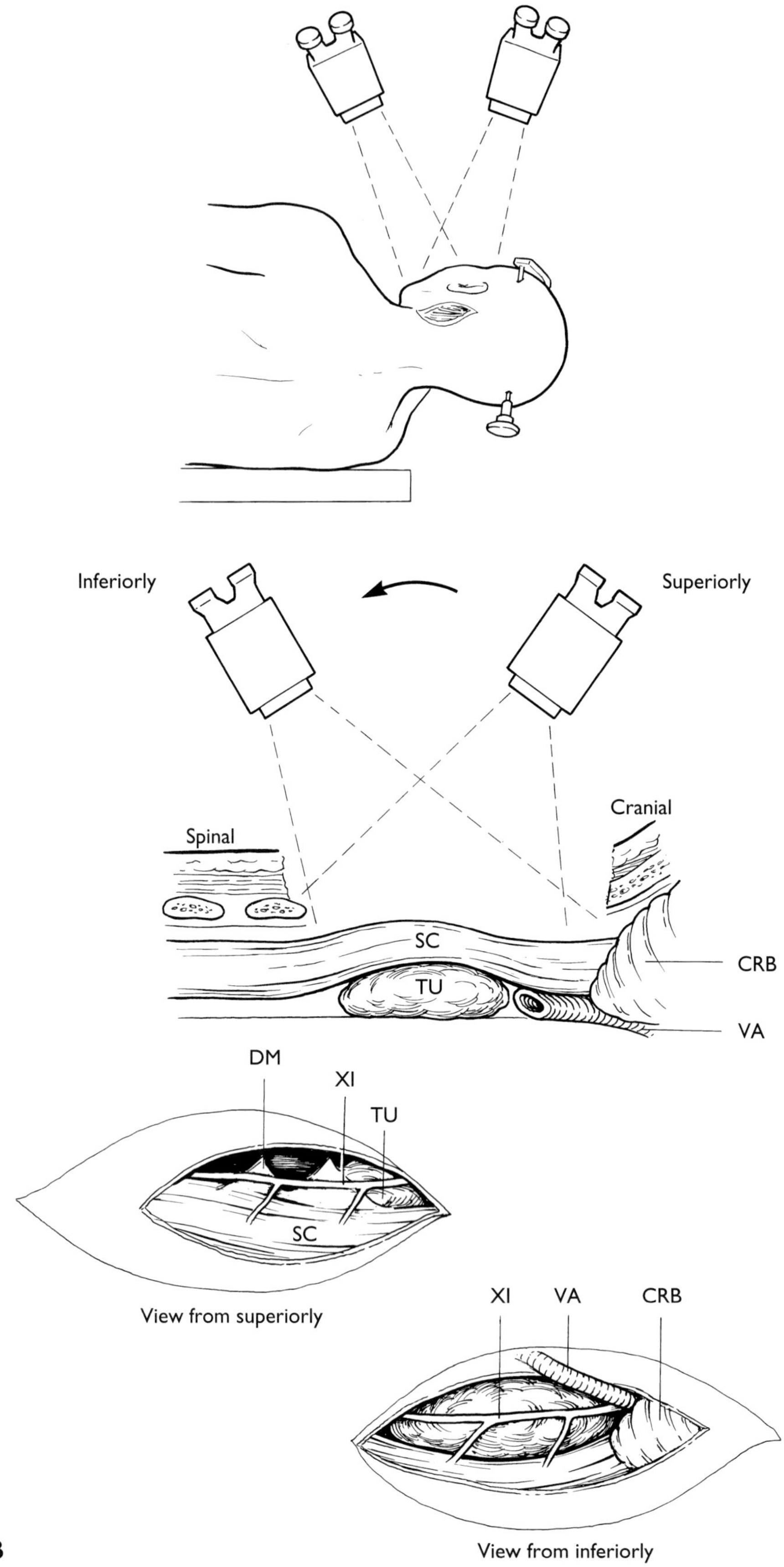

Figure 21-3 (Continued).

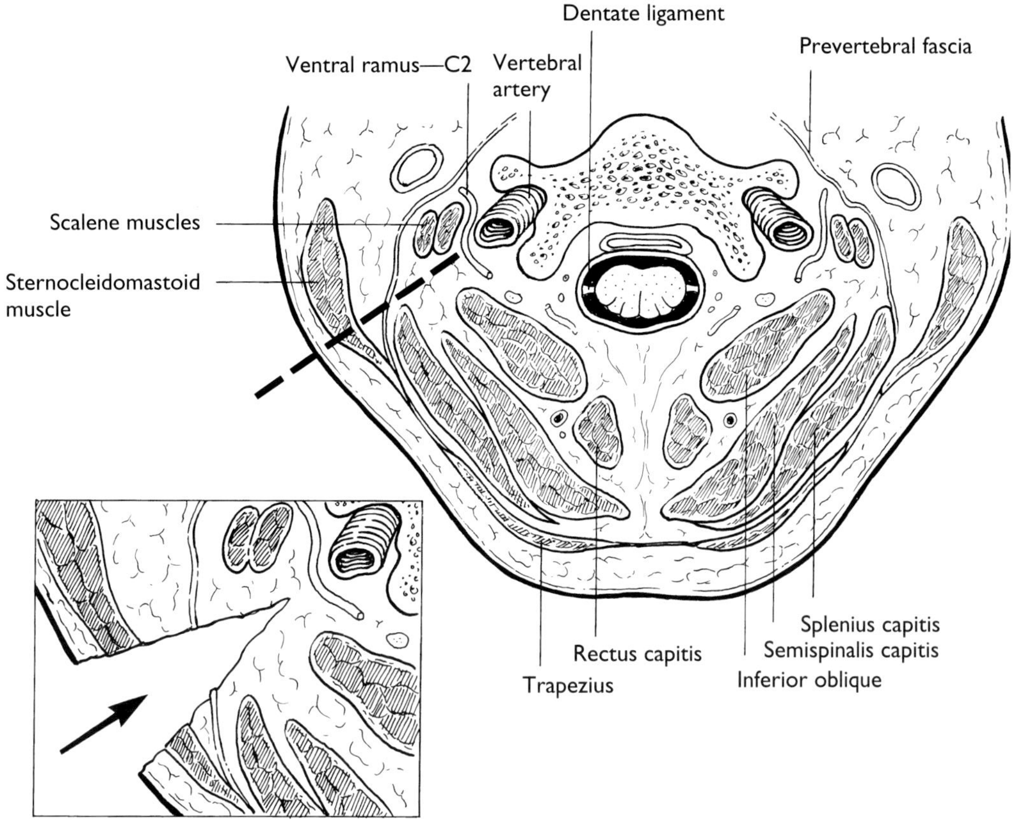

Figure 21-4. The fatty plane first described by Henry (1973), used for avascular exposure of the transverse processes of the upper cervical spine. Drawing of the axial plane. The plane is defined by dorsal musculature consisting of the splenius capitis, semispinalis, and longissimus capitis. The ventral musculature is composed of the levator scapulae and the scalene muscles. Blunt dissection carried through this plane provides free access to the transverse process of C1 and the lateral mass of the lower cervical vertebrae, while mobilizing the bulky dorsal musculature dorsomedially and providing a true lateral, unobstructed view to the craniovertebral junction.

appropriate spinal segments is performed. The foramen transversarium of C1 is unroofed with a drill to allow mobilization of the vertebral artery. With the artery protected, approximately 1 cm of suboccipital bone is removed from the foramen magnum. It is important to take this bony exposure far lateral to the junction with the occipital condyle. If the lesion is positioned very far ventrally, the dorsal one-third of the occipital condyle is removed with an air drill.

For lesions of the foramen magnum it is not necessary to perform a mastoidectomy, to expose the sinojugular bulb, or to perform a large craniotomy.

Intradural Pathology

After the vertebral artery has been isolated and the appropriate bone removal has been performed, the dura is opened dorsal to the entry of the vertebral artery. The dural edges are retracted with sutures and neurovascular structures are identified. The spinal accessory nerve is seen running parallel to the spinal cord, between the dorsal rootlets and the dentate ligaments. The hypoglossal nerve lies dorsal to the vertebral artery (Fig. 21-6). Greater ventral exposure is obtained after dividing the first two dentate ligaments.

With intradural pathology, delineation of the intracranial vascular supply to the tumor is the priority. The lesion is removed after the vertebral, anterior, and spinal arteries and PICAs are identified. When removing tumors, particularly meningiomas,

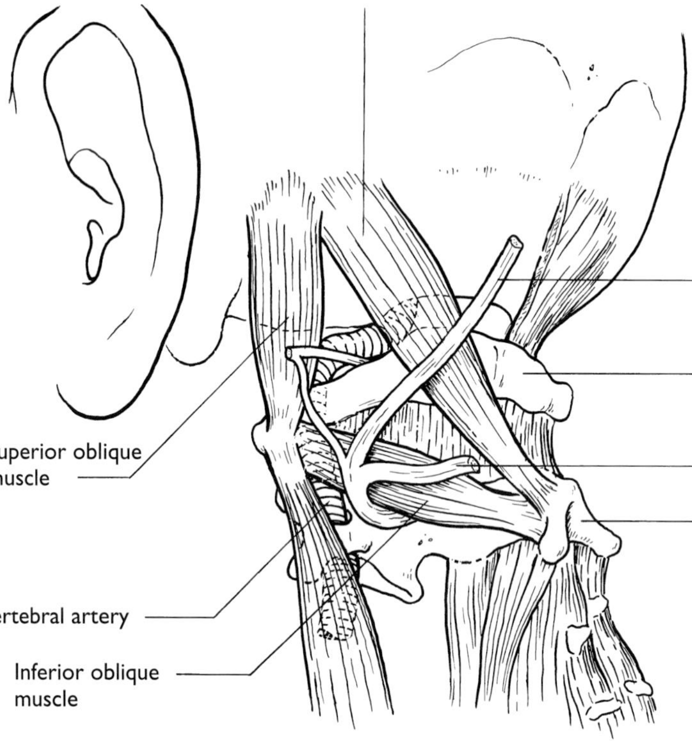

Figure 21-5. Location of the vertebral artery at the C1-C2 intertransverse space. The artery is found caudal to the inferior margin of the inferior oblique muscle and ventral to the ventral primary ramus of the C2 nerve root.

the vascular supply of the mass should be sacrificed early. This greatly reduces blood loss during tumor debulking and improves the maneuverability of the tumor by softening and shrinking the mass. The tumor may then be debulked with great care exercised to avoid retracting neurovascular structures (Fig. 21-6).

After tumor resection, the dura is approximated but rarely can it be closed in a watertight fashion. Instead, the defect is covered with Surgicel and thrombin glue (Tisseel).

Necessity of and Technique for Fusion

If the ventral two-thirds of the occipital condyle, the lateral mass of C1, of the C2 facet joint have not been removed surgically or destroyed by tumor, internal fixation and fusion are not necessary. If there is instability, a unilateral occipital-cervical fusion and fixation using autologous iliac crest is performed. First, the patient's head is placed in the neutral positioning by adjusting the Mayfield clamp. Then a bone strut is fashioned from autologous iliac crest. This is laid along the dorsolateral portion of the suboccipital bone to the first intact lateral masses (usually C3). The bone strut is secured with titanium miniplates and cancellous bone chips are placed under the strut to augment fusion (Fig. 21-7). There is no inherent stability with this construct until bone fusion has occurred, thus immobilization in a halo-body jacket is essential.

Closure and Postoperative Care

The muscle and skin are then meticulously closed in order to reduce the chance of a CSF leak. Postoperatively, the patients often remain intubated until lower cranial

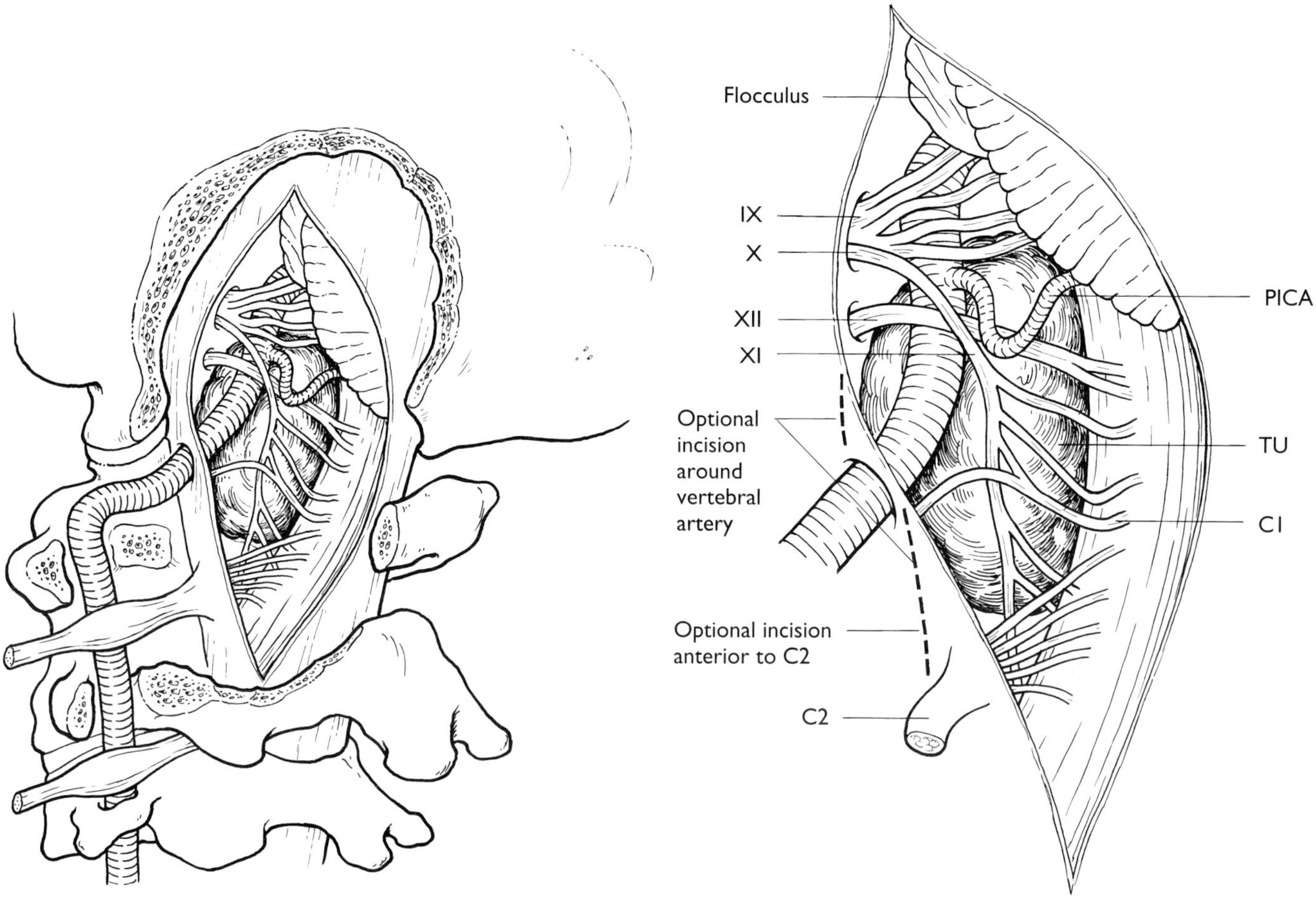

Figure 21-6. Illustration of a large ventrolateral intradural tumor, displacing the neuraxis dorsomedially. Foramen magnum and laminae of the axis and atlas have been removed. The dura was opened dorsal to the vertebral artery. The artery is displaced ventrally and the neuroaxis is pushed posteromedially. The spinal accessory nerve runs parallel to the spinal cord, dorsal to the lesion.

nerve function can be properly assessed. If there has been bulbar or lower cranial nerve compromise, a percutaneous gastrostomy, tracheostomy, or both may be needed for a few weeks postoperatively. Lumbar spinal drains are set at 10 to 15 cc/hr for 4 to 5 days postoperatively to prevent pseudomeningocele formation.

Complications

Intraoperative Complications

Through careful subperiosteal dissection, many venous structures can be avoided. However, brisk venous bleeding is sometimes encountered during vertebral artery dissection between the atlas and axis. This can be controlled with gentle packing and by elevating the patient's head using the tilt function on the operating table. If a vertebral artery injury occurs, direct repair should be attempted. If the injury is not primarily repairable, further measures are dictated by the preoperative angiogram. If the contralateral vertebral artery supply is absent or clearly diminished, an end-to-end primary anastomosis or the placement of a saphenous vein graft may be necessary. However, if there is adequate contralateral arterial supply and there is no significant medullary contribution from the injured segment, ligation of the artery without repair is recommended. From our own experience and in agreement with George we

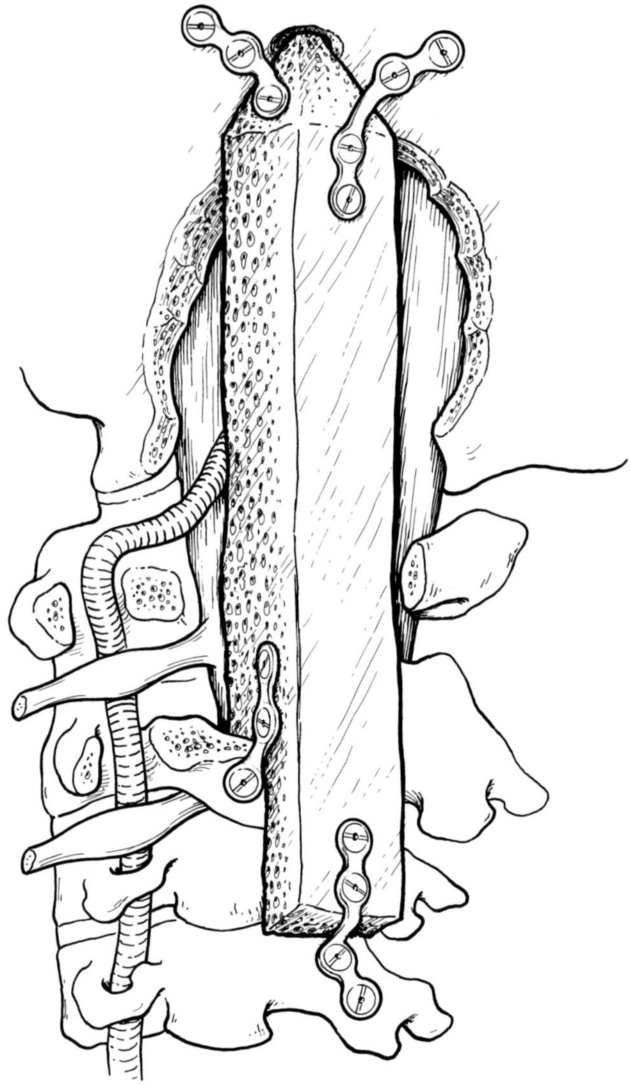

Figure 21-7. When necessary unilateral occipitocervical fusion can be performed concomitantly with the far lateral approach. The bone strut is fashioned from iliac crest and secured with titanium miniplates. Halo-vest immobilization is used postoperatively.

consider the use of vascular repair much less important than do Sen and Sekhar (1991) (George, 1989; Kratimenos and Crockard, 1994).

Early Postoperative Complications

Retraction of the neuraxis or arterial insult may lead to neurologic disability immediately postoperatively, but compromise to venous drainage may result in the delayed presentation of spinal cord or brain stem signs and symptoms (Henderson et al., 1993). Intradural lesions often involve the lower cranial nerves, and surgical manipulation can lead to transient or permanent difficulties with swallowing and airway protection in the immediate postoperative period. Because these possibilities exist, patients should remain intubated postoperatively until these functions can be thoroughly assessed. CSF leakage may compromise wound healing, lead to meningitis, or result in pseudomeningocele.

Patients frequently complain of significant posterior neck pain in the first few postoperative days. This is mostly related to the extensive muscular and bony dissection, but isolated posterior pain and numbness may be the result of C2 neuropraxia related to stretch injury.

Long-Term Complications

When neurologic deficits occur, their long-term effects may be devastating. However, most deficits that are not the result of arterial injury are transient. Lower cranial nerve function, specifically, often resolves after several months. Numbness or dysesthesias in the C2 distribution are usually transient.

In cases with primary bony pathology or extensive operative bone removal, instability may result. All patients complain of a dynamic neck pain for the first weeks to months postoperatively. This is infrequently related to instability and these symptoms eventually resolve (Sen and Sekhar, 1991; Spetzler and Grahm, 1990). If a patient complains of new or persistent dynamic neck pain several months after surgery, radiologic investigations should be performed and fusion considered.

References

Ashraf J, Crockard HA, Ransford AO, Stevens JM (1991) Transoral decompression and posterior stabilisation in Morquio's disease. Arch Dis Childhood 66:1318–1321

Bertalanffy H, Seeger W (1991) The dorsolateral, suboccipital, transcondylar approach to the lower clivus and anterior portion of the craniocervical junction. Neurosurgery 29:815–821

Calder I, Calder J, Crockard HA (1995) Difficult direct laryngoscopy in patients with disease of the cervical spine disease. Anaesthesia 50:756–763

Crockard HA (1993) Irreducible atlantoaxial subluxation. Anterior, lateral, and posterior approaches. pp. 137–149. In Garfin S, Northrup BE (eds): Surgery for Spinal Cord Injuries. Raven Press, New York

Crockard HA, Johnston F (1993) Development of transoral approaches to lesions of the skull base and craniocervical junction. Neurosurg Q 3:61–82

Crockard HA, Rogers MA (1995) Open reduction of traumatic atlanto-axial rotatory dislocation using the "extreme lateral approach." J Bone Joint Surg (in press)

Crockard HA, Sen CN (1991) The transoral approach for the management of intradural lesion at the craniocervical junction: review of 7 cases. Neurosurgery 28:88–97

Crockard HA, Sett P, Geddes JF et al. (1991) Damaged ligaments at the craniocervical junction presenting as an extradural tumour: a differential diagnosis in the elderly. J Neurol Neurosurg Psychiatry 54:817–821

DeOliveira E, Rhoton AL Jr, Peace D (1985) Microsurgical anatomy of the region of the foramen magnum. Surg Neurol 24:293–352

George B (1989) Lateral and lateral anterior approaches in tumors of the cervical vertebrate. Neurochirurgie 35:332–353

George B, Dematons C, Cophignon J (1988) Lateral approach to the anterior portion of the foramen magnum. Application to surgical removal of 14 benign tumors: technical note. Surg Neurol 29:484–490

George B, Laurian C (1987) The vertebral artery: pathology and surgery. Springer-Verlag, Wien

George B, Lot G, Velut S (1993) Pathologie tumorale du foramen magnum. Neurochirurgie, suppl. 39:1–89

Gilsbach JM (1991) Extreme lateral approach to the intradural lesions of the cervical spine and foramen magnum. Neurosurgery 28:779

Harkey HL, Crockard HA, Stevens JM et al. (1990) The operative management of basilar impression in osteogenesis imperfecta. Neurosurgery 27:782–786

Henderson FC, Crockard HA, Stevens JM (1993) Spinal cord oedema due to venous stasis. Neuroradiology 35:312–315

Henry A (1973) Extensile Exposures. pp. 58–82. Churchill Livingstone, Edinburgh

Heros RC (1986) Lateral suboccipital approach for vertebral and vertebrobasilar artery lesions. J Neurosurg 64:559–562

Kratimenos GP, Crockard HA (1993) The far lateral approach for ventrally placed foramen magnum and upper cervical spine tumours. Br J Neurosurg 7:129–140

Kratimenos GP, Crockard HA (1994) The lateral approach for anterior tumours of the foramen magnum. pp. 1095–1105. In Samii M (ed): Skull Base Surgery, Karger, Basel

Kuttner H (1917) Die verletzungen und traumatischen Aneurysmen der Vertebralgefasse am Halse und ihre operative Behandlung. Beitr Klin Chir 108:1–60

Lang J (1986) Craniocervical region, blood vessels. Neurorthopaedics 2:55–56

Lister JR, Rhoton AL Jr, Matsushima T, Peace DA (1982) Microsurgical anatomy of the posterior inferior cerebellar artery. Neurosurgery 10:170–199

Meyer FB, Ebersold MJ, Reese DF (1984) Benign tumours of the foramen magnum. J Neurosurg 61:136–142

Orrell RW, Marsden CD (1994) The neck-tongue syndrome. J Neurol Neurosurg Psychiatry 57:348–52

Perneczy A (1986) The posterolateral approach to the foramen magnum. pp. 460–466. In Sami M (ed): Surgery in and Around the Brain Stem and the Third Ventricle. Springer-Verlag, New York

Rhoton A, DeOliveira E (1991) Microsurgical anatomy of the region of the foramen magnum. pp. 434–460. In Wilkins R, Regnachary S (eds): Neurosurgery Update. McGraw-Hill, New York

Sen CN, Sekhar LN (1990) An extreme lateral approach to intradural lesions of the cervical spine and foramen magnum. Neurosurgery 27:197–204

Sen CN, Sekhar LN (1991) Extreme lateral approach to intradural lesions of the cervical spine and foramen magnum. Neurosurgery 28:779

Spetzler R, Grahm T (1990) The far lateral approach to the inferior clivus and the upper cervical region: technical note. Barrow Neurolog Ins Q 6:35–38

Stein M, Leds N, Taveras J et al. (1963) Meningiomas of the foramen magnum. J Neurosurg 20:740–751

Verbiest H (1968) A lateral approach to the cervical spine: technique and indications. J Neurosurg 28:191–203

22

Techniques of Skull Base Reconstruction

Ricardo Izquierdo

Reconstruction should be an integral part of skull base surgery and planning should begin with the decision to perform surgery. At our center, a surgical team consisting of a neurosurgeon, an otolaryngologist, and a plastic surgeon are routinely involved in the care of patients with basicranial tumors. Preoperative discussions are important between all members of the surgical team and should address patient positioning, surgical approach, expected operative findings, and possible pitfalls during the procedure. The reconstructive surgeon must take into account requirements for a secure and immunologically competent dural closure, sequestration of the cranial contents from the aerodigestive tract, adequate volumetric and three-dimensional reconstruction, and minimal morbidity at the donor and recipient site. If proper preparations are made, oncologic principles of resection should not be compromised. Likewise, a preoperative three-dimensional understanding of the structures to be excised and the expected defect can help in choosing the optimal choice for reconstruction. All options, from simplest to most complex, should be evaluated. This mental exercise becomes especially important if local tissues are to be used for reconstruction. Placement of incisions and identification of prior incisions must be carefully assessed in order to take advantage of regional tissues, should they be available. The judicious harvesting of these local flaps can sometimes avoid the need for more complex, and potentially difficult reconstruction.

The choice of grafts, regional flaps, or distant flaps alone or in combination should be assessed for each individual case. Despite this preparation, the requirements for reconstruction may evolve throughout the procedure due to unexpected findings or the need to excise other structures. The reconstructive surgeon should have several options available and executable if the need arises. This chapter focuses on reconstruction using flaps that have an identifiable vascular supply. Such tissues provide enhanced vascularity to the surgical site. This factor is important for adequate healing especially in areas that have been previously operated or irradiated.

History

Extensive tumors at the cranial base previously had been considered unresectable. Their location and proximity to vital vascular and neural structures prohibited conventional approaches and patients were frequently subjected to subtotal resection. However, the recent growth and progress in craniofacial and skull base surgery has allowed surgeons to safely approach these regions.

Prior to the advent of muscle flaps, reconstruction of the head and neck region was limited to local scalp flaps (Frederichs, 1956; Hanna et al., 1967; Kazanjian and Converse, 1940), and distant pedicled flaps such as the deltopectoral flap (Bakamjiam, 1965; Farrior, 1979). The explosion of anatomic knowledge of flaps in the last two decades has increasingly allowed safer and more complete reconstruction of tumor defects. The temporalis (Antonyshyn et al., 1988; Arden et al., 1987; Shagets et al., 1986), sternocleidomastoid (McGraw et al., 1979), trapezius (McGraw et al., 1979; Seyfer, 1988), and the pectoralis muscle flaps (Ariyan, 1979; Sasaki et al., 1985) helped make major advances in head and neck reconstruction. Subsequent identification of the galea and pericranium as hearty and dependable flaps added simple but effective local measures for adequate closure. The growth of microsurgical transplantation using free flaps has essentially made reconstruction of almost any defect possible and has allowed aggressive and complete removal of tumors without fear of inadequate tissue for reconstruction.

Grafts

One of the major elements in reconstruction of this region is an adequate appraisal of the resultant defect so that an effective method of reconstruction can be chosen. The site and volume of the tumor extirpation are important determinants in the method of reconstruction. Some tumors will require only excision of overlying dura, making reconstruction relatively simple with the use of autogenous tissue such as fascia lata (Thammavaran et al., 1990) or allografts (Prolo et al., 1980). However, the approach to tumors in the cranial base frequently requires ablation of surrounding structures for adequate access to the lesion and control of vascular structures. These approaches sacrifice more tissue than the tumor represents on preoperative radiographic studies.

Some tumors can be excised and the surrounding structures will collapse and obliterate the dead space. As more bony dissection is performed, there is less ability for collapse in this rigid remaining cavity. These areas will require the addition of bulk for adequate obliteration. Fat grafts have been used in "small" areas to obliterate these extirpation defects (Boyce et al., 1994; Conley and Clairmont, 1978). However, these grafts are devoid of vascular supply upon transplantation. Maintenance of their structure is dependent on revascularization from surrounding tissues and/or fibrosis during the healing process. It has been shown that significant resorption of the transplanted fat, up to 60 to 70 percent, can be expected (Billings and May, 1989; Carpaneda and Ribeiro, 1993). Necrosis is a potential problem if the mass of the graft exceeds the ability for vascularization. Aseptic meningitis has occurred in translabyrinthine excision of acoustic tumors (Reece et al., 1989). Therefore, this method of reconstruction should be limited to relatively small defects.

Flaps

Temporalis Muscle and Temporoparietal Fascia

There are several local flaps that can provide a well-vascularized closure, good sequestration for the intracranial contents, and moderate volume reconstruction. The temporalis muscle has long been a workhorse for head and neck reconstruction and is a suitable muscle for lateral and anterior defects (Shagets et al., 1986) (Fig. 22-1).

The vascular supply to the temporalis muscle is from the internal maxillary artery. This muscle can be used for defects in the infratemporal fossa as well as the anterolateral skull base, orbit, and maxillary regions. However, it will not dependably reach the midline. The flap can be split longitudinally, and only that part that is needed used. Rotation can be extended by subperiosteal dissection and fracturing of the coronoid process. It is important to maintain the muscular attachment to this insertion point so as to preserve added venous egress from the flap.

The temporalis muscle flap can be used in concert with the overlying temporoparietal fascia (Antonyshyn et al., 1988). This very well-vascularized tissue is dependent on the superficial temporal vessels and can incorporate the galea aponeurotica up to the midline (Arden et al., 1987; Horowitz et al., 1984). McCarthy and Zide (1984) have shown that the outer table of the parietal cranium can be transferred on this pedicle using the underlying pericranium as the vascular conduit. Large perforators from the superficial temporal artery system enter the underlying pericranium and arborize into a richly vascularized plexus (Habal and Maniscalco, 1981; Har-Shai et al., 1992; McCarthy and Zide, 1984) (Fig. 22-2). Although this flap cannot be extended beyond the midline, a bipedicled flap using both temporoparietal fascia and

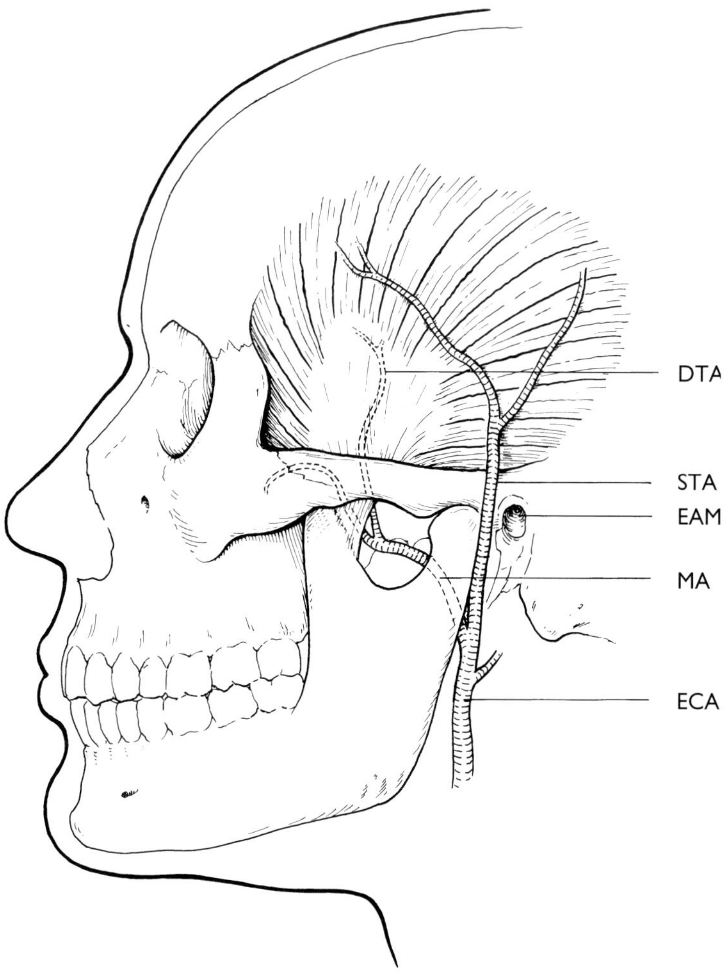

Figure 22-1. Temporalis muscle has its main blood supply from the internal maxillary artery, which runs on the deep surface of the muscle. Transposition of this flap will cover the temporal and anterolateral skull base. (For explanations of abbreviations see Appendix 1, p. 373.)

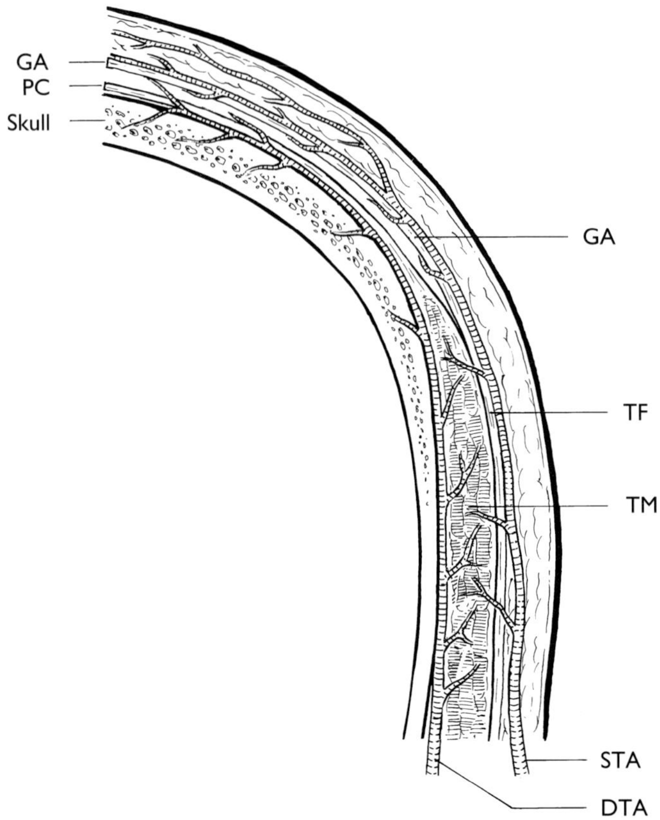

Figure 22-2. The rich vascular arborization between the superficial temporal artery and the deep temporal artery allows the dissection of longer flaps and can also transfer bone from the parietal area.

temporalis muscles can be harvested and transposed anteriorly. This is especially useful if the supraorbital vessels are damaged or if a previous bicoronal incision was placed low on the anterior hairline and compromises the length of an anteriorly based pericranial flap.

Pericranial Flap

The pericranial flap is composed of the periosteum of the skull and its overlying loose areolar tissue. The main vascular supply is via the supraorbital and supratrochlear vessels. This flap can be harvested as far posteriorly as the auricular plane, giving a length of 10 to 12 cm (Johns et al., 1981; Price et al., 1988; Wolfe, 1978) (Fig. 22-3). Because of its rich vascular plexus, longer flaps may be dissected. It can be used for coverage of the anterior cranial base, passing it through a slit in the craniotomy, either over or under the supraorbital bar.

When using this flap, it is easier to raise it initially during the elevation of the scalp. The bicoronal flap is elevated at the subgaleal-frontalis muscle level down to the supraorbital ridges. Care should be taken not to disturb the vascular supply that may penetrate the frontalis muscle above the orbital ridge. If a long flap is required, the posterior portion of the scalp can be elevated and the pericranial incision made where needed. Dissection then proceeds anteriorly under the pericranium down to the pedicles. At times, incision of portions of the frontalis muscle near the vessels is required to maintain the vascularity of the flap (Jackson et al., 1986). This flap should not be underestimated for its vigor, applicability, and dependability (Argenta et al., 1985). A variation of the flap can use one of the pedicles over the supraorbital and supratrochlear vessels and allow for a wider arch of rotation.

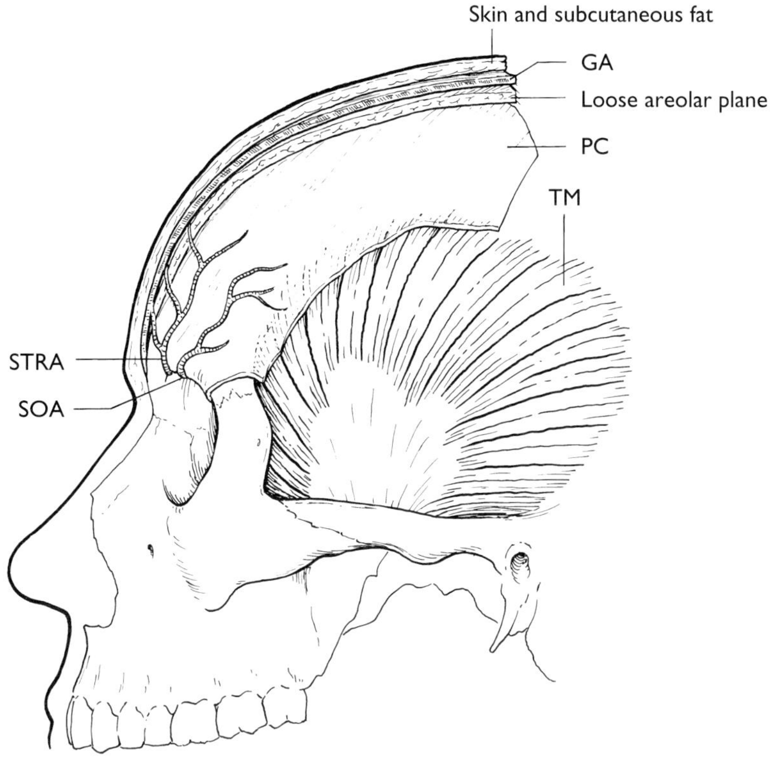

Figure 22-3. The pericranial flap is a versatile and robust flap. It can be used alone or in combination with the galea/frontalis muscle flap. The supratrochlear and supraorbital vessels supply both layers after dividing within 1 to 2 cm of the supraorbital ridge.

Pectoralis and Latissimus Muscles

The pectoralis muscle can be raised as a myocutaneous flap based on the thoracoacromial vascular pedicle as it crosses under the clavicle just medial to the pectoralis minor muscle. A line drawn from the midportion of the clavicle to the xiphoid delineates the path of the vessels. The perforators of the internal mammary artery will require ligation as the medial part of the muscle is being raised.

The latissimus muscle can be raised using the thoracodorsal vessels, which come off of the axillary artery. Several thoracolumbar perforators will require ligation near the posterior and inferior portion of the flap. At times, this distal area of the muscle has a less than optimal blood supply. Usually, the skin paddle is designed near the anterior border of the muscle where the vascularity can safely be assured.

Some authors have used pectoralis pedicled myocutaneous flaps to close craniofacial defects around the skull base (Sasaki et al., 1985). Various maneuvers have been described to extend the reach of these flaps to the upper reaches of the head and neck. The pectoralis myocutaneous flap can be extended by transecting the clavicle near the thoracoacromial pedicle to gain further upward distance near the cranial base. The clavicle can be plated. The latissimus myocutaneous flap can be extended by transection of the humeral insertion thus increasing the arc of rotation. However, despite these maneuvers, one should be aware that these flaps can deliver only a limited volume of tissue above the zygomatic arch and infraorbital rim.

Trapezius Muscle

The vertical trapezius myocutaneous flap is a versatile and hearty flap fed by the descending branch of the transverse cervical artery (Seyfer, 1988) (Fig. 22-4). Dis-

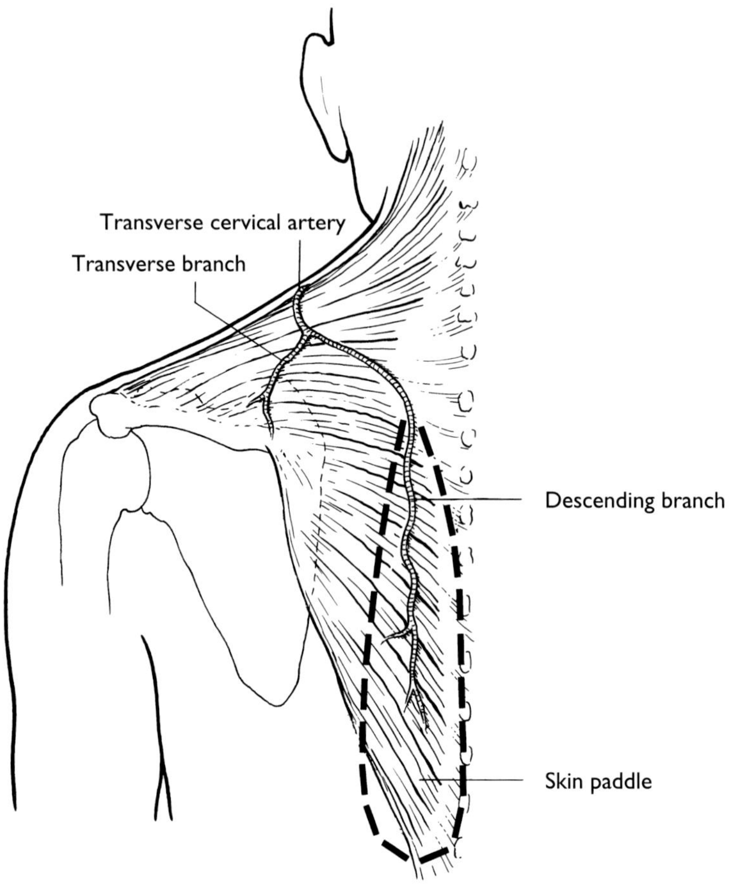

Figure 22-4. The trapezius myocutaneous flap can cover the posterior and lateral skull base. It usually cannot reach anterior to the auricle.

section of this muscle will yield a flap that can cover the posterior temporal fossa, lateral skull base, and posterior skull base. We have used it on occasion to reach as far as the cranial vertex without difficulty. Proper dissection will allow preservation of the transverse portion of the muscle and therefore maintain shoulder shrugging.

The trapezius muscle is a triangular-shaped muscle with "corners" at the occiput, scapula, and lumbosacral fascia. A secondary blood supply comes from paravertebral perforators that must be ligated when the vertical flap is harvested. The flap can be either muscle or myocutaneous. The myocutaneous flap transfers added bulk and length. It is preferable to use the myocutaneous flap in lesions that require coverage farther anterior than the occiput. The skin paddle is based over the muscle and can be extended past the end of the muscle in a random fashion for several centimeters giving extra length to the reach of the flap. Because the skin and underlying structures around the base of the posterior neck are tight, tunneling of this flap is not performed. This assures lessened pressure on the pedicle, and less risk of strangulating or kinking the blood supply.

Microsurgical Free Tissue Transfer

Small defects can often be repaired by transferring local or distant pedicled flaps to secure closure of the patient's cranial contents. Extirpation of larger lesions creates formidable defects of soft tissue, bone, and, at times, dura. Likewise, those undergoing craniofacial resection, extended transtemporal bone surgery, or excision of recurrent tumors often have large, geometrically complex defects. Some of these ablation defects require a large volume of tissue for reconstruction precluding the use of galeal flaps or pedicled muscle flaps. Free tissue transfer provides the solution for dependable reconstruction in these patients. The ability to transfer virtually any amount and combination of tissues for reconstruction has allowed cranial base surgeons to undertake the resection of increasingly larger and more complex tumors.

In choosing the donor for free tissue transfer, several important areas must be addressed. The site of the defect, position of the patient for harvesting, donor morbidity, recipient vasculature, and the need for an adequate pedicle length should be carefully assessed. Virtually every free tissue flap territory has been transferred for the skull base (Angel et al., 1992; Barrow et al., 1984; Bridger et al., 1986; Jones et al., 1986; Ueda et al., 1990, 1992, 1993). However, the requirements for closure depend on the defect (e.g., the need to repair the oropharynx, external skin deficit, volume replacement, thin tissue). Much of this can be appreciated prior to surgery and planned. Most moderate-to-large defects can be reconstructed using the rectus muscle/myocutaneous flap or the latissimus muscle or myocutaneous flap. They are adequate flaps with dependable anatomy.

Standard Free Flaps

If the patient is supine, the rectus muscle territory is a natural choice for transfer (Fig. 22-5). The rectus muscle free flap is based on the deep inferior epigastric vessels

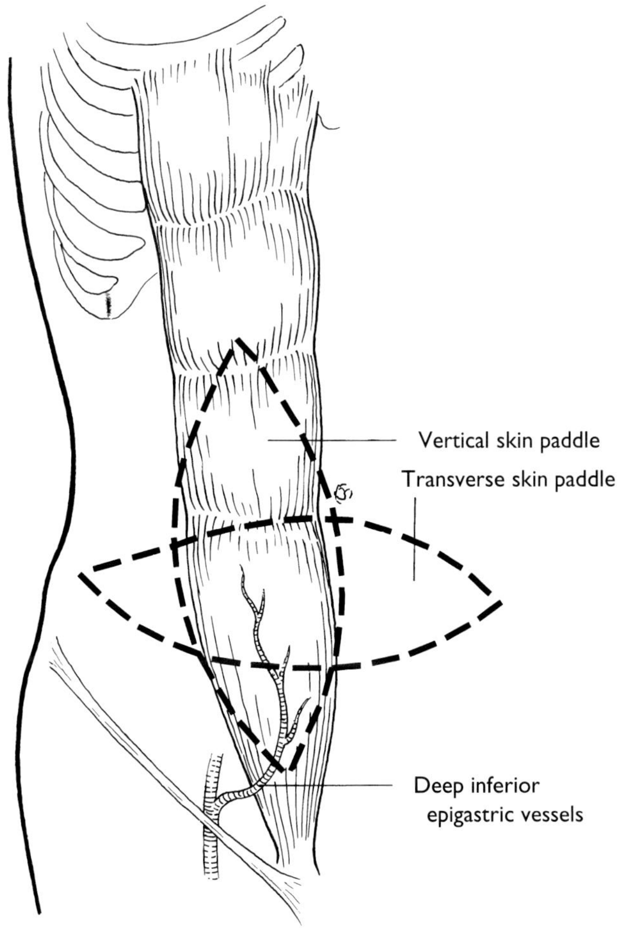

Figure 22-5. The rectus abdominis muscle can transfer the overlying skin and subcutaneous tissue in either a vertical or horizontal design.

that branch from the external iliac artery and vein proximal to the inguinal ligament. This muscle is easy to dissect in the supine position and has a dependable and relatively large pedicle. Usual lengths are 4 to 6 cm, with arterial diameters of 3 to 4 mm.

If bulk or skin is needed, the overlying skin and subcutaneous tissues can be harvested with the flap. We have used this variation of the flap with great success in dealing with intricate central defects. The overlying adipose tissue has an abundant blood supply for musculocutaneous perforators and allows easy sculpting and shaping of the flap for use in the central and sometimes irregular defects (Izquierdo et al., 1993a, 1993b).

When patients are placed in a lateral position, or if the rectus muscle is not available due to previous surgery or scarring, the latissimus muscle provides an equally good amount of tissue for transfer. This flap dissection is also straightforward. The thoracodorsal vessels provide up to an 8- to 10-cm pedicle with arterial diameters of 4 to 6 mm. The overlying skin can be taken with the flap if external skin or oral lining is required. However, there is less subcutaneous fat in this area as compared to the rectus myocutaneous flap.

Special Circumstances

On some occasions, pedicle length may need to be longer because of a paucity of available recipient vessels due to previous surgery or irradiation. Long pedicles are preferable to vein grafts to bridge the distance due to a higher complication rate with the latter (Miller et al., 1993). The radial forearm fasciocutaneous flap and the serratus anterior muscle flap can provide pedicle lengths of 10 to 12 cm.

The radial forearm flap is based on the radial artery septocutaneous perforators to the overlying forearm skin and fascia (Fig. 22-6). Sacrifice of this vessel usually does not require reconstruction of the radial artery due to the cross circulation from the ulnar artery via the superficial arch of the hand. Assessment of this anastomosis is readily made preoperatively with the use of the Allen's test.

The radial forearm free flap is ideal for defects requiring thin tissue and enhanced vascularity. Three-quarters of the circumference of the forearm skin and fascia can be transferred. Sizes of 12 × 20 cm can be harvested. The fascia can be taken alone and used for thin reconstruction. Also, this fascia free flap can be used for thin covering in areas where skin should not be buried. The skin of the fasciocutaneous flap can be used intraorally to seal the cranial cavity from the pharynx if needed.

If more bulk is desired, the lower three slips of the serratus muscle can be transferred based on the thoracodorsal vessels. Pedicle length can reach 10 to 12 cm with this flap (Fig. 22-7). Sacrifice of these lower slips preserves the neural supply from the long thoracic nerve to the remaining muscle and prevents winging of the scapula. These three muscle slips can also be transferred with their branches of the nerve and used for facial reanimation.

In large complex excisions, the aerodigestive tract may require sequestration from the intracranial cavity. A secure barrier can usually be achieved with any of the previous muscle free flaps. Some authors have allowed mucosalization of these muscle flaps at the interface of the two tissues, whereas others have transferred the cutaneous portions of flaps for accurate closure. When possible, I have transferred skin paddles for use at the brain-oral cavity interface. I believe that using a skin paddle provides precise closure of the defect and obviates the need to wait for mucosalization or risk suture line breakdown. Although either skin or muscle can be used intraorally safely, one should not depend on subcutaneous fat alone to adequately seal or close the oropharyngeal cavity.

Other authors have advocated using portions of the gastrointestinal tract for closure. Jejunum and greater curvature of the stomach provide ample mucosal recon-

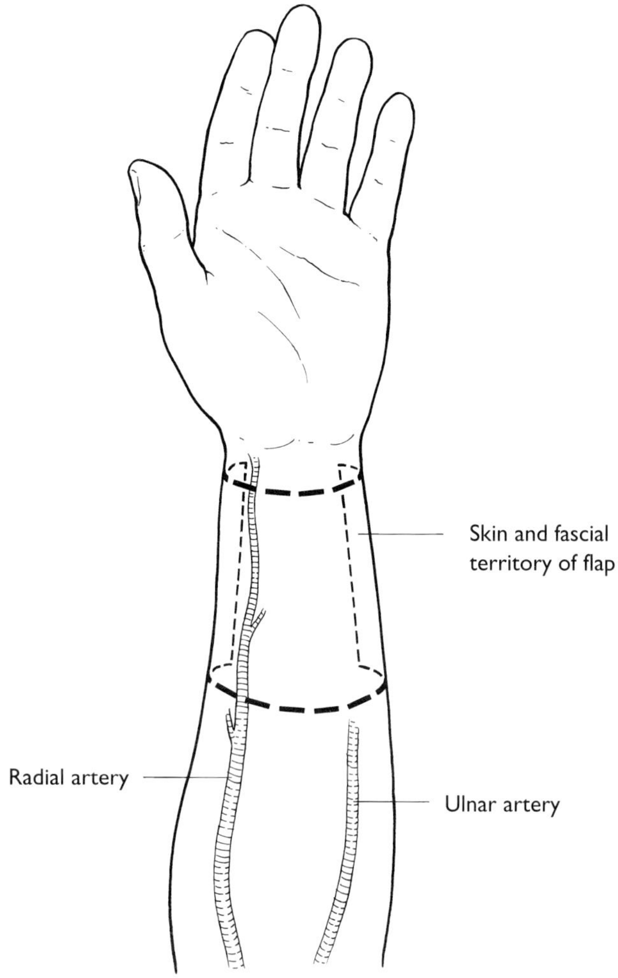

Figure 22-6. The radial forearm flap can be designed to transfer the skin or only the fascia. Three-quarters of the distal forearm circumference can be used. The pedicle length can be tailored for the defect by dissecting proximally to the origin at the brachial artery.

struction to the oronasopharynx as well as closure of the cranial base (Reece et al., 1994; Schramm, 1993, personal communication). The jejunum has been used successfully for the reconstruction of the cervical esophagus and upper pharynx. It can provide a 10- to 12-cm length of mucosal tissue based on a mesenteric vascular arcade. This can be opened longitudinally on the antimesenteric border to provide a rectangular flap. One drawback to the use of this flap transfer is the relatively short pedicle length (5 cm) and the usual high position of the cranial base in relation to vessels for anastomosis.

The greater curvature of the stomach can be harvested with the omentum providing both bulk and oral mucosal reconstruction. Pedicle lengths can be varied with the use of the right gastroepiploic vessels. Morbidity for both these forms of reconstruction may be increased due to the need for gastrointestinal tract manipulation. Laparotomy is also required, although with the advent of laparoscopic techniques, minimally invasive surgery may reduce this risk.

Complications

Complications are usually due to vascular compromise and flap necrosis. Failure of a flap may lead to catastrophic consequences. Therefore, accurate assessment and pro-

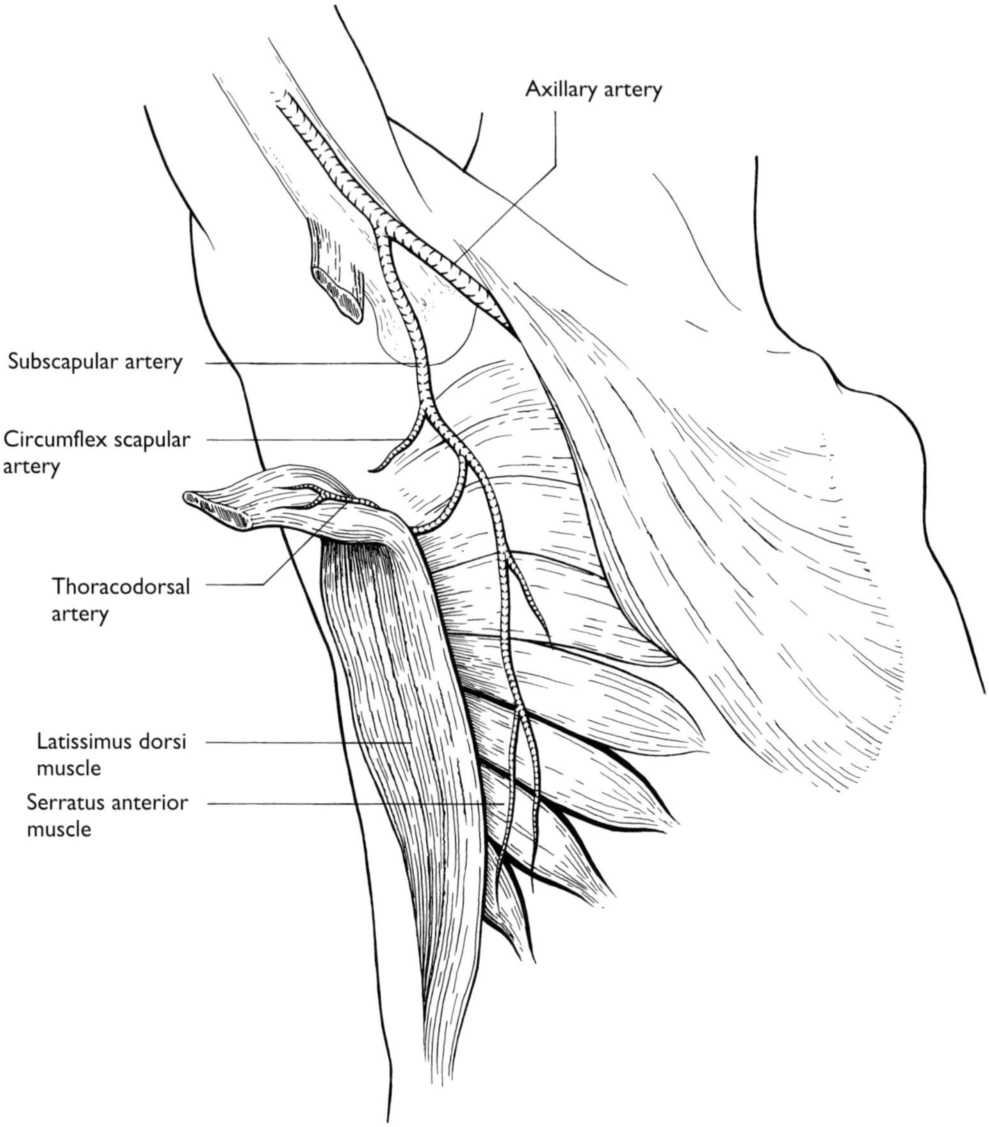

Figure 22-7. The three lower slips of the serratus anterior muscle can be transferred on the subscapular-thoracodorsal artery pedicle. Use of only these three slips will not cause winging of the scapula and can deliver good bulk with a long pedicle.

tection of the vascularity of the flap is mandatory. Proper care of the tissues during the procedure should include keeping the flap moist and warm, as well as minimizing extensive retraction and tension upon transfer.

Partial necrosis of some unburied regional pedicled flaps can sometimes be treated by conservative measures. Intermittent debridement and dressing changes can be performed while wound contraction and closure by secondary intention is accomplished. However, if the tissue necrosis overlies important structures (e.g., dura, vessels), more aggressive surgical revision is indicated to avoid reconstructive failure and possible increased morbidity and mortality.

If the flap is to be transferred by microsurgical techniques, anastomotic thrombosis may jeopardize the entire flap and reconstruction. Free tissue transfers are usually successful in greater than 97 percent (Khouri, 1992). However, vascular compromise may be difficult to assess if the flap is fully buried. If thrombosis occurs, the secondary ischemia time that a flap can tolerate is much less than the primary ischemia time that it underwent for the initial transfer and revascularization (Kerrigan et al., 1984). Therefore close postoperative monitoring is important in these particular patients.

Conclusions

The choice for reconstruction is dependent on many factors. With most moderate-to-large defects, previously operated patients, or irradiated areas, free tissue transfer offers excellent closure, obliteration of the defect, and, in most cases, minimal morbidity. Transfer of free flaps provides superior vascularity to the bed for healing. Most flaps can be tailored for the individual patient's problems or needs. Local flaps or grafts should be limited to small defects or primary cases that require minimal excision of tissue. This method of reconstruction may be used in defects where the surrounding structures are well vascularized and obliteration of a large space is not necessary.

It is imperative that the reconstructive surgeon have a sound understanding of the anatomy and knowledge of the requirements for secure repair of the dura, oral cavity, as well as obliteration of the defect. With these directives, a logical choice of regional or distant flaps can be made and help assure a successful patient outcome.

References

Angel MF, Bridges RM, Levine PA et al. (1992) The serratus anterior free tissue transfer for craniofacial reconstruction. J Craniofac Surg 3:207–212

Antonyshyn O, Gruss JS, Bist BD (1988) Versatility of temporal muscle and fascial flaps. Br J Plast Surg 41:118

Arden RL, Mathog RH, Thomas LM (1987) Temporalis muscle-galea flaps in craniofacial reconstruction. Laryngoscope 97:1336

Argenta LC, Friedman RJ, Dingman RO (1985) The versatility of pericranial flaps. Plast Reconstr Surg 76:695–702

Ariyan S (1979) The pectoralis major myocutaneous flap. A versatile flap for reconstruction in the head and neck. Plast Reconstr Surg 63:73–81

Bakamjiam VY (1965) A two-stage method for pharyngoesophageal reconstruction with a primary pectoral skin flap. Plast Reconstr Surg 36:173

Barrow DL, Nahai F, Tindale GT (1984) The use of greater omentum vascularized free flaps for neurosurgical disorders requiring reconstruction. J Neurosurg 60:305–311

Billings E, May JW (1989) Historical review and present status of free fat graft autotransplantation in plastic and reconstructive surgery. Plast Reconstr Surg 83:368–381

Boyce RG, Nuss DW, Kluka EA (1994) The use of autogenous fat, fascia, and nonvascularized muscle grafts in the head and neck. Otolaryngol Clin North Am 27:39–68

Bridger GP, Baldwin M, Gonski A (1986) Craniofacial resection for paranasal sinus cancer with free flap repair. Austral N Z J Surg 56:843–847

Carpaneda CA, Ribeiro MT (1993) Study of the histologic alterations and viability of the adipose graft in humans. Aesthet Plast Surg 17:43–47

Conley JJ, Clairmont AA (1978) Dermal fat-fascia grafts. Otolaryngology 86:641–649

Farrior RT (1979) Situational modification of regional flaps. Otolaryngol Head Neck Surg 87:497–514

Frederichs S (1956) External ear malignancy. Br J Plast Surg 9:136

Habal MB, Maniscalco JE (1981) Observations of the ultrastructure of the pericranium. Ann Plast Surg 6:103

Hanna DC, Richardson GS, Gaisford JC (1967) A suggested technique for resection of the temporal bone. Am J Surg 114:553

Har-Shai Y, Fukuta K, Collares MV et al. (1992) The vascular anatomy of the galeal flap in the inter parietal and midline regions. Plast Reconstr Surg 89:64–69

Horowitz JH, Persing JA, Nichter LS et al. (1984) Galeal-pericranial flaps in head and neck reconstruction: anatomy and application. Am J Surg 148:489

Izquierdo R, Leonetti JP, Origitano TC et al. (1993a) Refinements using free tissue transfer for complex cranial base reconstruction. Plast Reconstr Surg 92:567–574

Izquierdo R, Origitano TC, Al-Mefty O et al. (1993b) Use of vascularized fat from the rectus abdominis myocutaneous free flap territory to seal the dura of basicranial tumor defects. Neurosurgery 32:192–197

Jackson IT, Adham MN, March R (1986) Use of the galeal frontalis myofascial flap in craniofacial surgery. Plast Reconstr Surg 77:905

Johns ME, Winn HR, McLean WC, Cantress RW (1981) Pericranial flap for the closure of defects of craniofacial resection. Laryngoscope 91:952–959

Jones NF, Kekhar LN, Schramm VL (1986) Free rectus abdominis muscle flap reconstruction of the middle and posterior cranial base. Plast Reconstr Surg 78:471–479

Kazanjian VH, Converse JM (1940) Reconstruction after radical operation for osteomyelitis of the frontal bone. Arch Otolaryngol 31:94

Kerrigan CL, Zelt RG, Daniel RK (1984) Secondary ischemia of experimental skin flaps. Plast Reconstr Surg 74:522–526

Khouri R (1992) Free flap surgery: the second decade. Clin Plast Surg 19:757–761

McCarthy JG, Zide BM (1984) The spectrum of calvarial bone grafting: introduction of the vascularized calvarial bone flap. Plast Reconstr Surg 74:10

McGraw JB, Magee WP, Kalwaic H (1979) Uses of the trapezius and sternocleidomastoid myocutaneous flaps in head and neck reconstruction. Plast Reconstr Surg 63:49–57

Miller MJ, Schusterman MA, Reece GP, Kroll SS (1993) Interposition vein grafting in head and neck reconstructive microsurgery. J Reconstr Microsurg 9:245–251

Prolo DJ, Pedrotti PW, White DH (1980) Ethylene oxide sterilization of bone, dura mater, and fascia lata for human transplantation. Neurosurgery 6:529–539

Price JC, Lowry M, Carson B, Johns ME (1988) The pericranial flap for reconstruction of anterior skull base defects. Laryngoscope 98:1159–1164

Reece AT, O'Reilly B, Teasdale E, Todd NV (1989) Subarachnoid fat embolism complicating autologous fat grafting following translabyrinthine excision of acoustic neuroma. J Laryngol Otol 103:870–871

Reece GP, Bengston BP, Schusterman MA (1994) Reconstruction of the pharynx and cervical esophagus using free jejunal transfer. Clin Plast Surg 21:125–136

Sasaki CT, Ariyan S, Spencer D, Buckwalter J (1985) Pectoralis major myocutaneous reconstruction of the anterior skull base. Laryngoscope 95:162–166

Seyfer AE (1988) The lower trapezius flap for recalcitrant wounds of the posterior skull and spine. Ann Plast Surg 20:414–418

Shagets FW, Panje WR, Shore JW (1986) Use of temporalis muscle flaps in complicated defects of the head and neck. Arch Otolaryngol Head Neck Surg 112:60–65

Thammavaran KV, Benzel EC, Kesterson L (1990) Fascia lata graft as a dural substitute in neurosurgery. South Med J 83:634–636

Ueda K, Harashina T, Inoue T et al. (1993) Microsurgical scalp and skull reconstruction using a serratus anterior myo-osseous flap. Ann Plast Surg 31:10–14

Ueda K, Inoue T, Harada T et al. (1992) Dura and cranial base reconstruction by external oblique fascia and recturs abdominus muscle flap. J Reconstr Microsurg 8:427–432

Ueda T, Kashiwabara S, Imaizumi T et al. (1990) Reconstruction of skull base by omentum transplantation. No Shinkei Geka 18:339–346

Wolfe SA (1978) The utility of pericranial flaps. Ann Plast Surg 1:147

23

Alternative Methods for Reconstruction of Skull Base Bone Using Locally Available Materials

Atul Goel

With increasing surgical sophistication in skull base and craniofacial surgery, reconstructive efforts are challenged to provide a reliable means of compartmentalization. Preoperative planning of the reconstruction methodology leading to suitable alteration of the operating steps is important for success of a skull base surgical procedure. Reconstruction with local and regional flaps is an integral part of the operation and must be adequately planned and performed. There are various inherent difficulties involved in skull base reconstruction. The proximity of the skull base to potentially infective spaces such as paranasal sinuses, nasal, oral, and pharyngeal pathways, and the external ear canal; long duration of the surgical procedures; and involvement of multiple surgeons and extensive instrumentation adds to the risk of infection.

The basal dura is relatively thin and friable and densely stuck to the bone. Approximation of edges and watertight suturing often may not be possible especially in areas of vessel and nerve transit. Frequently there are large dead spaces that need to be filled in after basal bone, soft tissue, and tumor resection. The reconstruction begins at the end of a relatively long operation when the operative team may be exhausted and errors of omission may be made. Occasional cases of persistent postsurgical or traumatic cerebrospinal fluid fistula can pose a formidable surgical challenge and super-added infection can be a life-threatening condition. Familiarity with various methods of reconstruction and their satisfactory performance can be a gratifying surgical procedure.

All bone defects in the skull base do not require reconstruction. Because the questions of cosmesis, arthrodesis, and stability are not usually applicable in basal reconstruction, the principal purpose of reconstructing bone defects is to avoid possible herniation of the brain matter into the aerodigestive tracts, ear, orbit, or into the space resulting from a large tumor resection or after treating a basal encephalocele. The possibility of such an eventuality is rare and the decision regarding reconstruction of basal bone should be a calculated one. In the presence of intact basal dura, even large bone defects can be tolerated without any consequence. The author has observed that as much as one-third to one-half of the orbital roof can be removed without any problem of pulsating exophthalmos. Large clival, petrous, and sphenoid bone defects can safely be left unrepaired. Often it is safer not to perform bone reconstruction at the end of a long surgical procedure because of the possibility of infection complicating the entire surgical procedure.

Larger defects over the tegmen tympani and orbital roof should preferably be replaced with bone because the dura in this region is relatively thin and the region is deprived of large basal cerebrospinal fluid cisterns. Consequently, initially the brain pulsations can be transmitted and later the brain can herniate into these spaces. Support for brain tissue may be necessary where large bone defects are created following the operation.

Reconstruction of the bone is also carried out to support the dura and help in the provision of watertight sealing of the base and avoiding the formation of cerebrospinal fluid fistulas. Protection of the brain from future injury and restoration of a reasonable appearance and quality of life are other significant objectives.

Vascularized Bone Flaps

The size of the defect and its site, extent of the resection of the associated structures, history of previous operative procedures, and endovascular and radiation treatment are important variables that determine the appropriate reconstructive procedure. Various methods of reconstruction of basal bone have been described. Reconstruction of bone defects in the cranial base should preferably be done with the help of bone. In sterile fields free small or large bone pieces can be used for this purpose. Ribs, iliac crest, and scapular grafts have been successfully used. Acrylic and metal plates can also be used in such a situation. However in the potentially infected fields that are more frequently encountered after a skull base operation, the use of a bone flap based on a vascularized pedicle is recommended.

Vascularized Osteomyoplastic Flap

The reconstruction can be done by split or full thickness cranial bone pedicled on muscle flaps (Goel, 1994a). Temporalis muscle being in close proximity to the skull base and also the ease with which it can be rotated in various directions allow it to be used effectively for such an osteomyoplastic flap skull base reconstruction (Fig. 23-1). The temporalis muscle has an extensive blood supply to the calvarium through multiple perforators. Elevation of the bone flap with wide attachment to the muscle pedicle results in a well-vascularized flap. Vascularized bone flaps can also be based on muscles of the nape of the neck. Judicious use of split cranial grafts can fill up the resulting defects in the skull. Various experimental studies have been conducted on the evolution of temporalis osteomuscular flaps compared with calvarial free bone grafts (Antonyshyn et al., 1986; Combelles and Zadeh, 1984; Fasano et al., 1987). The studies confirmed that vascularized bone flaps remain viable and are characterized by normal evolution, whereas the free bone grafts show typical signs of necrosis and resorption. Such vascularized bone flaps based on a muscle pedicle have been used in cosmetic facial surgery and mandibular, maxillary, and palatal reconstruction and mastoid cavity obliteration (Bite et al., 1987; Choung et al., 1991).

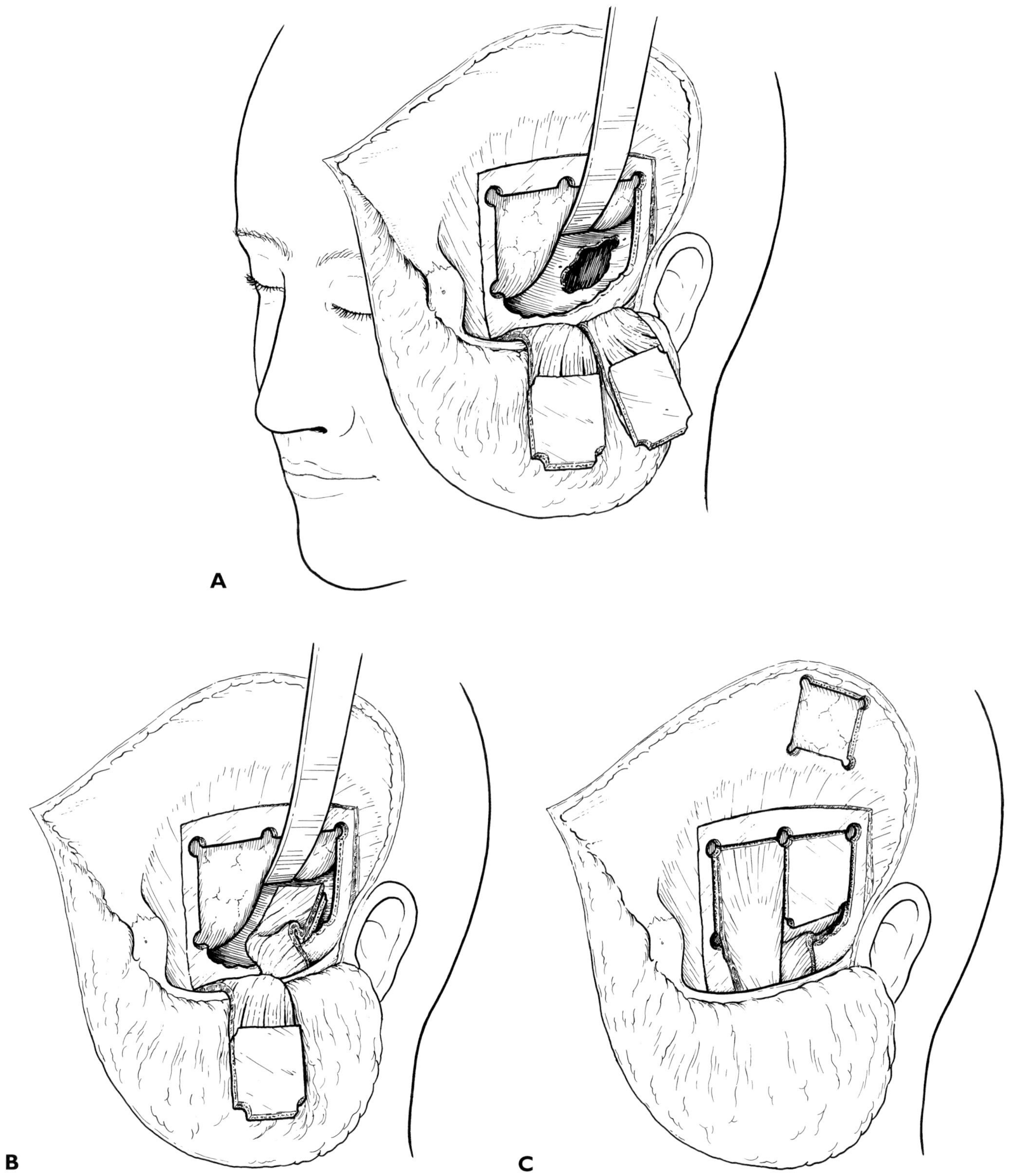

Figure 23-1. *(A)* The bone defect in the middle cranial fossa base on retracting the temporal brain. The temporal bone is split into two, each piece being placed on temporalis muscle pedicle. *(B)* The posterior piece of the temporal bone flap is rotated to fill up the defect. *(C)* The anterior piece of the temporal bone flap is replaced back in the convexity. The parietal bone is split, the outer table being placed in the temporal bone defect.

Osteomyoplastic flaps can be used for reconstruction of middle fossa and petrous bone defects with relative ease. The fascial layers covering the temporalis muscle can be used to seal the defects in the basal dura while the muscle and bone occupy the area of bone defect. Unlike the pericranial and galeal flaps, which can be raised either before or after the surgical resection, osteomyoplastic flaps, on most occasions, must be planned and fashioned in the exposure stage of the operation. The incisions and dissection in the muscle and fascial planes are modified to avoid transection of blood supply, which could be crucial to sustain the bone flap.

Pericranium-Based Bone Flaps

Pericranial and galeal flaps have been described for reconstruction of anterior cranial base and craniofacial deformities (Goel, 1994b). The pericranium is composed of an outer layer of loose areolar tissue and an inner layer of osteoblasts and contains an extensive vascular network. The pericranium derives its blood supply anteriorly from the supratrochlear and supraorbital arteries and laterally from the superficial temporal arteries. Pericranial layer pedicled flaps can be based on either of these vessels, and accordingly rotated anteriorly or laterally. The pericranium can sustain the calvarial flap by means of multiple small, vertical perforators. Studies have shown that the calvarial flaps can safely be pedicled on the pericranial layer or, galeo-pericranial layer (Casanova et al., 1986; Cutting et al., 1984; Goel, 1994c, 1996; Goel and Gahankari, 1995; Price et al., 1988; Snyderman et al., 1990; Watson, 1993).

Bone flaps of the calvarium can be either of full thickness or only of the outer table. A split thickness osteo-galeo-pericranial flap as shown in Figure 23-2 can be used to reconstruct the anterior cranial fossa base. Easy availability, rotational capability, long length, and close proximity to the operative area of such vascularized flaps

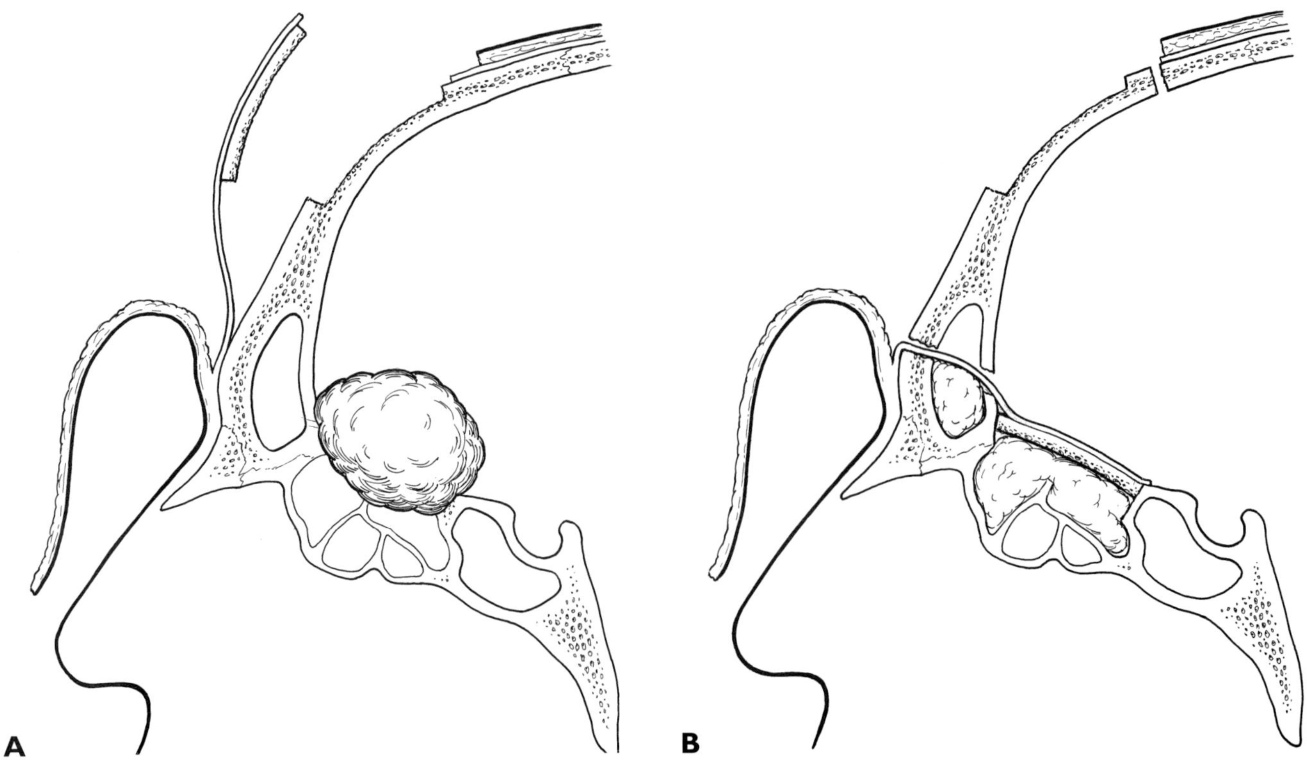

Figure 23-2. *(A)* The anterior cranial basal tumor. A split thickness calvarial graft pedicled on galeo-pericranial layer is taken. *(B)* The tumor has been resected. The bone graft is placed in the resultant basal defect. Fat occupies the opened sinuses.

make them ideally suited for skull base reconstruction. The bone piece can be pedicled on a large base of pericranium and can be additionally nourished by the galeal flaps. Whenever necessary, the bone flap can be turned upside down so that the bone surface is not directly exposed to the paranasal sinuses. The flap can even be sandwiched between the pericranial layers. In cases with extensive defects, an extended subgaleal fascia–pericranial temporalis flap can first be placed in the region of the defect (Goel and Gahankari, 1995) over which the described bone flap can be placed. The reconstruction can thus be with multiple layers of vascularized tissue. The bone piece can be fractured into two or more pieces retaining its attachment to the pericranium so that its contour can be adjusted to suit the local environment. Such vascularized flaps are more resistant to infection, tolerate radiation therapy better, are mechanically stronger, contract less, and survive better in poorly vascularized bed when compared with free bone grafts. It is presumed that such grafts would be ideal when treating basal encephaloceles.

Long Vascular Pedicle Composite Cranial Flap

The flap described (Goel, 1995a) is a split or full thickness cranial bone flap based on the pericranial layer, which receives its vascular nourishment from the temporalis muscle and its overlying fascial layers. Subgaleal elevation of the scalp is carried out. The temporalis muscle with its overlying fascial layers and the pericranial layer is retained with the skull. The outer table of the skull bone is split as shown in Figure 23-3, preserving overlying pericranium. A part of the temporalis muscle (and fascial layers) along with the pericranium is elevated and rotated as required (Figs. 23-3,

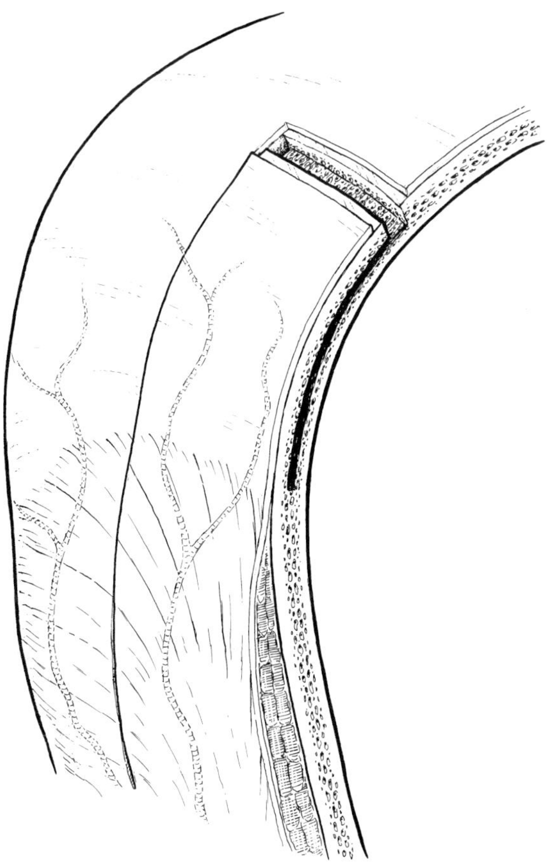

Figure 23-3. Splitting of the cranial bone to be based on the pericranium and the muscle.

and 23-4). Such flaps have been described in plastic surgery literature and used in malar reconstruction for the Treacher Collins syndrome (Horowitz et al., 1984; McCarthy and Zide, 1984).

The superficial fascial layer over the temporalis muscle is a part of the pericranial aponeurosis whereas the deep temporal fascial layer completely invests the superficial aspect of the temporalis muscle. The temporalis muscle, its fascial envelope, and the pericranium receive their blood supply from the anterior, middle, and posterior deep temporal and superficial temporal arteries. Subperiosteal elevation of the temporalis muscle along with the fascial layers preserves the integrity of all the major vascular supply. The split or full thickness cranial bone, based on the pericranial layer and the temporalis musculofascial layer as described, results in a viable flap with an abundant vasculature. Vertical splitting of the temporalis muscle into half or one-third would still preserve at least one or two of the main feeding vessels. This splitting would not adversely affect the circulation to the flap and could help in preservation of the function of the temporalis muscle. The skull bone is thicker superior to the temporal line, which marks the attachment of the temporalis muscle. Splitting of the skull bone is easier in the paramedian frontoparietal area bone due to the well-formed diploic channels. The split thickness graft can be broken into pieces and can be suitably contoured, preserving the attachment of the pericranium.

The long length, local availability, and maneuverability of the flap makes it versatile with great potential for reconstruction of skull convexity and basal defects. The other advantages of such a flap include harvesting of grafts of adequate size, ease of access within the same operative field, and no or minimal postoperative morbidity and discomfort for the patient. The described flap can be used particularly to recon-

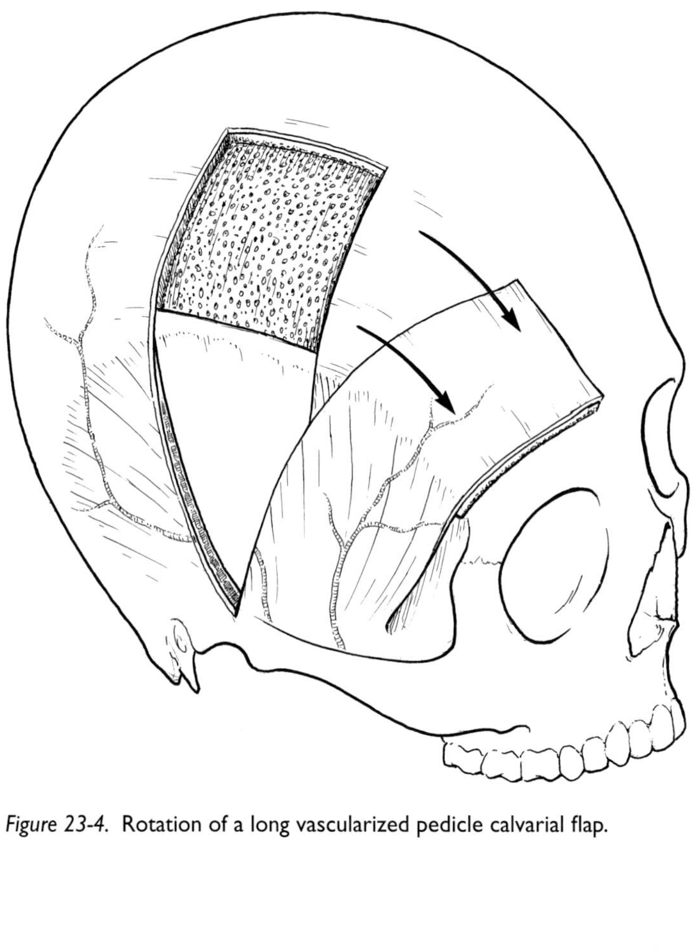

Figure 23-4. Rotation of a long vascularized pedicle calvarial flap.

struct cranial defects where there is poor local nourishment and potential infection and in areas that are cosmetically crucial.

Multilayered Basal Reconstruction

A multilayered vascularized pedicled flap was found to be useful in reconstruction of large bone and dural defects in the middle fossa base and the tegmen tympani in which brain matter communicated freely with the external ear (Goel, 1996). Such a situation has been encountered twice in the author's practice. In the first case (a 4-year-old boy) there was a large congenital encephalocele that extended widely into the infratemporal fossa and external ear canal through a large defect in the middle fossa base and tegmen. The child presented with a small swelling in the external ear canal and cerebrospinal fluid otorrhea. A similar problem was encountered in a 23-year-old man who developed three episodes of pyogenic meningitis within a period of 6 months, 18 years after a fall from height. A large middle fossa and petrous bone defect was detected on investigation. Brain matter had herniated into the middle and external ear. Air bubbles could be seen intracranially.

Both these patients required an elaborate reconstruction of the bone and dural defect. A large dead space created by the removal of herniated necrotic brain also had to be filled up. Due to the communication with the external ear the entire reconstruction had to be with vascularized pedicle flaps. The reconstruction is shown in Figure 23-5. The temporalis muscle was split into two. A 3 × 3 cm segment of squamous temporal bone was retained with the anterior half of the split temporalis muscle. This portion of the flap was a vascularized pedicle osteomyoplastic flap as described earlier. The posterior half of the temporalis muscle was reflected free of the bone by its subperiosteal elevation. An extended vascularized temporalis muscle–fascia flap was fashioned from this portion (Goel, 1994c). The deep layer of the temporalis fascia was everted partially over the temporalis muscle preserving its vascularity. A composite flap comprising temporalis muscle and its fascia attached along its superior border was now available for reconstruction. Partial eversion of the temporalis fascia over the muscle increased the length of the flap while retaining its vascular pedicle. The composite muscle fascia flap covers the region of the defect over which the anterior half of the osteomyoplastic flap is placed. Such a multilayered flap fashioned entirely with vascularized pedicles by virtue of its bulk and long length can be used to cover bone defects, may be folded for bulk, and may be used to carry blood supply to poorly vascularized recipient sites. In an occasional case of cerebrospinal fluid otorrhea, such an elaborate reconstruction could be a life-saving operation.

Other Techniques

Use of Bone Dust and Debris

With the use of modern power tools for making burr holes, a large amount of bone dust can be obtained. Figure 23-6 shows the amount of bone dust obtained after drilling one burr hole. This bone dust can be flattened and placed in the form of a sheet over the site of the defect. It provides a valuable source of live osteoblasts. These osteoblasts, being sandwiched between the vascularized dura underneath and covered by vascularized muscle, lay down bone that mimics cortical bone and thus provides a simple and reliable form of cranioplasty. Small bone chips and bone debris that are generally available during a craniotomy can be placed interspersed in the bone dust. This forms a template over which new bone and fibrous tissue is laid and a firm, strong, and resistant barrier is formed.

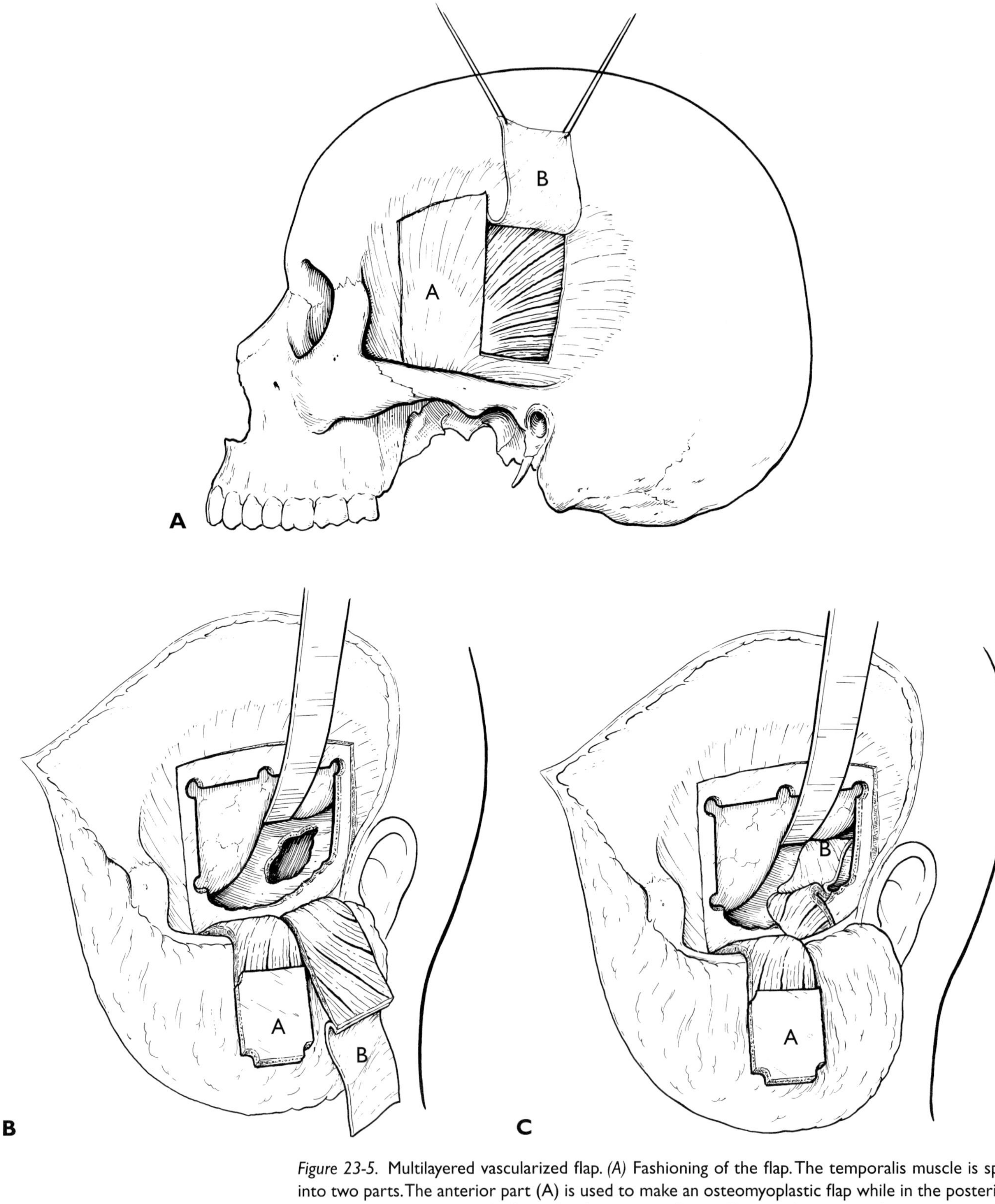

Figure 23-5. Multilayered vascularized flap. *(A)* Fashioning of the flap. The temporalis muscle is split into two parts. The anterior part (A) is used to make an osteomyoplastic flap while in the posterior part (B) the deep temporalis fascia has been everted partially over the temporalis muscle. *(B)* Part A of the flap is an osteomyoplastic flap whereas part B is an extended muscle fascia flap. *(C)* The composite temporalis muscle–fascia flap (part B) is rotated in the region of the defect in the region of the petrous bone. Temporal craniotomy has been done and the temporal lobe elevated off the base with the help of a retractor. *(Figure continues.)*

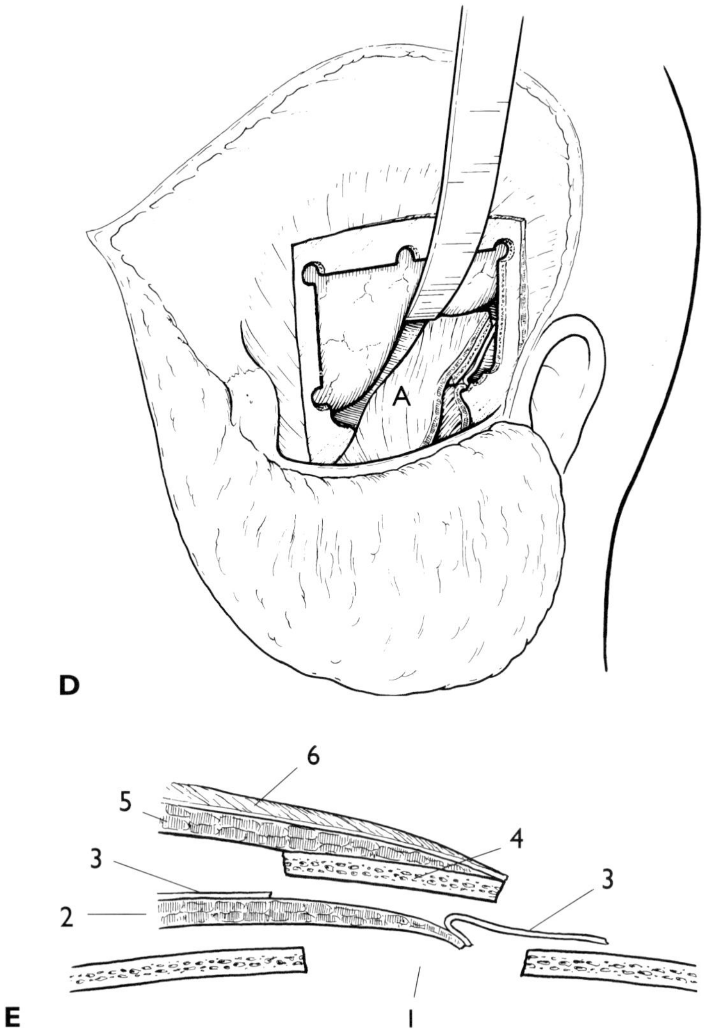

Figure 23-5 *(Continued)*. *(D)* The osteomyoplastic flap (part A) is rotated and placed over the composite muscle fascia flap (part B). *(E)* The multiple layers of the flap are shown diagramatically. 1, The region of the defect. 2, Layer of temporalis muscle. 3, Fascial layers of the temporalis muscle, the superior part of which is partially everted. 4, Temporal bone flap. 5, Temporalis muscle layer. 6, Fascial covering of the temporalis muscle.

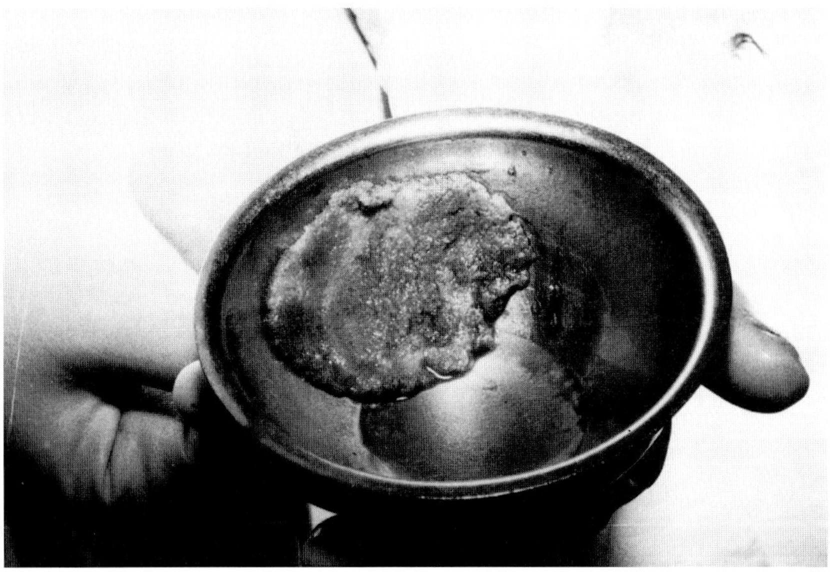

Figure 23-6. Bone dust obtained after drilling one burr hole has been taken in a bowl and spread into a sheet.

Reconstruction of Skull Base with Free Bone Graft

Whenever possible bone defects should be filled up with a vascularized pedicle bone flap. However, such a vascularized bone flap is sometimes not available and in this situation a free bone graft may be indicated. A free bone graft should preferably not be directly exposed to the paranasal sinuses or mucosal surfaces. Whenever such a free bone graft is placed in the skull base, it should be adequate in size and care should be taken that it be covered on both sides with vascularized and viable soft tissue. Such a "sandwich" free bone graft can be placed between muscle and fascial-pericranial layers. Postoperative collection of hematoma around the bone graft should also be avoided and whenever necessary external drains can be placed. Tenting scalp stitches should be used (Goel, 1992) whenever possible and indicated (see below).

Suturing of Bone Pieces

Suturing of the small bone pieces, like those obtained after zygomatic and orbital osteotomy, should preferably be carried out with thin wires, unbraided silk, or nylon stitches. Because no significant movements are expected in the basal cranial bones, use of miniplates, screws, and an excessive volume of metal can be avoided.

Placement of Soft Tissue in Place of Bone

Although not consistent with the generally taught principles of reconstruction, placement of soft tissue can form a firm barrier of fibrous tissue and serve the purpose in cases of basal bone defects. Rotation of a vascularized pedicle muscle, pericranial or fascia flap, or free fat graft or muscle can be performed to occupy the area of bone defect and empty spaces (Goel, 1994c, 1996; Goel and Gahankari, 1995).

Use of Outer Layer of Dura as a Pedicled Flap

Cranial dura is formed by two layers: the outer endosteal layer and the inner meningeal layer. These layers are well defined and "separable" by manual dissection, particularly in younger individuals. The dura is supplied by multiple small and medium-sized arteries circumferentially. The meningeal blood vessels are largely located in the endosteal layer. When preserved intact the outer endosteal layer can be rotated and used to cover defects in the proximity (Goel, 1995b). The principal advantage of using such a material is that it may be used as a vascularized pedicle flap or a free graft (Fig. 23-7). The consistency and quality of the material matches that of adjacent dura. Local availability and ease of rotation of this flap are the other advantages. Despite the limitations in using this flap due to technical difficulties in separating the layers, it can be useful in an occasional patient.

Subgaleal Preservation of Bone Flaps

In some rare situations like brain swelling, potentially infective operative field, and other such conditions, convexity and basal bone flaps can be removed preserved, and replaced at the original site after a period of time (Goel and Deogaonkar, 1995). Various techniques of preservation of bone flaps have been described both inside and outside the body. The flaps have been most frequently and successfully stored in the subcutaneous plane of the abdominal wall or in the thigh. External storage methods include deep freezing, autoclaving it before replacing, storing after radiation treatment, and using antibiotic solutions.

An alternative method of preservation of the skull bone flap in the subgaleal space was found to be effective. The method was used by the author in eight patients and the flap was successfully replaced to the original site in four of these cases. The sub-

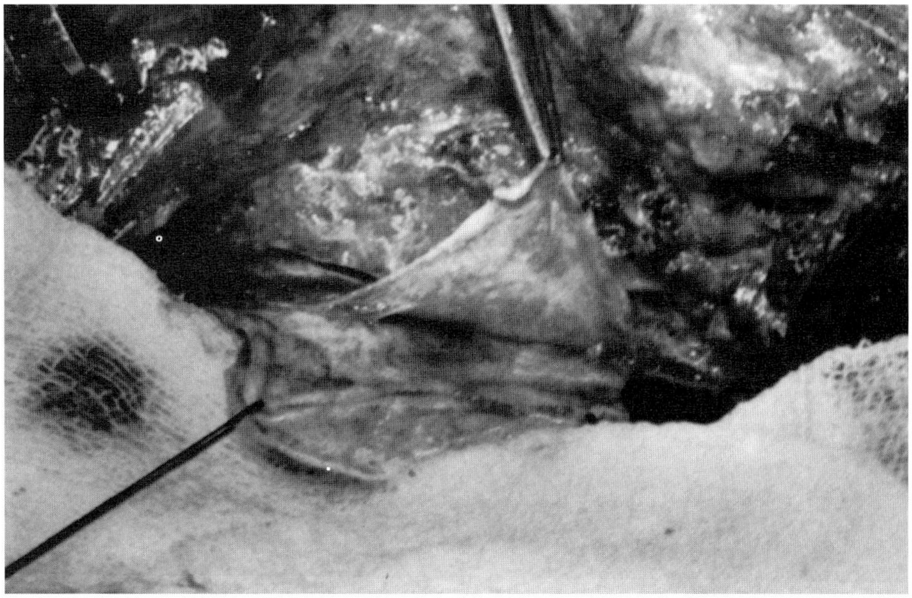

Figure 23-7. Operative picture showing the two split dural layers. Layer held by a stay suture is the cerebral layer, whereas that held by a forceps is the endosteal layer. The endosteal layer was rotated to cover the mastoid air cells.

galeal plane adjacent to the site of operation was exposed widely using blunt dissection. The bone flap was placed in this plane taking care that the curvature of the bone flap did not excessively elevate the scalp or cause tension over the scalp edges (Fig. 23-8). In cases where larger bone flaps were placed subgalealy the curvature necessitated fracturing of the bone flap in two or more pieces. The relative avascularity of the subgaleal plane helps in limiting the rate of resorption of the bone.

There was no significant bone resorption in any of the patients in the presented series during the period of observation, which varied from 3 to 16 months. The subgaleal space can be easily exposed widely providing a large area for bone placement. Such a large and avascular space is not available elsewhere in the body. Frequently the curvature of the bone flap matches that of the adjacent bone, which assists in the ease of placement. The flap is placed and replaced to the original site in one operative field. As no additional incision is necessary, the procedure is quick to perform. Whenever such bone preservation is not anticipated the abdomen or thigh is not shaved or adequately prepared. Such maneuvers at the termination of a surgical procedure may not be satisfactorily performed, adding to the risk of infection. None of the patients in the presented series complained of any discomfort due to the flap placement.

Use of Synthetic Material in Skull Base Bone Reconstruction

Synthetic material is rarely required to reconstruct truly basal bone. Issues of biocompatibility, corrosion characteristics and metallurgic properties of the implant, hardness and malleability, suitability of the host area to adjust to the foreign intrusion, and various other factors must be adequately analyzed prior to selection of such a material. Various substances including acrylic casts, plastics, glassionomer cement, silicone bars, Prolene mesh, stainless steel and titanium miniplates, and screws and wires have all been used. Such material is more commonly advocated for the reconstruction of cosmetically sensitive areas such as the orbital rim and zygomatic arch

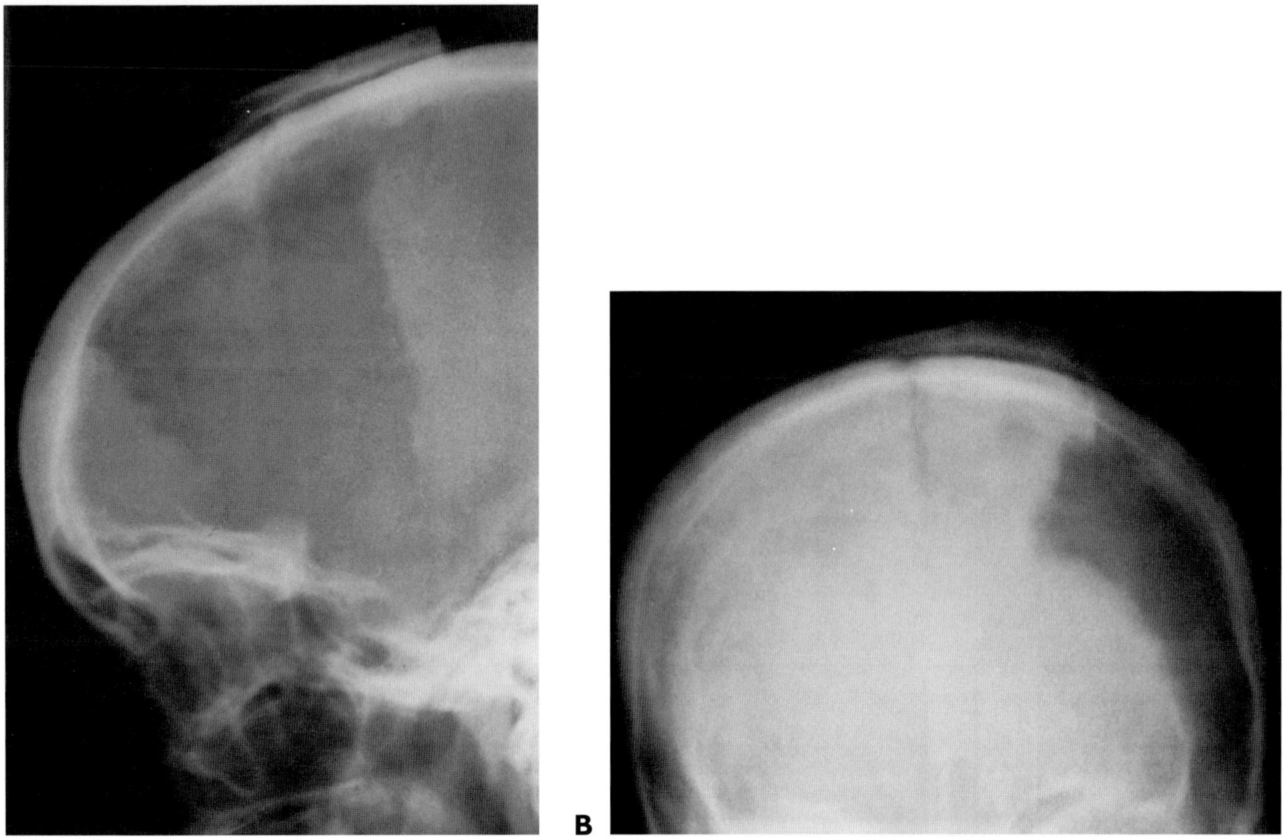

A B

Figure 23-8. (A) Lateral radiograph of the skull showing the subgaleal placement of the bone flap and the bone defect. *(B)* Anteroposterior radiograph showing the subgaleal bone flap and the bone defect.

and for facial contour defects. Patients with large and complex bone defects sometimes present with major functional and aesthetic disability. Adequate reconstructions or prosthesis is necessary and important to restore them to their accustomed way of life.

Tenting Scalp Stitches

Postoperative collections underneath the scalp are common, although usually no more than a nuisance to the surgeon and the patient. However, sometimes these collections can be a source of secondary complications such as wound breakdown and infection. Such complications are particularly relevant after a long skull base operation. The problem can occur after an osteoplastic craniotomy when the collection develops between the galea and the pericranium, or following free bone flap exposure in which case the collection is between the pericranial layer and the bone flap. Suction drains and tight head dressings are frequently used at the time of closure to avoid this problem. Occasionally, there is a need to drain the collection and approximate the scalp layers by a large bore needle and sometimes lumbar drainage of cerebrospinal fluid may be necessary. Suction or gravity drains often become clogged or only approximate the layers of the scalp in a limited area. They cannot be used for long periods because of the risk of infection. Tight head dressings loosen over a period of time, can be a source of discomfort to the patient, and occasionally compromise the blood supply of the skin flap.

"Tenting" sutures of the dura should be routine after every craniotomy (Goel, 1992). These stitches help to prevent the occurrence and expansion of extradural collections. The stitches shown in Figure 23-9 are similar in principle and action for the scalp. This is a simple and non–time-consuming technique. The sutures help to seal surgically created space between the layers of the scalp and act as internal compression. The closer approximation of the scalp to the bone improves the vascularity of the bone by providing an additional pathway for blood supply in the initial postoperative phase.

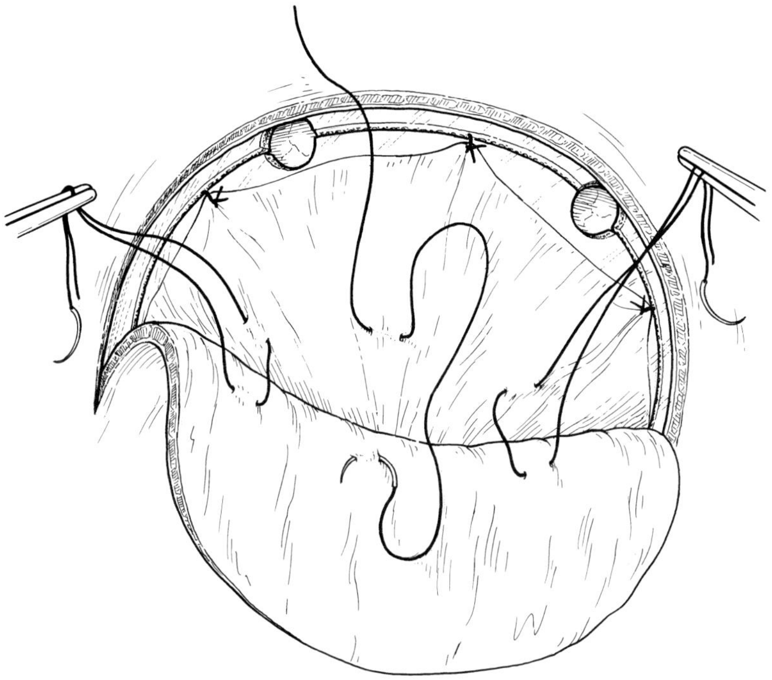

A

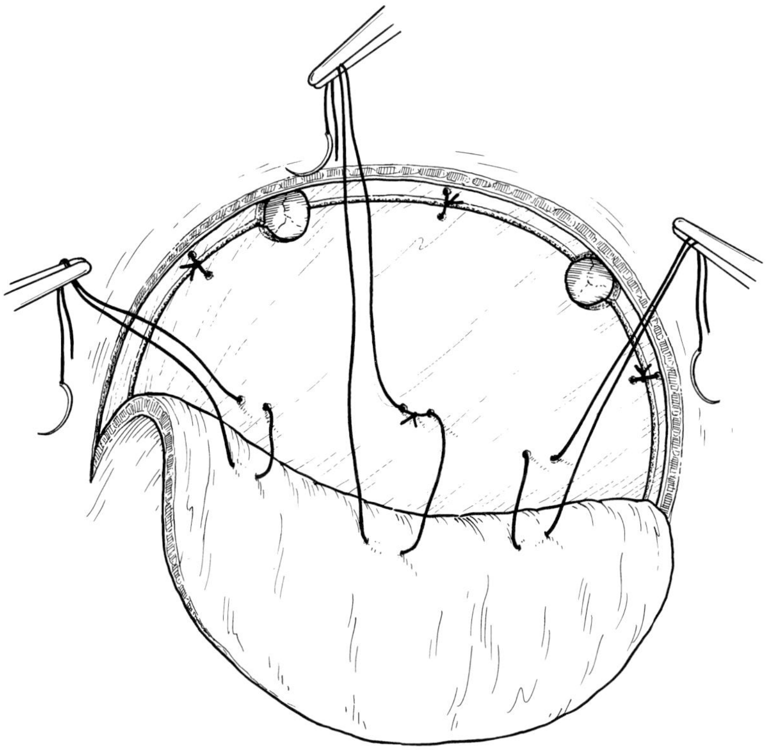

B

Figure 23-9. (A) The galea to pericranium stitches. *(B)* The galea-pericranial layer bone flap stitches. Note that the dural tenting sutures have already been placed and tied in the central bone holes.

After adequate hemostasis when the scalp is reflected back for closure, three to four (or more) sutures are placed between the galea and pericranium, as shown in Figure 23-9A. The site of the sutures is carefully judged so that the scalp wound can approximate closely. It is usually easier to place the sutures at a distance of about 5 cm from the scalp incision. The greater the number of sutures placed, the more compact is the closure of the layers. It is easier to tie knots after all the sutures have traversed the layers. In case of a free bone flap, the pericranial layer is sutured to the bone after drilling holes in the bone. The holes already used for "tenting" the dura in the center of the bone flap can be used for this purpose (Fig. 23-9B).

References

Antonyshyn O, Cocleugh RG, Hurst LN, Anderson C (1986) The temporalis myo-osseous flap: an experimental study. Plast Reconstr Surg 77:406–415

Bite U, Jackson IT, Wahner HW, Marsh RW (1987) Vascularized skull bone grafts in craniofacial surgery. Ann Plast Surg 19:3–15

Casanova R, Cavalcante D, Grotting JC, Vasconez LO (1986) Anatomic basis for vascularized outer-table calvarial bone flaps. Plast Reconstr Surg 78:300–308

Choung PH, Nam IW, Kim KS (1991) Vascularized cranial bone grafts for mandibular and maxillary reconstruction. The parietal osteofascial flap. J Craniomaxillofac Surg 19:235–242

Combelles R, Zadeh J (1984) Temporalis osteomuscular flap. Anatomical study and experimental and surgical technic. Rev Stomatol Chir Maxillofac 85:351–354

Cutting CB, McCarthy JG, Berenstien A (1984) Blood supply of the upper craniofacial skeleton: the search for composite calvarial bone flaps. Plast Reconstr Surg 74:603–610

Fasano D, Menoni V, Riberti C, Bacchini P (1987) The temporalis osteomuscular flap versus the free calvarial bone graft. An experimental study in growing rabbit. J Craniomaxillofac Surg 15:332–341

Goel A (1992) 'Tenting' stitches for the scalp. Br J Neurosurg 6:357–358

Goel A (1994a) Vascularized osteomyoplastic flaps for skull base reconstruction. Br J Neurosurg 8:79–82

Goel A (1994b) Vascularized bone flap for anterior skull base reconstruction. Acta Neurochir 128:166–168

Goel A (1994c) Extended vascularised temporalis muscle-fascia flap. Br J Neurosurg 8:731–733

Goel A (1995a) Long vascular pedicle cranial flap. Br J Neurosurg 9:667–670

Goel A (1995b) Use of outer layer of dura as a pedicled flap. Surg Neurol 44:92–93

Goel A (1996) Multilayer reconstruction of middle fossa floor Acta Neurochir (in press)

Goel A, Deogaonkar M (1995) Subgaleal preservation of calvarial flaps. Surg Neurol 44:181–183

Goel A, Gahankari D (1995) Extended subgaleal fascia-pericranial temporalis flap for skull base reconstruction. Acta Neurochir 135:203–205

Horowitz JH, Persing JA, Nichter LS et al. (1984) Galeal pericranial flaps in head and neck reconstruction: anatomy and applications. Am J Surg 148:489–493

McCarthy JG, Zide BM (1984) The spectrum of calvarial bone grafting: Introduction of the vascularized calvarial bone flap. Plast Reconstr Surg 74:10–17

Price JC, Loury M, Carson et al. (1988) The pericranial flap for reconstruction of anterior skull base defects. Laryngoscope 98:1159–1164

Snyderman CH, Janecka IP, Sekhar LN et al. (1990) Anterior cranial base reconstruction: role of galeal and pericranial flaps. Laryngoscope 100:607–614

Watson Jones R. (1993) The repair of the skull defects by a new pedicle bone-graft operation. BMJ 1:780

Appendix I

Abbreviations

ACA	anterior cerebral artery
ACh A	anterior choroidal artery
ACP	anterior clinoid process
AEA	anterior ethmoidal artery
AICA	anterior inferior cerebellar artery
AL	anterior loop (of ICA)
ANT	mastoid antrum
AOph V	accessory ophthalmic vein
ATN	auriculotemporal nerve
AZ	annulus of Zinn
BA	basilar artery
BM	buccal muscle
BN	buccal nerve
BS	brain stem
C	craniotomy
CAC	carotid artery canal
CC	common crus
CD	clival dura
CH	optic chiasm
ChT	chorda tympani
CMA	clival meningeal artery
CRB	cerebellum
CO	cochlea

COA	cochlear area
CON	cochlear nerve
CS	cavernous sinus
DG	digastric muscle
DGR	digastric ridge
DM	dura mater
DMA	dorsal meningeal artery
DR	distal ring (around ICA)
DS	diaphragma sellae
DTA	deep temporal artery
DTF	deep temporal fascia
E	eye
EA	arcuate eminence of temporal bone
EAM	external auditory meatus
ECA	external carotid artery
ES	ethmoid sinus
ET	eustachian tube
ETH	ethmoid bone
FAL	falciform ligament
FB	frontal bone
FC	facial nerve canal
FH	facial hiatus
FI	fossa incudis
FL	frontal lobe
FLO	flocculus
FM	foramen magnum
FN	frontal nerve
FO	foramen ovale
FR	foramen rotundum
FRS	frontal sinus
FS	foramen spinosum
GA	galea aponeurotica
GG	gasserian ganglion
GNG	geniculate ganglion
GWS	greater wing of sphenoid bone
HC	hypoglossal canal
HS	spine of Henle

I	incus
IAA	internal auditory artery
IAM	internal auditory meatus
ICA	internal carotid artery
ICA(h)	horizontal internal carotid artery
ICA(v)	vertical internal carotid artery
IDN	inferior dental nerve
IHA	inferior hypophyseal artery
IJV	internal jugular vein
IM	incisura mastoidea
IOF	inferior orbital fissure
IOM	inferior oblique muscle
ION	infraorbital nerve
IPS	inferior petrosal sinus
IRM	inferior rectus muscle
IVA	inferior vestibular area
IVN	inferior vestibular nerve
JB	jugular bulb
JF	jugular foramen
LA	lacrimal artery
LAC	lacrimal bone
LCT	lateral carotico–cavernous trunk
LG	lacrimal gland
LIN	lingual nerve
LN	lacrimal nerve
LPM	lateral pterygoid muscle
LPSM	levator palpebrae superioris muscle
LR	lateral ring (around ICA)
LRM	lateral rectus muscle
LSC	lateral semicircular canal
LV	vein of Labbé
LWS	lesser wing of sphenoid bone
M	malleus
MA	maxillary artery
MAS	mastoid process
MAX	maxillary bone
MC	Meckel's cave

MCA	middle cerebral artery
MCO	mandibular condyle
MHA	meningeal branch of MHT
MHT	meningohypophyseal trunk
MM	masseter muscle
MMA	middle meningeal artery
MPM	medial pterygoid muscle
MRM	medial rectus muscle
NIM	nervus intermedius
NN	nasociliary nerve
NLF	nasolacrimal fossa
NLP	nerve to levator palpebrae
NMH	nerve to mylohyoid muscle
NMP	nerve to medial pterygoid
NPC	nerve of pterygoid canal
OC	optic canal
OCO	occipital condyle
OF	optic foramen
ON	optic nerve
Oph A	ophthalmic artery
Oph V	ophthalmic vein
OT	oculomotor trigone
P	promontory
PA	petrous apex
PB	pituitary
PBS	pituitary stalk
PC	pericranium
PCA	posterior cerebral artery
PCom A	posterior communicating artery
PCP	posterior clinoid process
PCL	petroclinoid (petroclival) ligament
PD	parotid duct
PEA	posterior ethmoidal artery
Pf	periosteal flap
PFD	posterior fossa dura
PG	parotid gland

PH	pterygoid hamulus
PICA	posterior inferior cerebellar artery
PL	posterior loop (of ICA)
PMA	posterior meningeal artery
PN	petrosal nerve(s)
PR	proximal ring (around ICA)
PS	planum sphenoidale
PSC	posterior semicircular canal
PTF	petrotympanic fissure
PTP	pterygoid process
PV	petrosal vein
S	stapes
SAA	subarcuate artery
SAF	subarcuate fossa
SC	spinal cord
SCA	superior cerebellar artery
SDA	sinodural angle
SG	submandibular gland
SIN	singular nerve
SM	sternomastoid muscle
SMF	stylomastoid foramen
SML	sphenomandibular ligament
SOA	supraorbital artery
SOF	superior orbital fissure
SOM	superior oblique muscle
SON	supraorbital nerve
SPF	sphenopalatine fossa
SPG	sphenopalatine ganglion
SPH	body of sphenoid bone
SPS	superior petrosal sinus
SRM	superior rectus muscle
SS	sigmoid sinus
SSC	superior semicircular canal
SSP	spine of sphenoid
ST	stapedial tendon
STA	superficial temporal artery
STRA	supratrochlear artery

STRN	supratrochlear nerve
STV	superficial temporal vein
SVA	superior vestibular area
SVN	superior vestibular nerve
TA	tentorial artery
TE	tentorium
TF	temporalis fascia
TI	trigeminal impression
TL	temporal lobe
TM	temporalis muscle
TMJ	temporomandibular joint
TML	temporomandibular ligament
TRC	transverse crest
TS	tuberculum sellae
TT	tegmen tympani
TU	tumor
TYM	tympanic membrane
VA	vertebral artery
VAQ	vestibular aqueduct
VBJ	vertebrobasilar junction
VTC	vertical crest
ZA	zygomatic arch
ZM	zygomatic part of temporalis muscle
ZMS	zygomaticomaxillary suture
ZY	zygomatic bone
I	olfactory nerve
II	optic nerve
III	oculomotor nerve
IV	trochlear nerve
V	trigeminal nerve
V_1	ophthalmic division of V
V_2	maxillary division of V
V_3	mandibular division of V
VI	abducens nerve
VI(L)	left abducens nerve
VI(R)	right abducens nerve

VII	facial nerve
VIII	vestibulocochlear nerve bundle
IX	glossopharyngeal nerve
X	vagus nerve
XI	accessory nerve
XII	hypoglossal nerve

Appendix 2

Equipment Manufacturers

Aesculap AG, Tubingen, Germany (Fahlbusch pituitary instruments, Chapter 5)

Aloka Co., 6-22-1 Mure, Mitaka-shi, Tokyo 181, Japan (Microsonop ultrasonic surgical aspirator, Chapter 20)

Amsco-Hall Surgical, Santa Barbara, California 93101 (Zimmer Micro 100 reciprocating saw, Chapter 8)

Carl Zeiss, Germany, Tokyo, Japan, and 1 Zeiss Drive, Thornwood, New York 10594 (Contraves autofocus surgical microscope, Chapters 8 and 12)

Codman Shurtleff—Johnson and Johnson Medical (Hardy pituitary instruments, Chapter 5; transoral retractor system (Crockard type), Chapter 10; irrigating bipolar forceps, Chapter 12; Rhoton microdissector set, Chapter 16)

DP Medical Systems Ltd., Sutton Business Centre, Restmor Way, Wallington, Surrey SM6 7AH, England (Fujita microsucker, designed by Fukishima, Chapter 17)

Fehling Medizintechnik GMBH, Postfach 1109, Frankenstrasse 21, D-8757 Karlstein 1, Germany (nasal speculum, Chapter 6)

Howmedica Inc., 359 Veterans Blvd., Rutherford, New Jersey 07070-2584 (bone plating system, Chapter 8)

Immuno Ag, Vienna, Austria (Tisseel fibrin glue, Chapters 6, 16, and 21)

Koken Co., Meziro 3-14-3, Toyosima-ku, Tokyo 171, Japan (intravascular balloon catheter, Chapter 11)

Liebinger L. P., 14540 Beltwood Pkwy. East, Dallas, Texas 75244 (Fahlbusch curettes, Chapter 5; bone plating system, Chapter 8)

Magstim, Spring Gardens, Whitland, Dyfed, Wales (Neurosign nerve monitor, Chapter 17)

Midas Rex, 3001 Race St., Fort Worth, Texas 76111 (drills, Chapter 8)

Mizuho Medical Co., Fuse Building 2F 30-10, 3-chrome, Hango, Bunkyo-ku, Tokyo 113, Japan (skull base microsurgery forceps, Chapter 12; operating table MST-7200 and rotatable head holder, Chapter 12; Sugita brain retractor with hooks, Chapter 16)

Muranaka Medical Instruments Co., Higashi-kouraibashi 4-15, Chuoh-ku, Osaka 540-91, Japan (maxillary retractor, Chapter 11)

Nagashima Medical Instrument Co., 5-24-1 Hongo, Bunkyo-ku, Tokyo 113, Japan (illuminating fiber cable, illuminated mirror, Chapter 20)

Ohwa Tsusho, Tokyo, Japan (malleable tip spatulas, Chapter 12)

Synthes Maxillofacial, 1690 Russel Rd., P.O. Box 1767, Paoli, Pennsylvania 19301-1222 (bone plating system, Chapter 8)

Xomed Surgical Products, 19 Wellington Business Park, Crowthorne, Berks RG11 6LS, England (nerve integrity monitor, Chapter 17)

Index

Page numbers followed by *f* indicate figures; those followed by *t* indicate tables

F

K

L

M

T